Migration and Health

Migration and Health

A Research Methods Handbook

Edited by

Marc B. Schenker
Xóchitl Castañeda
Alfonso Rodriguez-Lainz

UNIVERSITY OF CALIFORNIA PRESS

University of California Press, one of the most distinguished university presses in the United States, enriches lives around the world by advancing scholarship in the humanities, social sciences, and natural sciences. Its activities are supported by the UC Press Foundation and by philanthropic contributions from individuals and institutions. For more information, visit www.ucpress.edu.

University of California Press
Oakland, California

Library of Congress Cataloging-in-Publication Data

Migration and health : a research methods handbook / edited by Marc B. Schenker, Xóchitl Castañeda, Alfonso Rodriguez-Lainz.
   p. cm.
   Includes bibliographical references and index.
   ISBN-13: 978-0-520-27794-6 (cloth : alk. paper)
   ISBN-10: 0-520-27794-5 (cloth : alk. paper)
   ISBN-13: 978-0-520-27795-3 (pbk. : alk. paper)
   ISBN-10: 0-520-27795-3 (pbk. : alk. paper)
   1. Immigrants—Health and hygiene—Research—Methodology.
   I. Schenker, Marc, editor.   II. Castañeda, Xochitl, editor.
   III. Rodriguez-Lainz, Alfonso, 1958-, editor.
   RA427.M47 2014
   613.086'912—dc23   2014019613

Manufactured in the United States of America

23 22 21 20 19 18 17 16 15 14
10 9 8 7 6 5 4 3 2 1

In keeping with a commitment to support environmentally responsible and sustainable printing practices, UC Press has printed this book on Natures Natural, a fiber that contains 30% post-consumer waste and meets the minimum requirements of ANSI/NISO Z39.48–1992 (R 1997) (*Permanence of Paper*).

To all those working to improve the health and health care of immigrants and migrants around the world, and to immigrants and migrants everywhere, all of whom deserve health equality.

CONTENTS

FOREWORD

Migrant health is central to socioeconomic development and will gain unprecedented importance in the years to come. . . . The future paradigm requires that governments take stock of the lessons learned to date, identify their specific capacity needs, and forge a more systematic approach towards managing the health aspects of migration.

—"FUTURE CAPACITY NEEDS IN MANAGING THE HEALTH ASPECTS OF MIGRATION," INTERNATIONAL ORGANIZATION FOR MIGRATION, 2010

The University of California Global Health Institute (UCGHI), established in 2009, addresses long-standing and emerging challenges to global health through its education, research, and partnership initiatives. Its three multicampus, cross-disciplinary Centers of Expertise comprise dozens of faculty across the ten-campus UC system who are using their vast knowledge and proficiency to address the increasingly complex global health problems and needs of the world's most vulnerable populations. The three Centers of Expertise are Migration and Health; One Health: Water, Animals, Food, and Society; and Women's Health and Empowerment.

The decision to establish a Center of Expertise on Migration and Health (COEMH) was a natural one for the University of California. California, one of the world's ten largest economies, attracts millions of new immigrants each year. More than 25% of California residents are foreign-born, with Hispanics constituting the largest group in that cohort. Migrant health is a major public health focus in California. The University of California's fifteen health sciences schools constitute the largest health science and medical training program in the United States and the fifth-largest health care delivery system in the state of California.

COEMH's mission is to improve health and eliminate health disparities among international migrants, refugees, and internally displaced people around the world through basic and action-oriented research, policy analyses, applied learning opportunities, and innovative dissemination activities. Forty UC faculty, all actively researching migration and health issues, many of them for decades, are joined in this collaborative effort.

This book, which exemplifies the vision and mission of the UCGHI, stems from and supports the work of the COEMH. One of its coeditors, Marc B. Schenker, is codirector of COEMH, and another coeditor, Xóchitl Castañeda, is one of COEMH's core faculty at UC Berkeley. They and the third coeditor, Alfonso Rodriguez-Lainz of the US Centers for Disease Control and Prevention, have been working on this book for more than three years, collaborating with more than forty contributing authors from around the globe. They envision that the book will be a core resource for academic programs that offer courses in migration and health, as well as for health professionals and researchers who are actively engaged in developing the systems and services needed by the world's ever-growing migrant populations.

Providing quality health care and prevention services to the growing proportion of the world's population that is uprooted, marginalized, and all too often without representation can only be done if there is a global cadre of researchers committed to defining the problems and proposing effective solutions in collaboration with migrant communities. Given the characteristics and health disparities of migrant populations and the limitations of most traditional study methodologies to capture information on migrant health issues, there is a pressing need to enhance awareness about novel and appropriate methodological approaches designed for the study of these populations. This book hopes to fill this compelling need by providing a comprehensive description of study methodologies for migrant populations.

Special thanks go to the Bill and Melinda Gates Foundation for its generous support of the establishment of the UC Global Health Institute and the Center of Expertise on Migration and Health. Funding from the foundation was essential for the development and publication of *Migration and Health: A Research Methods Handbook.*

Michael V. Drake, MD
Former Chancellor, University of California, Irvine
Founding Member, UC Global Health Initiative

Introductory Materials

Section Editor: Marc B. Schenker

1

Introduction

Marc B. Schenker

This book is intended to address a large and growing global health challenge—the health of migrant people around the world. It was written with the belief that the global health community can decrease the substantial health disparities that exist between migrant and nonmigrant populations by recognizing the unique needs of migrant populations and using the right tools to understand and improve their health. The primary goal of the book is to summarize in one reference the many methods available for health research on migrant populations and to address the unique issues involved in conducting research on health among migrants. Our focus in the book is on health outcomes, although the methods are applicable to other outcomes (e.g., economic, environmental, social). A secondary goal of the book is to increase attention to the health disparities and lack of health services available to migrants. Ultimately, we hope that the methods learned and applied will be used in research and public health programs to improve the health and quality of life of migrants around the world.

Existing books on global and public health generally have very little or no discussion of the association between human migration and health; or if they do consider the topic, their review is often limited to a narrow focus, such as the migration of health care workers. Similarly, books on specific diseases and health outcomes (e.g., tuberculosis, AIDS) generally address migration, if it is considered at all, as a cofactor in disease transmission risk and not as a characteristic defining a population at risk for multiple diseases. We believe that if we are to conduct valid research and develop effective intervention programs, migrants need to be viewed as a vulnerable population at risk for multiple diseases and a population needing unique approaches. This would make migrants similar to other vulnerable populations such as certain ethnic groups, women, children, and the elderly.

THE MAGNITUDE OF GLOBAL MIGRATION

The largest numbers of international migrants move from developing to developed countries, but a surprisingly large number (over 40%) migrate from one developing to another developing country. Geographically, migration from developing to developed countries is often realized as south-to-north migration and migration from one developing country to another is seen in south-to-south migration. Women represent almost half of global migrants. This is a marked change from a few years ago, when they were a distinct minority of global migrants.

The number of internal migrants (those who move from one region within a country to another region within the same country) dwarfs the global total of transnational migrants. The United Nations estimated that in 2010 there were 740 million internal migrants in the world (UNDP 2009); this number includes mostly internally displaced people and rural-to-urban migration. The number of internal migrants in China alone is nearly as large as the total number of international migrants in the world, and this trend of rural-to-urban internal migration shows no signs of slowing. Since many of the health and health care delivery issues affecting internal migrants are similar to those facing international migrants, and since there are similar considerations in studying these populations, they are considered together in this book.

Addressing migrant health, therefore, is not an academic exercise affecting a small number of people in the US and around the world. The percentage of the total US population that are immigrants is now approaching 13%, with eight states having over 15% of their population born outside of the country (US Department of Commerce 2010). California leads the nation in this regard, with 27.2% of its population foreign-born. The percentage of international migrants is expected to continue to increase as a greater percentage of population growth is made up of immigrants. Already some states are showing a 100–200% increase in their immigrant populations. In addition, there is a shift of immigrant populations from the traditional high immigrant states (California, New York, Texas, Florida, Illinois, and New Jersey) to other parts of the country. Around the world the percentages of immigrants in some countries and regions far eclipse the percentages seen in the US. In the Middle East, for example, the percentage of foreign-born people ranges from 27.8% in Saudi Arabia to 40.4% in Israel to a high of 86.5% in Qatar (Koser et al. 2010).

INTENDED AUDIENCES

We envision this book achieving these broad goals by reaching several different audiences. First, it is intended for academic researchers at universities around the world, who may be in public health or medical schools or in other disciplines. In the health sciences such researchers would most commonly be located in epidemiology or community health departments, but multiple other health-related departments could have a focus on migration and health research. For example, health policy and management and environmental science researchers may consider migrants as one focus of their research. Beyond the health sciences, there are diverse nonmedical departments and research institutions for which migration and health is a subject of research. Relevant disciplines include but are not limited to administration, anthropology, economics, education, ethnic studies, environmental science, law, political science, psychology, and sociology.

Another important audience for this book is public health practitioners in local, state, national, and international agencies and organizations. This includes policy analysts and staffers in these agencies and organizations. This group would benefit from a better understanding of the methods described in the book, either to conduct their own research or to understand the work of others. Whether for simple prevalence surveys or for evaluation of targeted intervention programs among immigrant populations, the approaches used by public health practitioners would benefit from understanding the crosscutting language, culture, legal, and psychological issues affecting migrant populations.

Students at all levels of secondary and postgraduate education will also benefit from this book. It is current students who will have the challenge, indeed the necessity, of addressing a world where immigrants comprise an increasingly larger and growing percentage of the population. Sensitizing them to this reality now and providing tools to study and improve the health of migrants will help direct their career paths to situations in which this can be accomplished.

BOOK ORGANIZATION

We have divided the book into four sections. The first section includes overview chapters and advances a conceptual model for migration and health research. Other sections address quantitative methods (section 2), qualitative methods (section 3) and crosscutting issues (section 4). While we recognize that most people work in a single discipline (e.g., epidemiology, sociology), we nevertheless strongly believe that understanding the health status and factors affecting health among immigrants requires both quantitative and qualitative approaches. In addition, unique vulnerabilities and limitations of migrant populations, such as language and legal status, apply to all research and programmatic interventions conducted among immigrants.

Quantitative methods such as classic epidemiological study designs (e.g., cross-sectional, case-control, and cohort designs) are most appropriate for estimating disease or risk factor prevalences, or for modeling associations of disease and risk factors. However, the nature of immigrant populations (mobile, lack of sampling frame, low education levels) makes it more challenging to conduct classic epidemiological studies. Because migration is a process of movement between two locations (often two countries), studies conducted in only one location (e.g., country of origin or receiving country) by definition limit the conclusions possible. The dynamic and selective nature of migration, such as nonrandom selection of who migrates and who returns to the place of origin, further limits conclusions possible from studies done in one location. Limited follow-up also compounds the challenges of conducting quantitative research. It is likely, too, that the most vulnerable migrants, for example, the undocumented, will be harder to reach or will decline participation in research studies.

The difficulty and expense in conducting longitudinal studies among migrant populations limits these studies among this hard-to-reach population. Easier and less expensive cross-sectional studies are more common, but have the inherent limitation of no temporality and difficulty in allowing interpretation of cause-effect associations. This is particularly significant when population selection may occur at many stages in the migration process. Despite these challenges, we believe that the research community should not avoid epidemiological studies of migrants but rather should use alternative and creative quantitative approaches to study health in this vulnerable population. Put another way, the perfect (study) should not be the enemy of the good, particularly when the need for studies and programs to improve the health of immigrants is so critical.

In section 2 we present chapters on classic epidemiological study designs and their use to understand health among immigrants, and we also provide some less common methods that are appropriate for studying immigrant populations. Some of these less common methods are actually used more frequently by demographers and other researchers who focus on hard-to-reach populations. For example, the chapters on respondent-driven sampling, time-space sampling, and prior enumeration address methods that are not commonly used by epidemiologists, but are useful for conducting research among harder-to-reach migrant populations.

The purpose of section 3 is to give an overview of how qualitative methodological approaches can be used to study the intersection of migration and health. More specifically, it addresses how qualitative research is employed in many different academic disciplines, traditionally in the social sciences, and how these approaches can complement and enrich findings from other disciplines.

In the field of migration and health, using qualitative instruments (such as key informant interviews, focus group discussion, photo voice, etc.), researchers aim to form an in-depth understanding of migrant human behavior and the variables that govern such behavior. Because immigrant populations often come from different cultures, standard epidemiological methods and instruments may miss important behaviors and exposures not seen in the dominant culture. For example, dietary practices, alternative medicines, and cultural beliefs may not be addressed in standard survey instruments.

Section 4, on crosscutting issues in migrant health research, addresses some of the common, and critically important, themes that should be considered in studies among immigrant populations. For example, migration is almost always associated with a change in the dominant language. In this context it is important to recognize that people who are not fluent in the dominant language need to be included in research, as they may be the population most in need. Traditional epidemiological studies tend to focus on the dominant population and exclude smaller groups that may differ in language ability or other characteristics. An associated challenge is that many immigrants have low educational levels and may not be able to understand or complete study instruments. Once again, the goal is to create study instruments that are more inclusive.

Another crosscutting issue is immigrant legal status. This sensitive topic must be handled carefully to avoid causing harm to the immigrants participating. It should also be recognized that undocumented migrants may have the most need of health services, but also may be reluctant to participate in any research. A closely related topic is research on political refugees. At a minimum, all research must be approved by the appropriate institutional review boards to protect the study subjects.

International migration research should ideally be done in the countries of origin and the receiving countries. This raises many crosscutting issues relevant to conducting research in foreign communities or binational research. We consider the methods to achieve host government acceptance for such research to be just as important as the research methods themselves. Indeed, without the appropriate approvals and acceptance, the research cannot be completed. This crosscutting issue is addressed in the chapters on working internationally and on binational collaborative research.

CAUSES OF GLOBAL MIGRATION

The largest cause of migration in the world today, both internal and international, is economic disparity. Lack of job opportunities in developing countries and low salaries for those that do have jobs constitute the major impetus for people moving from rural to urban areas, and from developing to developed countries. Closely related to this economic disparity are the low birth rates and aging populations in developed countries, in contrast to higher birth rates and younger populations in developing countries. Family reunification is another important cause of migration to some countries, like the United States.

A very different global cause of migration, requiring different expertise, is environmental-associated change. Acute natural disasters (e.g., earthquakes and floods) as well as chronic environmental pressures associated with global climate change (e.g., rising sea level and droughts) are forcing an increasing number of people around the world to move from their homelands. While the environmental causes of migration are generally different from the economic disparities, the human impacts on health are often the same, and research methods are similar.

Finally, forced migration due to conflicts and to political and other types of persecution (e.g., refugees and asylum seekers) are a constant reality, if not an increasing one, around the world. Understanding the cause of political migration and developing effective solutions raises many questions requiring an understanding, including having a firm legal foundation in the receiving country's regulations.

While understanding these different causes of migration requires very different expertise, the methods to study health outcomes in these different populations are quite similar. In addition, crosscutting issues such as language and legal status apply, at different levels, to all immigrant populations. Ultimately the improvement in health of migrant populations requires multidisciplinary solutions, whether the people are in refugee camps or settled into established communities in developed countries.

HEALTH ISSUES ASSOCIATED WITH MIGRATION

This is a methodology book and as such it does not go into detail on specific health problems associated with migration. However, it is worth pointing out here that there is a very large range of health issues caused or exacerbated by migration, and that the injuries and illnesses caused by migration are independent of reductions in health services commonly received by immigrants. Further, for this book we use the International Organization of Migration (IOM) definition of migration health, that is, the health of migrants and how migration affects people in countries of origin, transit, and destination, as well as how migration affects the offspring of migrants (IOM 2011). Given the breadth of populations and factors affecting health among migrants in their countries of origin and destination, a variety of approaches are needed to understand the complex web of causation among factors affecting the health of immigrants. It should also be recognized that many health outcomes are better among migrants than among the native population, the so-called healthy migrant paradox.

A primary consideration is an understanding of the conceptual models of migration and health. These models, discussed in chapter 3, set the frame for understanding the unique factors affecting health among immigrants. Foremost among these is a recognition that factors in the country and community of origin, in transit, and in the receiving country may all affect the health of immigrant populations. To focus exclusively on the conditions in the receiving country is a serious mistake that can lead to faulty conclusions or ineffective programs to improve the health of migrants. It should also be recognized that immigrants have some health advantages after immigration, although some of these advantages decline with increased time since migration (Franzini et al. 2001; Fennelly 2007).

A secondary consideration is to recognize that adverse health outcomes among immigrants cover the spectrum from acute infectious diseases and traumatic injuries to chronic diseases such as asthma, heart disease, and cancer. No longer is the focus on migrant health limited to infectious diseases that could, in theory, be stopped by screening and quarantine of new immigrants. The magnitude and speed of global movement has rendered that approach ineffective for preventing disease transmission, as was demonstrated by the global spread of SARS and the H1N1 influenza epidemic. Understanding the causes of the increase in chronic diseases among migrants with longer duration of stay in the host country requires careful etiologic studies, ideally involving the populations in both the countries of origin and those receiving. For example, the increase in asthma prevalence among Latino immigrants to the US may be related to some combination of factors including neonatal or childhood exposures in the country of origin, and/or diet, medication, occupational, or environmental factors in the receiving country. Underlying genetic and epigenetic factors may further influence the disease's occurrence, as can stress and health-related behaviors such as cigarette smoking. Similar situations exist for other chronic diseases.

A third theme is that immigration-associated effects on health occur over the life span and may have a different influence at different points in the immigration cycle. Thus, childhood exposures in the country of origin may have an important influence on health outcomes in the host country. Gene-environment interactions and epigenetic factors may also reflect exposures at different points in the immigration cycle. In addition, behaviors of the parents may be significant in shaping health outcomes among immigrant children.

MULTIDISCIPLINARY APPROACHES

A fundamental consideration that underlies this book is that multidisciplinary approaches are appropriate, indeed necessary, for understanding the causes of poorer health for some conditions among immigrants and for developing effective solutions to reduce the disparities in health and health care between immigrant and nonimmigrant populations. Multidisciplinary methods are necessary because of the complex factors that drive migration as well as the equally complex factors that cause the disparities that negatively impact the health of migrant populations (Koser et al. 2010).

ACHIEVING SOLUTIONS

The ultimate goal of this book, then, is to improve the health of migrant populations around the world. We believe that too little quality research has been done on health among immigrants, and this has in turn reduced the resources and efforts to improve their health. This situation has occurred in part because migrants have not been recognized as a large population with unique health needs, and in part because it is more difficult to study migrants than the dominant, nonmigrant population. Migrants are, by definition, mobile. They often don't speak the dominant language and education levels may be low. Legal fears may further inhibit participation in any research. Despite these challenges we know that such research is possible, and indeed it can and should form the basis for efforts to improve the health of individuals with some of the greatest need in the population.

It is time for a new paradigm in addressing the health of immigrants (WHO 2010). Instead of the old isolation mentality, in which countries thought they could protect their native populations by excluding or quarantining immigrants, we need new, multinational, inclusive approaches that recognize the reality of modern human mobility and disease epidemiology. The health of immigrant populations should be monitored, and health care systems need to be sensitive to the needs of migrants. Policy-legal frameworks should protect the rights of migrants to health, including equal access to health care. By developing such systems, and conducting research on disease causation and prevention among migrants, we can truly achieve better health for all.

We are not so naïve as to be unaware that this must be done in the context of a political environment that is often "anti-immigrant." However, diseases don't recognize national boundaries and modern public health should not, either. In the words of former secretary general of the United Nations Kofi Annan, "We now understand better than ever that migration is not a zero-sum game. In the best cases, it benefits the receiving country, the country of origin and migrants themselves."

REFERENCES

Fennelly, K. 2007. "The 'Healthy Migrant' Effect." *Minnesota Medicine* 90(3):51–53.
Franzini, L., J.C. Ribble, and A.M. Keddie. 2001. "Understanding the Hispanic Paradox." *Ethnicity and Disease* 11(3):496–518.
International Organization on Migration (IOM). 2011. Migration for the Benefit of All. Accessed July 30, 2012. http://www.iom.int/jahia/Jahia/about-migration/facts-and-figures/lang/en.
Koser, Khalid, and Frank Laczko, eds. 2010. *World Migration Report 2010—The Future of Migration: Building Capacities for Change.* Geneva: International Organization for Migration (IOM).
United Nations Development Program (UNDP). 2009. "Human Development Report 2009—Overcoming Barriers: Human Mobility and Development." Accessed December 22, 2012. http://hdr.undp.org/en/media/HDR_2009_EN_Complete.pdf.

United States Department of Commerce. 2010. US Census. Accessed July 30, 2012. http://www.census.gov/population/foreign/.

World Health Organization (WHO). 2010. *Health of Migrants: The Way Forward—Report of a Global Consultation, Madrid, Spain, 3–5 March 2010*. Accessed July 30, 2012. http://www.who.int/hac/events/3_5march2010/en/.

Dr. Alfonso Rodriguez-Lainz contributed to this book in his personal capacity. The views expressed are his own and do not necessarily reflect the views of the Centers for Disease Control and Prevention, the Department of Health and Human Services, or the United States government.

2

Studying Migrant Populations

General Considerations and Approaches

Alfonso Rodriguez-Lainz
Xóchitl Castañeda

MIGRATION RESEARCH

The increased diversity and volume of migration is one of the main factors shaping social, demographic, cultural, and economic processes in the twenty-first century. Because of its widespread impact, migration has become an increasingly contentious issue. The causes and consequences of migration for origin, transit, and destination communities are passionately debated in the public arena. On the one hand, pro-immigration groups emphasize migrants' human rights, the positive link between migration and economic development for origin and receiving countries, and the positive aspects of increased cultural diversity. Anti-immigrant groups, on the other hand, view migration as a threat to national sovereignty, security, and the prevalent culture. They also tend to see immigrants as a drain on limited social, educational, and health care resources. Attitudes toward migration typically get more extreme during times of conflict and economic hardship, which has certainly been the case since the onset of the global economic crisis that started in 2008.

Yet, despite migration's relevance, there are serious limitations to the amount and quality of evidence available to properly assess and manage migration flows and the complex issues associated with immigration. Likewise, the causes and consequences of migration are often poorly understood. According to a report by the Commission on International Migration Data, the quality of migration data that countries now collect and publish is so limited that "we are setting migration policies in the dark, ... based on anecdotes and emotion" (Center for Global Development 2009).

Historically, academic research on migration has been focused predominantly on its economic and social aspects (e.g., effects on labor markets, use of public resources by migrants, social integration processes, acculturation, economic impact of remittances, etc.). Although the association between migration and health has been recognized for centuries, quality research on this topic has been very limited until recent years (Ingleby 2009; Argeseanu Cunningham et al. 2008). Both the conceptual frameworks and appropriate study designs for migration health research are still in relatively early stages of development (see chapter 3 of this volume, by Spallek et al.).

Migration is considered a more difficult demographic phenomenon to measure than mortality and nativity (Massey, 2010). Migration is made up of two complementary population flows: immigration and emigration. In the case of international migration, there are challenges in harmonizing, coordinating, and sharing migration data across countries in the same migration system. Migration is also a very dynamic process. Both the numbers and characteristics of migrants in origin and destination countries change overtime. Sometimes that change can be dramatic, such as in massive population displacement due to wars or environmental disasters. People may migrate multiple times and for different durations during their lifetime. Over time, the same individual may belong to different migrant legal status categories (Massey 2010).

Migration can have effects at multiple levels. For instance, the determinants and consequences of migration are relevant not only to individual migrants but also to the communities in the countries of origin, transit, and destination. Finally, migration can have an impact on the health of migrants' offspring born in the host country and even later generations who may not ever have migrated themselves.

The absence of an internationally accepted definition of what constitutes a migrant is considered one of the main roadblocks in advancing migration research (Center for Global Development 2009). Countries and agencies within countries may use different definitions based on their own policies, regulations, data needs, and practices, limiting the comparability of migration statistics across countries and agencies. For example, in the United States, terms like "migrant," "immigrant," "undocumented," "minorities," "Latinos," and "farmworkers" are frequently not well described and/or are used interchangeably both in the media and in scientific and other publications (Loue and Bunce 1999). This happens despite the fact that these terms typically represent highly diverse populations, with different migration experiences or, in the case of some native minority groups, no migration at all. These practices reduce the interpretability of data and might also be a reason for the sometimes contradictory results reported in the migrant health literature.

The objective of this chapter is to provide the general theoretical and epistemological framework of this handbook. First, we will discuss several general limitations of available migration data sources. Second, we will describe characteristics common among migrant populations that need to be considered in the planning and conducting of migration research. These issues are relevant to most migrants to different degrees and require the adaption of study designs appropriate for the general population and/or the use of specialized study methodologies. The final section of the chapter provides general recommendations for conducting migration research. Although focused on international migrants, these recommendations can also apply to internal migrants, and similar approaches can also be adapted for the study of other minorities and hard-to-reach populations (e.g., homeless people, people with disabilities, sexual minorities, illegal drug users, sex workers).

LIMITATIONS OF MIGRATION DATA SOURCES

Before the initiation of any new research or data collection project it is important to assess the availability and quality of data on the population and topic of interest, a process that should include a thorough literature review. A variety of national data collection systems may collect information useful for migration research, including the following (UN 2007b, 2007c; Grieco and Rytina 2011):

a. Population census is the most viable data source in most countries for counting and describing the sociodemographic characteristics of international migrants. The census may also include some limited health data (e.g., disability and health insurance in the US).

b. (Continuous) population registers are maintained in many Western European countries and Japan. All residents, including immigrants, are required to register with the local community when they relocate. Some countries have a register dedicated only to foreigners in their territory. Population and foreigner registers are likely to have incomplete coverage of certain populations, such as unauthorized migrants.

c. Border statistics and admissions data collection systems collect information on individuals entering and, in a few countries, on those departing the national territory. These data systems collect information on events (e.g., admissions) rather than individuals (i.e., one individual can enter and depart a given country several times during a given period). Very limited demographic information is collected. Most admissions are visitors rather than migrants.

d. General purpose surveys are more likely to be useful to study migration if they have a large sample size (e.g., 50,000–100,000), if migrants constitute a relatively large share of the population in that region (e.g., 10% or more), if the survey has good coverage of migrants, and if it collects information that allows for the identification of migrants (e.g., country of birth, citizenship, or previous place of residence) (UN 1998).

e. Health information systems such as hospital discharge information systems, disease registries (e.g., cancer registries), and notifiable disease surveillance systems are focused on different health issues and may also collect some migration-related variables.

f. Demographic surveillance systems (DSS) consist of longitudinal monitoring of demographic and vital events (births, deaths, and migrations) of populations living in well-defined geographic areas. After a DSS site is selected, data collection starts with a baseline census followed by periodic data updates to assess changes in population dynamics and, in particular, in- and out-migration of individuals into and out of the area. In addition to core demographic data, DSS also collect detailed health, social, and economic characteristics of the target population. Study populations in current DSS sites range from 30,000 to more than 500,000 people. Most DSS sites are located in rural areas of less-developed countries in Africa, Asia, and the Americas (Ye et al. 2009; Collinson 2010). An international network of independent research centers, the INDEPTH Network (www.indepth-network.org), runs DSS. DSS have been used extensively to study the dynamic relationship of migration and health (Collinson et al. 2009; Welaga et al. 2009; Collinson 2010; Gerritsen et al. 2013).

Several national data collection systems in the European Union and the United States are discussed in detail in chapters 4 and 5 of this volume, by Levecque et al. and Singh, respectively. In general, the availability and quality of migration data varies greatly both among and within countries (Center for Global Development 2009), and may also vary with time, with more recent data often being of greater quality than older data. According to the United Nations, "Even the most basic data on the numbers of migrants continues to be weak and unreliable in many countries" (UN 2007a). Data sources are especially limited in statistics on temporary, recent, and unauthorized migrants. Most countries also lack a system to monitor people, whether native or foreign, who emigrate to another country (Massey 2010; Kahanec and Zimmermann 2008; UN 1998).

Although many countries already collect a wealth of data on the foreign-born, in many cases these data have not been fully analyzed or widely disseminated. This may be due to a combination of reasons, including limited interest in (or awareness about) migration issues among those responsible for the data system, limited awareness among researchers about the existence of those datasets and their usefulness for migration research, and restrictive data access policies or inadequate data access infrastructure by agencies and organizations with the responsibility for maintaining them (Center for Global Development 2009; Kahanec and Zimmermann 2008).

A major limitation is that many official data sources do not collect information on key migration variables. For example, in the US, hospital discharge data systems do not collect any migration-related data besides language preference. Other data systems only collect information on foreign birth and thus do not allow disaggregating data by country of origin. For datasets that only collect current citizenship information and not foreign birth, migrants who have acquired citizenship in their host country cannot be differentiated from native populations. Information on experiences and circumstances of migrants before migration (i.e., in their country of origin) is also generally not available even though those risk factors might be determinants for some of the health conditions identified in migrants after arrival in the host country. Available data usually provide very limited information about migration trajectories or history (Kahanec 2008), that is, the different countries where migrants have lived, and the durations and circumstances of their travel and stays (Bilsborrow et al. 1997). Other variables of interest that are not frequently collected include migration legal status, religion, preferred language, and proficiency in the host country's language.

Some migration-related variables are difficult to collect with accuracy and reliability. One example is "duration of stay in the host country." Most data sources estimate duration of stay by asking for the date the migrant arrived to reside in the country. Commonly, this date is interpreted as the most recent date of arrival. However, this interpretation does not allow for time spent in the country by individuals who have migrated several times to the same host country for different periods of time. According to Massey (2010), this is an especially important issue for migration research in the US because the majority of new legal immigrants have already spent time in the country in some other status and because the total duration of stay varies markedly from country to country.

Legal status (e.g., naturalized citizen, legal permanent resident refugee, temporary worker, undocumented) is another variable difficult to collect. The legal categories vary from country to country and can change over time for the same individual. A migrant's legal status is an important variable to collect because the different legal categories have different rights and access to government-funded benefits (e.g., education, economic assistance for low-income families, unemployment benefits) (Massey 2010), which may affect access to care and health outcomes. For example, undocumented migrants often have the least access to publicly funded health services and can suffer from greater discrimination, both of which can be associated with poorer health outcomes. Legal status is also very sensitive information to collect, especially in an anti-immigrant environment. Migrants are unlikely to provide honest answers about their legal status unless this information is collected by a trusted organization (Deren et al. 2005).

Other variables that are important to take into account, but are difficult to measure, are those related to what Rayna Rapp calls a "political economy of risk" (2000). That is, migrants face risks related to health (physical, emotional, and psychological) that are contingent upon their placement within the local economy and shaped by political and social forces. In this sense, it is important to take into account local expressions of transnational inequalities (Ginsburg and Rapp 1995; Martin 1995). According to these scholars, individuals (in this case, migrants) imagine and enact cultural logics and social formations through varied mechanisms—personal struggle, generational mobility, participation in social movements, or contestation of powerful religious and political ideologies. Globalization sets in motion capital, technology, popular culture, and/or sexually transmitted infections that cross national borders.

Overlapping with these class and social forces, racism is another factor that needs to be considered: when people (e.g., indigenous migrants from Guatemala) migrate to countries in which the dominant racial group is "white," they tend to be racially discriminated against in multiple ways, not just by the dominant population but by other minorities that are better situated (e.g., some Mexican contractors). That is, there are historic and socio-demographic meanings and practices that segregate these populations as racially inferior (Omi and Winant 1994). Racialization can be seen in the concentration of indigenous migrants in "brown-collar jobs" (Catanzarite 2000; Ibarra 2000) such as farm labor, which is considered to be at the bottom of the labor market in the US (Villarejo et al. 2000).

Official statistics on the second generation (i.e., children born in the US with one or both parents foreign-born) are generally limited because most data sources do not collect information on parental birthplace. In the US, for example, the decennial census stopped asking that question after 1970 (Massey 2010; Kahanec and Zimmermann 2008). This data limitation is important because of the higher fertility rate among immigrant women and the increasing share of second-generation children among all children in the country.

A sizable proportion of the migrant population (frequently those who are most vulnerable) is likely not captured by routine national information systems and research studies. This may be due to a combination of reasons, including distrust of government agencies, fear of deportation or of losing public benefits, language barriers, geographic or social isolation, and limited access to care. Migrants are also more likely to live in irregular housing units or have complex housing arrangements, be more mobile, have no access to a landline phone, or be out of the country at the time of data collection (Andresen et al, 2004; Deren et al, 2005; McKenzie and Mistien 2007). Outflows of migrants from the receiving country, voluntary or involuntary (i.e., deportation of unauthorized migrants), can be substantial and vary markedly by country of birth (Massey 2010; Kahanec and Zimmermann 2008; UN 1998). All of these factors limit the accuracy of data on the number of migrants in a particular region and time period and may also affect migrant health indicator data in ways that are difficult to assess and that result in biased information. For example, mandatory communicable disease surveillance systems may underestimate disease prevalence and risk factors among migrants because of their limited access to diagnostic and treatment services or lack of diagnostic tests and/or reporting requirements for certain diseases that are more prevalent among migrant populations (e.g., parasitic diseases). Or, if large numbers of migrants leave the country or study area, especially if they leave because of illness or old age, disease and mortality estimates will also be confounded. The lack of reliable data on the number of migrant subpopulations in many geographic areas also creates challenges to obtaining denominator data needed to calculate statistical rates and proportions used in health indicators.

Most data sources on migrants are cross-sectional (Massey 2010), with all of the advantages of this design, including efficiency and cost, but with limitations to studying a phenomenon that is intrinsically longitudinal, where important factors such as acculturation, immigration status, and policies change over time. Thus few data sources allow researchers to adequately examine changes in health outcomes, behaviors, or access to health care concurrent with changes in migration-related factors (Loue and Bunce 1999; Kahanec and Zimmermann 2008).

A common approach to studying changes in migrant health and social characteristics over time is to compare the outcome of interest across year-of-entry cohorts. As Massey (2010) points out, this approach can produce results that may represent actual changes over time (improvements or worsening of the outcome), but the results may also be due to selective return (i.e., those with better or worse health) or differences in the cohort of immigrants arriving over time. For example, the prevalence of obesity among Mexican adults has almost tripled between 1980 (12%) and 2011 (30%), close to the prevalence in the US (33.8%) (Mexico Secretariat of Health 2010). Similar cohort effects may also exist for social determinants of health (e.g., education, economic status). Both scenarios, that is, real changes and selective in- and out-migration, may occur simultaneously.

CHARACTERISTICS OF MIGRANTS

Migrants often share a number of key characteristics that are relevant to research; all of the following characteristics should be considered by those embarking upon a research project involving immigrant populations:

- self-selection
- diversity
- mobility
- geographic dispersion and local concentration
- rare (or low-frequency) populations
- hidden populations
- multinational and multilevel exposures and risk factors
- vulnerability

Self-Selection

Individuals and households who decide and succeed in migrating likely have different characteristics than those who do not migrate. Some of those characteristics are easier to observe (e.g., age, gender, ethnicity/race, education, income), while others are not (e.g., risk aversion, sexual conflicts, self-confidence, ambition). But, to paraphrase the twentieth-century Spanish liberal philosopher José Ortega y Gasset, "The individual is him/herself and his/her circumstances." Self-selection is not isolated from the social-economic-political causes that push individuals to leave their communities of origin and to migrate in search of a better life.

Differences in characteristics between migrants and nonmigrants may confound the effect of migration on health or other outcomes of interest and thus need to be addressed in the study design and/or data analysis. One method to limit this form of selection bias is to collect or analyze information about a migrant's characteristics and situation immediately prior to emigration. Multivariate regression models can then be used to statistically control for those potential confounders (Kahanec and Zimmermann 2008).

Immigrants residing in a country at a given point in time are a selective subset of all foreigners who might have ever migrated to the country. They do not include those who have died or left the area prior to the study or data collection. To the extent that either death or emigration is associated with the outcome of interest (e.g., health status, integration, language ability), and/or individuals who emigrate are systematically different from those who remain, estimates of the association of migration with those outcomes may be confounded (Massey 2010; Carletto and de Brauw 2008).

Diversity

Migrants are a very heterogeneous population in terms of culture, ethnicity, language, religion, education, reasons for migrating, and migration experiences, among other characteristics. This is the case even among migrants from the same country. For example, Mexican migrants in the US include highly educated professionals, agricultural workers, and indigenous people (some of them non-Spanish speakers). Migrants' diversity translates into a mosaic of beliefs, attitudes, and practices related to health that frequently contrasts with those of the native population (Ingleby 2009). Migrants' diversity is frequently ignored or missed in many studies and research reports. This is the case, for example, when data on African-born individuals in the US are included with the larger African American population statistics, or when Latino migrant subgroups (e.g., Mexicans, Salvadorians) are combined into one group. In another, more complex, example, the primary HIV transmission routes for Puerto Ricans is through injection drug use or through sex with an HIV-positive drug user, while for foreign-born Hispanics, and especially Mexicans, the primary HIV transmission route has been through sexual contact between men who have sex with men. At the same time, summary statistics on the foreign-born can be heavily influenced by a single country of birth if that is the predominant migrant group (e.g., Mexicans in the US) (Deren et al. 2005).

Migrants' cultural, educational, and linguistic diversity also needs to be considered in the development and use of data collection instruments. Currently there is limited information about the reliability and validity of data collection instruments being used with such diverse populations (Loue and Bunce 1999). These populations are not "pure," or monolithic. In the process of migration, they bring with them a complex background of "hybrid" cultures (García Canclini 1990). As inheritors of hybrid cultures, individuals represent fragments of traditions, modernity, and postmodernity in which social representations are being constantly reinvented against the background of earlier intersections and intermingling with vestiges of earlier cultures. For instance, some migrants might bring aspects of ancient Mesoamericans, the culture(s) of the Spaniards, modern Japanese technology, the fashions of the Bronx, and Brazilian soap operas *(telenovelas)*, along with other centuries-old beliefs and traditions.

Mobility

Migrants often have different migration and travel patterns than native populations (Mexico Secretariat 2010). For example, in the US, the foreign-born have been reported to be more mobile than natives (i.e., have lived in a different residence in the previous five years). The foreign-born have a higher rate of intracounty migration, while natives have a higher intrastate rate. Recent foreign-born arrivals and noncitizens have higher mobility rates than those who have resided longer in the US. Finally, mobility varies by region of origin, with Africans having the highest mobility rate and the European-born the lowest (US Department of Commerce 2003). Migrants also tend to travel regularly to their country of origin for extended periods of time to visit friends and relatives. This and other types of mobility may expose migrants and their offspring to environmental, transportation, and other health risks. As indicated earlier, migrants' mobility may also affect their likelihood of being included in national data systems and studies (Leder et al. 2006; Bilsborrow et al. 1997). The effects of in- and out-migration on the representativeness of study samples or datasets are usually difficult to quantify because of a lack of information about the numbers, reasons, and characteristics of those that move.

Geographic Dispersion and Local Concentration

Although the diversity of regions of origin and destination of migrants is increasing, migrants still tend to originate from specific areas in the origin country and to concentrate in specific areas in the destination country (UN 2007c). This is a useful characteristic for efficient data collection (especially for household surveys) and also for targeted program implementation. However, it is also important to keep in mind that migrants residing in nontraditional migration areas may have different characteristics from those living in more traditional destinations; for example, they may be more isolated, have less support from migrant-serving organizations, and have less access to cultural and linguistically appropriate services.

Rare (or Low-Frequency) Populations

In many geographic areas, migration is considered a *rare event*. Rare events are defined as statistical occurrences that happen infrequently. Migrants frequently represent a small fraction of the general population in many countries of origin and also in most countries or regions of destination, even in some of the traditional destination countries like the US (Center for Global Development 2009; UN 1998; Carletto and de Brauw 2008). For example, in the US, which has a population of 12 million Mexican-born residents (the predominant migrant population), most counties have a proportion of Mexican-born lower than 3%. That percentage would be even smaller if our population of interest is just recent immigrants (e.g., those who arrived in the last five years). Other populations considered rare or low frequency include some race/ethnic minorities, people with disabilities, and seniors.

There is no specific cutoff point that defines a "rare" population for research purposes. Andresen et al. (2004) suggest a 10% level. That is, if a subgroup composes less than 10% of the population in a geographic area, a random sample will likely only include a handful of members of that subpopulation, the consequence being a large sampling margin of errors in estimates for that subpopulation.

The rarity of migrants in some geographic locations is an important challenge in migration research because traditional sampling methodologies that are appropriate for the general population frequently fail to capture an adequate number of migrants. For example, the typical multipurpose nationally representative survey has a sample size between 5,000 and 10,000 households, which may not provide data on a sufficient number of migrants to obtain statistically reliable estimates. This limitation is even more extreme for smaller migrant subgroups. For that reason, specialized sampling designs are frequently required to ensure representativeness and adequate sample size of migrants in surveys (Carletto and de Brauw 2008; UN 2007c). The fact that immigrant populations are sometimes both rare and geographically dispersed can make research even more difficult.

Hidden Populations

Some migrant groups have been described as *hidden* populations in the sense that they prefer to remain incognito; they do not want to disclose their migration status to government agencies or researchers because of distrust, concerns about discrimination, or fear of immigration authorities, among other reasons. Some migrant groups are also hidden because they live in unsafe, unofficial, or difficult-to-reach areas, and thus are likely missed by researchers and government agencies (e.g., by the decennial census). As a result, sampling frames to survey migrants, if available, may be very incomplete and not include important migrant subgroups, which frequently are the most vulnerable (McKenzie and Mistien 2007; UN 2007c). For example, in the US some Guatemalan migrants in areas dominated by Mexican immigrants tend to "Mexicanize" as a survival strategy and are especially hard to identify (Castañeda et al. 2002). Furthermore, migrant populations that are both low frequency and hidden (e.g., victims of trafficking, unauthorized migrant sex workers) can also be extremely hard to reach (Andresen et al. 2004).

Multinational and Multilevel Exposures and Risk Factors

Health behaviors and outcomes among migrants are influenced by many complex and interrelated individual factors and environmental, social, and cultural exposures in the countries of origin, transit, and destination. In migrant health research, for example, it is ideal to consider health-related beliefs, attitudes, and practices; prevalent health conditions; and health infrastructure and access to health care before, during, and after migration. The migration experience itself may be an important determinant of health for migrants (e.g., travel-related injuries, sexual abuse, mental illness, etc.). Multinational and multilevel factors need to be considered both for data collection and analysis. However, many theoretical frameworks and studies focus only on specific factors or on conditions after migration and thus fail to take into account the inherent complexity of the migration experience for both migrants and their families (Deren et al. 2005).

Vulnerability

Migrants can be a highly vulnerable population that requires special protection strategies for research. Vulnerabilities associated with migration legal status, communication barriers, and lack of familiarity with the system and rights in the destination country must be considered (UN 1998). When living in an anti-immigrant social or political environment, even authorized immigrants can be exposed to discrimination, abuse, and xenophobia. In addition, migrants may also experience vulnerabilities similar to those of other ethnic, minority, and marginalized populations such as populations with low education level and low socioeconomic status. Extra attention is crucial in the study of migrant populations that tend to have little or no past experience with research and their rights as participants (Deren et al. 2005).

STRATEGIES FOR CONDUCTING RESEARCH AMONG MIGRANT POPULATIONS

This section includes some general strategies to address the issues discussed above. This is not intended to be an exhaustive list, nor is it an in-depth analysis. It is an introduction to the topics and strategies that are explored in greater detail throughout this book. Most of these strategies are also relevant for conducting research with other minority and hard-to-reach populations.

Harmonize Migration Definitions

The need for international harmonization of migration definitions and statistics has been recognized for many decades. One good example is the 1951 UN refugee definition, which most countries have adopted and incorporated into their national laws (see http://www.unhcr.org/3b66c2aa10.html). More recent initiatives include the UN's 1998 recommendations on statistics of international migration and follow-up implementation guidance reports (UN 2007a). In 2007 the European Parliament and the Council of the European Union adopted a new regulation requiring all EU member states to provide Eurostat harmonized statistics on migrant stocks (i.e., the number of migrants in a country at a specific point in time) and flows, and other migration-relevant data (EU 2007). A 2009 report by the Commission on International Migration Data proposes that the long-term objective of harmonizing migration data definitions should remain a priority. However, in the short term, a more pragmatic approach is for countries to disseminate migration data collected according to their own criteria, but to provide the specific definitions used (Center for Global Development 2009). This recommendation can also be extended to researchers.

Disseminate and Analyze Available Data

Agencies and other organizations maintaining databases with migration information should analyze and publish available data in a timely manner and facilitate public (including researchers) access to the datasets as anonymous individual microdata. National and agency regulations and practices need to be respected. However, aggregating data (e.g., countries of birth) to protect respondent confidentiality is not necessary as long as appropriate national regulations and international guidelines for anonymizing, storing, documenting, and disseminating microdata are established and followed (e.g., guidelines from International Household Survey Network).[1] There are some good examples of how this can be done, including the Integrated Public Use Microdata Series–International (IPUMS-I; https://international.ipums.org/international/), which provides the public with access through their website to large amounts of census microdata from many countries; the Mexican Migration Project (see mmp.opr.princeton.edu/), which has disseminated anonymous detailed microdata on thousands of individual migrants since the 1980s; and the US Census Bureau's census and labor force surveys, which can be freely downloaded from the organization's website (see www.census.gov/acs/www/data_documentation/data_main/ and www.census.gov/cps/data/). In cases where release of microdata is politically or legally infeasible, detailed disaggregated tables should be provided.

There is also a need to increase awareness among researchers about the existence of migration data sources, their strengths and limitations, and how to access them. For instance, the National Population Council of Mexico (CONAPO) has published in collaboration with the Mexican Ministry of Health and the Health Initiative of the Americas (HIA, a program of the UC Berkeley School of Public Health) a series of annual reports focused on data sources and various health topics (e.g., access and utilization of health services, health insurance access, disease-specific reports, etc.; see http://hia.berkeley.edu/index.php?page = migration-and-health-reports).

One area of great opportunity to increase the availability of migration data is the merging of datasets across agencies and even among countries. Different datasets can also be linked to yield new migration-related data; for example, a dataset that is rich in socioeconomic and health information but limited in migration information can be linked with another dataset that includes key migration data. Examples of this approach can be found in chapter 5, on US. information systems, by Singh.

Add Migration-Related Questions to Existing Data Sources

Before a new migration survey or other study is planned, current data systems must be assessed in terms of their content, sampling design, sample size, language of instruments, and the availability of any migration-related data (Carletto 2008). For data systems with larger sample sizes and coverage, but with limited or no migration data, adding a core "migration module" of migration-related variables can be a cost-effective alternative (Center for Global Development 2009; Kahanec and Zimmermann 2008). For example, this would be a good option for several ongoing large household surveys in countries of origin and destination, such as the Living Standards Measurement Study surveys by the World bank (see go.worldbank.org/IFS9WG7EO0) and Demographic and Health Surveys, by Macro International (see www.measuredhs.com/). This approach would also be feasible with many other large health and/or workforce surveys. Some large surveys are already implementing this recommendation, including the National Mexican Health Survey (ENSALUT), which has added migration-related questions to traditional sections of this periodic survey.

A number of key migration-related variables need to be considered by those conducting migration studies. In household and phone surveys, migration information should be recorded for all persons interviewed and ideally for all household members (UN 1998). In the case of surveys or other studies involving children, it is important to collect and analyze key migration information about their parents (e.g., place of birth, language spoken, immigration legal status). At a minimum, parental place of birth should be collected so the children of foreign-born parents (i.e., the second generation) can be identified and their health status assessed.

Significant variables of interest that should be considered in migration research include the following:

- place (country, state) of birth of respondents and their parents
- place (country, state) of residence at a specified time in the past (e.g., one or five years ago)
- current country, state of residence
- time of (first and last) arrival to live in the country/periodicity of travel back and forth
- total duration of residence in host country
- age at migration
- frequency of, duration of, and reasons for returns to origin country
- migrant's intentions to remain temporarily or permanently in the host country or plans for further moves (Kahanec and Zimmermann 2008)
- migration legal status (at least country of citizenship, including any change of citizenship and its timing, and that of immediate relatives, e.g., children)
- language(s) spoken at home
- ability to speak the predominant language of the host country
- ethnicity, especially if different from the predominant group in the country of origin; for example, specific ethnic groups from African countries, or migrants from indigenous communities in Latin America
- ancestry
- religion
- experience of suffering from racism and discrimination
- remittances, periodicity, and purposes

Some studies may choose to obtain a more detailed migration history to document all moves over a specified reference period (Carletto and de Brauw 2008). With proper training and by anchoring migration episodes to explicit time benchmarks such as political elections, natural disasters, or a personal life event (i.e., marriage, the birth of a child), reconstructing full migration histories may be feasible and highly productive. To facilitate recall, more detailed migration information could be collected for recent years (e.g., 5–10 years), or questions might be limited to longer-duration migration episodes. However, at a minimum it is worthwhile to collect the year of first migration, the most recent entry, and the estimated total duration of residence in the host country for everyone in the sample with any migration experience.

Researchers always need to consider that, given the complexities of migration laws, self-classification of specific immigrant status may not be straightforward for many migrants. Also, for individuals who have traveled multiple times to a destination country, it might be difficult to recall all visits or the total time living in that country (Massey 2010).

Addressing Low Frequency

Several approaches have been recommended when the migrant population of interest is rare, including the following (Center for Global Development 2009; Andresen et al. 2004; Bilheimer and Klein 2010, Bilsborrow et al. 1997):

a. *Aggregating data by geography and/or time:* Aggregating data will increase the sample size of migrants available for analysis, although the number still may be insufficient to provide adequate data for smaller immigrant groups. Special attention is needed when multiple years of data are combined or when immigrant cohorts from different time periods are compared. The definitions and quality of data may have changed over time, and/or there may have been changes in eligibility criteria for publicly funded benefits, for example.

b. *Use of exact statistics:* When the sample size of migrants in a dataset is too small to allow calculation of confidence intervals or statistical tests based on the assumptions of the normal distribution, exact statistical methods can provide better estimates. Exact statistics are available in most commercial statistical packages.

c. *Case-control studies:* Case-control studies allow for the study of risk factors for rare populations and/or rare conditions that might be more prevalent among migrant populations. For a detailed discussion on the use of case control in migration research please see chapter 11, by Pezzi and Kass, in this volume.

d. *Oversample migrant groups:* If it is feasible and resources are available, specific migrant groups of interest can be oversampled in a survey or other study in order to obtain adequate sample sizes for analysis. For example, one recommended strategy for household surveys is to oversample geographic areas where immigrants concentrate. Kalsbeek (2003) suggests sampling areas with a higher concentration of minorities up to about four times the rate of other areas to improve estimates from minorities. Greater oversampling is likely to have an adverse effect on overall population estimates. Appropriate weights to adjust the estimates will need to be used during data analysis.

e. *Specialized sampling methods:* A number of techniques have been proposed in the literature to sample rare populations. Two of those approaches are considered especially appropriate for migration household surveys, particularly if used in combination: disproportionate or oversampling of areas with higher proportions of migrants and two-phase sampling of households (UN 1998; Bilsborrow et al. 1997; Carletto and de Brauw 2008). This approach requires a way to (at least roughly) estimate the proportions of migrants by geographic or administrative areas. A major advantage of this approach is that it leads to some geographical concentration of fieldwork and thus is cost-effective. Oversampling can also be used with telephone-based surveys. For a detailed description, please see chapters 6 and 10 in this volume, by Marcelli and Grant et al., respectively.

Two other sampling techniques have been widely used with other hard-to-reach, hidden, and rare populations, and they are also promising for migration research: respondent-driven sampling and time-location sampling, which are discussed in chapters 7 and 8, by Johnston and Malekinejad and Semaan, respectively.

The decision to acquire more primary data or markedly change the completeness, quality, and detail of current data sources may require substantial funding, significant changes in data collection instruments and databases, and additional training of project personnel. The added benefits and costs of each strategy need to be carefully weighed (Andresen et al. 2004).

Use of Qualitative Methodologies

Qualitative methodological approaches have proved to be very useful and complementary for research among mobile populations due to the environmental and political issues that frequently impact these populations. Specifically in the migration and health arena, researchers using qualitative instruments aim to generate an in-depth understanding of human behavior and the processes through which such behavior is constructed and has meaning. Using the qualitative approaches listed below and discussed in section 3 of this volume, researchers can examine the "why and how" of decision making, besides the magnitude of the problem, that is, its prevalence, incidence, and other epidemiologic issues.

Ethnography, discussed in chapter 13, by Holmes and Castañeda, is a useful strategy in answering questions associated with health issues related to migration and their meanings, myths, norms, and gender attributes. Because of its strong emphasis on exploring the nature of social phenomena, ethnography is also helpful for analyzing the system of concepts, beliefs, and practices related to the health-seeking behavior, perception of risk and vulnerability, and other factors. Migration and health patterns, tendencies, and problems do not exist outside certain socio-economic, political, and historical conditions. In this sense, ethnography helps to contextualize and link local specificities with global perspectives, addressing migrant configuration, resettlement, social welfare characteristics, and health-seeking behaviors, as well as material and spiritual culture.

Participant observation, discussed in chapter 14, by Aguilera and Amuchástegui, is one of the earliest and most basic forms of research, and it is the most likely to be used in conjunction with others, such as interviewing. What differentiates research observations from those of everyday-life factors is the systematic and purposive nature of data collection. Through participant observation other sources of data, such as interviews or questionnaires, can be used for cross-checking and for triangulation of information.

Photovoice, discussed in chapter 17, by Langhout, is a methodology that provides insight into how migrant groups conceptualize their circumstances. For instance, migrants are asked to represent their personal point of view by taking photographs, discussing them together, and developing narratives to explain their photos. In this sense, photovoice attempts to make visible the perspectives of those who are "researched" and can help to identify local problems that are not necessarily obvious for a researcher who comes from another ethnic or socioeconomic background.

Focus groups/group qualitative interviews, discussed in chapter 15, by Zavella, obtain background information and insights into behavior, motivations, and trends from group interviews and can be highly useful for understanding the collective thinking and social consensus related to health problems. Group interviews have the potential to facilitate access to sensitive topics using local colloquial language. Insights gained through these instruments can serve as the basis of surveys through which hypotheses can be tested and generalized to a larger population.

Community-based participatory research has been embraced as a vital public health intervention and research technique (Andresen et al. 2004) and is fully discussed in chapter 19 of this volume, by Minkler and Chang. They highly recommend that, as with research with ethnic and cultural minorities, target migrant communities participate in the different stages of the research project, including determining the objectives, study design, implementation plan, and interpretation of results. The appropriate levels and strategies of community participation may vary depending on the specific target populations and circumstances. In general, it is important to request support from community leaders and advocates. When designing studies, researchers need to take into consideration issues that are a priority for the community.

The research team must also take the time, before data collection starts, to develop relationships of trust with the communities to be studied. It is especially important to provide assurances that researchers are not associated with immigration authorities. One approach is to work with migrant-serving organizations so they become the bridge between researchers and the community. Having contacts from the community can also help alert researchers when something may be going wrong with the study, for example, rumors about the objectives of the study (Deren et al. 2005). Such strategies will enhance recruitment of study participants and improve the quality of data collected. They will also increase the likelihood of the target community's acceptance of the study results and adoption of recommendations.

Appropriate Data Collection Personnel

Adequate training of staff is critical for the success of any study. Working with immigrant populations requires additional training on cultural awareness, language, and safety issues. For example, interviewers need to have knowledge and sensitivity about regional and national differences in language across subgroups (e.g., within Spanish-speaking populations) and interpersonal communication practices, as further discussed in chapter 24, by Gany et al. Formalities are particularly important to some migrant groups, especially traditional and rural cultures (Deren et al. 2005).

Matching interviewer characteristics to target population (e.g., country of birth, ethnic group, gender) has been recommended, especially for some traditional cultures where it is inappropriate for a male stranger to interview women or for young people to interview older community members. However, matching characteristics of interviewers and subjects may have negative consequences if community members become afraid of sharing sensitive information with individuals they perceive as being members of their own community. Many studies have successfully used trained community members to collect data, but professional bilingual and culturally aware interviewers can also succeed in collecting high-quality data from migrants. Safety issues in data collection are particularly relevant in migration studies because the target migrant population may live in unsafe and/or remote areas. This is often the case for studies of refugees and victims of trafficking (Deren et al. 2005; Andresen et al. 2004).

Developing and Validating Data Collection Instruments

In research it is very important to use validated data collection instruments or, if they are not available, to field-test all new instruments. However, data collection instruments are usually developed for the native population and are not necessarily valid for migrant and other minority cultural groups. Field tests should take place in a variety of target populations (Massey 2010). Qualitative methods such as focus groups and key informant interviews can be used to test the instruments. Techniques of cognitive interviewing are also becoming more widely used for cultural adaptation of instruments.

Developing or adapting instruments is time-consuming and expensive, and requires close collaboration between the design team, professional translators, and community members (see chapter 24, by Gany et al). The general recommendation of employing shorter questionnaires and only collecting information that is going to be used is especially applicable here. Another strategy is to use or adapt validated data collection instruments from multinational surveys (e.g., demographic and health surveys) or those conducted in the country of origin of the target migrant population (e.g., the census form or national health survey forms).

Direct translation is often not enough; the culture and literacy level of the target population also needs to be taken into consideration. It is important to be sensitive to differences in linguistic terms among migrants from different countries and regions, even among those who speak the same language. Sometimes, departure from "correct" or standard terms may be needed for migrant populations who might have adopted some vocabulary from the language in the host country or created hybrid terms (e.g., "Spanglish" terms spoken by Latin American migrants in the US). The use of vignettes can help address some translation and literacy issues. For some topics, measurement instruments need to be tailored to specific ethnic or cultural characteristics (e.g., dietary or illness treatment practices that are different from those of the native population).

Although all of the above recommended strategies to improve community participation, recruitment, and quality of data require more labor-intensive methods and increase the total survey costs, an increased response rate can decrease the cost per completed survey, and researchers can have more confidence that the information collected is an accurate representation of reality (Andresen et al. 2004).

Migrant-Targeted Studies and Information Systems

National or general population information systems cannot collect the type of detailed data necessary for in-depth studies of the determinants and/or consequences of migration. Migrant-targeted information systems and/or specialized studies are needed to complement general population data sources (UN 2007c; UN 1998). This strategy is particularly important for the most vulnerable and hard-to-reach migrant groups, such as new arrivals, temporary workers, asylum seekers, refugees, unauthorized migrants, and victims of trafficking.

Examples of migrant-targeted information systems include large longitudinal surveys[2] of new legal immigrants being conducted in several traditional migration destination countries (e.g., United States, Canada, Australia, and New Zealand) (UN 2007c; also see chapter 12, by Jasso, in this volume).

Adopting a Mixed-Methods Approach to Migrant Research

In general, a combination of qualitative and quantitative methods, or a mixed-methods approach, is highly recommended (see chapter 25, by Babu et al., for an extended case study of a mixed-methods approach being used to study internal migrants in India). As mentioned earlier, specialized sampling methodologies and data collection strategies will likely be needed (e.g., disproportionate sampling, respondent-driven sampling, time-space sampling) (UN 2007c), and these can often be combined to develop a more in-depth understanding of migration and health issues. For example, key issues related to migration and health that can be researched using a combination of qualitative and quantitative methodologies are the sense of belonging, cultural resiliency, and civic engagement.

The sense of belonging for immigrants goes beyond the geographic limits of the border. Even though proximity with the homeland is interrupted in the migratory process, communities, families, and people find mechanisms to keep intrinsically connected. The separation imposed by controlling the free circulation of individuals through borders (mainly for those who do not have the needed documentation to do so in a regular manner) is an impetus for creating new venues for sustaining relationships.

Cultural resiliency plays a major role on both sides of the migrant stream. People find mechanisms to invigorate the ties, vis à vis adversity, and to confront unfair regulations and restrictive sociopolitical mechanisms of control. A recent study conducted by the Mexican Population Council (CONAPO 2008) documents that 56% of Mexican immigrants in the US call their families in Mexico once a week or more, and another 31.7% call at least every two weeks. Also, the "absentee" makes him- or herself present by financially contributing to the household and local economies. In 2007, remittances, the money sent back from immigrants to the US to their families in Mexico, totaled $27 billion and was the third largest source of income in the country.

The emergence of hometown associations (HTAs) as a model of binational economic cooperation also illustrates cultural resiliency. HTAs are based on social networks established by community members of the same state or town of origin. They raise money through the organization of dances, beauty pageants, raffles, picnics, rodeos, membership dues, and private donations to support local development and improvement in their hometowns. Usually these HTAs invest in public infrastructure (e.g., construction or renovation of roads, bridges, parks, churches, schools, sport facilities, streets, etc.) and social projects (support of health care clinics, child-care centers, convalescent homes for the elderly; donation of ambulances, and medical and school supplies; educational grants, etc.).

Collection of Data on Comparison Groups of Nonmigrants

Too often migration and health research is based on information collected from migrants only. In most studies it is important to have information on a reference, or comparison, group to contrast migrants and nonmigrants at a certain point in time and/or over time in risk factors and/or health outcomes. The appropriate comparison group depends upon many factors, including the purpose of the study, the topic of interest, and the countries or migrant populations of interest. According to a UN report (2007c), the ideal study design to assess the determinants or consequences of migration for migrants would be to collect information from a sample of individuals before they migrate and collect follow-up information throughout their migration and settlement stages. However, this type of multi-country longitudinal, or panel, study is very complex and costly to implement. Since international migrants originate from a source population (in the country of origin) of individuals who are potential migrants themselves, the most relevant comparison group would be nonmigrant individuals and households from that source population, especially for studies on self-selection and the determinants and consequences of migration. Native populations in the destination country would be appropriate as a comparison group for the study of health inequities. This topic is further discussed in chapter 3, by Spallek et al.

As with other study design issues, it is important to emphasize that the "perfect should not be the enemy of the good." Study designs that do not include data on populations in the countries of origin and destination or do not include a comparison group from the source population can have enormous value, particularly for specific outcomes, especially when the limitations are recognized and noted.

Ethical Issues

Due to multiple and complex vulnerabilities, migrants should be considered at-risk populations and, as such, it is particularly important to abide by ethical research safeguards and standards that should be in place to protect such populations. For example, strict procedures are needed to ensure confidentiality of information, and researchers need to ensure that participants understand consent documents and their rights as research subjects. Sensitivity on the part of researchers to the cultural norms of specific migrant populations is also crucial. Many of these populations live peripheral lives and are not well integrated into the culture or society of their destination countries. They may also have lost their sense of belonging to communities in their country of origin.

Make sure that incentives are appropriate for the study population; consider social and economic situations when making incentive decisions. Incentives should not be so high as to "force" participation in the study. There is not much information in the literature about whether different incentive strategies work differently for different ethnic or migrant groups (Andresen et al. 2004). In Mexico, for example, it is less customary to provide economic incentives to participants in surveys or focus groups, while in the US incentives are standard practice. More research is needed in this area.

Research can itself be an intervention. For example, data collection teams can set aside time at the end of formal interviews to discuss questions and concerns and provide referrals to available health care or other services if needed. As Ingleby (2009) points out, this should be a standard component of research in migrant communities. Finally, efforts by researchers to share results with the community and the organizations serving them are a professional imperative (Ingleby 2009). These and other ethical issues are comprehensively considered in chapter 18, by Pottie and Gabriel.

International Coordination in Migration Data Collection

For international migrant research, it is highly recommended that coordinated studies of migrants and nonmigrants in origin and destination countries be conducted (Center for Global Development 2009). However, coordination of international studies is rarely done because of complexity and expense (UN 1998). International organizations have provided some support for these types of studies; examples of multinational migration household surveys include the Push-Pulls Survey project in seven origin and destination countries (UN 2007c) and the Migrations between Africa and Europe (MAFE) project (see www.mafeproject.com; Center for Global Development 2009).

Another strategy is to enhance information exchange among countries that are part of the same migration system. Further work is needed on international recommendations for migration data collection and harmonization.

Capacity Building for Migration Statistics

It is also important to enhance the capacity of government agencies and other organizations to collect, analyze, and use migration and health data and statistics. This is especially the case in origin (often developing) countries. A first recommended step, if not already completed, is to prepare a comprehensive report to catalogue and describe all administrative, census, and survey data systems pertinent to migration in origin countries, both from governmental and nongovernmental sources (Center for Global Development 2009). The European Union has recently finalized such an exercise, the PROMISTAT project (see www.prominstat .eu/drupal/?q = node/64).

Multilevel Conceptual Frameworks

Multilevel conceptual frameworks are needed in migration research to incorporate the many influences operating among migrant populations, such as structural-, social-, and individual-level factors from origin, transit, and destination locations (Deren et al. 2005). Many theoretical frameworks focus on individual factors and are not robust enough for migration research. The culture of migrants also evolves over time, with the adoption of new components from the destination country and the modification of old components from the origin country.

In comparisons of migrant and nonmigrant risk factors and outcomes, it is critical to statistically adjust/control for differences in other relevant characteristics (e.g., age, gender, education, income) associated with the outcome of interest to isolate the effect of migration per se, but this is often not done (UN 1998). New conceptual frameworks and recommendations in this area are discussed in chapter 3, by Spallek et al.

Multidisciplinary Research Teams

Besides health-specific information, there are other topics that affect the health of migrants, and it is important to collect such information to properly understand their effect on health outcomes and to inform decision making: number, origin, and characteristics of migrants; legal status; integration; nationality and citizenship; and public opinion and representations of migrants in the media are all important factors to consider. Poverty and marginalization are also factors that often affect migrants to a disproportionate extent. For that reason, it is important for researchers in the field of migrant health to collaborate with their colleagues in the social sciences (e.g., housing, education, legislation, security) and put together multidisciplinary research teams whenever possible (Ingleby 2009).

To improve analysis of migration data, it is recommended that the information be disaggregated by relevant variables such as gender, age, country of origin, and duration of residence. Such disaggregation would make it possible to assess the diversity of health issues among different migrant subpopulations (Center for Global Development 2009).

CONCLUSIONS

Both the number and diversity of origins of migrants are expected to continue expanding in the future. Migrants and their offspring are already a substantial proportion of the population in many countries. Important disparities in migrants' access to health care and health outcomes have been identified in the literature. However, in spite of a remarkable increase in the volume and quality of scientific publications in recent years, migration health still remains an emerging area of research with many unanswered questions (Ingleby 2009; Argeseanu Cunningham et al. 2008). High-quality and timely migration research is urgently needed to foster understanding of the dynamic causes and effects (including health) of migration and to implement evidence-based policies and interventions to protect and advance the health of migrants in the communities of origin and destination (Kahanec and Zimmermann 2008). The need for data is especially critical for the most vulnerable migrant populations (e.g., farmworkers, asylum seekers, unauthorized migrants, and victims of trafficking) and for smaller migrant subgroups (e.g., for certain countries of origin, occupations, and ethnic groups).

According to the Commission on International Migration Data, significant progress can be made in the short run, with limited resources, by implementing some of the simpler recommendations in this chapter, such as those related to harmonizing of migration definitions, better use of available data, and adding core migration variables to existing data sources. Another key strategy in that direction is to enhance sharing among countries and researchers of data and best practices in data collection. Broader access to data systems and dissemination of research results will not only better disseminate knowledge and best practices but also educate the media, politicians, and the public about migration issues. Greater availability of unbiased information may reduce negative stereotyping of migrants and facilitate their social integration.

Implementing some of the described recommendations may increase total cost of data collection; however, following the recommendations will likely result in an improvement in the quality and completeness of data as well as increased participation of migrants in research. Thus these research practices may actually reduce the cost per completed survey.

As described in this book, researchers now have a range of appropriate and promising methodologies available to study migrant populations. However, the relative efficiency and appropriateness of the various study methodologies has not been properly evaluated for these populations (Loue and Bunce 1999), and there is still a critical need for further advances in this area of research (Argeseanu Cunningham et al. 2008). We hope this book is a tool that will be used in support of such efforts.

NOTES

1. International Household Survey Network has developed guidelines for confidentiality of microdata around the world: http://www.surveynetwork.org/home/.

2. Longitudinal studies are especially well suited for determining changes in health status of migrants over time. However, they are more expensive than other study methodologies, and participating migrants have a higher likelihood of being lost to follow-up.

REFERENCES

Andresen EM, P Diehr, and DA Luke. 2004. "Public Health Surveillance of Low-Frequency Populations." *Annual Review of Public Health* 25: 25–52.

Argeseanu Cunningham S, JD Ruben, and KM Narayan. 2008. "Health of Foreign-Born People in the United States: A Review. *Health and Place* 14(4): 623–35.

Bilheimer LT, and Klein RJ. 2010. "Data and Measurement Issues in the Analysis of Health Disparities." *Health Services Research* 45(5 Pt 2): 1489–1507.

Bilsborrow, RE, G Hugo, AS Oberai, and H Zlotnik. 1997. *International Migration Statistics: Guidelines for Improving Data Collection Systems*. Geneva: International Labour Office.

Carletto, C, and A de Brauw. 2008. *Measuring Migration Using Household Surveys*. Migration Operational Vehicle Note 2. Washington DC: World Bank. http://siteresources.worldbank.org/INTMIGDEV/Resources/2838212–1237303771337/MigNote2_Carletto_de_Brauw_Measuring_Migration_Using_Household_Surveys.pdf.

Castañeda X, B Manz, and A Davenport. 2002. "Mexicanization: A Survival Strategy for Guatemalan Mayans in the San Francisco Bay Area." *Migraciones Internacionales* 1(3): 103–23.

Catanzarite, L. 2000. "'Brown Collar Jobs': Occupational Segregation and Earnings of Recent-Immigrant Latinos." *Sociological Perspectives* 43(1): 45–75.

Center for Global Development, Commission on International Migration Data for Development Research and Policy. 2009. "Migrants Count: Five Steps toward Better Migration Data." http://www.cgdev.org/content/publications/detail/1422146/.

Collinson MA. 2010. "Striving against Adversity: The Dynamics of Migration, Health and Poverty in Rural South Africa." *Global Health Action* 3: 5080. DOI: 10.3402/gha .v3i0.5080.

Collinson MA, K Adazu, MJ White, and SE Findley, eds. 2009. *The Dynamics of Migration, Health and Livelihoods: INDEPTH Network Perspectives.* Aldershot: Ashgate.

CONAPO. 2008. http://www.conapo.gob.mx/publicaciones/migra2.htm.

Deren S, M Shedin, CU Decena, and M Mino. 2005. "Research Challenges to the Study of HIV/AIDS among Migrant and Immigrant Hispanic Populations in the United States." *Journal of Urban Health* 82(2 Suppl 3): 13–25.

European Union. 2007. Regulation (EC) No. 862/2007 of the European Parliament and of the Council of 11 July 2007 on Community Statistics on Migration and International Protection and Repealing Council Regulation (EEC) No. 311/76 on the Compilation of Statistics on Foreign Workers. No. 862/2007. http://eurlex.europa.eu/LexUriServ /LexUriServ.do?uri = OJ:L:2007:199:0023:0029:EN:PDF.

García Canclini N. 1990. *Culturas híbridas.* Mexico City: CONACULTA-Grijalbo.

Gerritsen A, P Bocquier, M White, et al. 2013. "Health and Demographic Surveillance Systems: Contributing to an Understanding of the Dynamics in Migration and Health." *Global Health Action* 6: 10. DOI: 3402/gha.v6i0.21496.

Ginsburg FD, and R Rapp. 1995. "Introduction." In *Conceiving the New World Order: The Global Politics of Reproduction,* edited by FD Ginsburg and R Rapp, 1–18. Berkeley: University of California Press.

Grieco EM, and NF Rytina. 2011. "U.S. Data Sources on the Foreign Born and Immigration." *International Migration Review* 45(4): 1001–16.

Ibarra M. 2000. "Mexican Immigrant Women and the New Domestic Labor." *Human Organization* 59(4): 452–64.

Ingleby D. 2009. "European Research on Migration and Health: Background Paper." International Organization for Migration. http://www.migrant-health-europe.org/files /Research%20on%20Migrant%20Health_Background%20Paper.pdf.

Kahanec M, and KF Zimmermann. 2008. "Migration and Globalization: Challenges and Perspectives for the Research Infrastructure." Institute for the Study of Labor (IZA) Discussion Paper No. 3890.

Kalsbeek WD. 2003. "Sampling Minority Groups in Health Surveys." *Statistics in Medicine* 22: 1527–49.

Leder K, S Tong, L Weld, et al. 2006. "Illness in Travelers Visiting Friends and Relatives: A Review of the GeoSentinel Surveillance Network." *Clinical Infectious Diseases* 43: 1185–93.

Loue S, and A Bunce. 1999. "The Assessment of Immigration Status in Health Research." Centers for Disease Control and Prevention, National Center for Health Statistics. Vital and Health Statistics 2(127). http://www.cdc.gov/nchs/data/series/sr_02/sr02_127.pdf.

Martin E. 1995. *Flexible Bodies: Tracking Immunity in American Culture—From the Days of Polio to the Age of AIDS.* New York: Beacon.

Massey DS. 2010. "Immigration Statistics for the Twenty-First Century." *Annals of the American Academy of Political and Social Science* 631:124–40.

McKenzie DJ, and J Mistien. 2007. "Surveying Migrant Households: A Comparison of Census-Based, Snowball, and Intercept Point Surveys." World Bank, Development Research Group.

http://siteresources.worldbank.org/INTMIGDEV/Resources/2838212–1160686302996
/mckenziemistiaen.pdf.

Mexico Secretariat of Health. 2010. Acuerdo Nacional para la Salud Alimentaria. Estrategía
contra el sobrepeso y la obesidad, accessed August 28, 2012. http://www.promocion
.salud.gob.mx/dgps/descargas1/programas/Acuerdo%20Original%20con%20credi-
tos%2015%20feb%2010.pdf.

Omi M, and H Winant. 1994. *Racial Formation in the United States*. New York: Routledge.

Rapp R. 2000. *Testing Women, Testing the Fetus: The Social Impact of Amniocentesis in
America*. New York: Routledge.

United Nations, Department of Economic and Social Affairs, Statistics Division. 1998. "Rec-
ommendations on Statistics of International Migration–Revision 1." Statistical Papers
Series M, No. 58, Rev. 1, accessed March 17, 2013. http://unstats.un.org/unsd/publication
/SeriesM/SeriesM_58rev1E.pdf.

United Nations, Department of Economic and Social Affairs, Statistics Division. 2007a.
Report of the Expert Group Meeting on Measuring International Migration: Concepts
and Methods, accessed March 17, 2013. http://unstats.un.org/unsd/demographic
/meetings/egm/migrationegm06/FINAL%20REPORT%20L3.pdf.

United Nations, Department of Economic and Social Affairs, Statistics Division. 2007b.
United Nations Expert Group Meeting on the Use of Censuses and Surveys to Measure
International Migration—Part Two: Measuring International Migration through Population Censuses, accessed March 17, 2013. http://unstats.un.org/unsd/demographic
/meetings/egm/migrationegmsep07/TECHREP2_Part%20Two.pdf.

United Nations, Department of Economic and Social Affairs, Statistics Division. 2007c.
United Nations Expert Group Meeting on the Use of Censuses and Surveys to Measure
International Migration—Part Three: Measuring International Migration through
Sample Surveys, accessed March 17, 2013. http://unstats.un.org/unsd/demographic
/meetings/egm/migrationegmsep07/TECHREP3_Part%20Three.pdf.

United States Department of Commerce, Census Bureau. 2003. "Migration of Natives and
the Foreign Born: 1995–2000." Washington, DC: Government Printing Office, accessed
March 17, 2013. http://www.census.gov/prod/2003pubs/censr-11.pdf.

Villarejo D, D Lighthall, D Williams, A Souter, R Mines, B Bade, S Sarnules, and SA
Mccurdy. 2000. "Suffering in Silence: A Report on the Health of California's Agricultural
Workers." Davis: California Institute for Rural Studies.

3

Life Course Epidemiology

A Conceptual Model for the Study of Migration and Health

Jacob Spallek
Hajo Zeeb
Oliver Razum

INTRODUCTION

Both the absolute numbers of international migrants and their proportion of the total population are increasing in most western European countries and the US. In 2005, western and central European countries, for example, hosted a total of more than 44 million foreign-born persons (Razum 2007). The term "migrant" here comprises persons who cross national borders to reside in another country for extended time periods or permanently.

The health of some migrant groups has been extensively studied in the past. However, studies about health differences between migrants and majority populations still face a fundamental challenge: there is not yet a broadly accepted comprehensive model for the study of migrant health (Razum 2006a). Several conceptual models of migrant health exist, such as the model of the healthy migrant effect (Razum 2006b; Razum and Rohrmann 2002), the health transition model (Razum 2006a), and the model developed by Schenk (2007), which aims to structure and integrate some previous approaches.

We will describe the healthy migrant and the health transition models in this chapter and introduce several important aspects of each model. One major problem common to these models is that they do not offer an explicit life course perspective that takes into account the influence of health-related factors in the different life stages of migrants (Spallek and Razum 2008). In other words, they lack an explicit time axis. A crucial question arises from this lack of a time axis: Which factors and exposures in the life course of migrants do we have to consider in migrant studies to understand the current health situation of migrants adequately? To answer this question, we recommend a life course epidemiology approach and describe a new conceptual model for epidemiological migrant studies from Spallek et al. (2011), complemented by quantitative methodological considerations. Other forms of migrant studies, for example, qualitative studies, are not explicitly considered.

Life Course Epidemiology

Life course epidemiology can be defined as the study of physical or social exposures during gestation, childhood, adolescence, young adulthood, and adult life, with the aim of examining their long-term effects on later-life health or disease risk (Kuh and Ben Shlomo 2004; Kuh et al. 2003; Ben Shlomo and Kuh 2002). Life course epidemiology can help to construct models of disease etiology with an emphasis on timing (critical/sensitive periods), duration (accumulation), and temporal sequence (triggers/interactions) of exposures (Ben Shlomo and Kuh 2002). One concept of life course epidemiology states that adult chronic disease can be the result of biological programming during critical periods in childhood and in utero. Other concepts of life course epidemiology focus on analyzing the effects of accumulated exposures over the lifetime on health risks, including the temporal sequence of exposures during the life course. These different concepts are not mutually exclusive but can operate together (Kuh and Ben Shlomo 2004).

The health of migrants is determined in part by exposures during the life course (before, during, and after migration) that are not experienced by the majority population of the host country. A migrant background is frequently associated with different exposures during (critical) periods, for example, in utero or in childhood, as well as in different accumulation patterns and timing of exposures. Adopting a life course perspective can help us, as researchers, to better understand the health situation of migrants and the health differentials they experience.

Migrant Health

Strictly speaking, transnational migrants are persons who migrated across national borders. Frequently, their offspring are included in a broader definition of the term, although these persons may not have migrated themselves. The term "persons with migrant background," comprising both groups, is increasingly used. In this chapter we focus on both groups: (1) migrants who migrated themselves and (2) the increasing number and proportion of people with migrant backgrounds living in the US and Europe who are the offspring of migrants and are members of ethnic minorities living in the host countries for one or two generations.

Migrant populations—like other populations—are heterogeneous in terms of cultural identity, ways of living, social situation, health behavior, and health risks. In this chapter we try to draw some general conclusions while appreciating that individual migrant groups differ considerably from each other. Not all health differentials experienced by migrants can be attributed to socioeconomic inequalities, and not all differences are the expression of social deprivation or exclusion (Razum 2006a; Schenk 2007). The main emphasis of this chapter is on migrants who migrated from lower-income to higher-income countries. The situation of migrant groups migrating between high-income countries, for example, from western Europe to the US or Australia, or between low-income countries (e.g., migration in sub-Saharan Africa), will be different in some aspects.

THE HEALTHY MIGRANT EFFECT

The traditional model of the healthy migrant effect describes the often observed health advantages of migrants compared to the majority population. According to this model the causes of these health advantages, which can exist despite social deprivation, can be attributed to the positive self-selection of migrants, comparable to the well-known healthy worker effect. Persons who are particularly fit and healthy are more likely to be willing to cope with the risks of migration to a foreign country.

One of the problems associated with this theory is that the statement "particularly fit and healthy" may be true compared to the population of the country of origin, but not necessarily compared to the country to which the person migrates and where the healthy migrant effect is observed. Another weakness of the model is the expectation that the health advantages of migrants will decrease quickly after migration, due to poorer socioeconomic situations, as well as poorer working and living conditions compared to the majority population of the host country. The expectation is that social deprivation will result in an increase in health risks and mortality. However, as can be seen in many countries, increased risks often occur slowly and are not always empirically verifiable (Razum 2006a). Some migrant populations continue to have mortality advantages compared to the indigenous population of the host country even decades after their migration. In the traditional healthy migrant effect model the explanation for this phenomenon is the returning of sick and old migrants to their country of origin. It is assumed that due to this so-called salmon bias, the mortality of migrants is underestimated, because data about the number of people who die after returning to their country of origin are often not available (Hergenc et al. 1999). However, some recent studies have found no evidence for the "salmon bias" (Singh and Hiatt 2006; Ronellenfitsch et al. 2006; Abraido-Lanza et al. 1999; Razum et al. 1998). It seems just as reasonable that older and ill migrants wish to benefit from health care that they perceive to be of better quality and lower cost because of entitlements in the country of immigration. Also, older migrants may often prefer to stay with their immediate families in the host country rather than return to weakened family networks in their countries of origin.

Newer models have been developed more recently that expand the healthy migrant model and try to explain the health advantages of migrants with factors other than positive self-selection and the salmon bias, for example, the model of migration as health transition.

MIGRATION AS HEALTH TRANSITION

Some migrant populations experience lower mortality rates than indigenous populations despite typically having lower socioeconomic status. This mortality advantage can be substantial. Singh and Hiatt (2006) showed that migrants in the US tend to experience up to 30% lower mortality from common cancers, cardiovascular disease (CVD), and diabetes relative to the nonmigrant population (Singh and Hiatt 2006). Similarly, studies in Germany of migrant workers from southern Europe showed a lower overall mortality compared to the indigenous population (Razum et al. 1998).

These seemingly contradictory findings can be explained in terms of migration as a health transition: many migrants entering Europe or the US from economically less-developed countries move from a society in an earlier phase of the health transition to a society in a more advanced phase (Razum 2006a). These migrant populations thus experience an unusually rapid health transition, which affects their health situation. Two components of this health transition are relevant:

- Therapeutic component: Mortality due to infectious disease as well as maternal and child mortality decreases quickly after migration, due to better health care in the country of immigration, compared to the country of origin. (An exception may be the situation of Mexican immigrants in the US: due to the universal health care system in Mexico, they may have had better access to care, especially to preventive measures, than in the US.)
- Risk factor component: Risk of infectious disease decreases due to better hygiene and environmental conditions (e.g., safe drinking water supply, nutrition). At the same time, new risk factors for chronic diseases (cancer, cardiovascular disease, diabetes, etc.) emerge, for example, smoking, unhealthy nutritional habits, and physical inactivity. Chronic diseases become the major cause of death, but only after a lag period.

Migrants benefit from improvements in health care, hygiene, and nutritional conditions almost immediately after migration. They are thus experiencing a fast decline of some morbidity and mortality risks that were typical of their home countries. Other risks increase, but mostly over a longer time period. The typical mortality pattern in western countries is characterized by chronic diseases with a long lag time (latency period) between relevant exposures and the clinical disease manifestation. Risk factors for CVD, for example, act over a long time during the life course and show their effects mainly in middle and older age. Initially, migrant populations tend to have lower morbidity and mortality rates from such chronic diseases compared to the population of the host country, but this advantage decreases over time (usually decades) with the adoption of a western lifestyle.

Another consequence of the health transition is that migrant populations may experience an increased mortality from specific diseases. In the study by Singh and Hiatt (2006), for example, the mortality for stomach and liver cancer was higher among immigrants than in the nonimmigrant US population. Contributing causes of these increased risks could be that infections with *Helicobacter pylori* and hepatitis virus, respectively, are common in childhood in economically less-developed countries. Also, the risk for hemorrhagic stroke is increased among migrants from these countries (Leon and Davey Smith 2000), again associated with poorer living conditions before migration. Empirical findings such as these demonstrate that migrants might face specific exposures during childhood—a critical period—which contribute to health differentials in later life in the host country.

Not all empirical findings are perfectly in line with the model of migration as a health transition. An example is the increased risk (measured by mortality and health care utilization) for CVD among migrants from South Asia in the UK (Bhopal 2000; Wild and McKeigue 1997). Unexpectedly, this increase occurs rapidly after migration. A possible explanation is offered by the adipose tissue overflow hypothesis (Sniderman et al. 2006). It postulates a genetically determined higher risk for obesity in settings with calorically unrestricted nutritional intake. Here, a health transition does occur, but its effects are accelerated by a gene-environment interaction. Another example of rapid—negative—health transition is the mental health development of Mexican migrants in the US, in particular for those who migrated in childhood or adolescence.

In contrast to South Asian migrants, ethnic German re-settlers from eastern Europe *(Aussiedler)* have a lower CVD mortality compared to the indigenous German population (Ronellenfitsch et al. 2006). No marked increase over time is visible at present; however, the postmigration observation period is still somewhat short. Factors like social deprivation or high fat intake seem not yet to have an influence on CVD mortality in this migrant population.

Nurture Versus Nature and Socioeconomic Status

After immigration migrants often live in poorer socioeconomic conditions than the indigenous population of the host country, which may also increase disease risks as described above. Migrants can also face barriers to accessing the health care system, including language and legal barriers and racial/ethnic discrimination.

Nevertheless, it should not be overlooked that migrants might have specific health benefits and resources (Razum et al. 2004), for example, a high level of reciprocity in their communities (White 1997) or more favorable health behaviors such as healthier nutrition and lower levels of smoking and alcohol consumption

(Reeske et al. 2009). Additionally, they might benefit from certain exposures during childhood, for example, higher physical activity.

Besides the socioeconomic differences between migrants and the indigenous population, differences in biological and medical risk factors exist as well. Migrants face different exposures during their life course, for example, during childhood. Some of them will increase while others will decrease the risk for certain diseases. The differences migrants experience compared with the indigenous population of the host country in the areas of physical and social life conditions and environment can be summarized under the term "nurture."

Additionally, differences in genetic background or "nature" might exist due to geographic and ethnic variation in genetic makeup. Such polymorphisms can result in different disease risks. An example are differences in blood concentrations of high-density lipoprotein cholesterols (HDL-C) between people from northwest Europe and east Turkey (Hergenc et al. 1999; Mahley et al. 1995). Therefore, besides environmental factors, migrants can differ from the indigenous populations of the host countries in genetic factors, best summarized under the term "nature."

Studying the explanatory variables of the health of migrants is thus complex. The different factors of nature and nurture act on their own and in combination (interaction), for example, in a gene-environment interaction. Figure 3.1 shows a schematic overview of these factors, without a claim to being complete. The factors associated with migrant health act on different levels, from individual to environmental to societal levels. Social status, despite its importance, is thus only one aspect of a larger set of factors. It seems reasonable that the association between social status and health deprivations, which is already very complex to study in nonmigrated populations, cannot be studied for migrants without adequately taking into account these other factors.

In this context it is necessary to discuss how to assess unhealthy behaviors (e.g., specific nutritional habits) of migrants that are expressions of their culture. If such behavior is due to lack of knowledge or lack of possibilities to change living conditions, it would be the expression of a deprivation. Alternatively, if such behavior is understood as "informed voluntary otherness," it would reflect cultural heterogeneity.

The association between socioeconomic status and health deprivation among migrants becomes even more complex if the heterogenic distribution of health risks and resources in the migrant population is taken into account. This heterogeneity is the expression of different individual attributes and different rates of economic success within the group of migrants, differences that can also be found in the indigenous populations of the host countries. In addition, the different epidemiological situations in the countries of origin of the migrants have to be considered, as well as different cultural backgrounds and beliefs. The question is: what is the valid comparison group against which to measure possible health disadvantages of migrants? Comparisons with the indigenous population of the host

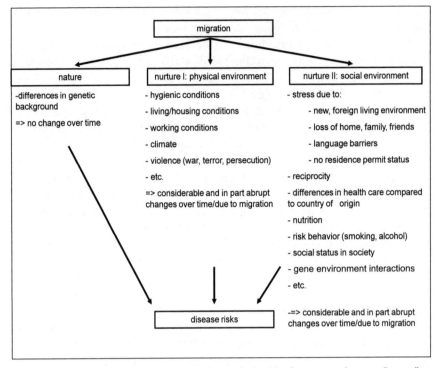

FIGURE 3.1. Possible positive and negative factors for health of migrants relating to "nature" and "nurture." (Adapted from Spallek and Razum 2006.)

country are problematic due to the differences in distribution of health risks stemming from different exposures during the life course, described later in this chapter. Differences in health could, but need not, be the expression of health deprivation. The other possible comparison group is the population of the country of origin. The question in this case is: do risks of migrants increase or decrease after migration compared to the population of the country of origin? This comparison does not take the specific situation of the migrants in the host country into consideration. Increases in risks compared to the country of origin could emerge without deprivation in the host country, for example, as a consequence of lower physical activity due to a better public transportation system or a job in an office.

When interpreting findings on the health situation of migrants, one should keep in mind that migrants are likely to have a differing genetic background and culture, lower socioeconomic resources in many cases, and differing health behaviors. It is an unacceptable simplification to generalize that migrants are poorer and therefore have a poorer health status than the population of their host country. In fact, a multidimensional network of factors shapes the health of migrants. Thus, the identification and quantification of the influence of particular factors may be even more difficult than in a nonmigrant population. Nevertheless, as questions on health inequalities and inequities continue to be raised, the objective of research about migrant health should be to identify the specific risks and resources of migrants, and which factors influence these risks. Such findings, ideally based on theoretically founded empirical research, could be used to improve existing health care systems and develop policies that are more adequate and fair.

In summary, the health situation of migrants is influenced by factors operating in the country of origin as well as in the host country—and in some cases in the transit countries—and acting at various phases in the lives of migrants. The nature and importance of these factors has been difficult to determine and to quantify empirically, as previous models of migrant health have lacked a crucial element, namely an explicit time axis. For this reason, we describe in the following section a new conceptual framework based on life course epidemiology published by Spallek et al. (2011). Such a concept should not only include the main factors acting on the health of migrant populations, but also make their temporal sequence explicit.

A LIFE COURSE MODEL FOR MIGRANT HEALTH

Periods of Migration

Migrant populations move through three basic phases of health transition during their life course: (1) the period before migration, including in utero exposure and the critical phase of early childhood, as well as other exposures in the country of birth to occupational, environmental, food, and infectious agents; (2) the period during the migration process itself; and (3) the period after migration.

In the first period migrants may be exposed to factors that are not—or only to a lesser degree—faced by the majority population in the host country. The resulting disease risks are constituted during critical periods in early childhood before migration and become manifest in later ages. Examples are higher risks for stomach cancer due to infection with *Helicobacter pylori*, or liver cancer due to hepatitis B or C. Another example may be the higher incidence of childhood leukemia, as observed among Turkish children in Germany (Spallek et al. 2008): there is evidence showing that infectious exposures due to unusual population mixing (populations usually separated coming in contact with each other) modify the risk of acute lymphoid leukemia (Kinlen 2004). In addition, factors might have existed that lead to the decision to migrate, for example, exposure to war, terrorism, natural disasters, political repression, and so forth. These factors can be substantial stressors and affect the physical and mental health of migrants in later life.

The second period—the process of migration itself, including sometimes long stays in transit countries—is a sensitive phase. The migration process produces stress, which might in turn increase the risks for specific psychiatric diseases or CVD. In the transit countries migrants at times face difficult living conditions, for example, food shortages, discrimination, or exposure to violence. In the third period, after the immigration process, migrants often live in poorer socioeconomic conditions than the indigenous population of the host country, which may increase disease risks by a process of accumulation. However, it is also possible that migrants have either specific health benefits and resources (Spallek and Razum 2008), for example, a high level of reciprocity in their communities (White 1997), or more favorable health behavior, for example, healthier nutrition, lower levels of smoking and alcohol consumption (Reiss et al. 2010; Reeske et al. 2009), which interact with the other risk factors and can result in lower risks for some diseases.

There is evidence that the risk of several chronic diseases is influenced by early childhood exposure, for example, stroke, allergies, and cancer (Reiss et al. 2010; Reeske et al. 2009; Grau et al. 2010). Migrants often face different exposures in their life course compared to the majority populations of the host countries due to the different situation in their home countries (nutrition, hygiene, prevalence of infectious diseases, etc.). The inclusive consideration of these influences and their time scale in a life course perspective, currently an important theme in public health/epidemiology (Ben Shlomo and Kuh 2002; Kuh and Ben Shlomo 2004; Lynch and Davey Smith 2005), is still missing in the research on migrant health.

Life Course Model

Figure 3.2 shows the conceptual model developed by Spallek et al. (2011) for migration and health, which integrate the influence of exposures that migrants face during their life course. This approach shows the different exposures of first-generation migrants along the three periods: in the country of origin, during migration, and in the host country. Depending on the age at migration, exposures and critical periods, for example, during early childhood, can fall into the period before, during, or after migration, and the accumulation of risk can take place in one period or over several periods. These different exposures, which act at different times during the life course, determine the disease risk of migrants. The model helps to understand why, for example, chronic diseases arise at different times and with different probability compared to the indigenous population of the host country. In particular, exposures in early childhood in the country of origin are included in the model. One example is the risk of obesity in adulthood, which is influenced by exposures in the prenatal phase: restricted fetal growth and low birth weight, both common problems in many low-income countries from which migrants originate, increase the risk for obesity in adulthood (Gillman 2004). The obesity risk of adult migrants thus is not determined solely by their nutritional behavior and physical activity in the host country. Another example is the possible

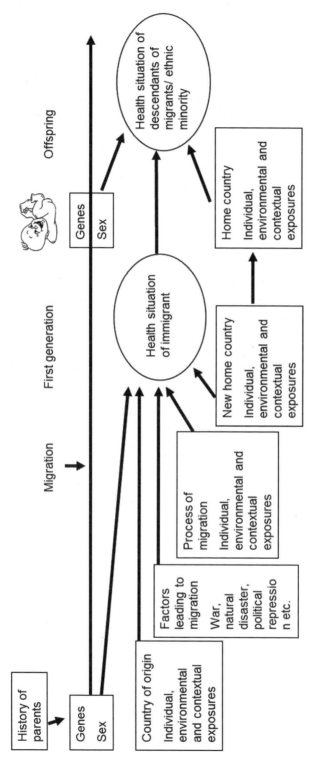

FIGURE 3.2. Different exposures during the life course on the health of migrants. (Adapted from Spallek et al. 2011.)

role of infections during childhood on the risks for specific cancers. For example, the increased risks for lymphatic leukemia among Turkish migrants in Hamburg, Germany, might be the result of a higher prevalence of exposure to Epstein-Barr virus in Turkey before migration (Spallek et al. 2009). In the same study, lower risks for gynecological cancers among women of Turkish origin might be explained by the lower prevalence of exposure to human papilloma virus in Turkey. The same might be true for Turkish women living in Sweden (Azerkan et al. 2008; Beiki et al. 2009) and in north Holland (Visser and van Leeuwen 2007). Conversely, in other situations, higher HPV prevalence in the country of origin may lead to increased cervical cancer risk over the life span of migrants, manifesting in a higher cervical cancer incidence among migrants, for example, from South American or south African countries in the respective host country.

Other important factors like family history, socioeconomic status, education, and living conditions, as well as health behaviors related to nutrition, physical activity, and alcohol and tobacco consumption, can come into play during different periods of migrants' lives. Accumulations and interactions of exposures in migrants can occur in several ways, for example, the accumulation of "pack years" can be changed by migration due to increased availability of cigarettes, targeted advertising, increased income, change in behavioral norms, or increased stress (Reiss et al. 2010; Reeske et al. 2009). Complex gene-environment interaction may result in changes in the accumulation of the high-calorie diet described in the adipose tissue overflow hypothesis (Bhopal 2000; Sniderman et al. 2006).

The health situation of the offspring of immigrants (the second generation) is influenced by specific exposures, too. Differences in genetic endowment can be passed from parent to offspring, for example, a darker skin type, and can result in specific health situations like lower risks for skin cancer or access barriers due to discrimination. Besides genetic factors, parents may pass on other aspects to their offspring. For example, cultural beliefs, health behaviors (nutrition, smoking and alcohol consumption), reproductive choices, and physical activity are influenced by the parents' lifestyle and behavior. Specific cultural beliefs and behaviors of ethnic minorities may persist over generations. Socioeconomic conditions of the parents determine the socioeconomic situation of offspring during childhood and can have a persisting influence in later life (Dragano and Siegrist 2006). The legal status of the parents can influence the health situation of their families and offspring, for example, due to lower access to health care or favorable living conditions. Thus, despite acculturation, the health situation of members of second-generation ethnic minorities may differ from that of the majority population. The health situation of the second-generation is different from the health situation of first-generation migrants because the former did not face the exposures in the country of origin and during the migration process. Moreover, they may to some extent be more acculturated or segregated than their parents. Higher disease risks of migrants might converge with the risks of the majority population in the second-generation or in younger birth cohorts, as studies about cancer risks among migrants in the Netherlands (Stirbu et al. 2006), British Columbia, Canada (Au et al. 2004), and Germany (Spallek et al. 2009) show, or remain stable, as demonstrated about the risk of skin cancer in a study among Turkish migrants in Hamburg, Germany (Spallek et al. 2009).

Acculturation can be a crucial factor for changes in health-related behavior after migration or between generations. With "dietary acculturation," for example, dietary habits of ethnic minorities and migrants often become less healthy due to increased intake of fat, sugar, salt, and processed food (Gilbert and Khokhar 2008). During "nutrition transition," dietary changes can be accompanied by changes in physical activity and obesity trends (Satia 2010). However, there are several different instruments and ways to measure acculturation depending on the different underlying conceptual models (Thomson and Hoffman-Goetz 2009). The relationship between acculturation and changing health behaviors might differ depending on the ethnic group examined and the measure of acculturation used (Gilbert and Khokhar 2008; Ayala et al. 2008).

The life course approach to migrant health research takes into consideration the different factors acting over the life span of migrants that researchers have to consider when describing and interpreting the current health status of migrants. So far, not all aspects of this framework have been empirically confirmed at an appropriate level of evidence, or specifically for migrants (in some cases, convincing evidence is available from studies of nonmigrants). For example, the influence of nutritional and hygienic conditions in early childhood on stroke and stomach cancer needs to be supported with further evidence from prospective migrant studies. Additional research on the associations and interactions of the environmental, genetic, and behavioral factors and their changes during the life course would allow a more detailed understanding of the health situation of migrants and how it changes over time—both in absolute terms and relative to the health of the majority population in the host country.

METHODOLOGICAL ISSUES

Ideally, an analysis of migrant health should include all aspects mentioned in Figure 3.1, that is, genetic background, situation in the country of origin, exposures during the migration process and in transit countries, the situation in the host country, and the attributes of the individual. Only if all interacting factors are understood (and controlled for, if necessary) can the influence of a single factor be analyzed appropriately. We need to better grasp these complex interactions and potential confounders to be able to analyze specific sets of factors in a more deterministic way.

Difficulties of Longitudinal Designs

Further studies about migrant health should aim to analyze the influence and interaction of factors falling in the "nature" and "nurture" categories when comparing disease risks of migrants to those of indigenous populations. A focus should be on the timing and dynamics of exposure. This will make it possible not only to describe point prevalences or risks of diseases but also to show periodic differences in disease development. Studies including all these factors require a longitudinal follow-up not only of the migrant population but also of the population in the country of origin and that in the host country. Such studies pose enormous methodological challenges (Razum and Twardella 2002; also see chapter 12, by Jasso, in this volume). An appropriate instrument to examine life course aspects are prospective birth cohorts; however, such studies are very difficult to implement with first-generation migrants because these persons would have to be included before migration, while still in their countries of origin, before they even know that they might migrate in the future. Given these obvious obstacles, a retrospective exposure assessment has so far been the most common method of choice in migrant studies. Clearly, studies attempting to retrospectively assess exposures and collect information about early childhood face several problems, such as recall bias, missing data, and so forth. These problems increase if data from an economically less developed country of origin are needed. However, in some countries of origin, such as Turkey, the quality and quantity of health data is improving. New mortality and disease registries are being set up, thus providing new opportunities for transnational migrant health research (Razum and Twardella 2002). In other countries of origin, there are still far too little data available for such studies.

The Challenge of Selecting Suitable Comparison Groups

Researchers need to consider which population(s) the health status of a migrant population should be compared to—in particular, when transnational epidemiological studies are possible. Comparisons can be made relative to

· the population of the host country,
· the second generation,
· the population of the country of origin (the general population or those of similar ethnic background as the migrant group), and
· migrant populations of the same origin that have migrated to other host countries.

Each comparison answers a different research question relevant to life course epidemiology.

Figure 3.3 provides an overview of the possible comparisons of the health status of a migrant population. The choice of the appropriate comparison population depends on the study question. Comparison 1 offers one way to study the possible

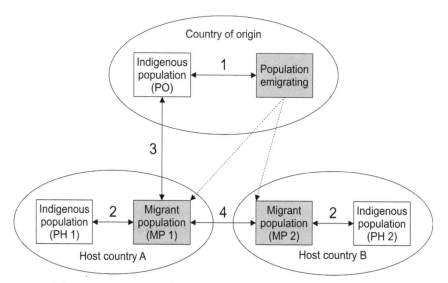

FIGURE 3.3. Four possibilities for comparing health of migrants with health of other populations. (Spallek et al. 2011.)

healthy migrant effect at the time of migration, that is, whether the population intending to emigrate is healthier than the general population of the country of origin (PO), a self-selection effect. Comparison 2 is the most common approach toward analyzing the health of migrants, namely a comparison of the health of an immigrant population (MP1) to the health of the majority population of the host country (PH1). This approach allows for the investigation of differences in exposure, behaviors, and in access to care. Comparisons 3 and 4 are approaches that are not used frequently at present. Comparison 3 investigates the health of a population who already has migrated (MP1) relative to the health of the population in the country of origin (PO), thus adding information about factors that are due to the migration process and the social and health situation in the host country. Comparison 4 adds information about the influence of factors specific to different host countries (MP1 vs. MP2), for example, differences in the structure of the respective health systems that might affect access of migrants to care, and thereby their health status.

Studies including all these factors and study populations are difficult to conduct, but they are useful for analyzing the influence and interaction of factors from "nature" and "nurture" categories on disease risks of migrants compared to indigenous populations. Such approaches will make it possible not only to describe point prevalences or risks, but also to show periodic differences in disease genesis. Such approaches could also provide opportunities to study questions such as the following:

- Is development of diseases determined, accelerated, or decelerated by specific exposures in specific periods of the life course?
- Does exposure A cause the outcome of interest only in conjunction with exposure B?
- To what degree do differences in the health of migrants relative to the health of the indigenous population of the host country originate from the situation in the country of origin, the migration process itself, or the situation in the country of immigration?

An ideal life course study of the health of migrants would comprise all four of these comparisons and so give new insights into the research questions raised. Furthermore, including additional comparison groups besides the population of the host country will contribute to producing more detailed information on the influence of exposures during the periods before, during, and after migration. While this ideal study is likely to remain elusive, some of its features may be feasible in new collaborative studies. As is common for observational epidemiological studies, the complete set of factors and confounders relevant for health in a migrant's life course cannot be investigated in one comprehensive study. In any case, researchers need to keep in mind possible effects of the unmeasured factors during analysis, interpretation, and dissemination of their results.

CONCLUSION

The health of migrants is determined by factors that operate in different phases of their life course and that may be considerably different from factors operating during the life course of members of the majority population of the host country. This strong temporal component has to be reflected by conceptual models of migrant health. Researchers studying migrant health should consider not only risks and exposures in the host country of migrants but also during the migration process and in the country of origin. Studies of members of the offspring and of ethnic minorities should consider exposures of the parental generation and the possibility that specific behaviors and risks are passed on to the next generation. Studies taking this life course framework into account will provide new insights into the development of disease and the health situation of migrants. For example, analyses of the change of cancer risks over time since migration or between migrant generations can provide new insights into the causes of cancer, critical periods during the life course, promoting factors (e.g., the stimulation of the immune system in early childhood), influence of genes and environment, and latency periods of the different processes (Arnold et al. 2010).

We believe that intense discussion is essential for further developing the theoretical framework and further adapting statistical methods (e.g., multilevel or cross-classified models) to the needs of migrant health research with the aim of improving future empirical studies. Our own research focuses on extending the proposed concept of life course epidemiology in such a way that it can be applied to the offspring of migrants and ethnic minorities who have not migrated themselves.

NOTE

This chapter is an adapted and extended version of J Spallek, H Zeeb, and O Razum, "What do we have to know from migrants' past exposures to understand their health status? A life course approach." *Emerg Themes Epidemiol* (2011) 8(1):6. Available at: http://www.ete-online.com/content/8/1/6.

REFERENCES

Abraido-Lanza AF, BP Dohrenwend, DS Ng-Mak, and JB Turner. 1999. "The Latino mortality paradox: A test of the 'salmon bias' and healthy migrant hypotheses." *American Journal of Public Health* 89:1543–48.

Arnold M, O Razum, and JW Coebergh. 2010. "Cancer risk diversity in non-Western migrants to Europe: An overview of the literature." *European Journal of Public Health* 46:2647–56.

Au WY, RD Gascoyne, RE Gallagher, N Le, RD Klasa, RHS Liang, C Choy, W Foo, and JM Connors. 2004. "Hodgkin's lymphoma in Chinese migrants to British Columbia: A 25-year survey." *Annals of Oncology* 15:626–30.

Ayala GX, B Baquero, and S Klinger. 2008. "A systematic review of the relationship between acculturation and diet among Latinos in the United States: Implications for future research." *Journal of the American Dietary Association* 108:1330–44.

Azerkan F, K Zendehdel, P Tillgren, E Faxelid, and P Sparen. 2008. "Risk of cervical cancer among immigrants by age at immigration and follow-up time in Sweden, from 1968–2004." *International Journal of Cancer* 123:2664–70.

Beiki O, P Allebeck, T Nordqvist, and T Moradi. 2009. "Cervical, endometrial and ovarian cancers among immigrants in Sweden: Importance of age at migration and duration of residence." *European Journal of Cancer* 45:107–18.

Ben-Shlomo Y, and D Kuh. 2002. "A life course approach to chronic disease epidemiology: Conceptual models, empirical challenges and interdisciplinary perspectives." *International Journal of Epidemiology* 31:285–93.

Bhopal R. 2000. "What is the risk of coronary heart disease in South Asians? A review of UK research." *Journal of Public Health Medicine* 22:375–85.

Dragano N, and J Siegrist. 2006. "Die Lebenslaufperspektive Gesundheitlicher Ungleichheit: Konzepte und Forschungsergebnisse." In *Gesundheitliche Ungleichheit: Grundlagen, Probleme, Perspektiven.* Edited by M Richter and K Hurrelmann. Wiesbaden: VS Verlag für Sozialwissenschaften: 255–70.

Gilbert PA, and S Khokhar. 2008. "Changing dietary habits of ethnic groups in Europe and implications for health." *Nutrition Review* 66:203–15.

Gillman MW. 2004. "A life course approach to obesity." In *A life course approach to chronic disease epidemiology.* Edited by D Kuh and Y Ben-Shlomo. Oxford: Oxford University Press: 189–217.

Grau AJ, C Urbanek, and F Palm. 2010. "Common infections and the risk of stroke." *Nature Reviews Neurology* 6:681–94.

Hergenc G, H Schulte, G Assmann, et al. 1999. "Associations of obesity markers, insulin, and sex hormones with HDL-cholesterol levels in Turkish and German individuals." *Artherosclerosis* 145:147–56.

Kinlen L. 2004. "Infections and immune factors in cancer: The role of epidemiology." *Oncogene* 23:6341–48.

Kuh D, and Y Ben Shlomo. 2004. *A life course approach to chronic disease epidemiology.* Oxford: Oxford University Press.

Kuh D, Y Ben-Shlomo, J Lynch, J Hallqvist, and C Power. 2003. "Life course epidemiology." *Journal of Epidemiology and Community Health* 57:778–83.

Leon DA, and G Davey Smith. 2000. "Infant mortality, stomach cancer, stroke, and coronary heart disease: Ecological analysis." *British Medical Journal* 320:1705–6.

Lynch J, and G Davey Smith. 2005. "A life course approach to chronic disease epidemiology." *Annual Review of Public Health* 26:1–35.

Mahley RW, KE Palaoglu, Z Atak, et al. 1995. "Turkish heart study: Lipids, lipoproteins, and apolipoproteins." *Journal of Lipid Research* 36:839–59.

Razum O. 2006a. "Commentary: Of salmon and time travellers—Musing on the mystery of migrant mortality." *International Journal of Epidemiology* 35:919–21.

Razum O. 2006b. "Migration, Mortalität und der Healthy-migrant-Effekt." In *Gesundheitliche Ungleichheit: Grundlagen, Probleme, Perspektiven.* Edited by M Richter and K Hurrelmann. Wiesbaden: VS Verlag für Sozialwissenschaften: 255–70.

Razum O. 2007. "Erklärungsmodelle für den Zusammenhang Zwischen Migration und Gesundheit." *International Journal of Public Health* 52:75–77.

Razum O, I Geiger, H Zeeb, and U Ronellenfitsch. 2004. Gesundheitsversorgung von Migranten. *Deutsches Ärzteblatt* 101:2882–87.

Razum O, and S Rohrmann. 2002. "Der Healthy-migrant-Effekt: Bedeutung von Auswahlprozessen bei der Migration und Late-entry-Bias." *Gesundheitswesen* 64: 82–88.

Razum O, and D Twardella. 2002. "Time travel with Oliver Twist—Towards an explanation for a paradoxically low mortality among recent immigrants." *Tropical Medicine and International Health* 7: 4–10.

Razum O, H Zeeb, HS Akgün, and S Yilmaz. 1998. "Low overall mortality of Turkish residents in Germany persists and extends into second generation: Merely a healthy migrant effect?" *Tropical Medicine and International Health* 3:297–303.

Reeske A, J Spallek, and O Razum. 2009. "Changes in smoking prevalence among first- and second-generation Turkish migrants in Germany—An analysis of the 2005 Microcensus." *International Journal for Equity in Health* 8:26.

Reiss K, J Spallek, and O Razum. 2010. "'Imported risk' or 'health transition'? Smoking prevalence among ethnic German immigrants from the Former Soviet Union by duration of stay in Germany—Analysis of microcensus data." *International Journal for Equity in Health* 9:15.

Ronellenfitsch U, C Kyobutungi, H Becher, and O Razum. 2006. "All-cause and cardiovascular mortality among ethnic German immigrants from the Former Soviet Union: A cohort study." *BMC Public Health* 6:16.

Satia JA. 2010. "Dietary acculturation and the nutrition transition: An overview." *Applied Physiology, Nutrition, and Metabolism* 35:219–23.

Schenk L. 2007. "Migration und Gesundheit—Entwicklung eines Erklärungs—Und Analysemodells für Epidemiologische Studien." *International Journal of Public Health* 52:87–96.

Singh GK, and RA Hiatt. 2006. "Trends and disparities in socioeconomic and behavioural characteristics, life expectancy, and cause-specific mortality of native-born and foreign-born populations in the United States, 1979–2003." *International Journal of Epidemiology* 35:903–19.

Sniderman AD, R Bhopal, D Prabhakaran, N Sarrafzadegan, and A Tchernof. 2006. "Why might South Asians be so susceptible to central obesity and its atherogenic consequences? The adipose tissue overflow hypothesis." *International Journal of Epidemiology* 36:220–25.

Spallek J, M Arnold, S Hentschel, and O Razum. 2009. "Cancer incidence rate ratios of Turkish immigrants in Hamburg, Germany: A registry based study." *Cancer Epidemiology* 33:413–18.

Spallek J, and O Razum. 2006. "Migrantensensible Studiendesigns in der Epidemiologie—Das deutsche Konzept 'Staatsangehörigkeit.'" In *Migrantensensible Studiendesigns zur Repräsentation des Migrationsstatus in der Gesundheitsforschung.* Berlin: Robert-Koch-Institut.

Spallek J, and O Razum. 2008. "Erklärungsmodelle für die Gesundheitliche Situation von Migrantinnen und Migranten." In *Health Inequalities: Determinanten und Mechanismen Gesundheitlicher Ungleichheit.* Edited by U Bauer, UH Bittlingmayer, and M Richter. Wiesbaden: VS Verlag: 271–90.

Spallek J, C Spix, H Zeeb, P Kaatsch, and O Razum. 2008. "Cancer patterns among children of Turkish descent in Germany: A study at the German Childhood Cancer Registry." *BMC Public Health* 8:152.

Spallek J, H Zeeb, and O Razum. 2011. "What do we have to know from migrants' past exposures to understand their health status? A life course approach." *Emerging Themes in Epidemiology* 8:6.

Stirbu I, AE Kunst, FA Vlems, O Visser, V Bos, W Deville, HG Nijhuis, and JW Coeberg. 2006. "Cancer mortality among 1st and 2nd generation migrants in the Netherlands: Convergence towards the rates of the native Dutch population." *International Journal of Cancer* 119:2665–72.

Thomson MD, and L Hoffman-Goetz. 2009. "Defining and measuring acculturation: A systematic review of public health studies with Hispanic populations in the United states." *Social Science and Medicine* 69:983–91.

Visser O, and FE van Leeuwen. 2007. "Cancer risk in first generation migrants in North-Holland/Flevoland, The Netherlands." *European Journal of Cancer* 43:901–8.

White JB. 1997. "Turks in the New Germany." *American Anthropology* 99:754–69.

Wild S, and P McKeigue. 1997. "Cross sectional analysis of mortality by country of birth in England and Wales, 1970–92." *British Medical Journal* 314:705.

Quantitative Methodological Approaches

Section Editor: Alfonso Rodriguez-Lainz

4

Use of Existing Health Information Systems in Europe to Study Migrant Health

Katia Levecque
Elena Ronda-Pérez
Emily Felt
Fernando G. Benavides

INTRODUCTION

Traditionally in public health research and practice, making health comparisons between migrant and native populations based on secondary data from routine health information systems has been useful for monitoring health problems, generating causal hypotheses, and distinguishing between the role of environmental and individual characteristics (MacMahon 1960). A very well known example is the study on gastric cancer using mortality data in which Japanese-born people living in the US were compared with native-born whites and Japanese descendants born in the US (Haenzel and Kurihara 1968). As noted by the authors, there were several possible explanations for why gastric cancer mortality rates among Japanese-born immigrants were greater than among the second generation of Japanese born in the US, and also greater than rates among whites born in the US. Differences in the induction period of disease, genetic characteristics, and cultural factors related to nutrition were some of the possible explanations. In any case, such studies could be carried out because of the availability of routine data like mortality and morbidity records, which include information that indicates migrant status, such as country of birth or nationality.

Today, with migration being a worldwide phenomenon (IOM 2010), we need more than ever to collect routine migrant health data, including data on health determinants such as housing, work, nutrition, and health-related behavior, for monitoring and explaining migrant use of health services and migrant health status. The premise is simple: before embarking on any new study of migrant populations, we must assess whether some of the information of interest has already been collected by routine health information systems and whether the data is available and sufficient for research purposes. In this chapter, our aim is to identify the health information systems in European countries that are most useful for migrant health studies. For a discussion of US health information systems see chapter 5 in this volume, by Singh. Here we look at both official registry datasets and major health surveys. Official registers such as birth and death registers, but also cancer and other morbidity registry-based information systems, offer an excellent opportunity for migrant health research, at least in some countries. As an example of such registry-based research, we take a close look at a Spanish study on mortality within an immigrant population shortly after arrival in Spain. In terms of the use of surveys as health information systems, in addition to national surveys it is notable that an increasing number of international surveys have emerged that contain valuable information on migrant health status. We illustrate migrant health research based on survey data by looking at a recent study on migrant health that uses data from the European Working Conditions Survey (EWCS) of 2005. Subsequently, we review the major strengths and weaknesses of using existing datasets for migrant health research and formulate recommendations that might help counter some of the limitations. We then provide a response to the question of how to find a data source that can be used to answer a specific research question. We end with some concluding remarks and highlight two fundamental recommendations on the use of existing health information systems for grasping insights into the issue of migrant health.

TYPES OF HEALTH INFORMATION SYSTEMS FOR MIGRANT STUDIES

Countries differ considerably in the availability of health information systems that allow for migrant health research: while countries like the US and Australia generally have a substantial amount of relevant information, in the majority of European countries health data by migrant status or ethnic group is rarely collected, with the United Kingdom, Sweden, and the Netherlands being important exceptions (Mladovsky 2007). Health information systems can be of different types: (1) birth and death registers, (2) cancer and other morbidity registers, (3) health care utilization data, and (4) health surveys and other surveys concerned with broader issues such as living standards or work/labor characteristics, which also often include data on health status and social determinants of health. Within these information systems, migrant status may be indicated in several ways: by foreign birth, by foreign citizenship, or by indicators of movement into a new country to stay temporarily (sometimes for as little as a year) or to settle for the long term or permanently. Unfortunately, migrant status is often conflated with race, membership in an ethnic or religious minority group, or indigenous minority status, or it is restricted to the specific category of asylum seekers and refugees. However, none of these indicators of migrant status are equivalent, and the use of different indicators and nonstandardized or poorly defined indicators poses a particular problem for consistency in scientific research and within larger public policy debates. For a deeper discussion of the question of how migrant status is indicated, see chapter 2 in this volume, by Rodriguez-Lainz and Castañeda.

Registers

Registers are formed by a continuous and systematic collection of data on all individuals or issues of interest. Birth registers, for example, include all people born in a geographic or administrative area, while death registers are made up of information on all of the deceased. Some of these registers collect data on all individuals that have experienced a specific form of morbidity, such as cancer. Such morbidity registers can be population based or hospital based.

Birth registers can be important tools for exploring the issues of perinatal morbidity and mortality because low birth weight and preterm delivery are important predictors of sickness, illness, and death during the first months or early years of life. Several studies have examined these reproductive outcomes in foreign and migrant women, showing that there are differences in both the direction and strength of the association in comparison with native populations (Guendelman et al. 1999; Agudelo-Suárez et al. 2009). For example, some studies suggest that newborns of immigrant mothers have better outcomes than children born of native parents (Singh and Yu 1996), and it has been argued that there is a "healthy immigrant effect" (i.e., migrants having better health outcomes compared to natives, despite lower socioeconomic status and limited access to health care). But there might be additional protective factors, such as genetic makeup or healthy behaviors during pregnancy, that are linked to the country of origin. Such hypotheses, however, can rarely be fully explored because such detailed information is not typically included in birth registers. When using birth registers, we must take such limitations into account. Furthermore, the quality of the data in birth registers must be closely evaluated. For example, some authors have reported that birth weight information is often more incomplete for migrants compared to natives and that such discrepancies in the quality of the data can be regionally specific (Rio et al. 2009).

In addition to birth registers, mortality statistics are probably the most common basic health data that can be used for migrant health research. For example, in one study mortality data was used to determine and quantify variations in diabetes mortality by migrant status in different European countries (Vandenheede et al. 2011). This study indicates that the overall pattern is one of higher diabetes mortality among migrant groups and that there are important differences in this disease according to the country of origin (the highest rate is observed for migrants from South Asia). The authors bring to light some methodological considerations related to registration issues. For instance, data from some countries were obtained from population censuses linked with the mortality registers (Belgium, the Netherlands, and Denmark), whereas data from other countries were unlinked. The unlinked data are susceptible to numerator-denominator bias; for example, differences between measurements of the country of origin in both sources (population census and mortality register). Another possible source of error may be under-registration of resident migrant groups either in the population census or in the mortality register. Underregistration of migrants in the census is rather unlikely in most European countries due to rigorous data collection—with the exception of specific areas where there are large numbers of unauthorized migrants or asylum seekers—but underregistration of deaths may be more substantial due to the return of many older migrants to their countries of origin prior to death.

In relation to specific causes of death, in Canada and Australia, also using data from individual mortality records, Kliewer and Smith (1995) found that breast cancer mortality rates among women in the majority of migrant groups shifted over time from the rate observed in their country of origin toward the rate of the native-born population in the destination country. These findings indicate, once again, that environmental and lifestyle factors associated with the new place of residence influence the health of migrants. A recent mortality study on cardiovascular disease in six European countries (Bhopal et al. 2011), using country of birth as an indicator of migrant status, highlights the relevance of cross-country comparisons. For instance, circulatory mortality was similar, for men and women, across countries for migrants born in India. However, for other groups (i.e., those born in China, Pakistan, Poland, Turkey, and Yugoslavia) there were substantial between-country differences. While health information systems in most European countries are not designed to identify people by migration status, death registers maintained in many countries are the exception to the rule. A study on the availability of large-scale epidemiological data on cardiovascular diseases and diabetes among migrants and ethnic minorities in the EU found that national death registers that allowed for disaggregation according to ethnicity or migrant status were available in twenty-four countries. Country of birth was used as an indicator in fifteen countries, citizenship in eight countries, and nationality in seven countries (some countries used more than one indicator) (Rafnsson and Bhopal 2009).

Surveys

The second category of health information systems that can be used for migrant health research are surveys of representative samples of a country or region's entire population. Because of the absence of indicators of migrant status in official registers in many countries in Europe, researchers are often dependent on survey data. While migrant health research using survey data has a longer tradition in countries such as the US (see chapter 5, by Singh), in Europe such research has not been undertaken until recently. Migrant health research can be based on health surveys (including health interview surveys and health examination surveys), but also on surveys of broader issues such as living standards or working conditions that include some limited information on health status or health care use. Sometimes, more general surveys are supplemented by targeted surveys aimed at hard-to-reach population groups and qualitative investigations (WHO 2010a). Since many of these surveys, such as the European Working Conditions Survey and a number of National Health Surveys, are carried out periodically, they could—in addition to registers—be considered as routine data collection systems for monitoring migrant health (see sidebar 4.1).

SIDEBAR 4.1 CASE STUDY INVOLVING THE USE OF SURVEY INFORMATION FOR MIGRANT HEALTH RESEARCH

This first case study attempts to illustrate an example of research in the field of occupational health and migration by the use of existing survey databases (Working Condition Surveys) (see Ronda-Pérez et al. 2012).

Rationale

International migrants were estimated at 214 million in 2010. Migrant workers (those who migrate for employment) and their families account for about 90% of all migrants. However, very few studies have critically evaluated the occupational health issues of migrant workers.

First Aim of the Research

The primary aim of the research was to describe and compare employment arrangements in migrant and nonmigrant workers in Europe.

Method

1. Source of data: Fourth European Working Conditions Survey 2005
2. Request of the dataset: the data is available free to all registered users intending to use it for not-for-profit purposes at http://www.eurofound.europa.eu/surveys/availability/index.htm
3. Format data: SPSS
4. Scope of the survey: 29,766 European workers were interviewed in 31 countries (all EU25 member states plus Bulgaria, Croatia, Norway, Romania, Turkey, and Switzerland), answering 103 items on a wide range of issues regarding their employment situation, working conditions, safety, training, and work-related health problems. All interviews were conducted face-to-face in the respondent's own

household. Response rate ranged from 67% (Czech Republic) to 28% (Netherlands).
5. Indicator of migration: nationality (<1% of the information is missing)
6. Analysis: prevalence rates adjusted for age, gender, and education level

Potential Benefits of the Use of the Working Conditions Survey

Conducting an international survey in many different countries and languages is demanding in terms of organizational planning and procedures. This survey provides a unique source of information on the conditions of work in all European countries and a source that is entirely comparable (the same questionnaire was used in all countries covered). It can be used to carry out detailed analysis of working conditions according to different employment characteristics or sectors of activity. It also allows for analysis of the current situation in the context of the last fifteen years as this is the fourth time this survey has been conducted. Moreover, most of the published studies only use information about those work-related health problems in workers affiliated with social security systems, leaving out of reach some specific groups such as those who are self-employed and workers in the informal economy, who are included in this survey.

Limitations of the Dataset

First, the small number of migrants surveyed makes subclassifications difficult, precluding the possibility of carrying out an analysis by region of origin and giving rise to wide confidence intervals in the estimations.

Second, there remain issues around the validity of comparing self-reported measures of working conditions across different countries with distinct cultures, attitudes, and regulations.

Third, nationality has been used as an indicator of migrant status. Migrants may take the nationality of the country in which they reside, which makes the groups under consideration heterogeneous and does not avoid possible bias due to poor classification. Important information not included in the survey, such as length of migrants' residence in the host country, is another limitation.

Finally, the migrant sample might not be representative of migrant workers in Europe in general. Specifically, the undocumented could be underrepresented. In many cases individuals working illegally may be exposed to worse working and employment conditions and may experience more serious discrimination and exploitation, and thus the associations could be underestimated.

However, countries differ considerably in the availability of survey data that allows for migrant health research. For a valuable overview of available health and migration data collected in surveys at the national level in several European countries, see the research note "Migration and Health in the EU" written for the European Commission by Mladovsky (2007) and updated overviews reported in Juhasz et al. (2010) and Rechel et al. (2011). Another valuable overview of existing surveys that might be considered for migrant health and health care usage research is the Migrant and Ethnic Minority Health Observatory (MEHO) atlas (http://www .meho.eu.com). The MEHO atlas contains twenty-three maps that depict the availability of information both in registries and in surveys on migrant status in different health fields in European countries.

Comparison of migrant health status between countries offers valuable insights into the way the sociopolitical environment might act upon the link between migrant status and health. Such comparisons require the availability of multicountry datasets containing comparable information. In recent years, several international surveys have been set up that include useful information on both migrant demographics and health. Some of these datasets are restricted to European countries, while others have a broader frame of reference and include information on the US and other nation-states. The European international datasets are often funded through the European Commission's Framework Programs, the European Science Foundation, and national funding bodies. For some of the surveys, comparability is achieved with centralized support and coordination of the national surveys by Eurostat, the Europe Union's statistical office. In the US, the Joint Canada/United States Survey of Health (JCUSH) of 2002–2003 constituted the first effort to collect information on health status using a standardized approach and a single survey across the two countries. Though the survey took place only once, the results have been useful for making migrant health comparisons; for example, the survey results were used to compare health disparities in access to care, receipt of health services, and health status based on race and immigrant status (Lasser et al. 2006).

In Table 4.1, we provide a description of some of the key surveys from the European Union that are useful for migrant health research. It should be noted that the list is not exhaustive. In the European Union cross-national comparisons among member states are of primary importance due to shared policy targets related to social issues. In the United States, surveys that would provide for such cross-national comparisons are more limited.

In some survey-based European datasets, the number of participating immigrants is large enough to allow analyses of migrant health at the national level. For each of the datasets listed in table 4.1, we describe characteristics of relevance to migrant health research. For each of the datasets listed in table 4.1, we report the objective and focus of the survey, the mode of data collection, including whether

TABLE 4.1 Description of Key EU/International and North America–Based Surveys Collecting Health and Migration Information

Survey	Health indicators	Migration indicators	Remarks
European Community Household Panel (ECHP) ECHP is an annual panel survey based on a representative panel of households and individuals in 15 EU countries covering a wide range of topics (health, income, housing, etc.). The data gathering was yearly, starting in 1994 and ending in 2001.	Self-perceived general health Being hampered in daily activities Temporary reduction of activity because of health problems Hospitalization in past 12 months Healthy lifestyle indicators (e.g., smoking)	Last foreign country of residence before coming to present country Foreign country of birth Citizenship	Sample permits analysis of cohorts of immigrants that reached western Europe before the mid-1990s. Because of the arrival of new immigrants, nonrandom sample attrition, and the absence of refreshments samples, the cross-sectional representativeness of the ECHP tends to deteriorate over time, negatively affecting its utility for immigrant health. Last foreign country of residence and foreign country of birth data are unavailable for Germany, the Netherlands, and Spain. Citizenship data is unavailable for the UK.[a]
European Working Conditions Survey (EWCS) EWCS aims at providing a comprehensive picture of the everyday reality of men and women at work. The survey was conducted in 1990 (12 countries), 1995 (15 countries), 2000 (29 countries), 2005 (31 countries), and 2010 (34 countries)	Work-related health problems (e.g., ear problems, backache, muscular pain in arms or legs, respiratory difficulties, etc.)	EWCS 1990, 1995, and 2000: nationality EWCS 2005: citizenship EWCS 2010: country of birth	Change of health indicators over time EWCS 2005: in some languages "citizenship" is translated as "inhabitant," which is not an equivalent
Survey of Health, Ageing and Retirement in Europe (SHARE) SHARE is a multidisciplinary and cross-national panel database of microdata on health, socioeconomic status, and social and family networks of more than 45,000 individuals aged 50 or over. The study was conducted in 2004 (12 countries), 2006 (15 countries), and 2008 (13 countries).	A diversity of self-reported health indicators regarding • cognitive function, • mental health (EURO-D scale), • physical health, • behavioral risk, • grip strength, and • walking speed.	Year of arrival in country Country of birth Citizenship	Questions on childhood illness are included. Wording of questions varies in the consecutive waves.

Survey	Health indicators	Migration variables	Notes
European Social Survey (ESS) ESS is a cross-sectional biennial survey that aims at charting and explaining the interaction between Europe's changing institutions and the attitudes, beliefs, and behavior patterns of its diverse populations. Cross-sectional data was gathered in 2002 (22 countries), 2004 (26 countries), 2006 (25 countries), 2008 (30 countries), and 2010 (20 countries). The questionnaire includes a core module that remains relatively constant from round to round, plus two or more rotating modules, repeated at intervals.	Self-perceived general health Being hampered in daily activities Center for Epidemiologic Depression Scale (CESD-8)	Year of arrival in country Country of birth (own, mother and father) Citizenship Member of an ethnic minority group	ESS 2002 contains a rotating module on migration. ESS 2004 and 2008 contain a rotating module on work, family, and health/well-being. ESS 2006 contains a rotating module on personal and social well-being.
European Union Statistics on Income and Living Conditions (EU-SILC) EU-SILC aims at collecting timely and comparable cross-sectional and longitudinal multidimensional microdata on income, poverty, social exclusion, and living conditions. The EU-SILC was launched in 2006 in 7 countries. As of March 2011, data for 29 countries were available.	Self-perceived general health Chronic illness or health problem Limitations in activity due to health problem Healthy lifestyle indicators (e.g., smoking)	Country of birth Citizenship	Limited sample size for migration analysis
Generations and Gender Survey (GGS) GGS aims at improving the knowledge base for policy making in UNECE countries. The GGS is a panel survey of a nationally representative sample of the 18- to 79-year-old resident population in each participating country with at least three panel waves and an interval of three years between each wave. Wave 1 was conducted in 2008–2010 (12 countries).	Self-perceived general health Chronic conditions Limitations in daily activities Emotional well-being	Date of arrival in country Age at which permanent residence in country was obtained Country of birth (own and of mother) Nationality Nationality at birth Naturalization	The questionnaires for the first wave may contain substantial differences in the various participating countries.

(Continued)

TABLE 4.1 *Continued.*

Survey	Health indicators	Migration indicators	Remarks
Eurobarometer (EB) The EB is a series of surveys on European public opinion, conducted for the European Commission since 1973. Topics investigated, include social conditions, health, culture, information technology, environment, and currency. There is great variation in participating countries depending on the topic of consideration.	Health questions are not included in all surveys, while some surveys specifically address health (e.g., EB73.2, organized in 2005, addresses mental health in 27 countries).	The information varies across the surveys, but is usually based on country of birth (own, sometimes also of mother and father).	Different wording across surveys
European Health Interview Survey (ECHiS) The ECHiS monitors health status and health care utilization in EU member states. Its basic survey, the European Core Health Interview Survey, is performed Europe-wide under the responsibility of Eurostat and covers about 130 questions. The first wave was conducted in 2007–2009.	Covers a variety of health conditions	Country of birth Nationality	
WHO Health Surveys (WHOHS) The WHO has developed and implemented a survey program and a world health survey to compile comprehensive baseline information on the health of populations and on the outcomes associated with the investment in health systems; baseline evidence on the way health systems are currently functioning; and ability to monitor inputs, functions, and outcomes. The WHO health surveys are not restricted to Europe, but cover about 61 countries.	Covers a variety of health conditions	The information varies across survey years (e.g., 2002, ethnic group; 2001, country of birth [own, mother and father])	Different indicators across the years

Survey			
Current Population Survey (CPS) The CPS documents the main labor force characteristics of the civilian population in the United States. It is a monthly survey of approximately 50,000 households; information pertaining to immigration is available from 1994 on. In addition to routine demographic data, periodic supplements contain information on health, income, and specific labor characteristics.	Health insurance coverage Health insurance type	Place of birth Parents' place of birth US citizenship status Time in the US (2007)	
American Community Survey (ACS) The ACS provides estimates of the foreign-born population annually in the United States; surveys 3 million households each year.	Disability status (e.g., hearing, cognitive, ambulatory) Health insurance coverage and type	Ancestry (since 1996) US citizenship status at birth	Survey does not ask about immigration status. Citizenship can be compared across years and also to the Census Decennial Survey. Health insurance coverage introduced in 2008.
National Health Interview Survey (NHIS) The US Census Bureau is the data collection agent for the NHIS. This survey has been collecting health data since 1957 on the health of the US civilian population. It is a cross-sectional household interview survey of about 35,000 households; sampling and interviewing occur continuously throughout the year. The survey has a core component and supplements. Estimates from the NHIS are used to produce the CDC's Vital and Health Statistics.	Contains data on a wide range of health topics	Ethnicity Country of birth	
National Health and Nutrition Examination Survey (NHANES) The NHANES provides information on the health and nutrition status of adults and children living in the United States. Since 2007 all Hispanics have been oversampled.	Numerous health conditions Dietary indicators	Country of birth (US, Mexico, other) Time lived in the US (2006)	Migration-related indicators not available for all years

(Continued)

TABLE 4.1 *Continued.*

Survey	Health indicators	Migration indicators	Remarks
National Survey of Children's Health (NSCH) The NSCH gathers data on the emotional and physical health and well-being of children ages 0–17 in the US.	Overall health Health conditions Health insurance coverage Health service access and utilization Medical home Community/neighborhood characteristics	Nativity Parent's nativity Time in the US Parent's time in the US	Migration-related indicators not available for all years
Survey of Income and Program Participation (SIPP) SIPP is a longitudinal survey (US) that collects information on demographic, income, employment characteristics, and health insurance. Each sample follows a stratified multistage probability sampling design. Core content is included in every wave (every 4 years), and topical content is included at varying frequency and timing.	Health, disability, and physical well-being included in topical modules: • Health and disability • Health and disability • Health status • Health service use • Work disability and medical expenses	Migration history topical module: • Place of birth • Places of residence • Time of residence • Citizenship status	
Canadian Community Health Survey CCHS The CCHS collects demographic and health information on the Canadian population. The CCHS is a cross-sectional survey that takes place annually (biannually until 2007). The instrument collects information about Canadians over age 12. It is made up of three components (common, optional, and rapid response).	Health conditions Social conditions Health care services Workplace injuries Other	Country of birth Citizenship (Canadian) at birth Year of arrival Language spoken at home	

SOURCE: Migration-related measurement information for US based on State Health Access Data Assistance Center 2009, "Data availability for race, ethnicity, and immigrant groups in federal surveys," Issue Brief #17, Minneapolis: University of Minnesota.

[a]Adapted from Mladovsky 2007.

it is a one-time, repeated, or panel survey, the number of countries covered, and some remarks that are specifically relevant for migrant health research. We also list the available health indicators and the different indicators of migrant status or ethnicity for each survey.

STRENGTHS AND WEAKNESSES IN THE USE OF ROUTINE HEALTH INFORMATION SYSTEMS FOR MIGRANT HEALTH RESEARCH

The challenges of conducting health research with migrant populations are huge (see chapter 2 of this volume). Here, we look specifically at the major strengths and weaknesses of using routine health information systems for national and international migrant health research. Throughout we also formulate some recommendations. For an additional and more extensive consideration of challenges more specifically related to the European context, we refer to Levecque et al. (2012).

When health information systems gather the same information on health and migrant status at different points in time, research into the dynamics of the link between migration and health becomes possible. One way of approaching these dynamics is to look into health trajectories of individuals. A health trajectory refers to the pattern of health experienced by an individual over time, which is assumed to result from multiple factors operating in genetic, biological, behavioral, social, cultural, environmental, political, and economic contexts that change as a person develops. Understanding the course and causes of change in health over time allows anticipation of those at greatest risk for adverse trajectories and events and creates the possibility for control by influencing the trajectory itself. In addition to health trajectories, the dynamics of the link between migration and health may also be approached from a trend perspective. Trend analysis is a method of time series data (information in sequence over time) analysis that is useful in (1) detecting general patterns of a relationship between associated factors or variables and (2) projecting the future direction of this pattern. A trend analysis might, for example, reveal how the strength of the link between migrant status and health changes over time in a specific country or for a specific migrant population. In addition, if there is comparable data for different regions or nations, comparative analyses of health information systems might also reveal how meso and macro features, such as specific health care system arrangements or specific migration and integration policies, might impact migrant status, health, and possible inequities in comparison to the native population. If the number of migrants is large enough in registers or surveys, important between-group differences within the migrant population might also be revealed.

In many European countries, information that allows for the study of the health of migrants is simply lacking. When data on migrant status is available, migrant indicators and definitions used in registers and surveys often differ from country to country, thereby limiting the possibility for conducting comparative studies on migrant health and health care use (Rechel et al. 2011; Levecque et al. 2012). The diversity in available registry-based migrant health data for health care in Europe for example, has been reported recently by Smith et al. (2009). In their overview, it is shown that only eleven of twenty-seven European countries have registry data on health care use that enable identification of migrants. The picture is somewhat different for migrant health research based on surveys, since in recent years several international surveys have become available that enable migrant health research both from a national and a cross-national comparative perspective. When the focus on migrant health (and health care use) is not primarily at the national, but at the cross-national level the scientific endeavor is yet more complex, reflecting—among other things—additional methodological costs (Levecque et al. 2012).

When registers or surveys contain the necessary information on health, migrant status, and their determinants, another common problem encountered in migrant health research based on existing health information systems is related to the small sample size of migrants, or in the case of registers, population size. In registers, especially clinical ones, small population size is often related to barriers in access to health services (Ingleby 2009). In survey research, this might be due to the relatively small size of migrant communities in many geographic areas, but also to usually low response rates among migrants (Mladovsky 2009; Juhasz et al. 2010). These low response rates may have several causes, a major one being language problems or distrust of government or other institutions (Levecque et al. 2009). For specific migrant groups such as asylum seekers or undocumented migrants, information is often completely lacking. As oversampling is often required in surveys or clinical studies in order to yield statistically relevant information on smaller subgroups of the population, and as researchers tend to be from the ethnically dominant, "native" population, mainstream medical research has for a long time favored homogenous samples, excluding migrants and ethnic minorities (Ingleby 2006). Small sample or population sizes can lead to inefficient estimates as well as biased estimates if the "not covered" migrant population has a significantly different sociodemographic and health (or health care use) profile. One way of dealing with small sample size is to pool datasets from several years, as, for example, Levecque et al. (2009) did when analyzing migrant health based on the Belgian Health Interview Surveys of 2001 and 2004. This pooling strategy is of course only an option when the same required information is available in the datasets one wishes to pool. However, when trying to address the problem of low sample or population sizes, researchers should recognize that the link between participation and survey error is not completely straightforward and studies with low response rates may in fact be less biased than studies with high response rates (Levecque et al. 2009). Whether rates are biased or not, a consequence that is inherent in the case of small sample or population sizes is that comparison between subcategories of migrants is often not possible. Small sample size could thus lead to an inaccurate picture of migrant health when significant differences within migrant groups exist.

Another weakness in migrant health research based on existing health information systems is related to what has been called the "denominator problem." Censuses and municipality registers of the population form datasets that are crucial to getting insight into the size of the migrant population in a specific location (e.g., country) at a specific point in time. Such information is necessary for data collection or statistical analyses, but a common problem in migrant health research is that migrant population size is often unknown or based on inaccurate estimates (WHO 2010a). One consequence of the denominator problem is that even when health information is available, data might be misleading if not adjusted for age, sex, socioeconomic, and migrant status. This also raises the question of which groups migrants should be compared to: is it the host population, other groups of migrants, or the population in the country of origin? Thus far the latter comparison has hardly been addressed through research, but may yield particularly valuable information on how migration has affected those who have moved from one country to another (Rechel et al. 2011).

Especially for migrant health research based on survey data, validity is an issue that needs serious consideration. While survey data in general have the advantage of containing a large number of indicators and are not generally restricted to specific health outcomes such as mortality, one of the major challenges with population-based surveys is that, as with health interview surveys, they are often confined to subjective measures of health such as self-reported health, which brings up concerns about cross-cultural differences (Ingleby 2009). However, this can be addressed to some extent by the use of anchoring vignettes, in which respondents are asked to indicate the health status they would attribute to a hypothetical person (Salomon et al. 2004).

As for migrant health research on mortality more specifically, a complicating factor in such studies is that migrants often return home when they become old or sick (Ingelby 2009). This may lead to a significant underestimation when migrant mortality statistics are based on death registers (Mladovsky 2007). Sidebar 4.2 presents a case study illustrating the use of register data provided by the Spanish Institute of Statistics to estimate mortality from cardiovascular diseases among recent immigrants in Spain.

HOW TO FIND A DATA SOURCE TO RESPOND TO A SPECIFIC QUESTION

Let us suppose that we have a research question on migrant health and we want to answer it using the data found in existing information sources. One suitable

SIDEBAR 4.2 CASE STUDY INVOLVING THE USE OF REGISTER
INFORMATION FOR MIGRANT HEALTH RESEARCH

This second case study illustrates the use of mortality data to compare the pattern of cardiovascular disease in migrant and nonmigrant populations (see Regidor et al. 2009).

Rationale

The magnitude of mortality from cardiovascular diseases varies widely in different parts of the world. The genetic and environmental factors that explain these patterns of mortality are not well known. Studies of mortality in immigrants can provide some clues to help identify these factors. One type of investigation of immigrants that can provide relevant information is the study of migrant populations that refer to a recent period, shortly after their arrival in the host country. As time passes, immigrants may adopt health-related attitudes and behaviors of the host country, such as tobacco use, dietary practices, and physical exercise.

Aim

The primary aim of this study was to estimate mortality from cardiovascular diseases among recent immigrants in Spain.

Method

1. The source of data was the municipal population register and the cause-of-death register, 2000–2004.
2. The data were provided by the Spanish Institute of Statistics.
3. The indicator of migration was country of birth.
4. The analysis focused on relative differences (ratios) in the mortality rates by cause of death according to birthplace

Results

Immigrants from sub-Saharan Africa had the highest mortality rate ratio for cardiovascular diseases overall (2.04), while those from South America had the lowest (0.64). These groups of immigrants also showed the highest (1.95) and lowest (0.60) mortality rate ratio from ischemic heart disease. Immigrants from eastern Europe also had higher mortality from ischemic heart disease than did the Spanish population. Immigrants from Central America and the Caribbean were the only group in which the rate of mortality from cerebrovascular disease differed significantly from that of the Spanish population, whose mortality rate was 1.97.

Limitations

Information about population and deaths was taken from different sources; therefore a numerator/denominator information bias could exist with regard to the country of birth. No information was available on the duration of residence in Spain.

approach to finding the databases tailored to a specific research question is the one proposed by Grady and Hearst (2007). Specifically, these authors suggest that after reviewing the specialized literature, the researcher must make a list of predictor variables (possible causes) and outcome variables (damage to health) whose relation could help answer the research question. Then it is necessary to identify the databases that may contain these variables and assess the migrant-specific data available in those databases. In this assessment, it is critical to know the different institutions that may have databases of interest for migrant health issues and related topics. Sometimes these data sources do not contain the specific variables of interest; nevertheless, they may contain variables that approximate the phenomenon one wishes to study, and it must be determined if these approximations are sufficient for addressing the research question. Finally, population sizes and the limitations regarding quality of data must also be considered.

A good strategy to reduce the time it takes to select databases is to consult researchers or administrators who have knowledge of and/or experience with different datasets, such as key experts for the European Commission or European Council on specific topics (e.g., migration), or to contact persons working for institutions that finance the organization of population surveys (e.g., the Research Council Flanders in Belgium). These experts can evaluate the suitability of different databases to the proposed research questions. Once the best database has been identified, the next step, if necessary, is to formally request access to the database from the responsible person in the institution that owns it. Finally, once the data are available, the researcher must establish the specific hypotheses, define the statistical methodology, and analyze the data.

Another option for studying the relation between a predictor variable and a specific outcome is to combine two or more databases. That is, one data source may contain information on an individual characteristic and another data source may contain information on some health measure like morbidity or mortality. As has been mentioned previously, this possibility depends on the data sources having a personal identifier for each individual, so that the sources can be linked. This also presupposes that the problems of confidentiality that are sometimes raised by this type of linkage have been resolved.

RECOMMENDATIONS AND CONCLUSIONS

The forementioned strategies address the limitations of migrant health research based on existing health information systems; in this section, we would like to stress two issues more specifically.

The first is evident and has already been well formulated by many others before us (e.g., Juhasz et al. 2010; WHO 2010b): countries need to step up efforts to address the current lack of data. There is a need for standardized definitions and the inclusion of relevant questions on migration and health in existing data collection sources such as censuses, national statistics, and health surveys, as well as in the collection of routine health information. Ideally, minimal additional requirements should be added to existing data collection systems. Such systems should allow duration of stay to be assessed (in European countries, for example), include the descendants of migrants, and be uniform across Europe (Razum 2006) and internationally. At the same time, these efforts must ensure respect for the principles of confidentiality, informed consent, and voluntary self-identification (Rechel et al. 2011).

The second recommendation is related to the first, and stresses the possibility of linkage between datasets, such as health surveys with census forms, population registers and statistical data systems (which combine administrative sources and population registers) in order to obtain the necessary information for migrant health research. In the European Union, such data sources are recognized as "official statistics sources" by the Council of Europe (INED 2007). In the official statistics sources of the 27-EU countries, for example, information on country of birth is available in all countries but Latvia and on citizenship in all countries but Latvia, Slovenia, and the UK. Data on ethnicity/nationality is available in thirteen countries and religion in fourteen countries (MEHO atlas).

Another prerequisite for linkage of datasets in the EU is the availability of personal identification numbers, such as government issued IDs. However, many countries are reluctant to implement a transnational identification system due to historical, political, and ethical concerns (Smith Nielsen et al. 2009; Levecque et al. 2012). In some countries, for example, in Belgium, the use of personal identification numbers enables linkage of official datasets in theory, but at the moment, the Belgian Commission for the Protection of Privacy is implementing privacy laws so strictly so that in practice it looks very unlikely that researchers would be given permission to analyze linked data on migrant health, even if it is sufficiently anonymous. In some countries, such as the UK, migrant health research is rapidly developing (e.g., Fischbacher et al. 2007; Hippisley-Cox et al. 2008) through the linkage of primary and secondary care datasets, with linkage to census data being the next challenge. The potential for linking European datasets is considerable (Bhopal 2009). Major advances have already been made in using linkage to explore ethnicity and health in the Netherlands (Bos et al. 2002), Sweden (Hedlund et al. 2008), and Denmark (Norredam et al. 2011).

The unique opportunities to study migration, ethnicity, and health by linkage of register-based datasets in Denmark have been very well demonstrated by Norredam et al. (2011), who linked the Danish Cancer Registry, Psychiatric Research Register, National Patient Register, National Health Service Register, Injury Register, and Medical Birth Register with registers of Statistics Denmark and the Civil Registration System. These linkages were enabled by a unique individual identification number (CPR number). The study shows that register-based research on migration and ethnicity requires well-defined categories and that objective definitions are most often based on data about one's own and/or parents' country of birth and date of arrival in Denmark. These variables facilitate follow-up over time and comparisons between generations. In addition, the Danish Immigration Service registers data on migration status, nature of residence permit, and length of asylum procedure, which can be used to distinguish refugees from family reunification immigrants (Norredam et al. 2011).

In summary, though health data by migrant status is sometimes available in US, Australian, Canadian, and New Zealand health information systems, various methodological challenges exist for its effective use. In Europe, some countries do not routinely collect health data by migrant status (Juhasz et al. 2010). While the Netherlands and the UK have significant experience in conducting population-based surveys that also contain information on migration status or ethnicity, countries such as Belgium, Germany, and Spain have only recently started to include such variables in health surveys of the general population. The newer EU member states generally do not include variables on migration status in their health registries or surveys (Rechel et al. 2011; Levecque et al. 2012). The need for better health information systems on migrants has not been unrecognized, as can be seen, for example, in the conclusions of the European Council (Council of Europe 2010) and declarations and recommendations of the Council of Europe (Committee of Ministers 2006; Council of Europe 2007). Until recently, however, these calls for more accurate migrant health data failed to elicit improvements in health information systems in many European countries (Rechel et al. 2011).

The sources described here are tools that can be very useful in improving knowledge about the health status of migrant populations and in developing strategies to improve their health. Moreover, the availability and relative ease of use of these tools make it possible to obtain a high return on the information they provide. However, some considerations must be taken into account. Using previously collected data makes it necessary to work with the variables contained in the databases. Further, in some cases the databases come from records that have been collected for administrative purposes, which can create some obstacles to access. With respect to the sample size of surveys, we have explored the frequent problems that can arise from the small number of migrants included and that can limit the validity of the analysis. In this regard, it is important to promote the development of mechanisms to obtain more representative samples of migrant health.

REFERENCES

Agudelo-Suárez, Andres, Elena Ronda-Pérez, Diana Gil-González, Laura González-Zapata, and Enrique Regidor. 2009. "Relationship in Spain of the length of the gestation and the birth weight with mother's nationality during the period 2001–2005." *Revista Española de Salud Pública* 83: 331–37.

Bhopal, Raj. 2009. "Chronic diseases in Europe's migrant and ethnic minorities: Challenges, solutions and a vision." *European Journal of Public Health* 19: 140–43.

Bhopal, Raj, Snorri Rafnsson, Charles Agyemang, Anne Fagot-Campagna, Simona Giampaoli, Niklas Hammar, Seeromanie Harding, Ebba Hedlund, Knud Juel, Johan Mackenbach, Paola Primatesta, Gregoire Rey, Michael Rosato, Sarah Wild, and Anton Kunst. 2011. "Mortality from circulatory diseases by specific country of birth across six European countries: Test of concept." *European Journal of Public Health.* doi: 10.1093/eurpub /ckr062. First published online 20 May 2011.

Bos, Vivian, Anton Kunst, Ingeborg Keij-Deerenberg, and Johan Mackenbach. 2002. "Mortality amongst immigrants in the Netherlands." *European Journal of Public Health* 12: S41.

Committee of Ministers. 2006. Recommendation 18 of the Committee of Ministers to member states on health services in a multicultural society. Strasbourg: Council of Europe.

Council of Europe. 2007. Bratislava declaration on health, human rights and migration. Eighth Conference of European Health Ministers, Bratislava, 23 November 2007.

Council of Europe. 2010. Council conclusions on equity and health in all policies: Solidarity in health. 3019th Employment, Social Policy, Health and Consumer Affairs Council meeting, Brussels, 8 June 2010.

Fischbacher, Colin, Raj Bhopal, Chris Povey, Markus Steiner, Jim Chalmers, Ganka Mueller, Joan Jamieson, and David Knowles. 2007. "Record linked retrospective cohort study of 4.6 million people exploring ethnic variations in disease: Myocardial infarction in South Asians." *BMC Public Health* 7: 142.

Guendelman, Sylvia, Pierre Buekens, Beatrice Blondel, Monique Kaminski, Francis Notzon, and Godelieve Masuy-Stroobant. 1999. "Birth outcomes of immigrant women in the United States, France, and Belgium." *Maternal and Child Health Journal* 3: 177–87.

Grady, Deborah, and Norman Hearst. 2007. "Utilizing existing databases." In Stephen Hearst, Steven Cumming, Warren Browner, Deborah Grady, and Thomas Newman, eds., *Designing clinical research: An epidemiologic approach.* Philadelphia: Lippincot Williams and Wilkins: 207–20.

Haenzel, William, and Malaysia Kurihara. 1968. "Studies of Japanese migrants: Mortality from cancer and other diseases among Japanese in the United States." *Journal of National Cancer Institute* 40: 43–68.

Hedlund, Eva, Kenneth Pehrsson, An Lange, and Niklas Hammar. 2008. "Country of birth and survival after a first myocardial infarction in Stockholm, Sweden." *European Journal of Epidemiology* 23: 341–47.

Hippisley-Cox, Julia, Carol Coupland, Yana Vinogradova, John Robson, Rubin Minhas, Sheikh Aziz, and Peter Brindle. 2008. "Predicting cardiovascular risk in England and Wales: Prospective derivation and validation of QRISK2." *British Medical Journal* 336: 1475–82.

INED—Institut National d'Etudes Démographiques. 2007. "'Ethnic' statistics and data protection in the Council of Europe countries." Study report. Strasbourg: Council of Europe.

Ingleby, David. 2006. "Getting multicultural health care off the ground: Britain and the Netherlands compared." *International Journal of Migration, Health and Social Care* 2: 4–14.

Ingleby, David. 2009. "European research on migration and health." Background paper developed within the framework of IOM Project Assisting Migrants and Communities (AMAC): Analysis of Social Determinants of Health and Health Inequalities. Geneva: International Organization for Migration.

International Organization for Migration. 2010. *World Migration Report 2010—The future of migration: Building capacities for change.* Geneva: International Organization for Migration.

Juhasz, Judith, Peter Makara, and Agnes Taller. 2010. "Possibilities and limitations of comparative research on international migration and health." Promoting Comparative Quantitative Research in the Field of Migration and Integration in Europe (PROMIN-STAT). Working paper no. 09. Brussels: European Commission.

Kliewer, Erich, and Ken Smith. 1995. "Breast cancer mortality among immigrants in Australia and Canada." *Journal of National Cancer Institute* 87: 1154–61.

Lasser, Karen, Steffie Himmelstein, and David Woolhandler. 2006. "Access to care, health status, and health disparities in the United States and Canada: Results of a cross-national population-based survey." *American Journal of Public Health* 96: 1300–1307.

Levecque, Katia, Ina Lodewyckx, and Piet Bracke. 2009. "Psychological distress, depression and generalised anxiety in Turkish and Moroccan immigrants in Belgium. A general population study." *Social Psychiatry and Psychiatric Epidemiology* 44: 188–97.

Levecque, Katia, Fernando G. Benavides, Elena Ronda, and Ronan Van Rossem. 2012. "Using existing health information systems for migrant health research in Europe: Challenges and opportunities." In David Ingleby et al., eds., *Health inequalities and risk factors among migrants and ethnic minorities.* Antwerp: Garant. 53–68.

MacMahon, Brian. 1960. *Epidemiology: Principles and methods.* Boston: Little, Brown.

Mladovsky, Philippa. 2007. "Migration and health in the EU. Research note." European Commission—Directorate-General, Employment, Social Affairs and Equal Opportunities Unit E1-Social and Demographic Analysis.

Mladovsky, Philippa. 2009. "A framework for analyzing migrant health policies in Europe." *Health Policy* 93: 55–63.

Norredam, Marie, Marianne Kastrup, and Karin Helweg-Larsen. 2011. "Register-based studies on migration, ethnicity and health." *Scandinavian Journal of Public Health* 39: 201–5.

Rafnsson, Snorri, and Raj Bhopal. 2009. "Large-scale epidemiological data on cardiovascular diseases and diabetes in migrant and ethnic minority groups in Europe." *European Journal of Public Health* 19: 484–91.

Razum, Oliver. 2006. "Commentary: Of salmon and travellers—Musing on the mystery of migrant mortality." *International Journal of Epidemiology* 35: 919–21.

Rechel, Bernd, Philippa Mladovsky, and Walter Devillé. 2011. "Monitoring the health of migrants." In Bernd Rechel, Philippa Mladovsky, Walter Devillé, Barbara Rijks, Roumyana Petrova-Benedict, and Martin McKee, eds., *Migration and health in the European Union*. Berskshire: Open University Press McGraw-Hill. 73–90.

Regidor, Enrique, Elena Ronda, Cruz Pascual, David Martínez, Calle Elisa, and Vincente Domínguez. 2009. "Mortality from cardiovascular diseases in immigrants residing in Madrid." *Medicina Clínica* 132: 621–24.

Rio, Isabel, Adela Castello, Mireia Jané, Ramón Prats, Carmen Barona, Rosa Mas, Marisa Rebaliagto, Oscar Zurriaga, and Francisco Bolumar. 2009. "Quality of data used to calculate reproductive and perinatal health indicators in native and migrant populations." *Gaceta Sanitaria* 24:172–77.

Ronda-Pérez, Elena, Fernando G. Benavides, Katia Levecque, John G. Love, Emily Felt, and Ronan Van Rossem. 2012. "Differences in working conditions and employment arrangements among migrant and non-migrant workers in Europe." *Ethnicity and Health* 17: 563–77.

Salomon, Joshua, Ajay Tandon, and Christopher Murray. 2004. "Comparability of self-rated health: Cross-sectional multi-country survey using anchoring vignettes." *British Medical Journal* 328: 258.

Singh, Gopal, and S. M. Yu. 1996. "Adverse pregnancy outcomes: Differences between US and foreign-born women in major US racial and ethnic groups." *American Journal of Public Health* 86(6): 837–43.

Smith Nielsen, Signe, Allan Krasnik, and Aldo Rosano. 2009. "Registry data for cross-country comparisons of migrants' healthcare utilization in the EU: A survey study of availability and content." *BMC Health Services Research* 9: 210.

Vandenheede, Hadewijch, Patrick Deboosere, Irina Stirbu, Charles O. Agyemang, Seeromanie Harding, Knud Juel, Snorri Björn Rafnsson, Enrique Regidor, Grégorie Rey, Michael Rosato, Johan P. Mackenbach, and Anton E. Kunst. 2011. "Migrant mortality from diabetes mellitus across Europe: The importance of socio-economic change." *European Journal of Epidemiology* 14, PMID:22167294.

World Health Organization (WHO). 2010a. "Health of migrants—The way forward. Report of a global consultation." Madrid, Spain, 3–5 March 2010.

World Health Organization (WHO). 2010b. "How health systems can address health inequities linked to migration and ethnicity." Copenhagen: WHO Regional Office for Europe.

5

Use of National Data Systems to Study Immigrant Health in the United States

Gopal K. Singh

INTRODUCTION

The US immigrant population has grown considerably in the last four decades, from 9.6 million in 1970 to 40 million in 2010 (US Census Bureau 2011). Immigrants currently represent 12.9% of the total US population, the highest percentage in eight decades (Walters and Trevelyan 2011; US Census Bureau 2011). The rapid increase in the immigrant population since 1970 reflects large-scale immigration from Latin America and Asia (Walters and Trevelyan 2011; Grieco and Trevelyan 2010; Grieco 2010). Over half (53%) of all US immigrants are from Latin America and another 28% of immigrants come from Asia (Walters and Trevelyan 2011). Europeans, who accounted for 75% of immigrants in 1960, currently represent 13% of the total US immigrant population (Walters and Trevelyan 2011; Grieco and Trevelyan 2010; Grieco 2010). There are currently 29 million immigrants in the prime workforce (ages 25–64 years), making up about 17.5% of the total US population (Walters and Trevelyan 2011; US Census Bureau 2011). Increases in the immigrant child population have also been substantial. The number of US children in immigrant families more than doubled in the past two decades, from 8.2 million in 1990 to 17.1 million in 2010. In 2010, nearly a quarter of US children had at least one foreign-born parent (US Census Bureau 2011; FIFCFS 2011).

Despite the marked increase in the immigrant population, the systematic monitoring of health, mortality, and disease patterns among US immigrant populations of various ethnic and national origins remains relatively undeveloped. Most national data systems in the United States do not routinely report and analyze health statistics by immigrant status. Moreover, immigrant health analysis is hampered by difficulty in obtaining relevant population denominator data or by an incomplete reporting of immigrant status in national surveillance databases. The substantial ethnic, cultural, and linguistic diversity of the US immigrant population makes it even more difficult to monitor immigrant health and well-being on a systematic basis (Singh and Hiatt 2006; Singh and Miller 2004).

Although reduction of health inequalities among various socioeconomic and demographic groups remains the primary focus of the national health initiative Healthy People, this initiative in health promotion and disease prevention lacks data and policy objectives that explicitly target the health of US immigrants (DHHS 2012, 2006, 2000). Moreover, the nation's premier and most comprehensive annual report on health statistics, *Health, United States,* does not include any data on the US immigrant population (NCHS 2011a).

In this chapter, I describe eight major federal data systems that can be used to study the health of immigrants in the United States in some detail. These data systems vary considerably in their coverage of health and behavioral characteristics, identification of major immigrant groups, and availability of time periods. A secondary objective is to provide, by using these data systems, current estimates of some of the most important health and behavioral indicators for both immigrant and US-born populations across the life course, including life expectancy; infant mortality; low birth weight; mortality from major causes of death such as cancers, cardiovascular disease (CVD), homicide, suicide, and unintentional injuries; self-assessed physical and mental health; disability; health insurance coverage; and health risk factors such as obesity, smoking, poor nutrition, and physical inactivity. Each of the data systems is described below with illustrative results and interpretation.

The strengths, limitations, and characteristics of each data system are summarized in table 5.1. Survival and logistic regression models, prevalence, age-specific and age-adjusted death rates, and standard life table methodology are used to examine nativity/immigrant differentials. Since all health surveys discussed in this study have complex sampling designs, SUDAAN software is used to estimate prevalence, standard errors, and regression models (SUDAAN 2009).

The remainder of the chapter is organized with presentation of the complete-count administrative data systems first, followed by the national sample surveys, broadly adopting a life course perspective. The chapter ends with a discussion of the relative significance of each data system for carrying out immigrant health analyses in the US and offers suggestions and new directions for strengthening and/or developing databases for immigrant health assessment.

I begin with the National Vital Statistics System, which has been the cornerstone of health monitoring among social groups and geographic areas in the US for over a century (Minino et al. 2011; Martin et al. 2011; Hoyert et al. 1995; Singh 2000; Kitagawa and Hauser 1973).

TABLE 5.1 National Data Systems for Studying Immigrant Health in the United States

Data system	Data collection and design	Government or sponsoring agency	Immigration variables	Period of data availability	Number of records or sample size	Subnational analysis	Advantages	Disadvantages
National Vital Statistics System (NVSS)	Period data; temporal; death and birth registration; complete-count administrative data	National Center for Health Statistics, Centers for Disease Control and Prevention (CDC)	Decedent's nativity/ immigrant status; maternal nativity status derived from the place-of-birth variable; detailed country-of-birth information for mothers in the birth file	1900 through 2009	2.5 million deaths and 4.25 million births annually	Regions, census divisions, states, counties, metro and nonmetro areas	Large number of vital records; race/ethnicity detail; geographic detail; long-term time trend; various health, mortality, and birth outcome measures	No data on several key immigration-related variables, e.g., duration of US residence, naturalization, English-language proficiency
National Linked Birth and Infant Death Data	Longitudinal; cohort; complete-count administrative records	National Center for Health Statistics, Centers for Disease Control and Prevention (CDC)	Mother's nativity/ immigrant status	1985 to 2008	30,000 to 40,000 infant deaths linked to a cohort of more than 4 million births each year	Regions, census divisions, states, and counties	Large population size; ethnic detail; extensive infant mortality analysis by age, cause of death, and medical risk	No data on duration of US residence, naturalization, language, or legal status
National Longitudinal Mortality Study (NLMS)	Longitudinal; census and CPS records linked prospectively to deaths by cause of death and cancer incidence records	National Institutes of Health, US Census Bureau, and National Center for Health Statistics, CDC	Nativity/ immigrant status; country/ region of birth	1973 to 2008	2.3 million CPS records at baseline and nearly 500,000 deaths during the 25-year mortality follow-up	State-level analysis possible for selected cohorts	Large sample size; self-reported race/ethnic detail; longitudinal; mortality by cause of death	Only a subset of the dataset is available as public-use file

(Continued)

TABLE 5.1 *Continued.*

Data system	Data collection and design	Government or sponsoring agency	Immigration variables	Period of data availability	Number of records or sample size	Subnational analysis	Advantages	Disadvantages
National Survey of Children's Health (NSCH)	Cross-sectional; sample survey; telephone survey	Health Resources and Services Administration (HRSA) and National Center for Health Statistics, CDC	Parents' and children's nativity/ immigrant status; duration of residence in the US; English-language proficiency	2003, 2007, and 2011	Approximately 100,000 children under age 18 in 2003 and 93,000 children in 2007	Regions, census divisions, and states	Large sample size; state-specific analyses; large number of health and behavioral indicators	All data based on parental reports; ethnic detail not available in the public-use file
National Survey of Children with Special Health Care Needs (NS-CSHCN)	Cross-sectional; sample survey; telephone survey	Health Resources and Services Administration (HRSA) and National Center for Health Statistics, CDC	English-language use	2001, 2005–2006, and 2009–2010	Over 40,000 children with special health care needs screened from a sample of 375,00 children aged <18	Regions, census divisions, and states	Household language use; state-specific analysis; extensive health services data for CSHCN	No nativity/ immigrant status variable; sample size too small for ethnicity detail
National Health Interview Survey (NHIS)	Cross-sectional; temporal; sample survey; in-person interview data	National Center for Health Statistics, Centers for Disease Control and Prevention, CDC	Children's and adults' nativity/ immigrant status; duration of residence in the US; naturalization/ citizenship status	1957 to 2010; immigrant status first became available in the 1976 survey	Approximately 100,000 children and adults annually	Four broad census regions only (Northeast, Midwest, South, and West)	Large sample size; race/ ethnicity detail; long-term time trend; extensive sociodemographic, behavioral, health, and morbidity indicators	No geographic detail; data on most Asian subgroups suppressed in public-use file; no language variables; no information on immigrants' legal or refugee status

National Health and Nutrition Examination Survey (NHANES)	Cross-sectional; temporal; sample survey; in-person interview data	National Center for Health Statistics, Centers for Disease Control and Prevention, CDC	Children's and adults' nativity/ immigrant status; duration of residence in the US; naturalization/ citizenship status	1976 to 2010; periodic survey from 1976 to 1998; and continuous survey since 1999	Approximately 10,000 children and adults in each wave	None	Clinical examination data; medical and lab test results; measured height and weight; interview data on health status, morbidity, diet and nutrition	Small sample size; limited ethnic detail; no geographic detail; no language variables; no immigrants' legal or refugee status variable
American Community Survey (ACS) Public-Use Microdata Sample	Cross-sectional; sample survey; in-person interview	US Census Bureau	Nativity/ immigrant status; parents' nativity status; detailed country of birth information; duration of residence in the US; naturalization status; English language ability; languages spoken at home	From 2000 through 2010	More than 3 million records in the annual sample	Regions, census divisions, states, and counties (on summary files)	Large sample size; extensive race/ethnicity detail; detailed country of birth information; language; naturalization status; duration of US residence	No health variables other than disability and health insurance coverage

NATIONAL VITAL STATISTICS SYSTEM (NVSS)

The NVSS is a vital registration system of all births and deaths occurring in the United States (Minino et al. 2011; Martin et al. 2011). The system is maintained by the CDC's National Center for Health Statistics (NCHS). The national mortality data are available on an annual basis in published form from 1900 to the present and on public-use microdata files from 1968 to the present (Minino et al. 2011; Hoyert et al. 1995). This data system allows the examination of mortality differentials by cause of death according to individual characteristics, including nativity/ immigrant status and geographic areas such as state, metropolitan/nonmetropolitan areas, and counties. The national mortality data system is one of the very few administrative sources of health statistics in the United States that is routinely available, that covers all events, and that is comparable at the international, national, state, and local levels (Hoyert et al. 1995; Singh 2000).

The national mortality files are based on information from death certificates of every death occurring in the United States each year. In 2009, 2,437,163 deaths were reported in the United States (NCHS 2012a). The *US Standard Certificate of Death,* revised most recently in 2003 by the US Department of Health and Human Services, is the basis for the national mortality data (Minino et al. 2011; NCHS 2012a). The *US Standard Certificate of Death* serves as the model for state death certificates in an effort to establish uniform certificates. Most state certificates conform closely to the national standard, with modifications to meet particular state needs or legislation. Although the principal responsibility for data collection, data processing, and data quality maintenance rests with the states, the federal government is required to collect and publish national vital statistics data (Minino et al. 2011; Hoyert et al. 1995; Singh 2000).

For the study of mortality differentials, the following variables are available on the death certificate: sex, race/ethnicity, age at death, place or country of birth (US- or foreign-born), place of residence (state, county, and metropolitan/nonmetropolitan area), educational attainment, occupation, industry, and marital status, underlying and multiple causes of death (coded according to the *International Classification of Diseases*), autopsy status, place of death (hospital, clinic, nursing home, residence, etc.), and injury at work (Minino et al. 2011; NCHS 2012a).

Nativity/immigrant status in the mortality file is determined by decedent's state/country of birth (Singh and Hiatt 2006; Singh and Miller 2004; NCHS 2012a). The place-of-birth variable includes codes for the fifty states; the District of Columbia (DC); the US territories of Puerto Rico, the Virgin Islands, Guam, American Samoa, and the Northern Marianas; and those born in Canada, Mexico, Cuba, and remainder of the world (NCHS 2012a). For mortality analysis, those born outside the fifty states, DC, and US territories are considered foreign-born (Singh and Hiatt 2006; Singh and Miller 2004). In 2009, 202,307 deaths occurred among the foreign-born, representing 8.3% of all US deaths. About 13,000 deaths occurred among those born in Canada, while 33,445 deaths occurred among those born in Mexico (NCHS 2012a). In 2009, 3.6% of the death records were missing information on state/country of birth.

The most current national mortality data available in electronic form are for the 2009 calendar year (NCHS 2012a). For computing mortality rates, relevant population (denominator) data on immigrant status (US- or foreign-born), race/ethnicity, and sociodemographic characteristics can be obtained from the decennial censuses or the American Community Survey (Singh and Hiatt 2006; Singh and Miller 2004; Minino et al. 2011).

The major advantages of the national mortality file are its size, geographic and ethnic detail, and the fact that the information on individual death records dating from 1968 is available electronically (Singh and Hiatt 2006; Hoyert et al. 1995; Singh 2000). Moreover, the availability of published information since 1900 on an annual basis makes the national mortality file especially useful for analyzing long-term national and state trends in mortality, survival, and life expectancy (Minino et al. 2011; Hoyert et al. 1995; Singh 2000).

The natality component of the NVSS includes birth certificate data for the over 4 million births that occur in the United States each year (NCHS 2011a; Martin et al. 2011; NCHS 2012b). Birth certificate data are available on an annual basis in published form from 1915 to present and in electronic form on public-use data files from 1968 to 2009 (Martin et al. 2011; NCHS 2012b). The *US Standard Certificate of Live Birth,* revised most recently in 2003, is the basis for the national birth data (Martin et al. 2011).

Nativity/immigrant status of infants and mothers in the natality file is defined according to mother's place (state/country) of birth. The place-of-birth variable in the natality file is identical to that in the mortality file. However, for birth data, detailed codes for the mother's country of birth are also available (NCHS 2012b). Out of 4.13 million US births in 2009, nearly a million births occurred among foreign-born mothers. In 2009, 401,861 births occurred among mothers born in Mexico, 28,850 births among mothers born in India, 21,288 births among mothers born in China, 20,851 births among mothers born in the Philippines, and 11,226 births among mothers born in Canada (NCHS 2012b). In 2009, 0.3% of US birth records lacked state/country of birth information.

Besides nativity/immigrant status, the variables available for analyzing fertility and birth outcomes include maternal and paternal age, race/ethnicity, marital status, education, birth weight, gestational age, tobacco and alcohol use during pregnancy, prenatal care utilization, maternal weight gain during pregnancy, method of delivery (vaginal or c-section), pregnancy history, and a variety of medical risk factors and complications such as gestational diabetes, pregnancy-induced hypertension, eclampsia, uterine bleeding, and placenta previa (Martin et al. 2011; NCHS 2012b).

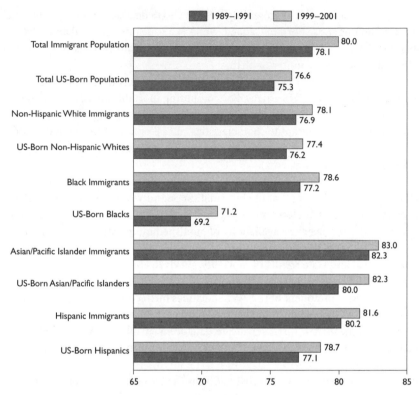

FIGURE 5.1. Life expectancy at birth (average lifetime in years) by race/ethnicity and immigrant status, United States, 1989–2001. (Based on data from the US National Vital Statistics System, 1989–2001. Also see GK Singh and RA Hiatt, *International Journal of Epidemiology* [2006] 35[4]:903–19.)

Life expectancy based on US mortality data is shown in figure 5.1. During 1999–2001, US immigrants had a life expectancy of 80.0 years, 3.4 years longer than the life expectancy of the US-born population. The immigrant differential in life expectancy increased between 1989 and 2001. In all racial/ethnic groups, immigrants had a higher life expectancy than their US-born counterparts. The nativity differential was greatest for black immigrants, who had 7.4 years longer life expectancy than US-born blacks. Among the foreign-born population, Asian/Pacific Islander immigrants had the highest life expectancy (83.0 years), followed by Hispanic immigrants (81.6 years), black immigrants (78.6 years), and white immigrants (78.1 years) (Singh and Hiatt 2006).

During 1999–2001, male and female immigrants experienced 23% and 16% lower all-cause mortality than their US-born counterparts, respectively. This pattern held for whites, blacks, Asian/Pacific Islanders, and Hispanics. Ethnic-nativity patterns in CVD and all-cancer mortality were generally similar to those in all-cause mortality. Immigrants had substantially higher rates of stomach and liver cancer mortality rates than the US-born, with the absolute risk of stomach and liver cancer mortality being particularly high among immigrant and US-born Asians, Hispanics, and blacks. Higher liver and stomach cancer mortality rates in these groups have been partly attributed to their higher incidence of hepatitis B virus and *Helicobacter pylori* infection (Singh and Hiatt 2006). Detailed ethnic-nativity differentials in mortality from other major causes of death are reported elsewhere (Singh and Hiatt 2006; Singh and Miller 2004).

The NVSS can be used to analyze all-cause and cause-specific mortality of immigrants in any age group. Besides data for broad ethnic groups such as Asian/Pacific Islanders, Hispanics, blacks, and whites, the NVSS allows analyses of immigrant mortality and life expectancy differentials for detailed Asian and Hispanic subgroups such as Chinese, Japanese, Filipino, Asian Indian, Koreans, Vietnamese, Mexican, Cuban, Puerto Rican, and Central and South American (Singh and Hiatt 2006; Singh and Miller 2004).

NATIONAL LINKED BIRTH AND INFANT DEATH DATA

National linked birth and infant death files are prepared by the NCHS and are a by-product of the natality and mortality components of the NVSS (Mathews and MacDorman 2012). They are available as public-use data files for the 1983 through 2002 US birth cohorts and as period-linked files from 2003 to 2008 (Mathews and MacDorman 2012; Singh and Yu 1996; Hummer et al. 1999a). In this dataset, the death certificate is linked with the corresponding birth certificate for each infant who dies in the United States. For each national birth cohort, approximately 30,000 infant deaths are linked to a cohort of more than 4 million births each year (Mathews and MacDorman 2012; Singh and Yu 1996).

The purpose of the linkage is to use many additional variables available from the birth certificate in infant mortality analysis (Mathews and MacDorman 2012). Information on all of the 4.25 million births in the US each year is also included. For the 2002 birth cohort, more than 98% of US infant death certificates were successfully matched to birth certificates. In the 2008 period-linked file, 1,034,416 live births and 5,228 infant deaths occurred among foreign-born mothers (Mathews and MacDorman 2012).

Besides nativity/immigrant status, the variables available for infant mortality and perinatal outcomes analyses include maternal age, race/ethnicity, marital status, education, place of residence, cause of death, age at death, birth weight, gestational age, tobacco and alcohol use during pregnancy, prenatal care utilization, maternal weight gain during pregnancy, and a variety of medical risk factors (Mathews and MacDorman 2012).

Nativity/immigrant status in the linked file is determined according to the mother's place of birth as described in the natality file. The data in table 5.2 indicate the sort of immigrant health analyses that can be supported by the linked file. Infants born to immigrant mothers have significantly lower risks of infant mortality, low birth weight, and preterm birth than those born to US-born mothers. Even after controlling for various infant and maternal risk factors, immigrants in all racial/ethnic groups experience lower risks of infant mortality than natives. However, nativity patterns in birth outcomes and associated risk factors vary widely across racial/ethnic groups (table 5.2).

NATIONAL LONGITUDINAL MORTALITY STUDY (NLMS)

The National Longitudinal Mortality Study (NLMS) is a longitudinal dataset for examining socioeconomic, occupational, and demographic factors associated with all-cause and cause-specific mortality in the United States (Hoyert et al. 1995; Singh 2000; Sorlie et al. 1995; USCB 2007; Singh and Siahpush 2001, 2002). The NLMS is conducted by the National Heart, Lung, and Blood Institute in collaboration with the US Census Bureau, the National Cancer Institute, the National Institute on Aging, and the NCHS (Rogot et al. 1992; Sorlie et al. 1995; USCB 2007; Singh and Siahpush 2001). The NLMS consists of thirty Current Population Survey (CPS) and census cohorts between 1973 and 2002 whose survival (mortality) experiences were studied between 1979 and 2003 (USCB 2007). The CPS is a sample household and telephone interview survey of the civilian non-institutionalized population in the United States and is conducted by the US Census Bureau to produce monthly national statistics on unemployment and the labor force. Data from death certificates on the fact of death and the cause of death are combined with the socioeconomic and demographic characteristics of the NLMS cohorts by means of the National Death Index (Rogot et al. 1992; Sorlie et al. 1995; USCB 2007; Singh and Siahpush 2001). Detailed descriptions of the NLMS have been provided elsewhere (Rogot et al. 1992; Sorlie et al. 1995; USCB 2007; Singh and Siahpush 2001).

The NLMS consists of data on more than 3 million individuals drawn from thirty CPS and census cohorts whose mortality experience has been followed from 1979 through 2003. The total number of deaths during the twenty-four-year follow-up exceeds 500,000 (USCB 2007). Cancer incidence, stage of disease at diagnosis, and cancer survival data from eleven SEER (Surveillance, Epidemiology, and End Results) cancer registries have also been linked to the various NLMS cohorts to prospectively study the risk of cancer incidence and mortality according to baseline individual-level socioeconomic and demographic characteristics (Clegg et al. 2009; Du et al. 2011; Howlader et al. 2011).

TABLE 5.2 Infant Mortality Rate per 1,000 Live Births and Prevalence (%) of Selected Sociodemographic and Medical Risk Factors for Selected Ethnic-Immigrant Groups, United States, 1999–2002 (N = 16,022,367 Live Births)

Ethnic-nativity group	Teen birth (maternal age ≤ 19 years)	Maternal education ≥ 16 years	Delayed or no prenatal care	Smoking during pregnancy	Low birth weight	Preterm birth	Gestational diabetes	Chronic/pregnancy hypertension	Infant mortality rate	Unadjusted infant mortality risk ratio[a]	Adjusted infant mortality risk ratio[b]	95% confidence interval
Total population												
US-born[c]	12.5	26.2	3.2	14.3	8.0	12.2	2.9	5.1	7.2	1.39*	1.26	1.23–1.29
Foreign-born[d]	8.0	20.3	5.6	2.1	6.5	10.2	3.6	2.8	5.2	Reference	1.00	Reference
Non-Hispanic white												
US-born	8.8	32.4	2.2	16.0	6.8	10.8	2.9	5.2	5.7	1.25*	1.21	1.16–1.26
Foreign-born	3.3	41.3	3.5	5.7	6.0	9.3	3.1	3.9	4.6	Reference	1.00	Reference
Non-Hispanic black												
US-born	21.1	10.6	6.4	10.1	13.6	18.0	2.6	5.6	13.8	1.43*	1.41	1.36–1.48
Foreign-born	5.6	23.5	6.8	1.3	9.8	14.0	4.3	4.9	9.7	Reference	1.00	Reference
Asian Indian[e]												
US-born	6.2	60.7	3.6	4.0	10.0	11.0	4.0	2.9	7.3	1.81*	1.58	1.05–2.36
Foreign-born	1.1	54.7	3.9	0.3	9.5	9.9	8.0	2.4	4.0	Reference	1.00	Reference
Mexican												
US-born	24.1	7.8	4.7	5.2	6.9	12.2	2.6	3.5	6.1	1.25*	1.30	1.25–1.35
Foreign-born	12.3	3.7	7.3	0.8	5.6	10.6	3.1	2.5	4.9	Reference	1.00	Reference

SOURCE: Data derived from the 1999–2002 US National Linked Birth and Infant Death data files.

[a]Risk ratio = ratio of the infant mortality rate or risk for the US-born in each ethnic group to that for the corresponding immigrant group.

[b]Adjusted for maternal age, marital status, birth order, infant sex, plurality, maternal education, prenatal care, and smoking during pregnancy.

[c]US-born are those born in the 50 states and the District of Columbia.

[d]Foreign-born are those born outside these territories.

[e]Data for Asian Indians were available for only 11 states: CA, HI, IL, MI, MO, NJ, NY, TX, VA, WA, WV.

*$p < 0.05$.

In the NLMS, place of birth (born in the 50 states, DC, US territories, Canada, Cuba, Mexico, or rest of the world) is the basis for defining nativity/immigrant status (US- or foreign-born) (USCB 2007; Singh and Siahpush 2001, 2002). The NLMS does not include other immigration-related variables collected by CPS, such as citizenship/naturalization status and duration of residence in the US. For immigrant differentials in all-cause and cause-specific mortality, covariates such

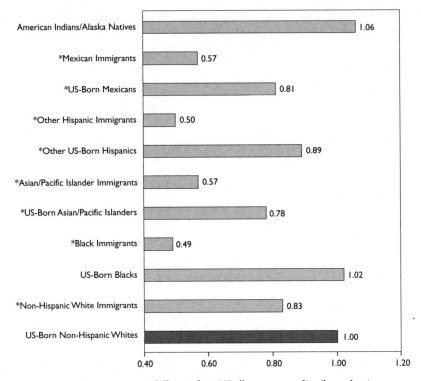

FIGURE 5.2. Ethnic-immigrant differentials in US all-cause mortality (hazard ratio or relative risk): The US National Longitudinal Mortality Study, 1980–1998 (*N* = 304,594). Adjusted by Cox regression for age, sex, marital status, household size, education, family income, employment status, and rural/urban residence. *p < 0.05. US-born non-Hispanic whites were the reference group. (Updated analysis of data presented in GK Singh and M Siahpush, *Human Biology* [2002] 74 [1]:83–109.)

as age, race/ethnicity, marital status, rural/urban residence, education, occupation, employment status, family income, and housing tenure can be used (USCB 2007; Singh and Siahpush 2001, 2002). The NLMS also permits analyses of the effects of early childhood social conditions as well as labor force transitions on risks of mortality from different causes of death.

According to the 1980–1998 NLMS, black, Asian/Pacific Islander, Mexican, and white immigrants aged ≥25 years had, respectively, 51%, 43%, 43%, and 17% lower risks of all-cause mortality than US-born non-Hispanic whites of equivalent socioeconomic and demographic background (figure 5.2). Immigrants had significantly lower mortality rates than natives from all cancers combined and from lung, colorectal, prostate, and breast cancers. However, immigrants had substan-

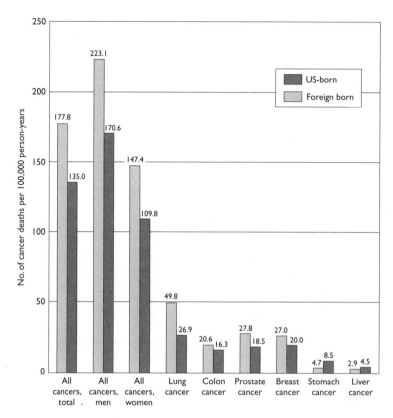

FIGURE 5.3. Site-specific US cancer mortality rates by nativity/immigrant status: The US National Longitudinal Mortality Study, 1980–1998 (N = 304,594). Mortality rates are age-adjusted to the 2000 US standard population. Differences in mortality rates between US- and foreign-born individuals were statistically significant at the 0.05 level. (Updated analysis of data presented in GK Singh and M Siahpush, *American Journal of Public Health* [2001] 91[3]:392–99.)

tially higher age-adjusted mortality rates than natives from stomach and liver cancers (figure 5.3). The linked NLMS-SEER data indicate similar immigrant patterns in site-specific cancer incidence rates (figure 5.4).

NATIONAL SURVEY OF CHILDREN'S HEALTH (NSCH)

The NSCH is conducted by the NCHS/CDC, with funding and direction from the Health Resources and Services Administration's Maternal and Child Health Bureau (MCHB) (HRSA 2009; NCHS 2009). The purpose of the survey is to

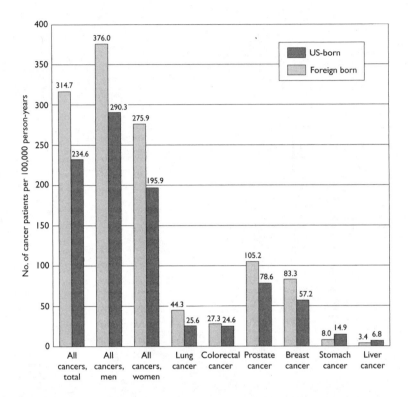

FIGURE 5.4. Site-specific US cancer incidence rates by nativity/immigrant status: The US National Longitudinal Mortality Study linked with eleven SEER cancer registries, 1980–1998. SEER = Surveillance, Epidemiology, and End Results. Incidence rates are age-adjusted to the 2000 US standard population. Differences in incidence rates between US- and foreign-born individuals were statistically significant at the 0.05 level for all cancers combined, lung, prostate, breast, and stomach cancers. The eleven SEER registries include Iowa, Hawaii, Seattle, Connecticut, Detroit, Utah, Los Angeles, San Francisco/Oakland/San Jose/Monterey, Greater California, Louisiana, and Kentucky.

provide national and state-specific prevalence estimates for a variety of children's health and well-being indicators (HRSA 2009; NCHS 2009). The survey also includes an extensive array of questions about the family, including parental health, stress, and coping behaviors; family activities; and parental concerns about their children (HRSA 2009; NCHS 2009).

The NSCH has been conducted twice thus far, in 2003 and 2007. A third round of the survey was completed in April 2012, with the data becoming available in early 2013. The 2007 NSCH was a telephone survey conducted between April 2007 and July 2008, and the 2003 NSCH was conducted between January 2003 and July 2004 (HRSA 2009; NCHS 2009; Singh et al. 2007, 2008, 2009). The 2007 survey had a total sample size of 91,642 children under 18 years of age, including a sample of about 1,800 children per state (HRSA 2009; NCHS 2009). The total sample size of the 2003 NSCH was 102,353 (Singh et al. 2007, 2008, 2009). In the two surveys, a random-digit-dial sample of households with children under 18 years of age was selected from each of the fifty states and DC. One child was selected from all children in each identified household to be the subject of the survey. Interviews were conducted in English, Spanish, and four Asian languages. The respondent was the parent or guardian who knew the most about the child's health status and health care. The interview completion rate was 66.0% in 2007 and 68.8% in 2003 (HRSA 2009; NCHS 2009; Singh et al. 2007, 2008, 2009). Substantive and methodological details of the two surveys are described elsewhere (HRSA 2009; NCHS 2009; Singh et al. 2007, 2008, 2009; Blumberg et al. 2012).

In NSCH, the children's immigrant status (US- or foreign-born) can be defined by both children's own nativity and that of their parents (Singh et al. 2007, 2008, 2009). In the 2007 survey, 12,539 children (20.1%) were born to immigrant parents. The NSCH also includes data on the child's and parents' length of stay in the United States and primary language spoken in the home (NCHS 2009).

Table 5.3 provides an example of the kind of analysis that can be undertaken to examine child health disparities between immigrants and natives. Immigrant children are defined here as those born to one or both immigrant parents. Thus, the overall immigrant group includes foreign-born children with both immigrant parents (first generation) and US-born children with one or both immigrant parents (second generation). US-born children with both US-born parents (third or higher generation) are considered native-born. Immigrant children and adolescents aged 10–17 years are 10% more likely to be overweight than their native-born counterparts. Immigrant children are less likely than native-born children to engage in sports and physical activity. Immigrant children are less likely than native children to be diagnosed with behavioral problems, autism, asthma, and other chronic conditions. However, despite the lower prevalence of these health conditions, immigrant parents are more likely than US-born parents to assess their children's general health as fair/poor. Immigrant parents are also more likely to report their own physical health and mental health as fair/poor compared to US-born parents.

NATIONAL SURVEY OF CHILDREN WITH SPECIAL HEALTH CARE NEEDS (NS-CSHCN)

The 2005–2006 NS-CSHCN was conducted by the NCHS, with funding and direction from MCHB (HRSA 2007; NCHS 2012c; Yu and Singh 2009). This

TABLE 5.3 Weighted Prevalence (%) of Selected Behavioral and Health Indicators among Immigrant and Native-Born Children <18 Years: The 2007 National Survey of Children's Health (N = 91,642)

Behavioral or Health indicator	Immigrant children[a]		Native-born children[b]	
	%	SE	%	SE
Obesity (BMI ≥95th percentile)[c]	17.8	1.6	16.1	0.5
Overweight (BMI ≥85th percentile)[c]	34.2	2.0	31.1	0.6
No physical activity	16.4	1.2	8.9	0.3
Lack of sports participation	48.9	1.5	40.0	0.5
Fair or poor overall health status	5.9	0.5	2.9	0.2
Behavioral/emotional health problem	3.0	0.5	6.5	0.2
Autism spectrum disorder	0.7	0.2	1.2	0.1
Asthma	4.4	0.4	10.2	0.3
One or more chronic conditions	13.1	0.7	24.6	0.4
Maternal breastfeeding rate	88.9	1.1	71.7	0.7
Mother in fair/poor health	14.6	0.9	10.2	0.3
Mother in fair/poor mental health	7.8	0.7	7.2	0.2
Father in fair/poor health	12.6	0.9	6.2	0.3
Father in fair/poor mental health	6.3	0.7	4.6	0.3

NOTE: Nativity differences in prevalence were statistically significant at $p < .05$ for all indicators except obesity.
[a]US-born and foreign-born children of immigrant parents.
[b]US-born children of US-born parents.
[c]Defined for children and adolescents aged 10–17 years.

random-digit-dial telephone survey used the State and Local Area Integrated Telephone survey platform to assess the health care needs and experiences of children with special health care needs (CSHCN), using approximately equal sized samples of CSHCN from each state and DC (HRSA 2007). From April 2005 to February 2007, all children under 18 years of age in 191,640 households were screened for special health care needs. One child with special needs was randomly selected from households with CSHCN to be the target of the detailed interview. The survey respondent was the parent or guardian who knew the most about the health care experiences of the CSHCN. Interviews were conducted in English, Spanish, and four Asian languages. The overall response rate was 61.2%. Substantive and methodological details of the survey are described elsewhere (HRSA 2007). The first round of the NS-CSHCN survey was conducted in 2001, and the third round of the survey was released in December 2011 (HRSA 2007; NCHS 2012c).

The 2005–2006 survey included 40,773 CSHCN, who were screened from a sample of 363,183 children aged <18 years. The 2009–2010 survey includes detailed interview data for 40,242 CSHCN who were screened from a sample of 371,671 children. CSHCN are defined as those "who have or [are] at increased risk for a chronic physical, developmental, behavioral, or emotional condition and who also require health and related services of a type or amount beyond that required by children generally" (HRSA 2007; Yu and Singh 2009).

The NS-CSHCN does not include a direct question on immigrant status of children or their parents. Rather, household language use (primary language spoken) is used to infer immigrant status of CSHCN (Yu and Singh 2009). In 2005–2006, 4.5% of children in non-English-speaking households were identified as having special health care needs, compared with 15.2% of children in English-speaking households. In 2009–2010, the weighted CSHCN prevalences for the two groups were 7.8% and 16.3%, respectively. In the 2009–2010 survey, of 30,998 children in the non-English-speaking households, 2,565 were identified as having special health care needs (NCHS 2012c).

Children in non-English-speaking households are more likely than children in English- speaking households to lack access to a medical home, usual source of care, personal doctor/nurse, family-centered care, and insurance coverage. Families of children in non-English-speaking households are more likely to experience financial hardship and to stop working because of the child's condition (Yu and Singh 2009).

NATIONAL HEALTH INTERVIEW SURVEY (NHIS)

The NHIS is a national sample household survey in which data on socioeconomic, demographic, behavioral, morbidity, health, and health care characteristics are collected via personal household interviews (Singh and Hiatt 2006; Schiller et al. 2012; Bloom et al. 2011; Singh et al. 2011). Data collected in the survey are based on self-reports. The survey uses a multistage probability design and is representative of the civilian non-institutionalized population of the United States. The NHIS is one of the longest running annual federal health surveys and is conducted by the NCHS (Singh and Hiatt 2006; NCHS 2011a; Schiller et al. 2012). Detailed descriptions of the NHIS can be found elsewhere (NCHS 2011a; Schiller et al. 2012; Bloom et al. 2011). The NHIS covers a broad range of health topics for both children and adults, including physical and mental health status; activity limitation; asthma; learning disability; attention deficit hyperactivity disorder; school absence; chronic conditions such as heart disease, cancer, diabetes, kidney disease, and liver disease; health-risk indicators such as obesity, smoking, diet, physical inactivity, and alcohol use; health insurance coverage; and use of preventive health services such as cancer screening. Besides the core survey, the NHIS often includes supplemental surveys on special topics such as child health, mental health, cancer control, occupational health, child and adult immunization, complementary and alternative medicine, HIV, and diabetes (NCHS 2011a; Schiller et al. 2012; Bloom et al. 2011).

In the NHIS, nativity/immigrant status is determined via place-of-birth information (Singh and Hiatt 2006; Singh and Miller 2004; Singh et al. 2011). Besides immigrant status (US- or foreign-born), the public-use dataset includes geographic region of birth (US; Mexico, Central America, Caribbean Islands; South America; Europe; Russia/former USSR; Africa; Middle East; Indian subcontinent; Southeast Asia; and Asia), duration of residence in the United States, and citizenship status (table 5.1). In 2010, out of a sample of 89,976 children and adults, 17,658 were identified as immigrants.

The NHIS can be used to examine socioeconomic and demographic profiles of various ethnic-immigrant groups (Singh and Hiatt 2006; Singh et al. 2011). It is particularly useful for estimating immigrant differentials in chronic-disease risk factors (Singh and Hiatt 2006; Singh et al. 2011). For example, there is considerable variation in obesity and overweight prevalence among various ethnic-immigrant groups. Although immigrants in each racial/ethnic group have lower prevalence than their US-born counterparts, immigrants' risk of obesity and overweight increases with increasing duration of residence in the United States. In 2003–2008, obesity prevalence ranged from 2.3% for recent Chinese immigrants to 31% or higher for American Indians, US-born blacks, Puerto Ricans, US-born Mexicans, and long-term Mexican immigrants (Singh et al. 2011).

Current smoking rates vary widely among ethnic-nativity groups, with immigrants considerably less likely to smoke than the US-born (table 5.4). Black immigrants are two-thirds less likely to smoke than US-born blacks (8.2% vs. 22.7%), while Mexican immigrants are one-third less likely to smoke than US-born Mexicans (11.6% vs. 18.4%). Immigrants' risk of smoking increases with increasing duration of residence in the US. Even after controlling for various sociodemographic factors, ethnic-immigrant differentials remain, with all Asian, Hispanic, and black immigrant groups reporting substantially lower smoking rates.

Immigrants are more likely to be at a higher risk of physical inactivity than the US-born (figure 5.5). This pattern holds for all racial/ethnic groups except blacks. Rates of physical inactivity decline with increasing length of stay in the US. For example, the prevalence of physical inactivity is 76% among Cuban immigrants to the US in the past 15 years, 69% among Cuban immigrants who have been in the US for more than 15 years, and 41% among US-born Cubans.

Immigrants in all racial/ethnic groups are substantially more likely to be without health insurance coverage than their US-born counterparts. Almost 60% of Mexican immigrant children and adults lack health insurance coverage (data not shown).

NATIONAL HEALTH AND NUTRITION EXAMINATION SURVEY (NHANES)

During the past four decades, the NHANES surveys have been conducted periodically by the NCHS to obtain data on chronic-disease prevalence and risk fac-

TABLE 5.4 Weighted Prevalence and Adjusted Odds of Current Smoking among US Adults Aged 18+ from 26 Ethnic-Immigrant Groups: The National Health Interview Survey, 2004–2009

Duration of residence and ethnic-immigrant group	Smoking prevalence		Adjusted odds ratio[a]	
	%	SE	OR	95% CI
Duration of residence in the US (years)				
<5	13.2	0.8	0.60	0.52–0.70
5–9	11.7	0.6	0.49	0.43–0.56
10–14	11.6	0.7	0.47	0.41–0.55
15+	12.7	0.3	0.64	0.59–0.69
US-born	22.2	0.2	1.00	Reference
Ethnic-immigrant group				
Non-Hispanic white, US-born	22.3	0.2	1.00	Reference
Non-Hispanic white, immigrant	15.9	0.7	0.78	0.70–0.88
Non-Hispanic black, US-born	22.7	0.4	0.68	0.65–0.72
Non-Hispanic black, immigrant	8.2	0.7	0.22	0.18–0.27
American Indian/Alaska Native	33.4	2.6	1.20	0.94–1.53
Asian Indian, US-born	8.7	2.8	0.38	0.18–0.79
Asian Indian, immigrant	6.4	0.8	0.33	0.25–0.43
Chinese, US-born	4.3	1.4	0.24	0.13–0.47
Chinese, immigrant	6.3	0.8	0.30	0.23–0.39
Filipino, US-born	18.6	2.2	0.90	0.67–1.22
Filipino, immigrant	12.6	1.4	0.65	0.49–0.85
Hawaiian/Pacific Islander, US-born	26.4	4.6	1.06	0.71–1.59
Pacific Islander, immigrant	19.1	5.7	0.64	0.30–1.35
Other Asians, US-born[b]	13.6	1.5	0.72	0.55–0.94
Other Asians, immigrant[b]	15.1	1.0	0.61	0.51–0.72
Mexican, US-born	18.4	0.6	0.52	0.48–0.57
Mexican, Immigrant	11.7	0.5	0.21	0.19–0.23
Puerto Rican, Mainland US-born	21.8	1.5	0.60	0.50–0.72
Puerto Rican, Puerto Rico-born	19.2	1.5	0.56	0.46–0.68
Cuban, US-born	21.6	2.8	0.86	0.60–1.23
Cuban, Immigrant	13.9	1.4	0.47	0.38–0.59
Central and South American, US-born	12.5	1.4	0.40	0.31–0.52
Central and South American, immigrant	11.3	0.7	0.25	0.21–0.29
Other Hispanics, US-born	27.1	1.7	1.05	0.88–1.25
Other Hispanics, immigrant	12.5	3.3	0.37	0.20–0.68
All other groups	16.9	2.4	0.66	0.45–0.95

NOTE: OR = odds ratio; SE = standard error; CI = confidence interval.

[a]Adjusted by logistic regression model for survey year, age, gender, ethnic-immigrant status (or race/ethnicity and length of immigration), region of residence, education, marital status, poverty status, and occupation.

[b]This category includes Koreans, Vietnamese, Japanese, Cambodians, Laotians, Hmongs, Thais, Pakistanis, and other Asians.

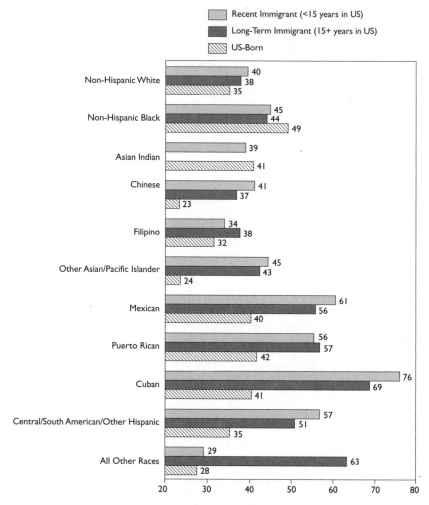

FIGURE 5.5. Physical inactivity prevalence (%) by race/ethnicity and immigrant status, US adults aged 18 years and older. (The 2002–2007 National Health Interview Survey.)

tors such as obesity, smoking, hypertension, cholesterol levels, and diet and nutritional factors (NCHS 2011a, 2011b). Beginning in 1999, the NHANES became a continuous annual survey using a complex, stratified, multistage probability clustered sample design, collecting data for a representative sample of the US civilian population. The NHANES data are based on clinical examinations, selected medical and laboratory tests, and in-home person interviews (NCHS 2011a, 2011b).

The overall response rate in the NHANES for both interview and examination components was at least 76% in each of the six waves, 1999–2000, 2001–2002,

TABLE 5.5 Obesity and Overweight Prevalence (Weighted) among US Children and Adolescents Aged 2–19 (*N = 16,717*) and Adults 20+ Years (*N = 18,391*) by Immigrant Status: The 1999–2006 National Health and Nutrition Examination Survey (NHANES)

Immigrant status	Childhood obesity prevalence		Childhood overweight prevalence		Adult obesity prevalence		Adult overweight prevalence	
	%	SE	%	SE	%	SE	%	SE
Total population	15.4	0.5	31.3	0.9	31.8	0.7	65.7	0.6
US-born	15.7	0.5	31.6	0.8	33.4	0.7	66.6	0.7
Foreign-born	12.2	1.1	24.9	1.5	22.9	1.0	60.9	1.1
Non-Hispanic white								
US-born	13.5	0.8	29.5	1.2	31.1	0.7	64.8	0.8
Foreign-born	10.0	2.5	16.8	3.6	24.2	2.3	57.8	2.5
Non-Hispanic black								
US-born	19.4	0.7	35.2	0.8	44.2	1.0	74.0	0.9
Foreign-born	13.8	2.4	24.3	2.8	21.9	2.5	61.4	2.1
Mexican American								
US-born	21.9	1.0	38.3	1.2	40.2	1.7	73.5	2.0
Foreign-born	16.8	1.2	35.6	1.5	28.7	1.4	70.7	1.2
Other Hispanic								
US-born	20.4	2.1	37.8	2.3	38.3	4.4	72.3	3.7
Foreign-born	12.2	3.2	26.9	4.5	26.8	1.9	70.8	2.6
All other ethnic groups								
US-born	13.4	1.6	26.9	2.5	42.1	4.1	73.3	3.0
Foreign-born	4.9	2.2	12.8	3.7	6.5	1.7	35.2	2.6

NOTE: Childhood overweight and obesity are defined as body mass index (BMI) at or above the gender and age-specific 85th and 95th percentile cutoff points from the 2000 CDC growth charts. Adult overweight is defined as body mass index (BMI) $\geq$25 and obesity as BMI $\geq$30. Obesity and overweight prevalence in NHANES are based on measured height and weight data.

2003–2004, 2005–2006, 2007–2008, and 2009–2010. Substantive and methodological details of the NHANES are described elsewhere (NCHS 2011a, 2011b).

Immigrant status in the NHANES is derived from the country-of-birth variable (born in 50 US states or DC, Mexico, other Spanish-speaking country, or non-Spanish-speaking country). In the 2009–2010 NHANES, out of a total sample of 10,537 individuals, only 1,991 were foreign-born. The other immigration-related variables in the NHANES include naturalization/citizenship status and length of time in the US (NCHS 2011b).

Because of small sample sizes, several years of NHANES data need to be pooled in order to conduct detailed ethnic and immigrant analyses such as those presented in table 5.5. Obesity and overweight prevalence estimates for children, adolescents, and adults in NHANES (unlike the NSCH and the NHIS) are based on measured height and weight data. The data in table 5.5 show lower obesity and overweight prevalence among foreign-born children aged 2–19 and adults aged 20+ years compared to their US-born counterparts. Regardless of nativity, childhood and adult obesity prevalence among both US-born and foreign-born Mexicans and other Hispanics ranks among the highest in the world (Singh et al. 2011). In terms of nutritional characteristics, immigrants in each racial/ethnic group have significantly lower total calorie and fat intake than the US-born. Moreover, immigrants' likelihood of excess calorie and fat intake increases with increasing length of residence in the US (Singh et al. 2011).

AMERICAN COMMUNITY SURVEY (ACS)

Decennial censuses conducted by the US Census Bureau have long been the source of detailed socioeconomic and demographic information for the immigrant population in the United States (Walters and Trevelyan 2011; Larsen 2003; Singh and Hiatt 2006; Singh and Miller 2004; USCB 2003). With the discontinuation of the long-form questionnaire in the 2010 decennial census, the American Community Survey (ACS) has become the primary census database for collecting data on socioeconomic, demographic, and housing characteristics of various population groups, including the immigrant population at the national, state, county, and local levels (USCB 2003, 2009, 2011). The advantage of the ACS is that it is conducted annually with a sample size of over 3 million records, as compared with the decennial census long-form data, which were only available every 10 years (USCB 2009, 2011).

In the ACS microdata sample, nativity/immigrant status is defined based on the place-of-birth variable, which provides extensive details on individuals' US state of birth and country of birth (table 5.1) (Grieco and Trevelyan 2010; USCB 2011). Additionally, nativity of parents is available for children under 18 years of age. Duration of residence in the United States, naturalization/citizenship status, English-language ability, and an extensive list of languages spoken at home are the other immigration-related variables available in the ACS (USCB 2011). By pooling multiple years of microdata samples, the ACS can be used to study socioeconomic, demographic, disability, and health insurance characteristics of various immigrant subgroups in the US by cross-classifying nativity status with the extensive race/ethnicity groupings that are available in the dataset. Weighted statistics for select variables from the ACS can also be obtained from the web-based American FactFinder (USCB 2012).

The 2010 microdata sample contains data on 347,945 immigrants, including information on 144,341 children born to immigrant parents. As mentioned above, numerous linguistic groups are represented in the 2010 sample, including

TABLE 5.6 Rates (Weighted %) of Disability and No Health Insurance Coverage among US Children, Working-Age Adults, and Elderly According to Nativity/Immigrant Status and World Region of Birth: The 2010 American Community Survey, Public Use Microdata Sample ($N = 3,061,692$)

Nativity/immigrant status	Disability			No health insurance coverage		
	<18 years	18–64	≥65	<18 years	18–64	≥65
Foreign-born	2.7	5.3	36.1	31.2	39.0	5.7
US-born	4.1	11.2	39.0	7.1	18.4	0.3
World region of birth						
US-born (50 states and DC)	4.1	11.2	38.9	7.1	18.3	0.3
Puerto Rico and US Island Territories	9.1	16.8	46.2	7.2	22.2	0.6
Latin America	2.9	5.8	38.9	43.9	53.3	8.6
Asia	2.5	4.6	33.7	12.9	20.7	6.2
Europe	3.9	6.5	35.9	7.5	17.6	1.5
Africa	2.0	4.5	30.2	14.5	27.7	10.9
Northern America (Canada and Mexico)	2.8	6.4	34.0	11.8	11.5	1.3
Oceania	2.2	4.9	33.0	12.8	18.6	1.8

(unweighted frequency) data on 26,806 Chinese- (Mandarin- and Cantonese-) speaking and 5,345 Hindi-speaking individuals aged ≥5 years. According to the data in table 5.6, foreign-born children and working-age adults are, respectively, 33% and 52% less likely to have a disability (hearing, vision, cognitive, ambulatory, and self-care difficulties) than their US-born counterparts. Child and adult disability rates are highest among those born in Puerto Rico and other US territories and lowest among those born in Asia and Africa. Immigrant children are four times more likely and working-age adults two times more likely than the US-born to lack health insurance. Approximately 44% of children, 53% of working-age adults, and 9% of the elderly born in Latin America do not have health insurance coverage.

DISCUSSION AND DIRECTIONS FOR FUTURE RESEARCH

In this chapter, eight major federal datasets have been described for assessing trends and differentials in the health of immigrants in the United States. These data systems vary substantially in their coverage of health and behavioral characteristics, identification of ethnic and immigrant groups, time periods, data collection methodologies, and the types of data analyses that can be supported for

studying immigrant health. Given the availability of a wide range of health variables and the inclusion of various ethnic-immigrant groups, the NVSS and NHIS
are the two most important data systems for studying and monitoring immigrant
health in the United States. These two data systems allow health, mortality, and
morbidity estimates for some of the smallest and newest immigrant groups, reliable data for whom are not available elsewhere. The new and updated health, mortality, morbidity, and health care access data for immigrants presented herein
should serve as the benchmark for setting up national health objectives for various
immigrant groups in the US and for conducting comparative analyses.

Health, life expectancy, mortality, and morbidity patterns for immigrants and
natives vary considerably in the United States. Overall, immigrants have better
infant, child, and adult health, higher life expectancy, and lower disability and mortality rates than the US-born (Singh and Hiatt 2006; Singh and Miller 2004; Singh
and Yu 1996; Hummer et al. 1999a; Singh and Siahpush 2001 and 2002; Singh et al.
2007, 2009, 2011). Nativity/immigrant patterns in several health outcomes, including those in mortality from major causes of death, vary across different racial/eth-
nic groups (Singh and Hiatt 2006; Singh and Miller 2004). Inequities in health care
access and utilization between immigrants and natives are very marked, with
nearly 60% of Mexican immigrant children and adults reporting having no health
insurance coverage. Acculturation, crudely measured by duration of residence
since the time of immigration, plays a major role in modifying the social, behavioral, and health characteristics of immigrants, particularly of Asian and Hispanic
immigrant groups; acculturation generally leads to a decline in their health and
mortality advantage over time (Singh and Hiatt 2006; Singh and Miller 2004; Singh
and Siahpush 2002; Singh et al. 2007, 2009, 2011; Arcia et al. 2011).

A number of explanations have been suggested for higher life expectancy, better
health, and lower mortality rates among immigrants. First, people immigrating to
the US may be healthier than those who remain in their countries of origin. This is
referred to as the "healthy immigrant effect," or positive immigrant selectivity
(Singh and Hiatt 2006; Singh and Miller 2004; Singh and Siahpush 2001, 2002;
Singh et al. 2011). Second, as shown here and elsewhere, immigrants have a lower
prevalence of health-risk behaviors than natives, including lower rates of smoking,
alcohol consumption, obesity, and poor nutrition (Singh and Hiatt 2006; Singh and
Miller 2004; Singh and Siahpush 2002; Singh et al. 2009, 2011). Third, immigrants
appear to have higher levels of social and familial support and social integration
compared to the native-born (Singh and Hiatt 2006; Singh and Miller 2004; Singh
and Yu 1996). Fourth, socioeconomic characteristics might partly account for the
immigrant differentials in health outcomes. Although immigrants are generally
better educated, they have higher unemployment and poverty rates and lower rates
of health insurance coverage than the US-born (Singh and Hiatt 2006; Singh et al.
2011). However, previous studies as well as analyses in the present chapter indicate

only a modest contribution from socioeconomic factors in explaining nativity differentials (Singh and Hiatt 2006; Singh and Miller 2004; Singh and Yu 1996; Singh and Siahpush 2001, 2002; Singh et al. 2011). Lastly, inconsistencies in the coding of immigrant status in the numerator (mortality) and denominator (population) data may contribute to the reported life expectancy and mortality differentials between immigrants and the native-born (Singh and Hiatt 2006; Singh and Miller 2004). However, the NLMS and longitudinal cohort studies have produced mortality patterns consistent with the cross-sectional patterns based on the NVSS (Singh and Hiatt 2006; Singh and Miller 2004; Singh and Siahpush 2001, 2002).

Monitoring the health and well-being of immigrants is important not only in the United States, but also in other industrialized countries with sizable immigrant populations such as Canada, Australia, the United Kingdom, Germany, France, Spain, Italy, and the Netherlands (Singh and Hiatt 2006). While the absolute number of immigrants in these countries is much smaller than that in the United States, the proportion of the foreign-born population is higher in Canada (20%), Australia (22%), and Spain (14%) than in the US (13%) (Statistics Canada 2012). Data sources for studying immigrant health in Canada have been well documented (Chen et al. 1996a; Perez 2002; Chen et al. 1996b; Dunn and Dyck 2000; Hyman 2004; Ali et al. 2004); chapter 4 of this volume, by Levecque et al., provides a comprehensive review of health information systems that are most useful for migrant health studies in Europe.

Vital records and other administrative health databases in the United States generally do not contain several key immigration-related variables, such as duration of residence or recency of immigration, parental nativity status, citizenship/naturalization status, legal or refugee status, and English-language proficiency, any of which might affect both immigrant health and its determinants (Singh and Hiatt 2006; Singh and Miller 2004). General population-based sample surveys can be a good source for facilitating in-depth analyses of these characteristics and other factors that influence immigrant health; however, they are not particularly useful for monitoring the health of the many immigrant groups that represent a small proportion of the total population (Singh and Hiatt 2006; Singh and Miller 2004). Vital records, cancer registries, and other disease surveillance systems are important for identifying significant health problems and disease risks among various ethnic-immigrant groups, monitoring changes in their health status over time, and conducting etiological analyses (Singh and Hiatt 2006; Singh and Miller 2004). In the SEER cancer registries, more than 45% of all cancer patients' place-of-birth information is missing (Howlader et al. 2011). Analysis of immigrant differentials in cancer incidence, disease stage, and survivorship based on cancer registries is biased because completeness of birthplace data in cancer registries varies systematically according to patient characteristics, including vital status (Lin et al. 2002; Gomez et al. 2004). Clearly, such surveillance databases need to be strengthened and augmented with more complete reporting of birthplace data and additional information on the immigration process (Singh and Hiatt 2006; Singh and Miller 2004). Large national surveillance systems such as the Behavioral Risk Factor Surveillance System and the Youth Risk Behavior Survey do not include nativity or place-of-birth information for respondents; the inclusion of the nativity/immigration variable in these datasets would greatly improve the capacity to analyze a wide range of health, quality-of-life, and behavioral data on immigrants at the national, state, and local levels (Chowdhury et al. 2010; Eaton et al. 2008). The California Health Interview Survey, the largest state health survey in the United States, is a good example of a state-based surveillance system that provides comprehensive health, health care, and behavioral data for a number of immigrant groups in California (UCLA 2012). Similar surveillance data systems can be developed in other US states (e.g., New York, Texas, New Jersey, Florida, and Illinois) that have a sizable and ethnically diverse immigrant population. Additionally, the data systems that link records from the major national population surveys with vital records and disease registries are particularly useful in this regard. Two national databases that use record linkages of population surveys with administrative sources such as the National Death Index (NDI) and the population-based cancer registries are the NLMS and NHIS-NDI record linkage studies, which allow for complex analyses of immigrant health and mortality patterns (Singh and Miller 2004; USCB 2007; NCHS 2011c; Ingram et al. 2008; Hummer et al. 1999b). With the continuation of long-term mortality follow-up, these longitudinal databases offer an exciting opportunity to analyze temporal changes in and determinants of immigrant health and mortality patterns.

REFERENCES

Ali JS, S McDermott, and RG Gravel. 2004. "Recent Research on Immigrant Health from Statistics Canada's Population Surveys." *Canadian Journal of Public Health* 95(3):I9–I13.

Arcia E, M Skinner, D Bailey, et al. 2011. "Models of Acculturation and Health Behaviors among Latino Immigrants to the US." *Social Science and Medicine* 53(1):41–43.

Bloom B, RA Cohen, and G Freeman. 2011. "Summary Health Statistics for U.S. Children: National Health Interview Survey, 2010." *Vital and Health Statistics* 10(250):1–82.

Blumberg SJ, EB Foster, AM Frasier, et al. 2012. "Design and Operation of the National Survey of Children's Health, 2007." *Vital and Health Statistics* 1(55):1–149.

Chen J, R Wilkins, and E Ng. 1996a. "Health Expectancy by Immigrant Status, 1986 and 1991." *Health Reports* 8(3):29–38.

Chen J, E Ng, and R Wilkins. 1996b. "The Health of Canada's Immigrants in 1994–95." *Health Reports* 7(4):33–45.

Chowdhury P, L Balluz, M Town, FM Chowdhury, W Bartoli, W Garvon, et al. 2010. "Surveillance of Certain Health Behaviors and Conditions among States and Selected Local Areas—Behavioral Risk Factor Surveillance System, United States, 2007." *Morbidity and Mortality Weekly Report* 59(SS-1):1–222.

Clegg LX, ME Reichman, BA Miller, BF Hankey, GK Singh, YD Lin, et al. 2009. "The Impact of Socioeconomic Status on Cancer Incidence and Stage at Diagnosis: Selected Findings from the Surveillance, Epidemiology, and End Results: National Longitudinal Mortality Study." *Cancer Causes and Control* 20(4):417–35.

Department of Health and Human Services (DHHS). 2000. *Tracking Healthy People 2010.* Washington, DC: US Government Printing Office.

Department of Health and Human Services (DHHS). 2006. *Healthy People 2010: Midcourse Review.* Washington, DC: US Government Printing Office.

Department of Health and Human Services (DHHS). 2012. *Healthy People 2020.* Available at http://www.healthypeople.gov/2020/default.aspx. Accessed May 30, 2012.

Du XL, CC Lin, NJ Johnson, and S Altekruse. 2011. "Effects of Individual-Level Socioeconomic Factors on Racial Disparities in Cancer Treatment and Survival: Findings from the National Longitudinal Mortality Study, 1979–2003." *Cancer* 117(14): 3242–51.

Dunn JR, and I Dyck. 2000. "Social Determinants of Health in Canada's Immigrant Population: Results from the National Population Health Survey." *Social Science and Medicine* 51(11):1573–93.

Eaton DK, L Kann, S Kinchen, S Shanklin, J Ross, J Hawkins, et al. 2008. "Youth Risk Behavior Surveillance—United States, 2007." *Morbidity and Mortality Weekly Report* 57(SS-4):1–131.

Federal Interagency Forum on Child and Family Statistics (FIFCFS). 2011. *America's Children: Key National Indicators of Well-Being, 2011.* Washington, DC: US Government Printing Office.

Gomez SL, SL Glaser, JL Kelsey, and MM Lee. 2004. "Bias in Completeness of Birthplace Data for Asian Groups in a Population-Based Cancer Registry (United States)." *Cancer Causes and Control* 15(3):243–53.

Grieco EM. 2010. *Race and Hispanic Origin of the Foreign-Born Population in the United States: 2007.* American Community Survey Briefs. Washington, DC: US Census Bureau.

Grieco EM, and EN Trevelyan. 2010. *Place of Birth of the Foreign-Born Population: 2009.* American Community Survey Briefs. Washington, DC: US Census Bureau.

Health Resources and Services Administration (HRSA), Maternal and Child Health Bureau. 2007. *The National Survey of Children with Special Health Care Needs Chartbook, 2005–2006.* Rockville, MD: US Department of Health and Human Services.

Health Resources and Services Administration (HRSA), Maternal and Child Health Bureau. 2009. *The National Survey of Children's Health 2007: The Health and Well-Being of Children, a Portrait of States and the Nation.* Rockville, MD: US Department of Health and Human Services.

Howlader N, AM Noone, M Krapcho, et al. 2011. *SEER Cancer Statistics Review, 1975–2008.* Bethesda, MD: National Cancer Institute. http://seer.cancer.gov/csr/1975_2008/.

Hoyert DL, GK Singh, and HM Rosenberg. 1995. "Sources of Data on Socioeconomic Differential Mortality in the United States." *Journal of Official Statistics* 11(3):233–60.

Hummer RA, M Biegler, PB De Turk, et al. 1999a. "Race/Ethnicity, Nativity and Infant Mortality in the United States." *Social Forces* 77(3):1083–1118.

Hummer RA, RG Rogers, CB Nam, et al. 1999b. "Race/Ethnicity, Nativity and US Adult Mortality." *Social Science Quarterly* 80(1):136–53.

Hyman I. 2004. "Setting the Stage: Reviewing Current Knowledge on the Health of Canadian Immigrants: What Is the Evidence and Where Are the Gaps?" *Canadian Journal of Public Health* 95(3):I4–I8.

Ingram DD, KA Lochner, and CS Cox. 2008. "Mortality Experience of the 1986–2000 National Health Interview Survey Linked Mortality Files Participants." *Vital and Health Statistics* 2(157):1–39.

Kitagawa EM, and PM Hauser. 1973. *Differential Mortality in the United States: A Study in Socioeconomic Epidemiology.* Cambridge, MA: Harvard University Press.

Larsen LJ. 2003. *The Foreign-Born Population in the United States: 2003.* Current Population Reports, P20–551. Washington, DC: US Census Bureau.

Lin SS, CA Clarke, CD O'Malley, and GM Le. 2002. "Studying Cancer Incidence and Outcomes in Immigrants: Methodological Concerns." *American Journal of Public Health* 92(11):1757–59.

Martin JA, BE Hamilton, PD Sutton, et al. 2011. "Births: Final Data for 2009." *National Vital Statistics Reports* 60(1):1–72.

Mathews TJ, and MF MacDorman. 2012. "Infant Mortality Statistics from the 2008 Period Linked Birth/Infant Death Data Set. *National Vital Statistics Reports* 60(5):1–49.

Minino AM, SL Murphy, JQ Xu, and KD Kochanek. 2011. "Deaths: Final Data for 2008." *National Vital Statistics Reports* 59(10):1–128.

National Center for Health Statistics (NCHS). 2009. *The National Survey of Children's Health (NSCH), 2007: The Public Use Data File and Documentation.* Hyattsville, MD: US Department of Health and Human Services. Available at http://www.cdc.gov/nchs/slaits/nsch.htm. Accessed February 27, 2012.

National Center for Health Statistics (NCHS). 2011a. *Health, United States, 2010 with Special Feature on Death and Dying.* Hyattsville, MD: US Department of Health and Human Services.

National Center for Health Statistics (NCHS). 2011b. *The National Health and Nutrition Examination Survey (NHANES), 1999–2010 Public Use Data Files.* Hyattsville, MD: US Department of Health and Human Services. http://www.cdc.gov/nchs/nhanes/nhanes_questionnaires.htm. Accessed May 29, 2012.

National Center for Health Statistics (NCHS). 2011c. *The National Health Interview Survey 1986–2004 Linked Mortality Files.* Hyattsville, MD: US Department of Health and Human Services. Available at http://www.cdc.gov/nchs/data_access/data_linkage/mortality/nhis_linkage.htm. Accessed May 30, 2012.

National Center for Health Statistics (NCHS). 2012a. *National Vital Statistics System, Mortality Multiple Cause-of-Death Public Use Data File Documentation.* Hyattsville, MD: US Department of Health and Human Services. Available at http://www.cdc.gov/nchs/nvss/mortality_public_use_data.htm. Accessed May 28, 2012.

National Center for Health Statistics (NCHS). 2012b. *National Vital Statistics System, 2009 Natality Public Use File and User Guide.* Hyattsville, MD: US Department of Health and Human Services. Available at ftp://ftp.cdc.gov/pub/Health_Statistics/NCHS/Dataset_Documentation/DVS/natality/UserGuide2009.pdf. Accessed May 30, 2012.

National Center for Health Statistics (NCHS). 2012c. *The National Survey of Children's Health with Special Health Care Needs, 2005–2006 and 2009–2010: The Public Use Data*

Files. Hyattsville, MD: US Department of Health and Human Services. Available at http://www.cdc.gov/nchs/slaits/cshcn.htm. Accessed May 29, 2012.

Perez, CE. 2002. "Health Status and Health Behavior among Immigrants." *Health Reports* 13 (Supplement): 1–12.

Rogot E, PD Sorlie, NJ Johnson, and C Schmitt. 1992. *A Mortality Study of 1.3 Million Persons by Demographic, Social, and Economic Factors, 1979–85 Follow-Up: U.S. National Longitudinal Mortality Study.* Washington, DC: Public Health Service. NIH publication 92–3297.

Schiller JS, JW Lucas, BW Ward, and JA Peregoy. 2012. "Summary Health Statistics for U.S. Adults: National Health Interview Survey, 2010." *Vital and Health Statistics* 10(252): 1–207.

Singh GK. 2000. "Socioeconomic and Behavioral Differences in Health, Morbidity, and Mortality in Kansas: Empirical Data, Models, and Analyses." In *The Society and Population Health Reader, Volume II: A State and Community Perspective,* edited by AR Alvin, R Tarlov, and RF St. Peter, 15–56. New York: The New Press.

Singh GK, and RA Hiatt. 2006. "Trends and Disparities in Socioeconomic and Behavioral Characteristics, Life Expectancy, and Cause-Specific Mortality of Native-born and Foreign-born Populations in the United States, 1979–2003." *International Journal of Epidemiology* 35(4):903–19.

Singh GK, MD Kogan, and DL Dee. 2007. "Nativity/Immigrant Status, Race/Ethnicity, and Socioeconomic Determinants of Breastfeeding Initiation and Duration in the United States, 2003." *Pediatrics* 119:S38–S46.

Singh GK, MD Kogan, and SM Yu. 2009. "Disparities in Obesity and Overweight Prevalence among US Immigrant Children and Adolescents by Generational Status." *Journal of Community Health* 34(4):271–81.

Singh GK, and BA Miller. 2004. "Health, Life Expectancy, and Mortality Patterns among Immigrant Populations in the United States." *Canadian Journal of Public Health* 95(3):I14–I21.

Singh GK, and M Siahpush. 2001. "All-Cause and Cause-Specific Mortality of Immigrants and Native Born in the United States." *American Journal of Public Health* 91(3):392–99.

Singh GK, and M Siahpush. 2002. "Ethnic-Immigrant Differentials in Health Behaviors, Morbidity, and Cause-Specific Mortality in the United States: An Analysis of Two National Data Bases." *Human Biology* 74(1):83–109.

Singh GK, M Siahpush, RA Hiatt, and LR Timsina. 2011. "Dramatic Increases in Obesity and Overweight Prevalence and Body Mass Index among Ethnic-Immigrant and Social Class Groups in the United States, 1976–2008." *Journal of Community Health* 36(1):94–110.

Singh GK, and SM Yu. 1996. "Adverse Pregnancy Outcomes: Differences between US- and Foreign-born Women in Major US Racial and Ethnic Groups." *American Journal of Public Health* 86(6):837–43.

Singh GK, SM Yu, M Siahpush, and MD Kogan. 2008. "High Levels of Physical Inactivity and Sedentary Behaviors among US Immigrant Children and Adolescents." *Archives of Pediatrics and Adolescent Medicine* 162(8):756–63.

Sorlie PD, E Backlund, and JB Keller. 1995. "US Mortality by Economic, Demographic, and Social Characteristics: The National Longitudinal Mortality Study." *American Journal of Public Health* 85(7):949–56.

Statistics Canada. 2012. *2006 Census: Immigration in Canada: A Portrait of the Foreign-Born Population, 2006*. Ottawa, Canada. http://www12.statcan.ca/census-recensement/2006 /as-sa/97–557/index-eng.cfm. Accessed May 30, 2012.

SUDAAN. 2009. *Software for the Statistical Analysis of Correlated Data, Release 10.0.1*. Research Triangle Park, NC: Research Triangle Institute.

UCLA Center for Health Policy Research. 2012. *California Health Interview Survey (CHIS)*. http://www.chis.ucla.edu/default.asp. Accessed May 28, 2012.

US Census Bureau (USCB). 2003. *2000 Census of Population and Housing, Summary File 3, Technical Documentation*. Washington, DC: US Department of Commerce.

US Census Bureau (USCB). 2007. *National Longitudinal Mortality Study, Reference Manual*. Washington, DC: US Census Bureau. http://www.census.gov/did/www/nlms /publications/reference.html

US Census Bureau (USCB). 2009. *A Compass for Understanding and Using American Community Survey Data: What Researchers Need to Know*. Washington, DC: US Government Printing Office.

US Census Bureau (USCB). 2011. *The 2010 American Community Survey*. Washington, DC: US Census Bureau. http://www.census.gov/acs/www/. Accessed May 28, 2012.

US Census Bureau (USCB). 2012. *American FactFinder*. Washington, DC: US Census Bureau. http://factfinder2.census.gov/faces/nav/jsf/pages/wc_acs.xhtml. Accessed May 28, 2012.

Walters LP, and EN Trevelyan. 2011. *The Newly Arrived Foreign-Born Population of the United States: 2010*. American Community Survey Briefs. Washington, DC: US Census Bureau.

Yu SM, and GK Singh. 2009. "Household Language Use and Health Care Access, Unmet Need, and Family Impact among CSHCN." *Pediatrics* 124(4):S414–19.

6

The Community-Based
Migrant Household Probability
Sample Survey

Enrico A. Marcelli

INTRODUCTION

For at least three reasons, international migrant health is perhaps the most difficult demographic phenomenon to study dispassionately and methodically. First, migrant health is relatively difficult to measure because, unlike fertility and mortality, it is not a tangible biological event (Carletto and de Brauw 2007; Davis 1974; Redstone and Massey 2004; Zlotnick 1987), and researchers employ numerous definitions of health (Cutler 2004; Pol and Thomas 2001; Young 2005). Second, even when probabilistic household sample survey data—the standard by which all social scientific findings are judged (Deaton 1997; Groves et al. 2004: 6)—include information regarding migration and health outcomes, they often fail to include variables on potentially important individual and sociogeographic sources of health such as premigration experience, current health behaviors, socioeconomic status (SES), home environment, neighborhood context, workplace or school environment, social networks, and civic engagement (Berkman and Kawachi 2000; Bilsborrow et al. 1997; Evans and Stoddart 1990; Link and Phelan 1995; Lorant et al. 2008; Marcelli et al. 2009b; Marcus 2009; McKenzie and Mistiaen 2007).[1] And third, it is not uncommon for researchers, politicians, and others to have strong negative or positive feelings about immigration that may influence their use or interpretation of available data (Best 2001; Handlin 2002 [1951]; Heer 1996; Huff 1993 [1953]; Huntington 2005 [2004]; Kuznets and Rubin 1954; Ramos 2010; Simon and Alexander 1993). In short, even if data include little sampling (e.g., nonprobabilistic subject selection) and nonsampling (e.g., interviewer, researcher) bias, they rarely permit a systematic investigation of factors influencing migrant health.

The main purpose of this chapter is to provide a practical guide for how community-based organizations (CBOs) and researchers can use an in-person area-based probability household sample survey to collect comprehensive, representative and up-to-date information about foreign-born residents of a host nation at various geographic scales (e.g., census block group, tract, zip code, county, region, state). Other nonprobabilistic data collection methods (e.g., censuses and registers, case studies, snowball samples, passenger lists) and general- and special-purpose random household surveys including relatively small numbers of migrants, focusing only on a subset of foreign-born residents, or employing telephone, mail, or Internet data collection modes have been used worldwide and are reviewed elsewhere (Beauchemin and González-Ferrer 2011; Bilsborrow et al. 1997; Carletto and de Brauw 2007; McKenzie and Mistiaen 2007; Thomas 1959; United Nations 2007). Here, I focus on what many scholars think is the gold standard for migrant research: the in-person area-based probabilistic household sample survey.

The first section of this chapter provides a brief history of the methodological limitations of collecting representative information in any nation until the mid-twentieth century. The second section reviews six recent general-purpose and special-purpose surveys (some discussed by other authors in this volume), arguing that there is a fundamental need for area-based probability migrant household sample surveys. And lastly, with reference to the 2007 Harvard-UMASS Boston Metropolitan Immigrant Health and Legal Status Survey (Holmes and Marcelli 2012; Marcelli et al. 2009a; Marcelli and Holmes 2012), the three phases of an in-person area-based probabilistic migrant household survey are discussed: (1) housing unit sample frame development and questionnaire design, (2) survey implementation, and (3) data cleaning and analysis. Important choices must be made within each phase; we will consider, for instance, how to select census blocks to be canvassed when developing a sample frame of housing units, why it is important to collaborate with a CBO, and how to "reduce" subject responses to digital format.

The chapter concludes with a discussion of several ongoing limitations of the area-based migrant household sample survey approach (e.g., locating hard-to-reach migrant populations efficiently) and suggests that future research would benefit from (1) collecting data from the same subjects over time, (2) collecting retrospective and current data on a subject's characteristics, behaviors and place of origin, (3) collecting biological health data, and (4) employing computer-assisted interviewer software in the subject's home.

THE HISTORIC MARCH TOWARD PROBABILISTIC HOUSEHOLD SAMPLE SURVEYING

The first known household surveys date back at least two millennia and were population counts undertaken for the purpose of raising taxes and revenues, apportioning political representation, or mustering soldiers from residents of particular geographic areas (Anderson 1988; Converse 1987; Wolfe 1932). During the eighteenth and nineteenth centuries (Hacking 2009 [1975]; Laplace 2007; Porter 1986), there were significant advances in probability theory and diffusion of statistical thinking, with subsequent efforts to describe statistically the effects of youth out-migration from rural US regions (Bowers 1974) and foreign-born in-migration to US metropolitan areas (Addams 1910; DuBois 1996 [1899]) using administrative records, expert informants, participant observation, and nonsampling interviewing. Probabilistic sampling was initially used in a 1912–1913 survey of four English towns (Bowley and Burnett-Hurst 1915). It was only after a 1930s study of unemployment by the Russell Sage Foundation, however, that random household sampling procedures became widely understood (Hogg 1930, 1932; Kruskall and Mosteller 1980; Neyman 1934; Seng 1951; Stephen 1948; Stouffer 1935). Counts of the number of foreign-born entrants into, residents of, and emigrants from the United States using nonsampling (e.g., census, steerage passenger shipping, population registry, border crossing, "social survey") methods predate the depression years (Bogardus 1928; Commons 1908; Edmonston and Michalowshi 2004; Ferrie 1999; Kuznets and Rubin 1954; Thomas 1959; Thomas and Znaniecki 1996 [1918–1920]). For example, the number of nonnaturalized foreign-born US residents was first counted as part of the fourth (1820) census, nativity (place-of-birth) data was first collected in the seventh (1850) census, and questions on parental nativity (ancestral place-of-birth) were included in the ninth (1870) through nineteenth (1970) censuses (Gauthier 2002; Gibson and Lennon 1999). Kuznets and Rubin (1954) provide a useful summary of efforts in the US, as does Thomas (1959) for all nations, to estimate net immigration leading up to the mid-twentieth century.[2] But it would take another four decades—as we shall see in the next two sections—before social demographers would begin collecting and making available individual-level health and other sensitive data from foreign-born US residents using household probability sampling techniques.

ONGOING NEED FOR IN-PERSON AREA-BASED PROBABILISTIC MIGRANT HOUSEHOLD SAMPLE SURVEY

General-Purpose Household Sample Surveys with Nativity Information: CPS and ACS

Unfortunately, although general-purpose area-based probabilistic household sample surveys such as the Current Population Survey (CPS) and the American Community Survey (ACS) provide some of the most important information regarding population characteristics at national and various subnational geographies (e.g., state, county, public use microdata area), they typically (1) suffer from a crude definition of international migrant (e.g., foreign-born, noncitizen) and view migration as an event rather than a process (Redstone and Massey 2004); (2) lack information concerning health outcomes, premigration experience, emigration, generation, and legal status that may influence health; and (3) mostly ignore health behaviors and various sociogeographic contexts that may influence health (Berkman and Kawachi 2000; Easterlin 1999; Evans and Stoddart 1990; Kawachi and Berkman 2003; Link and Phelan 1995). These limitations emanate from the fact that the main purpose of both surveys is to provide basic demographic and economic information about the entire US population rather than in-depth health information about foreign-born US residents, and that data on sensitive health and migration issues are difficult to obtain by telephone. The March CPS, for example, is a nationally representative voluntary household (telephone and in-person) survey that was first implemented in 1940 ($n \approx 65{,}000$ annually), and its main purpose is to enable researchers to study demographic and labor market characteristics of the entire US population regularly (US Census Bureau 2006). Although questions regarding access to health insurance, medical care, and various public assistance programs are asked, very few data are collected on health behaviors, health, or factors influencing these, and no information on nativity was collected until March 1994. Health-related variables are limited, for instance, to those for self-rated health and whether one retired or left a job due to an injury. Furthermore, given the survey in- and out-rotation of CPS respondents and the relatively small sample sizes for particular metropolitan areas, researchers interested in studying one the few health-related topics available by nativity need to concatenate several years of data. Marcelli and Heer (1998), for instance, applied migrant legal status predictors generated from their 1994 Los Angeles County Mexican Immigrant Legal Status Survey (LAC-MILSS) to foreign-born Mexican adults included in the combined 1994 and 1995 March CPS data to compare unauthorized Mexican migrant use of public assistance programs to that of other ethno-racial-nativity groups residing in Los Angeles County. Thus, while the general-purpose March CPS data may be used to study access to health insurance and medical care, as well as use of various "welfare" programs, by nativity, they feature few health behaviors or outcomes, rarely include information on emigration, do not have information about migrant legal status, and include very limited data on sociogeographic environments (e.g., home, neighborhood, work) that may influence health behaviors and outcomes.

A second prominent example of a general-purpose area-based probabilistic household sample survey with limitations similar to those of the CPS concerning health and migration—the ACS (Citro and Kalton 2007; Rampell 2012; US Census Bureau 2009)—collects data from about 3 million respondents annually (this is discussed further in chapter 5 of this volume, by Singh). Respondents are asked whether they were born in another country, and if they were, whether they are a US citizen, when (year) and how this occurred (born abroad to at least one US-citizen parent, or naturalized), and when they came live in the US. Although it is possible to separate foreign-born or US-citizen residents from others and to estimate how long they have resided in the US since coming to live, researchers cannot credibly separate migrants by legal status without using a probability sample survey-based imputation method similar to that developed by demographers in the 1990s and discussed below (Marcelli and Heer 1997), and it is questionable whether these data can provide useful estimates of the total amount of time migrants have spent in the US because questions regarding earlier visits and exits are not asked (Redstone and Massey 2004). Data concerning health behaviors and outcomes are also quite limited in the ACS. For instance, information collected includes whether an individual had health insurance, had a hearing problem, or was blind. For those who are at least five years old, questions are asked to assess whether they had difficulty concentrating, remembering, or making decisions due to a physical, mental, or emotional condition, as well as whether they had difficulty walking or climbing stairs, dressing or bathing, or doing errands alone such as shopping. And lastly, information on whether females between the ages of fifteen and fifty gave birth during the previous year is collected. Beyond these items, however, almost no other health-related data are collected. In other words, very little research on the health or health behaviors of international migrants residing in the US can be generated employing either of the two most prominent general-purpose area-based US household sample surveys available. Other national-level general-purpose surveys with similar or more restrictive health or nativity limitations include the General Social Survey (GSS) and the Panel Study of Income Dynamics (PSID).

Special-Purpose Household Health Surveys with Nativity Information: NHIS and NHANES

Whereas US general-purpose household surveys continue to offer relatively limited information on health behaviors and outcomes for either US or foreign-born subpopulations, special-purpose household health surveys have historically collected and continue to collect little on nativity. For example, the National Health Interview Survey (NHIS), which was launched in 1957, is an in-person annual state-stratified area-probability sample of about 100,000 individuals (90,000 adults and 10,000 children) residing in some 40,000 US households, and collects information on access to medical care, various health behaviors and outcomes from a subset of respondents (slightly more than 30,000 annually). However, NHIS did not begin collecting information on nativity until 1985, year of entry until 1989, and US citizenship until 1998 (Carter-Pokras and Zambrana 2001; Centers for Disease Control and Prevention 2012b). Specifically, for just a little more than two decades NHIS has enabled researchers to study various self-reported health outcomes at the national and state levels by basic nativity metrics.

However, as will be illustrated in the next section, applying demographic legal status predictors generated from area-based probabilistic migrant household sample survey data (e.g., age, sex, education, time residing in the US) to foreign-born residents enumerated in NHIS or other publicly available data provides a method for estimating the health of legal (e.g., US citizen, green-card holding, temporary visitor) and unauthorized (e.g., "undocumented," "illegal") migrants for some foreign-born subgroups separately (Marcelli 2007). NHIS is further discussed by Singh in chapter 5 of this volume.

Similarly, the National Health and Nutrition Examination Survey (NHANES) began in 1959 but did not start collecting ethnicity or nativity data until the early 1980s with the introduction of the Hispanic Health and Nutrition Examination Survey (HHANES). And it was not until NHANES III (1988–1994) that information regarding place of birth, US citizenship, and year of first US entry for Mexicans, the largest minority ethno-racial group in the US, first became available and researchers were able to distinguish these from all other Spanish-speaking subpopulations (Carter-Pokras and Zambrana 2001). The NHANES is designed to assess the nutrition and health of the US population, and although featuring a much smaller sample size ($n \approx 5{,}000$) than the NHIS, it includes both self-reported and biometric data (CDC 2012a). Singh discusses NHANES in chapter 5 of this volume. And, as was the case with the two general-purpose household surveys discussed above, there are other special-purpose household health surveys such as the Behavioral Risk Factor Surveillance System (BRFSS) that do not collect information which allows researchers to study the health of individuals by nativity, and those such as the California Health Interview Survey (CHIS) that only recently have begun collecting data allowing such analyses at particular subnational geographies (Brown et al. 2005).

Special-Purpose Household Surveys of Foreign-born US Residents: NIS and LACPS

Most special-purpose surveys of foreign-born US residents have focused on the behaviors and characteristics of a foreign-born subpopulation (e.g., legal permanent residents, foreign-born Mexicans) residing either in the entire US or in a particular location (e.g., Los Angeles County). The New Immigrant Survey (NIS), a prominent example of a representative prospective-retrospective household panel study of legal permanent residents (LPRs) residing in the US that is discussed by Jasso in chapter 12 of this volume, provides a public-use database on newly legalized US immigrants and their children that permits researchers to analyze factors influencing individual health and socioeconomic status. While cross-sectional data do not permit researchers to see relationships between potential (e.g., behavioral, familial, neighborhood, work- or school-related, social network) causal factors and individual outcomes due to an inability to control for unobserved intra-individual fixed characteristics (Menard 2002), panel data offer multiple observations on each immigrant in a sample through time and thus permit researchers to estimate causality (Hsiao 1999; Rindfuss et al. 2007). Jasso and colleagues (2004), for instance, employed the 1996 NIS pilot data and found that the increase in pre- to postmigration earnings (μ = \$21,000) had a large and statistically significant positive effect on self-reported health. The analytical advantages of panel data should not be ignored by migrant health researchers, but it is important to note that nonrandom attrition (e.g., subject refusing to participate in a subsequent wave of a survey) may diminish the attractiveness of panel data. Furthermore, even if panel data on migrant health exist, a focus on one particular segment of the foreign-born population (e.g., legal permanent residents) may miss what is most important for public policy purposes. For example, data from the US Census Bureau, the Department of Homeland Security, and the Pew Hispanic Center suggest that LPRs represent less than one-third (29%) of the approximately 40 million foreign-born residents of the US. Alternatively, naturalized US citizens represent about 40%, nonimmigrant visa holders ("temporary visitors") constitute some 5%, and about one-in-four are unauthorized migrant residents. Thus, while the NIS data offer valuable information regarding one major segment of the foreign-born US resident population, they do not provide any insight whatsoever regarding the health of most foreign-born residents.

Perhaps the first probabilistic (albeit not area-based) household sample survey in the US to obtain representative health and socioeconomic data from all foreign-born US residents of any country of birth and any legal status was the 1980–81 Los Angeles County Parents Survey (Heer 1990). The LACPS used Los Angeles County birth certificates to define its *universe* (Mexican-origin adults residing in Los Angeles County) and consisted of two *sample frames*—one including households with at least one parent who reported Mexican ethnicity and one foreign-born adult mother of a relatively healthy baby, and another including households with at least one parent who reported Mexican ethnicity and one US-born adult mother of a relatively healthy baby. A *systematic probabilistic household sample* is one in which the researcher randomly selects a first household and then skips a certain number of addresses in a frame before selecting another. Such a sample was initially drawn from each sample frame: 700 households from the first and 300 from the second. After confirming that each numeric address was associated with the reported street name using a Thomas Brothers Street Atlas for Los Angeles County, interviewers were instructed to approach each household for a possible interview no more than three times, and to vary these visits (i.e., weekday, weekday evening, weekend). Questionnaires were prepared not only for respondent mothers (n = 857) and fathers (n = 724), but also for unmarried brothers 18 to 44 years old (n = 194) and childless sisters age 18 to 29 years old (n = 131) residing in Los Angeles County. Due to cost constraints, interviewing of households with only US-born mothers was halted and interviewing of households with foreign-born Mexican mothers was slightly expanded toward the end of survey implementation. The weighted nonresponse rate was about 49% for the frame of foreign-born mothers and 53% for the frame of US-born mothers; and, importantly, although this early probabilistic migrant household sample survey was not an area-probability sample, the estimated number of legal and unauthorized Mexican migrants residing in Los Angeles County and their demographic profile were consistent with that extrapolated from the other leading legal status estimation methodology—the so-called residual method (Heer and Passel 1987). Yet this innovative systematic migrant household sample survey focused only on adult Mexican parents and siblings of circumscribed ages residing in one US county, and did not permit any subsequent interviewing of initial respondents because interviewers had to leave the address associated with a given questionnaire with the respondent upon interview completion. In other words, no identifying information was kept that would permit the household or respondent to be contacted again as in the NIS.

None of the above probabilistic household survey methodologies are adequate for studying the sources of health among all foreign-born US residents from even one sending nation (the "target population") because (1) they exclude important health (e.g., CPS, ACS) or nativity (NHIS, NHANES) questions, (2) the sample frames employed ignore certain segments of the target population (NIS, LACPS), or (3) they do not permit the collection of data on the same individuals over time or from a migrant's country or community of origin. Conversely, there are two main potential advantages of special-purpose area-probability migrant household sample surveys over those discussed directly above (Bilsborrow et al. 1997; Carletto and de Brauw 2007; DaVanzo et al. 1994; Edmonston 1996; Fowler 2002; Groves et al. 2004; McKenzie and Mistiaen 2007; United Nations 2007). First, similar to the NIS and LACPS, area-probability migrant household sample surveys permit researchers to collect more information than a census or general-purpose survey (e.g., biological, retrospective childhood and community-of-origin characteristics, emigration, census participation, health, legal status, social networks, neighborhood, workplace). And second, unlike clinical or laboratory data, which typically only offer information regarding proximate causes of health, household sample survey data can provide information about more distal or fundamental causes (Berkman and Kawachi 2000; Evans and Stoddart 1990; Link and Phelan 1995).

THE IN-PERSON AREA-BASED PROBABILISTIC MIGRANT HOUSEHOLD SAMPLE SURVEY METHODOLOGY

Collecting representative data that can be used to study individual and sociogeographic factors influencing migrant health (Cunningham et al. 2008; Dey and

Lucas 2006; Lorant et al. 2008; Singh and Siahpush 2001) requires demographers, survey statisticians, and other researchers to collaborate directly with a CBO that has good rapport among the foreign-born population of interest because some migrants (e.g., unauthorized residents) may be less willing to answer interviewers' questions in their homes or elsewhere (Marcelli et al. 2009a). Phase 1 includes creating a list of housing units in which migrants may reside and developing a questionnaire. The second phase involves selecting and training interviewers, establishing screening, consent and other survey protocols, and collecting data. In the final phase, researchers evaluate and prepare the data for analysis and decide how they will be studied using statistical software. The 2007 Boston Metropolitan Immigrant Health and Legal Status Survey (BM-IHLSS) provides a recent example of such a migrant household survey, and below we consider this to illustrate each of three phases and their constitutive components (Figure 6.1).

Phase 1: Creating a Sample Frame of Housing Units and Developing the Questionnaire(s)

Phase 1 has two distinct components on which researchers and their community partners should work simultaneously: (1) defining the sample frame of housing units and (2) developing the questionnaire.

Creating a Sample Frame of Housing Units.   After articulating reasons why available data do not permit one to understand the health of a migrant population of interest or its sources, researchers must ask what geographically circumscribed population ("universe") the data collected should represent. Figure 6.2 provides an example from the 2007 BM-IHLSS of two universes within metropolitan Boston: (1) four clusters of 100 randomly selected census blocks located in 10 census tracts with at least 7% of their respective populations having been born in Brazil, and (2) two clusters of 100 randomly selected census blocks with at least 25% of their populations having been born in the Dominican Republic.

If a representative picture of some population is desired, as is often the case, then there are three key steps that should be taken. First, it is necessary to build a sample "frame" of housing units within randomly selected subareas (e.g., census blocks) thought to include members of the migrant population of interest. However—because of new construction, demolition, or the conversion of unconventional spaces such as garages and porches into housing units since the last census—adequate housing unit lists may not be available and must be created. To take an example, the universe for the 2007 Brazilian BM-IHLSS was all foreign-born Brazilian adults and their children (regardless of nativity) residing in the Boston-Cambridge-Quincy Metropolitan Statistical Area (BCQ-MSA). In an effort to obtain a representative sample of this population in a relatively cost-effective manner, researchers developed a multistage area-probability sample frame by merging the 2000 tract-level Census

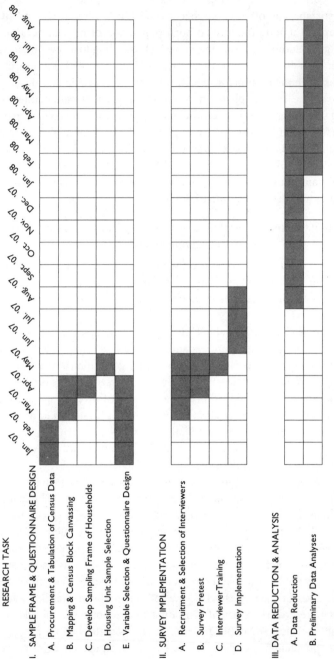

FIGURE 6.1. Example of an in-person area-based probabalistic migrant household sample survey design and implementation schedule. (2007 Boston Metropolitan Immigration Health and Legal Status Survey [BM-IHLSS].)

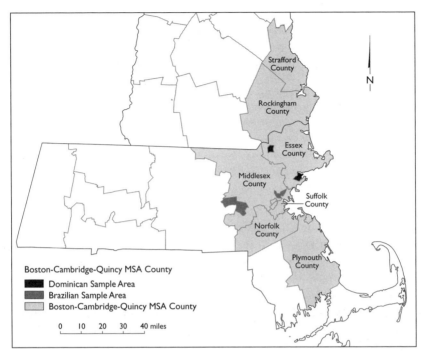

FIGURE 6.2. BM-IHLSS sample areas: 100 census blocks randomly selected from 10 tracts with at least 7% of their population born in Brazil, and 100 census blocks randomly selected from 10 tracts with at least 25% of their populations having been born in the Dominican Republic.

Summary File 3 (SF3) and block-level Summary File 1 (SF1) data[3] by tract, randomly selecting 100 (of 580) blocks within 10 (of 12) tracts in which at least 7% of population was born in Brazil, and listing every identifiable housing unit by walking through each block ("neighborhood"). This approach is "multistage" and "area-based" because it seeks to locate each migrant subject in his or her home, which is located in a census block, which in turn is part of a census tract within metropolitan Boston. And if housing units and individual subjects within them are also randomly selected, the sample will be probabilistic because the probability that an individual will be selected for a possible interview can be computed. This will be explained momentarily. But once the housing unit lists are completed, how do interviewers know which units to approach for possible interviews? Before determining the housing unit selection design, researchers must decide on the desired sample size. Although the details of how to compute a sample size that is adequate for describing a population are beyond the scope of this chapter, a general principle of random survey methodology is that only a small fraction of a migrant population is needed to approximate the mean and standard deviation of a variable of interest (e.g., income, sex ratio) fairly well regardless of how large the population is. Also, as shown below, larger sample sizes and variables with proportions of a sample with some characteristic closer to 50% will yield smaller estimated ranges within which a "true" population mean falls (Fowler 2002).

SAMPLE SIZE	ERROR (+/-): 50/50 RATIO	ERROR (+/-): 5/95 RATIO
100	10%	4%
300	6%	3%
500	4%	2%
1,500	2%	1%

For example, if about half a migrant population is female, and a random sample of 300 subjects generates an estimate of 46%, then one could say with 95% confidence that between 40% and 52% of the population is female. Alternatively, if the sample size were 500 rather than 300 and the same estimate were generated (46%), then one could assume a narrower range within which the true proportion rests with 95% confidence—between 42% and 50% of the population is female. To take another example, if a sample of 100 US adults suggests that about five percent are gay, then one would be 95% confident that the actual range is between 4% and 6%. If the sample size were 1,500 instead, then one could be 95% confident that the estimated range within which the real proportion rests is between 4% and 6%. Larger sample size translates into a tighter estimated range. Because we wished to minimize estimation error due to sampling for all BM-IHLSS variables within budget constraints, it was decided that a sample size of 300 adult Brazilian migrants would suffice. The estimated value of any variable could be expected to have a margin of error of +/-3% (best case) to +/-6% (worse case).

A third step involves sampling design. Rather than a simple random sample, we decided to employ a "systematic" sampling approach that randomly selected a starting housing unit within each block and then had interviewers knock on the door of every other housing unit. This was done because (1) there were 8,247 housing units listed by BM-IHLSS canvassers in the 100 blocks, (2) the mean proportion of foreign-born Brazilian residents in selected tracts was 11.5%, (3) we knew from previous in-person area-based representative migrant household sample surveys of legal and unauthorized migrant residents in Los Angeles County (Marcelli 2004; Marcelli and Heer 1997) that approximately one in four or five eligible housing units contacted completed a questionnaire,[4] and (4) it is almost always possible to design systematic samples that will produce results similar to those of a simple random sample (Fowler 2002). The decision to first knock on every other door was straightforward. If we approached at least 50% of all housing units listed (4,363 of 8,247),

12% of these had at least one foreign-born Brazilian adult resident, and, if we worked hard to ensure that at least 50% (rather than 25%) of eligible households completed a questionnaire, then our sample size would come close to our desired sample size of 300 (4,363 x 0.12 x 0.50 = 262). In the end, we were fortunate that 307 households had a foreign-born Brazilian who agreed to complete a questionnaire. Since 2011—four years following the completion of the BM-IHLSS—it has become possible to select blocks to create a migrant housing unit sample frame for any county, metropolitan area, or state by (1) randomly selecting tracts with particular characteristics (e.g., percent foreign-born Mexican) from five-year (e.g., 2006–2010) ACS data,[5] (2) merging these tracts with census blocks available from the US Census Bureau's Summary File 1 (SF1) data[6] using geographic-matching file software,[7] and (3) randomly selecting blocks within selected tracts. It is important to highlight, however, that because it is not possible to determine the extent to which migrants residing in tracts with relatively small proportions of compatriots (e.g., less than 10%) are different from those residing in the entire sample frame, estimated characteristics from a sample using this method may not reflect those of the entire migrant population (the universe). Fortunately, this was not a problem in the BM-IHLSS or earlier Mexican migrants surveys in Los Angeles County employing this methodology—that is, the systematic area-probability household sample survey data generated estimated counts and characteristics that are supported by other researchers' estimates (Heer and Passel 1987; Marcelli and Heer 1997; Marcelli et al. 2009a, 2009b; Marcelli and Lowell 2005). Figure 6.3 is an example of a block-level map in which canvassers identified housing units on a small street not listed by the US Census Bureau, suggesting that a benefit of the community-based migrant household probability sample survey methodology being described here is that it may offer an estimate of the target migrant population that differs from official statistics. Figure 6.4 shows a typical canvassing form that may be used to list housing units.

It should be noted that the sampling procedure described above may be prohibitively expensive for foreign-born populations that are not somewhat concentrated geographically. Two common methods for increasing sample size and reducing survey costs that have been discussed elsewhere but can only be mentioned in passing here are geographic stratification and disproportionate sampling (Bilsborrow et al. 1997; Carletto and de Brauw 2007). An example of "stratification" associated with the BM-IHLSS example discussed above would be to first separate census tracts into three groups ("strata") according to the percent foreign-born Brazilian residents (e.g., 25%, 10–25%, 10%), and then draw a systematic sample of housing units from canvassed blocks within each stratum in equal proportion to the percent foreign-born Brazilian. Alternatively, if a larger sample size is desired within budget constraints and there is no need to compare migrants across strata, then increasing the proportions of units approached in the two more highly concentrated strata ("disproportionate sampling") might work.

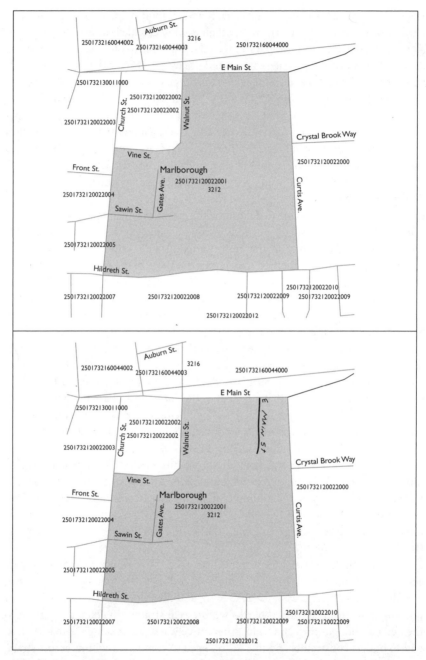

FIGURE 6.3. Example of a census block map that canvassers found was missing a small street (examine top right-hand corner of both maps).

TRACT	BLOCKGROUP	BLOCKı

STREET NAME	STREET NO.	APARTMENT NO.	COUNT	
Vine St.	11	1	1	
	17	1	②	
	23	1	3	
	31	1	④	
Walnut St.	36	1	5	
	32	1	⑥	
	28A	1	7	
	26A	1	⑧	
	26	1	9	
	22	1	⑩	
	12	1	11	
E. Main St.	183	1	⑫	
	191	1	13	
	193	1	⑭	
		60	15	
		61	⑯	
		62	17	
		63	⑱	
		64	19	
		65		
		66	⑳	11
		67	21	
		68	㉒	
		69	23	
		70	㉔	
		71	25	
		72	㉖	
		73	27	
		74	㉘	
		75	29	
		76	㉚	
		77	31	
		78	㉜	16
		79	33	
		80	㉞	17
		81	35	
		82	㊱	
		83	37	
		84	㊳	19
		85	39	
		86	㊵	20
		87	41	
		88	㊷	21
	211	1	43	
		2	㊹	22
	208	1	45	
		3	㊻	
	207	1	47	

FIGURE 6.4. Example of a canvassers' census block housing unit list (including units on segment of E. Main St. not shown in original census map in figure 6.2), and units that were systematically selected for possible interviews.

Developing the Questionnaire(s). While researchers should have the technical capacity to make the decisions discussed above, collaborating directly with a reputable CBO working with a targeted foreign-born population is necessary for designing a questionnaire that will permit interviewers to collect useful health, demographic, and socioeconomic information. Collaboration should ideally begin months or years before survey implementation, with researchers and community leaders discussing what topics are of most concern to migrants, CBOs, and policy makers. The 2007 BM-IHLSS, for instance, officially began in January 2007,[8] but researchers and community leaders of the Brazilian and Dominican migrant communities had been working together to find funding to study health among this population since 2005. Early and frequent contact between researchers and community leaders is essential because the former are more likely to know how standard demographic, health, and other questions are asked in national surveys as well as standard surveying protocols, and the latter are more likely to know about pressing issues migrants are facing that are not covered in conventional surveys. For instance, in addition to questions concerning what topics should be covered in a questionnaire, a household and subject screening protocol should be discussed and developed (the first component of a survey instrument). This is the purview of survey methodologists, and typically it is good to have interviewers approach an address up to three times and record one of several outcomes for each visit (no one home, no adult home, no adult migrant resident, interview rescheduled, refused, interview completed, cannot find address, vacant building, could not enter). The first part of the questionnaire (the second instrument component) is a household roster, which is used to collect basic demographic information for each household member (e.g., age, sex, place of birth) and to randomly select a foreign-born adult (e.g., Brazilian adult who last had a birthday, youngest Brazilian adult). Sometimes it is used to select other household members, such as a child. The second part of the questionnaire often focuses on the selected adult subject. The BM-IHLSS, for example, separated questions for adults into five sections (i.e., Migration, Socioeconomic Status, Social Capital, Health, Sociopolitical Identity). A final part of the questionnaire will sometimes focus on a randomly selected child, and regardless of the part or section in which a particular question appears, attention to reliability (ensuring that differences in respondents' answers to the same questions reflect actual differences) and validity (accuracy of responses) is important. One way of increasing the likelihood of high reliability and validity, as well as being able to compare estimated population size and characteristics, is to use questions that have been tested and employed in national surveys such as the ACS and NHIS. Comparing the estimated foreign-born population residing in the BCQ-MSA from BM-IHLSS data with that of 2007 ACS data was possible, for instance, because the BM-IHLSS asked questions regarding place of birth, age, sex, year of first entry into the US, US citizenship, educational attainment, labor force participation, and others in similar—and in some cases exact—ways as the ACS. Ultimately, deciding how many questions, question wording and placement, and who will translate questions needs to be done by both researchers and community leaders (Brown et al. 2005; Marcelli et al. 2009a; Wallerstein and Duran 2003).

Phase 2: Survey Implementation

I have briefly addressed methods for trying to limit sampling error and one component of nonsampling error (the questionnaire). But much nonsampling error also, and often, emanates from survey implementation. Survey implementation may be designed in many different ways, and is usefully separated into four tasks: interviewer selection and training, and survey pretesting and fieldwork. Interviewers are mainly hired to inform potential subjects, and gain their trust and cooperation if they are eligible to participate in the survey. Ideally, interviewers should (1) be mature and able to communicate well verbally and in writing, (2) understand that interviewing is a part-time job often for college students that is best suited for those who are more interested in acquiring research experience than in making money, (3) be flexible in terms of availability to work, and (4) be physically mobile (Fowler 2002). Past migrant household survey research also suggests that women who are fluent in the migrant population's language and were born in the same country of origin are more successful interviewers. But regardless of interviewer characteristics, if not trained well (e.g., questionnaire content, how to approach housing units, how to motivate subject participation, procedures for collecting biological data), interviewers will not likely succeed in collecting useful data. BM-IHLSS investigators and several of their assistants, for instance, interviewed over fifty foreign-born Brazilian college students and various older members of the Brazilian population residing in the BCQ-MSA, selecting twenty-four to form twelve interviewer teams and three to be field supervisors. Interviewers and supervisors were taught how to find neighborhoods and approach housing units, how to motivate participation, how to ask questions on the questionnaire and record responses, and how to measure height and weight as well as blood pressure. They were also taught how to collect saliva and blood samples. All of these protocols were taught by a research team consisting of an applied demographer/economist, an anthropologist, the director of a CBO working with Brazilians, and a neuroscientist. Interviewers were also required to complete an online course on research involving human subjects and were taught how to deliver self-reported and biometric data safely and securely to field supervisors for storage. Also, interviewers were required to do all fieldwork with their assigned partner and never after dusk, and each interviewer had to wear a picture identification badge that listed the participating CBO and universities. These procedures have contributed to representative and sensitive data being successfully collected three times from both legal and unauthorized Mexican migrants in Los Angeles County (1994, 2001, and 2012), and from legal and unauthorized migrants from Brazil and the Dominican Republic who resided in metropolitan Boston in 2007. Furthermore, the 2007 BM-IHLSS was the first in-person area-based probability household sample survey to collect biological data from a representative sample of legal and unauthorized migrants hailing from any nation. This is unsurprising given that only recently has it become possible for nonmedically trained interviewers to collect such data in household surveys (Christensen 2000; Crimmins et al. 2007, 2005; Holmes and Marcelli 2012; McDade 2007; McDade et al. 2007).

Between June 10 and September 17, 2007, the Harvard-UMASS BM-IHLSS collected self-reported data from 307 foreign-born Brazilian adult subjects, biological data from about two-thirds of these, and demographic and health information concerning 120 children born in Brazil and (mostly) the US. No subjects were compensated in any way; the average amount of time they spent completing a questionnaire and/or providing biological data was two hours, and the mean cost per completed questionnaire was $250. Additional funding was eventually secured to assay and analyze the data.[9]

The BM-IHLSS response rate of 44% was not dissimilar to the rates of other surveys, such as the ACS and LACPS, that attempt to collect data from various vulnerable populations (Diffendal 2001; Heer 1990), and the estimated number of foreign-born Brazilian adults and children (weighted by the inverse of the probability of having been selected in BM-IHLSS tracts, blocks, and housing units) was 64,000 (about 29% higher than the 2007 ACS estimate for the BCQ-MSA).[10]

Phase 3: Data Reduction and Analysis

The third and final phase of a household survey project involves "reducing" (digitizing and cleaning) and analyzing the data. Responses to the BM-IHLSS questions were written directly on the printed questionnaires and then had to be typed manually into several tabs of a spreadsheet before being converted into a format that could be analyzed using statistical software. It is best if data are entered as soon as questionnaires are returned from the field so that data entry personnel can check with interviewers when and if any uncertainties regarding responses emerge. It is also important to have written the computer code that will be used to check responses for valid response values (including those that should not have been answered due to predetermined skip patterns on the questionnaire), and to replace those that are invalid. BM-IHLSS staff used Stat/Transfer to convert Excel spreadsheet tabs into STATA-formatted files, and wrote STATA code to check responses to every question on the BM-IHLSS questionnaire. Before discussing four ways in which migrant household surveys could be improved in future research, I present results from an estimation of how BM-IHLSS interviewer characteristics and behaviors may have influenced whether foreign-born adult subjects from Brazil (1) answered a question about how many sex partners they had had in the previous year, (2) permitted interviewers to measure height, weight and blood pressure, (3) provided a saliva sample, and (4) allowed interviewers to collect blood droplets.

Figure 6.5 shows one surprising and one unsurprising result. Unsurprisingly, a larger proportion of an estimated 61,000 foreign-born Brazilian adults residing in metropolitan Boston (according to the weighted 2007 BM-IHLSS data[11]) were

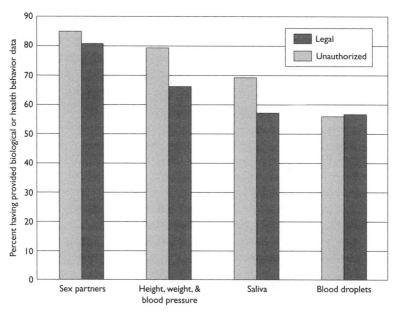

FIGURE 6.5. Percent foreign-born adult Brazilian migrants that responded to a sexual behavior question and provided various biological data by legal status, 2007 BM-IHLSS.

more likely to have responded to the question, "How many sexual partners (those with whom you have had vaginal, oral, or anal sex) have you had in the last 12 months?" (84%) than to have stepped on a scale, permitted interviewers to use a height rod to measure their height, or allowed them to take their resting blood pressure three times with a wrist monitor (75%); to have provided saliva on a swab of cotton (66%); or to have let interviewers use a finger prick technique to obtain blood droplets (56%). Surprisingly, however, unauthorized migrants were more likely than their legal compatriots to provide data for three of the four. In general, potential explanations (hypotheses) for subject item nonresponse can be usefully separated into seven categories: (1) questionnaire design, (2) data collection mode, (3) interviewer characteristics and behaviors, (4) subject characteristics, (5) home environment, (6) neighborhood, and (7) social capital (Groves 1987; Groves et al. 2004; Tourangeau and Smith 1996). We employed the Brazilian BM-IHLSS data to test the "deference" and "experience" hypotheses using several variables found within the third category. The first hypothesis suggests that subjects are more willing to provide biological and other sensitive health data if an interviewer is, or is perceived to be, of a higher socioeconomic status (e.g., college degree, lighter skin pigmentation). The second suggests that subjects are more willing to provide

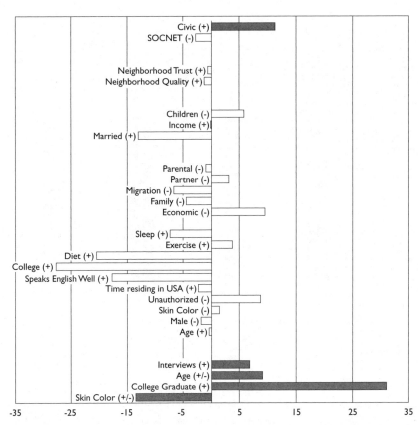

FIGURE 6.6. Percentage change in probability that a foreign-born Brazilian adult provided a saliva sample in the 2007 BM-IHLSS.

biological and other sensitive health data if the interviewer is, or is perceived to be, more experienced or mature (e.g., completed more interviews, older). We controlled for other factors typically placed within all except the first and second explanatory categories listed above because the same questionnaire and data collection mode (in-person within a subject's home) were used for all BM-IHLSS interviews. Figure 6.6 reports results from logistically regressing whether an adult Brazilian respondent provided a saliva sample (one of the four outcomes shown in Figure 6.5) on various factors separated in the five relevant explanatory categories listed above (3–5).

While all variables listed on the vertical axis were included in the analysis, there are two take-home points: (1) only variables associated with the shaded bars are estimated to have been statistically related (at a 90% confidence level or above) to

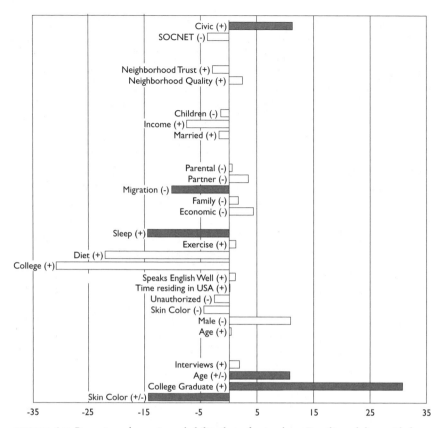

FIGURE 6.7. Percentage change in probability that a foreign-born Brazilian adult provided blood droplets in the 2007 BM-IHLSS.

a Brazilian subject having agreed to provide a saliva swab, and (2) while these results support both the subject deference and interviewer experience hypothesis, the former has more support than the latter. Specifically, a Brazilian subject was about 30% more likely to provide a saliva sample to an interviewer who had graduated from college, and about 13% more likely to provide a saliva sample to someone who had slighter lighter skin pigmentation—supporting the deference hypothesis. Also, a subject was approximately 10% more likely to do so if the interviewer was about ten years older, and about 7% more likely if the interviewer had completed about ten more interviews before attempting the current one—lending some (but less) support to the interviewer experience hypothesis.

Although there is insufficient space here to report regression results regarding how these factors may have influenced subject willingness to provide answers to the sexual partner question or the request for height, weight, and blood pressure data, results are consistent with those just reported for saliva, and available upon request from the author (Marcelli 2008). Figure 6.7 shows almost identical results for what appears to have been the datum Brazilian migrants were least likely to provide. That is, the probability of a subject having provided blood droplets was, except for prior number of interviews completed by an interviewer, estimated to be statistically associated with the remaining three variables representing the subject deference and interviewer experience hypotheses (i.e., age, education, skin color). Interviewer characteristics and experience are both important for the likelihood that migrant subjects will provide biological data and answer sensitive questions, but characteristics seem to be more important than experience. These results suggest it is possible, as demographers and survey researchers have recently learned, to collect biological data in random household sample surveys from a relatively vulnerable migrant population such as Brazilian migrants, among whom fully 70% were unauthorized US residents (Marcelli et al. 2009a). These results also suggest that having interviewers with higher socioeconomic status characteristics is more important than having interviewers with interviewing experience. These results are consistent with past household survey projects that demonstrated the value of hiring mature adult female interviewers who were born in the same country as the target population. In short, the demographic profile of interviewers appears to be more important than interviewing experience for collecting sensitive biological and other health data from legal and unauthorized foreign-born residents of the US.

DISCUSSION

This chapter began by asserting that even when data include little sampling (e.g., nonprobabilistic subject selection) bias, they rarely permit a systematic investigation of factors influencing international migrant health. This is because migration is difficult to measure even if clearly defined, available health data seldom include information regarding various sociogeographic domains of life that may influence health, and researchers and others interested in migrants often have strong feelings about them and their effects on society that may affect the data they employ or how these are interpreted. It is precisely these potential biases that an in-person area-based probability migrant household sample survey methodology has the potential to overcome, and this chapter has offered a practical guide for how CBOs and researchers can use such an approach to collect comprehensive, representative, and up-to-date information about the health of legal and unauthorized foreign-born residents of a host nation at various geographic scales (e.g., census block group, tract, zip code, county, region, state). Indeed, since the mid-1990s demographers have been (1) developing adequate area-based sample frames and household- and individual-level questionnaires, (2) successfully training interviewers without medical backgrounds to collect health, legal status, and other sensitive data from migrants, and (3) using survey data to estimate the number and characteristics of foreign-born residents of the US. But as this chapter illustrates, this type of survey is a costly endeavor and requires researchers to work directly with migrants from the target population and to partner with a reputable CBO.

Benefits of an area-probability migrant household sample survey include the acquisition of information that can help answer pressing questions regarding migrant health and its sources, as well as data that permit estimates of the number and characteristics of migrants that may differ from official government statistics. It is also the case that researchers can generate legal status prediction equations that may be applied to various public-use data (e.g., ACS, NHIS) to estimate international migrant health and socioeconomic status. For example, applying (1) age, (2) sex, (3) educational attainment, and (4) time residing in the US coefficients (generated by logistically regressing unauthorized legal status on these four variables using the 2001 Los Angeles County Mexican Immigrant Legal Status Survey) to 1998–2005 NHIS data for foreign-born Mexican migrants, for instance, suggests foreign-born Mexican adults were healthier on seven of fifteen available health outcomes (Marcelli 2007). Specifically, they were less healthy than most other ethnoracial-nativity groups when self-rated health, psychological distress, obesity, diabetes, kidney problems, tuberculosis, or activities of daily living were analyzed. And they were similarly healthy when hypertension was the focal outcome. But they were healthier on seven outcomes (cardiovascular disease, cancer, respiratory disease, liver condition, hepatitis, joint and other pain, annual bed days). Only on psychological distress were unauthorized Mexican migrants estimated to be less healthy than their legal compatriots. These and other results are available upon request from the author.

Yet there are some limitations to the survey methodology presented in this chapter, and at least four ways in which future surveying of migrants using area-probability household sample surveys might be improved. The most glaring potential limitation is that such an approach may not succeed among non-Latino migrant populations. How would foreign-born Chinese or recent Iraqi refugees respond to their compatriots showing up at their doorstep asking for sensitive health and other information? Another potential limitation is logistic. When migrants are not highly concentrated, it is more costly to find them. Thus, as noted in a previous section, if some migrants residing in suburban or rural areas with relatively low proportions of migrants are missed, the portrait of the target population may be distorted. Of course, this is likely to be the case, regardless of urban, suburban, or rural location, for foreign-born groups with small numbers.

Still, there are a number of promising paths forward. First, in addition to collecting data concerning current individual and sociogeographic factors that may influence current health, future surveys should make an effort to collect migrant subject contact information in order to reach them later to create panel datasets such as the NIS (but including migrants with both legal and unauthorized statuses) (Rindfuss et al. 2007). Second, researchers should attempt to collect information regarding subjects' family members, friends, neighbors, and social network members residing in the country of origin. A personal relationship with someone residing back home may have more influence on a migrant's health and well-being than is commonly suspected. Such information might be quite useful, for instance, in helping to explain the disparities reported above in psychological distress by legal status. And it is important to note that if the goal is to understand how such country-of-origin factors influence health among foreign-born residents of the US, then the best approach is to begin by randomly sampling migrants in the US and then collecting data in the migrant home country rather than the other way around (Beauchemin and González-Ferrer 2011; Bilsborrow et al. 1997). Third, because foreign-born residents of a host nation tend to be younger and therefore healthier, on average, it is more difficult to estimate their long-term health trajectories compared to those of native-born residents, and would it be useful to collect biological data such as saliva, blood, hair, height, weight, and blood pressure in addition to health behavior data. Indeed, evidence presented in this chapter and elsewhere suggests this is possible even among the most vulnerable migrants (Christensen 2000; Crimmins et al. 2005; Hayes-Bautista 2002; Holmes and Marcelli 2012; Marcelli and Holmes 2012). Lastly, to date interviewers using the methodology outlined here have simply recorded subject responses on a printed questionnaire and these, as well as results from assayed biological data, have been converted into digital format manually. There are considerable efficiency gains to be had from using computer-assisted personal interviewing (CAPI) software in the field, but this will need to be tested and evaluated along with how subjects of a vulnerable target population might respond to use of this technology in the context of sensitive questions.

NOTES

1. "Probabilistic" implies that each individual of a target population has a known positive probability of being included in a sample, and "household" refers to the level at which information is collected regardless of data collection mode (e.g., in-person face-to-face, telephone, mail, Internet).

2. Thomas (1959) identifies four historic phases of collecting data on worldwide international migration: (1) when newly formed nations did not systematically restrict migration (1800–1875), (2) when national regulation was initiated in Europe and the US in the late nineteenth century, (3) when nations established mechanisms for differentiating migrants from certain nations and with specific characteristics (early twentieth century), and (4) when the International Labor Organization (ILO) and Population Commission of the

United Nations (UN) summarized the different ways in which nations were attempting to measure international migration (mid-twentieth century).

3. http://www.census.gov/main/www/cen2000.html.

4. It is more complicated to compute conventional response rates than to compute questionnaire completion rates, as will be explained below. But in general, doing so requires one to know the probability of block selection, probability of housing unit selection, and the probability of household member selection once an eligible unit has been identified.

5. http://www.census.gov/acs/www/data_documentation/pums_data/.

6. http://2010.census.gov/2010census/data/.

7. http://mcdc.missouri.edu/websas/geocorr12.html.

8. In response to a call for proposal by the Dana Farber-Harvard Cancer Center/University of Massachusetts Boston Comprehensive Cancer Partnership Program (NCI Grant #5U56CA118635–03).

9. In addition to funding received from the National Cancer Institute (NCI), I am thankful for additional support from the University of Massachusetts Boston's Office of the Vice Provost for Research and the Blue Cross Blue Shield of Massachusetts Foundation.

10. The response rate (44%) was computed by first computing the percent of housing units for which interviewer teams could determine whether at least one foreign-born Brazilian adult was residing there (3,621/4,090), and then multiplying this by the percent of housing units with at least one foreign-born Brazilian adult resident providing a completed questionnaire (307/620). The first rate was quite high, the second not as high as desired.

11. Sample weights are computed for the purpose of estimating the number and characteristics of a target migrant population (universe). In general, this equals one divided by the probability of having been selected into the sample, and the first step is to compute the probability that a census block was selected (e.g., 100 blocks divided by 12,476 in the 10 BM-IHLSS census tracts with 7% or more of their populations having been born in Brazil). The second step is to compute the probability of a housing unit being selected into the sample by multiplying this block selection probability by the probability of a housing unit being selected within a block (e.g., 50% if the within-block skip pattern is every other housing unit). A "household-level" weight is then computed by dividing the inverse of the probability of a housing unit having been selected by the block response rate. The block response rate equals the percent eligible housing units (eligible housing units/housing units with at least one eligible resident) multiplied by the percent eligible housing units interviewed (housing units that were successfully interviewed/housing units with at least one foreign-born Brazilian adult). This household-level weight is not, however, corrected for biases that may exist at the block or housing unit level. Computing person-level sample weights requires correcting for these, and doing so for the block level involves multiplying the household-level weight by the inverse of the number of people interviewed in a block/total block population. Correcting for housing-unit-level bias involves multiplying the household-level weight that has been corrected for block-level bias by the inverse of the number of individual-level questionnaires completed in a housing unit/total number of household residents. Population size is then computed by multiplying each subject by his or her person-level weight. The mean person-level weight for the 2007 Brazilian BM-IHLSS was about 200, implying that each subject represented about 200 other foreign-born adult Brazilians residing in metropolitan Boston. These weights ranged from 42 to 668, however.

REFERENCES

Addams, Jane. 1910. *Twenty Years at Hull-House.* New York: Macmillan.

Anderson, Margo J. 1988. *The American Census: A Social History.* New Haven, CT: Yale University Press.

Beauchemin, Cris, and Amparo González-Ferrer. 2011. "Sampling International Migrants with Origin-Based Snowballing Method: New Evidence on Biases and Limitations." *Demographic Research* 25:101–34.

Berkman, Lisa F., and Ichiro Kawachi. 2000. *Social Epidemiology.* New York: Oxford University Press.

Best, Joel. 2001. *Damned Lies and Statistics: Untangling Numbers from the Media, Politicians and Activists.* Berkeley and Los Angeles: University of California Press.

Bilsborrow, R. E., Graeme Hugo, A. S. Oberai, and Hania Zlotnik. 1997. *International Migration Statistics: Guidelines for Improving Data Collection Systems.* Geneva: International Labour Office.

Bogardus, Emory S. 1928. *Immigration and Race Attitudes.* Boston: D. C. Heath.

Bowers, William L. 1974. *The Country Life Movement in America: 1900–1920.* Port Washington, NY: Kennikat Press.

Bowley, A. L., and A. R. Burnett-Hurst. 1915. *Livelihood and Poverty: A Study in the Economic Conditions of Working-Class Households in Northampton, Warrington, Stanley, and Reading.* London: G. Bell and Sons.

Brown, E. Richard, Sue Holtby, Elaine Zahnd, and George B. Abbott. 2005. "Community-based Participatory Research in the California Health Interview Survey." *Preventing Chronic Disease: Public Health Research, Practice, and Policy* 2:1–8.

Carletto, Gero, and Alan de Brauw. 2007. "Measuring Migration Using Household Surveys." The World Bank, Washington, DC.

Carter-Pokras, Olivia, and Ruth Enid Zambrana. 2001. "Latino Health Status." Pp. 23–54 in *Health Issues in the Latino Community,* edited by M. Aguirre-Molina, C. W. Molina, and R. E. Zambrana. San Francisco: Jossey-Boss.

Centers for Disease Control and Prevention. 2012a. "National Health and Nutrition Examination Survey (NHANES)." http://www.cdc.gov/nchs/nhanes.htm/.

———. 2012b. "National Health Interview Survey (NHIS)." http://www.cdc.gov/nchs nhis .htm.

Christensen, Kaare. 2000. "Biological Material in Household Surveys: The Interface between Epidemiology and Genetics." Pp. 43–63 in *Cells and Surveys: Should Biological Measures Be Included in Social Science Research,* edited by C. E. Finch, J. W. Vaupel, and K. Kinsella. Washington, DC: National Academies Press.

Citro, Constance F., and Graham Kalton. 2007. *Using the American Community Survey: Benefits and Challenges.* Washington, DC: National Academies Press.

Commons, John R. 1908. *Races and Immigrants in America.* London: Macmillan.

Converse, Jean M. 1987. *Survey Research in the United States: Roots and Emergence, 1890–1960.* Berkeley and Los Angeles: University of California Press.

Crimmins, Eileen M., Jung Ki Kim, Dawn E. Alley, Arun Karlamangla, and Teresa Seeman. 2007. "Hispanic Paradox in Biological Risk Profiles." *American Journal of Public Health* 97:1305–10.

Crimmins, Eileen M., Beth J. Soldo, Jung Ki Kim, and Dawn E. Alley. 2005. "Using Anthropometric Indicators for Mexicans in the United States and Mexico to Understand the Selection of Migrants and the 'Hispanic Paradox.'" *Social Biology* 52:164–77.

Cunningham, Solveig Argeseanu, Julia D. Ruben, and K. M. Venkat Narayan. 2008. "Health of Foreign-born People in the United States: A Review." *Health and Place* 14:623–35.

Cutler, David M. 2004. *Your Money or Your Life: Strong Medicine for America's Health Care System.* New York: Oxford University Press.

DaVanzo, Julie, Jennifer Hawes-Dawson, E. Burciaga Valdez, and Georges Vernez. 1994. "Surveying Immigrant Communities: Policy Imperatives and Technical Challenges." RAND, Santa Monica, CA.

Davis, Kingsley. 1974. "The Migrations of Human Populations." *Scientific American* 231:92–105.

Deaton, Angus. 1997. *The Analysis of Household Surveys: A Microeconomic Approach to Development Policy.* Baltimore, MD: Johns Hopkins University Press.

Dey, Achintya N., and Jacqueline Wilson Lucas. 2006. "Physical and Mental Health Characteristics of US- and Foreign-Born Adults: United States, 1998–2003." *Advance Data from Vital and Health Statistics* 369:1–20.

Diffendal, Gregg. 2001. "The Hard-to-Interview in the American Community Survey." *Proceedings of the Annual Meeting of the American Statistical Association,* August 5–9, 2001.

DuBois, W. E. B. 1996 [1899]. *The Philadelphia Negro.* Philadelphia: University of Pennsylvania Press.

Easterlin, Richard A. 1999. "How Beneficent Is the Market? A Look at the Modern History of Mortality." *European Review of Economic History* 3:257–94.

Edmonston, Barry. 1996. *Statistics on US Immigration: An Assessment of Data Needs for Future Research.* Washington, DC: National Academies Press.

Edmonston, Barry, and Margeret Michalowshi. 2004. "International Migration." Pp. 455–92 in *The Methods and Material of Demography,* 2nd ed., edited by David A. Swanson and Jacob S. Siegel. San Diego, CA: Elsevier Academic Press.

Evans, Robert G., and Gregory L. Stoddart. 1990. "Producing Health, Consuming Health Care." *Social Science and Medicine* 31:1347–63.

Ferrie, Joseph P. 1999. *Yankees Now: Immigrants in the Antebellum United States, 1840–1860.* New York: Oxford University Press.

Fowler, Floyd J., Jr. 2002. *Survey Research Methods.* 3rd ed. Thousand Oaks, CA: Sage.

Gauthier, Jason G. 2002. "Measuring America: The Decennial Censuses from 1790 to 2000." Washington, DC: US Census Bureau, Department of Commerce.

Gibson, Campbell, and Emily Lennon. 1999. "Historical Census Statistics on the Foreign-born Population of the United States: 1850–1990." US Census Bureau, Department of Commerce, Washington, DC.

Groves, Robert M. 1987. "Research on Survey Data Quality." *Public Opinion Quarterly* 51:S156–72.

Groves, Robert M., Floyd J. Fowler, Mick P. Couper, James M. Lepkowski, Eleanor Singer, and Roger Tourangeau. 2004. *Survey Methodology.* Hoboken, NJ: Wiley.

Hacking, Ian. 2009 [1975]. *The Emergence of Probability: A Philosophical Study of Early Ideas about Probability, Induction and Statistical Inference.* New York: Cambridge University Press.

Handlin, Oscar. 2002 [1951]. *The Uprooted: The Epic Story of the Great Migrations That Made the American People.* Philadelphia: University of Pennsylvania Press.

Hayes-Bautista, David E. 2002. "The Latino Health Research Agenda in the Twenty First Century." Pp. 215–35 in *Latinos: Remaking America,* edited by M. M. Suárez Orozco and M. M. Páez. Cambridge, MA: Harvard University Press.

Heer, David M. 1990. *Undocumented Mexicans in the United States.* New York: Cambridge University Press.

———. 1996. *Immigration in America's Future: Social Science Findings and the Policy Debate.* Edited by S. McNall and C. Tilly. Boulder, CO: Westview Press.

Heer, David M., and Jeffrey S. Passel. 1987. "Comparison of Two Methods for Computing the Number of Undocumented Mexican Adults in Los Angeles County." *International Migration Review* 21:1446–73.

Hogg, Margaret H. 1930. "Sources of Incomparability and Error in Employment Unemployment Surveys." *Journal of the American Statistical Association* 25:284–94.

———. 1932. *The Incidence of Work Shortage.* New York: Russell Sage Foundation.

Holmes, Louisa M., and Enrico A. Marcelli. 2012. "Neighborhoods and Systemic Inflammation: High CRP among Legal and Unauthorized Brazilian Migrants." *Health and Place* 18:683–93.

Hsiao, Cheng. 1999. *Analysis of Panel Data.* Edited by J.-M. Grandmont and C. F. Manski. New York: Cambridge University Press.

Huff, Darrell. 1993 [1953]. *How to Lie with Statistics.* New York: Norton.

Huntington, Samuel P. 2005 [2004]. *Who We Are? The Challenges to America's National Identity.* New York: Simon and Schuster.

Jasso, Guillermina, Douglas S. Massey, Mark R. Rosensweig, and James P. Smith. 2004. "Immigrant Health—Selectivity and Acculturation." Pp. 227–66 in *Critical Perspectives on Racial and Ethnic Differences in Health in Late Life,* edited by N. B. Anderson, R. A. Bulatao, and B. Cohen. Washington, DC: National Academies Press.

Kawachi, Ichiro, and Lisa F. Berkman. 2003. "Neighborhoods and Health." New York: Oxford University Press.

Kruskall, William, and Frederick Mosteller. 1980. "Representative Sampling, IV: The History of the Concept in Statistics, 1895–1939." *International Statistical Review* 48:169–95.

Kuznets, Simon, and Ernest Rubin. 1954. *Immigration and the Foreign Born.* New York: National Bureau of Economic Research.

Laplace, Pierre-Simon. 2007. *A Philosophical Essay on Probabilities.* New York: Cosimo.

Link, Bruce G., and Jo Phelan. 1995. "Social Conditions as Fundamental Causes of Disease." *Journal of Health and Social Behavior* 35:80–94.

Lorant, Vincent, Herman Van Oyen, and Isabelle Thomas. 2008. "Contextual Factors and Immigrants' Health Status: Double Jeopardy." *Health and Place* 14:678–92.

Marcelli, Enrico A. 2004. "The Unauthorized Residency Status Myth: Health Insurance Coverage and Medical Care Use among Mexican Immigrants in California." *Migraciones Internacionales* 2:5–35.

———. 2007. "Legal Status and the Health of Mexican Immigrants Residing in the United States." In Migration Working Group Seminar, Department of Sociology, UCLA and El Colegio de la Frontera Norte (COLEF) Migration Seminar, Los Angeles.

———. 2008. "Collecting Biological and Other Sensitive Health Data from Legal and Unauthorized Migrants in Household Surveys." In *Southern Demographic Association Annual Meetings,* Greenville, SC.

Marcelli, Enrico A., and David M. Heer. 1997. "Unauthorized Mexican Workers in the 1990 Los Angeles County Labour Force." *International Migration* 35:59–83.

———. 1998. "The Unauthorized Mexican Immigrant Population and Welfare in Los Angeles County: A Comparative Statistical Analysis." *Sociological Perspectives* 41:279–302.

Marcelli, Enrico A., and Louisa M. Holmes. 2012. "Blood Pressure." Pp. 289–93 in *Encyclopedia of Immigrant Health,* vol. 1, edited by S. Loue and M. Sajatovic. Berlin: Springer Science+Business Media.

Marcelli, Enrico A., Louisa Holmes, David Estella, Fausto da Rocha, Phillip Granberry, and Orfeu Buxton. 2009a. "(In)Visible (Im)Migrants: The Health and Socioeconomic Integration of Brazilians in Metropolitan Boston." San Diego State University, San Diego, CA.

Marcelli, Enrico A., Louisa Holmes, Magalis Troncoso, Phillip Granberry, and Orfeu Buxton. 2009b. "Permanently Temporary? The Health and Socioeconomic Integration of Dominicans in Metropolitan Boston." Center for Behavioral and Community Health Studies, San Diego State University, San Diego.

Marcelli, Enrico A., and B. Lindsay Lowell. 2005. "Transnational Twist: Pecuniary Remittances and Socioeconomic Integration among Authorized and Unauthorized Mexican Immigrants in Los Angeles County." *International Migration Review* 39:69–102.

Marcus, Alan Patrick. 2009. "(Re)creating Places and Spaces in Two Countries: Brazilian Transnational Migration Processes." *Journal of Cultural Geography* 26:173–98.

McDade, Thomas W. 2007. "Measuring Immune Function: Markers of Cell-Mediated Immunity and Inflammation in Dried Blood Spots." Pp. 181–207 in *Measuring Stress in Humans: A Practical Guide for the Field* (Cambridge Studies in Biological and Evolutionary Anthropology), edited by G. H. Ice and G. D. James. New York: Cambridge University Press.

McDade, Thomas W., Sharon Williams, and J. Josh Snodgrass. 2007. "What a Drop Can Do: Dried Blood Spots as a Minimally Invasive Method for Integrating Biomarkers into Population-Based Research." *Demography* 44:899–925.

McKenzie, David J., and Johan Mistiaen. 2007. "Surveying Migrant Households: A Comparison of Census-Based, Snowball, and Intercept Point Surveys." The World Bank, Washington, DC.

Menard, Scott. 2002. *Longitudinal Research.* 2nd ed. Thousand Oaks, CA: Sage.

Neyman, Jerzy. 1934. "On the Two Different Aspects of the Representative Method: The Method of Stratified Sampling and the Method of Purposive Selection." *Journal of the Royal Statistical Society* 97:558–625.

Pol, Louis G., and Richard K. Thomas. 2001. *The Demography of Health and Health Care.* 2nd ed. New York: Kluwer Academic/Plenum.

Porter, Theodore M. 1986. *The Rise of Statistical Thinking, 1820–1900.* Princeton, NJ: Princeton University Press.

Ramos, Jorge. 2010. *A Country for All: An Immigrant Manifesto.* New York: Vintage Books.

Rampell, Catherine. May 15, 2012. "The Beginning of the End of the Census?" *New York Times.*

Redstone, Ilana, and Douglas S. Massey. 2004. "Coming to Stay: An Analysis of the US Census Question of Immigrants' Year of Arrival." *Demography* 41:721.

Rindfuss, Ronald R., Toshiko Kandea, Arpita Chattopadhy, and Chanya Sethaput. 2007. "Panel Studies and Migration." *Social Science Research* 36:374–403.

Seng, You Poh. 1951. "Historical Survey of the Development of Sampling Theories and Practice." *Journal of the Royal Statistical Society* 114A:214–31.

Simon, Rita, and Susan H. Alexander. 1993. *The Ambivalent Welcome: Print Media, Public Opinion and Immigration.* Westport, CT: Praeger.

Singh, Gopal K., and Mohammad Siahpush. 2001. "All-Cause and Cause-Specific Mortality of Immigrants and Native Born in the United States." *American Journal of Public Health* 91:392–99.

Stephen, Frederick F. 1948. "History of the Uses of Modern Sampling Procedures." *Journal of the American Statistical Association* 43:12–39.

Stouffer, Samuel A. 1935. "Statistical Induction in Rural Social Research." *Social Forces* 13:505–15.

Thomas, Brinley. 1959. "International Migration." Pp. 510–43 in *The Study of Population: An Inventory and Appraisal,* edited by Phillip M. Hauser and Otis Dudley Duncan. Chicago: University of Chicago Press.

Thomas, William I., and Florian Znaniecki. 1996 [1918–1920]. "Introduction." Pp. iv–xvii in *The Polish Peasant in Europe and America: A Classic Work of Immigration History,* edited by E. Zaretsky. Urbana and Chicago: University of Illinois Press.

Tourangeau, Roger, and Tom W. Smith. 1996. "Asking Sensitive Questions: The Impact of Data Collection Mode, Question Format, and Question Context." *Public Opinion Quarterly* 60:275–304.

US Census Bureau. 2006. "Current Population Survey: Design and Methodology." Technical paper no. 66. Washington, DC: US Government Printing Office.

———. 2009. "American Community Survey: Design and Methodology." Washington, DC: US Government Printing Office.

United Nations. 2007. "Measuring International Migration through Sample Surveys." In *United Nations Expert Group Meeting on the Use of Censuses and Surveys to Measure International Migration.* New York: Department of Economic and Social Affairs, Statistics Division, United Nations Secretariat.

Wallerstein, Nina, and Bonnie Duran. 2003. "The Conceptual, Historical, and Practice Roots of Community Based Participatory Research and Related Participatory Traditions." Pp. 27–52 in *Community-Based Participatory Research for Health,* edited by M. Minkler and N. Wallerstein. San Francisco: Jossey-Bass.

Wolfe, A.B. 1932. "Population Censuses before 1790." *Journal of the American Statistical Association* 27:357–70.

Young, T. Kue. 2005. *Population Health: Concepts and Methods.* 2nd ed. New York: Oxford University Press.

Zlotnick, Hania. 1987. "Introduction: Measuring International Migration: Theory and Practice." *International Migration Review* 21:v–xii.

7

Respondent-Driven Sampling for Migrant Populations

Lisa Johnston
Mohsen Malekinejad

OVERVIEW

Imagine wanting to conduct a large (100+) quantitative survey of the health conditions of sub-Saharan migrants in Morocco, the living situations of Chinese students studying in Ukraine, the working environment of Polish people residing in Norway, the migration patterns of Central American females in Houston, or the vulnerability of Cambodian migrants crossing into Thailand. Because of their particular circumstances, it is difficult to generate a sampling frame from which to gather a representative sample from these populations. In addition, migrants are sometimes stigmatized or are in irregular administrative situations, which, in turn, makes them difficult to access and unwilling to participate in research efforts. They are, therefore, considered hard-to-reach populations for survey research purposes. At the same time, they are potentially networked (i.e., they know each other), such that you may be able to find a handful of group members, through their contacts with governmental and nongovernmental organizations and other sources, who are willing to recruit their peers. Over the past decade, respondent-driven sampling (RDS) has been highlighted as a robust and effective method to recruit hard-to-reach populations that are connected through social networks. This chapter provides an introduction to sampling migrant populations using RDS, including several key concepts and definitions needed to understand RDS recruitment and analysis, underlying assumptions, and practical guidance for implementation. By the end of this chapter readers should be able to

- identify and explain some differences between RDS and a *convenience* chain referral sample,

- explain how RDS works,
- describe why RDS is appropriate for migrant populations,
- describe the assumptions needed for RDS recruitment and analysis, and
- understand some of the challenges of and advantages to RDS.

In addition, the chapter provides references for obtaining more information about the specifics of using RDS.

CHARACTERISTICS OF CHAIN REFERRAL SAMPLING

RDS is a form of chain referral sampling that incorporates numerous methodological and statistical elements to mitigate the biases in chain referral sampling (Heckathorn 2002, 2007; Salganik and Heckathorn 2004). Chain referral sampling, a nonprobability method in which hard-to-reach populations are asked to provide referrals to other members of their group, has been commonly used as an easy and low-cost method to recruit hard-to-reach populations (Atkinson and Flint 2001; Biernacki and Waldorf 1981). Chain referral sampling is a nonprobability method in which hard-to-reach populations are asked to provide referrals to other members of their group. Typically, this method continues until the final sample size is attained or when an entire network of the population is sampled (Biernacki and Waldorf 1981; Sudman and Kalton 1986; Sudman et al. 1988). Although this method can easily and rapidly identify numerous respondents, it is prone to sampling biases because certain groups tend to be either over- or underrepresented depending on the number of connections they have to other population members (Atkinson and Flint 2001; Biernacki and Waldorf 1981; Erickson 1979).

RDS: AN IMPROVEMENT OVER CHAIN REFERRAL SAMPLING

RDS attempts to overcome the limitations associated with chain referral sampling while retaining several of its advantages, including

- the ability to recruit populations that usually cannot be studied using conventional sampling methods due to the lack of a sampling frame,
- relative ease of implementation given that it does not require intensive formative assessment and mapping, and
- relatively rapid recruitment given that initial recruits are asked to refer their peers.

RDS comprises two parts: a recruitment strategy and an analysis component. It is critical to carefully collect two pieces of data from respondents in order to make statistical adjustments when data are analyzed: (1) information about the personal network size and (2) who recruited whom. Without the necessary analytical adjustments, RDS is no different from a structured chain referral sample. When conducted and analyzed correctly, RDS estimates will be representative of the network of the population from which the sample was drawn.

RDS recruitment is initiated with a small, diverse, and influential group of "seeds" (eligible respondents) purposefully selected by the researchers. Each seed receives a set number of recruitment coupons to recruit his or her peers, who then redeem the coupons at a fixed site to enroll in the survey. Eligible recruits who finish the survey process are also given a set number of coupons to recruit their peers. The recruited peers of seeds who enroll in the survey become wave 1 respondents, and the recruits of wave 1 respondents become wave 2 respondents. This process of recruitment continues through successive waves until the calculated sample size is reached. In the end, the waves produced by effective seeds make up recruitment chains of varying lengths. The goal is to acquire long recruitment chains made up of multiple waves.

APPROPRIATENESS OF RDS FOR MIGRANT POPULATIONS

Used for the first time in 1994 in the United States (Heckathorn 1997), RDS has most widely been used in epidemiological surveys of HIV populations at higher risk of HIV, such as high-risk youth, sex workers, men who have sex with men, and people who inject drugs (Johnston et al. 2008; Malekinejad et al. 2008; Johnston, Thurman, et al. 2010; Montealegre et al. 2013; Johnston 2013a). Useful information from the wide range of manuals, materials, and published literature based on these surveys can be adapted for surveys of migrants. Only recently has RDS been seen as an effective method to sample migrant populations (Tyldum and Johnston, 2014; Montealegre, Johnston, and Sabin 2011). For instance, RDS has been widely used in Europe to sample Polish migrants in Oslo (Friberg and Tyldum 2007; Friberg and Eldring 2013), Copenhagen (Hansen and Hansen 2009), Dublin (Mühlau et al. 2011), and Reykjavík (Þórarinsdóttir and Wojtyńska 2011), and Brazilian, Moroccan, and Ukrainian migrants in The Netherlands, Norway, Portugal, and the United Kingdom (http://www.imi.ox.ac.uk/research-projects/themis). In the United States, RDS has been used to sample Latino first- and second-generation migrant males in Chicago (Ramirez-Valles et al. 2005), Nigerian migrants in New York City (Rodriguez 2009), undocumented migrant workers in Chicago, Los Angeles, New York City (Bernhardt et al. 2009), and San Diego (Zhang 2012), and Central American migrant women in Houston (Montealegre et al. 2012; Montealegre, Risser, et al. 2011). In Asia, RDS was used to sample Cambodian and Myanmar migrants in Thailand (Khamsiriwatchara et al. 2011) and, in Africa, RDS was used to sample Anglophone and Francophone sub-Saharan African migrants in Rabat, Morocco (Johnston 2013b).

RDS peer-to-peer recruitment relies on populations being connected through social networks. A *social network* in the context of RDS is a social structure of individuals who are connected by one or more specific attributes yielding interdependency between members of the network, such as relationships (sexual, work), friendship, kinship, and common interests. Many migrant populations are appropriate for sampling with RDS because they

- share similar cultural backgrounds (e.g., language, ethnic group, religion, country of origin),
- may be part of a migration network linking communities in the region of origin and destination,
- tend to rely on each other to transition into a new culture and settle down in the new society (e.g., finding jobs, housing, schools, etc.), and/or
- may face common social barriers that impede their assimilation into the larger society (e.g., stigma, discrimination, stereotyping) (Tyldum and Johnston 2014).

PREPARING FOR AN RDS SURVEY: FORMATIVE ASSESSMENT

Survey implementers should gather information through a formative assessment before conducting a survey using RDS. One of the most important questions to answer during a formative assessment is whether a population is sufficiently socially networked to sustain recruitment chains (Johnston, Whitehead, et al. 2010). Collecting data can be done through focus groups or interviews with the target population or with persons who work with the target population. Questions to consider include the following:

- Do population members recognize each other? Are they linked by a preexisting contact pattern, and are these relationships reciprocal? "I know you as a member of the target population and you know me as a member of the target population." For instance, working migrants returning to their country of origin do not necessarily know each other. Migrants arriving in a country at different times or for different reasons may not know each other (e.g., Polish migrants moving to Western Europe in the 1980s after the fall of the Soviet Union vs. those who moved in 2004 after Poland's accession to the EU) (Friberg 2007; Friberg and Horst 2014).
- How many individuals do they have in their personal social networks?
- Do they form diverse social network ties (strong and weak), and are they connected to different subpopulations?
- Are they made up of one social network or several isolated social network clusters? For instance, males and females may not form social networks in

some populations and therefore will not recruit across these subgroups. If this is the case, it is worth considering including just one of these groups in the sample. This is the same for subgroups based on tribal, country-of-origin, or language differences.

- If given as many coupons as they wanted, how many peers could they recruit?
- How quickly could they distribute their coupons?
- If given three coupons today, could they find three individuals to recruit who would enroll in the survey?

The ideal target population in RDS surveys is a category of people that can be clearly defined by the researcher as well as by respondents and that also has the characteristics of a social group in that they identify and interact with each other. Formative assessment is also helpful for finding seeds, for determining acceptability of RDS and research in general, and for planning the survey logistics (Johnston, Whitehead, et al. 2010; Johnston 2013a; Montealegre et al. 2014).

STEPS TO IMPLEMENT RDS

Once the preliminary steps of obtaining approval for research with human subjects (ethics review), and formative research are complete, it is time to gather a sample using RDS. The RDS recruitment steps are as follows:[1]

1. Researchers select a location accessible and acceptable to the survey population. They ensure that the site is neutral (e.g., not an organization that serves one subgroup in the network, not a stigmatized location, etc.), discreet, accessible, comfortable, and that it will not attract undue governmental or community attention.
2. Researchers identify and recruit a handful of *seeds* from the survey population. Past surveys of several hard-to-reach populations have typically used anywhere from three to fifteen seeds (Malekinejad et al. 2008). Seeds need not be selected randomly, but a diverse selection of seeds will help ensure reaching diverse members of the population more quickly. For instance, if the target population comprises different tribal groups, then seeds should also comprise these groups. Seeds are usually found through organizations working with the target population, but they can also be recruited through outreach from places in their community where they congregate (for more information about seeds see Johnston 2013a; Kubal et al. 2014).
3. Seeds complete the survey process and receive a set number of recruitment *coupons* (see Figs. 7.5, 7.6, below) to use in recruiting their peers.
4. Recruits are asked to go to the survey site for an interview. Easy access to the survey site is especially relevant for migrants because they may have transportation limitations, fear leaving their homes because of immigration

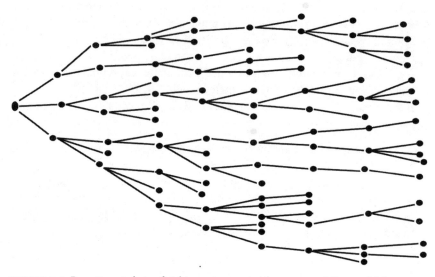

FIGURE 7.1. Recruitment chain of eight waves generated from one seed. Source: L Johnston and K Sabin, "Échantillonnage déterminé selon les répondants pour les populations difficiles à joindre" (Sampling hard-to-reach populations with respondent driven sampling). (*Methodological Innovations Online* [2010] 5[2]: 38–48; www.methodologicalinnovations.org.)

enforcement activities, and work several jobs at nontraditional hours. In some cases, cultural norms may prohibit women from traveling by themselves.

5. Membership in a target population needs to be ascertained through a screening process, preferably by someone who is familiar with or part of the target population.

6. The recruits of the seeds produce wave 1; the recruits of wave 1 produce wave 2, and so on. This process continues until the calculated sample size is reached (Fig. 7.1).

7. All respondents receive an incentive for completing the interview (primary incentive) and another incentive for recruiting their peers to participate in the survey (secondary incentive).

The objective in RDS is to generate long recruitment chains made up of several recruitment *waves* of respondents while limiting the number of recruits per each respondent (i.e., usually two to four). The combination of limiting the number of recruits per respondent (i.e., using a set number of coupons) and producing long recruitment chains increases the likelihood that the final sample characteristics will be independent of the purposefully selected seeds.

Example: An RDS survey was conducted in the summer of 2009 to estimate the proportion of long-term (LT; more than six months of stay) and short-term (ST; less than six months of stay) Cambodian and Myanmar immigrants in Thailand. The survey was implemented in three provinces near the Thai-Cambodia border, where there are many migrant workers. Recruitment started with a total of 30 seeds (18 Cambodian and 12 Myanmar). Seeds were given three traceable coupons to recruit other migrants. Respondents received approximately US$10.00 for each recruit. During eight weeks of recruitment, 1,719 respondents were recruited through 2–10 waves of recruitment. Cambodian migrant seeds (12 LT and 6 ST) recruited a total of 828 Cambodian migrants (350 LT, 475 ST, and 3 undetermined). Myanmar migrant seeds (11 LT and 1 ST) recruited a total of 891 migrants (871 LT and 19 ST) (Khamsiriwatchara et al. 2011).

For a larger survey, if there is an initial selection of twelve seeds and each of these seeds recruits two peers, then each of the two peers recruits two more peers over three waves; the sample will geometrically expand as follows:

12 SEEDS

Wave 1: 12 seeds select 2 peers each = 24 peers

Wave 2: 24 peers select 2 peers each = 48 peers

Wave 3: 48 peers select 2 peers each = 96

This example creates recruitment chains totaling 180 individuals (12 seeds + 24 + 48 + 96).[2]

DATA COLLECTION REQUIREMENTS FOR RDS

The following information must be collected from each respondent in order to analyze RDS data:

- Personal social network size—This is the number of individuals the respondent knows, and they know the respondent, within the target population based on the eligibility criteria (Heckathorn 2007).[3]
- Respondent's coupon number—This is the number on the coupon with which the respondent was recruited. Seeds are selected by survey staff and, therefore, do not get a coupon. However, seeds should be assigned a unique coupon number.[4]
- Coupon numbers of recruits—These are the numbers given to the recruits of each respondent. They are used to link the recruiter to his or her recruits.

RDS METHOD ASSUMPTIONS

Researchers must understand the assumptions underlying RDS before conducting an RDS survey. There are two types of assumptions: functional and analytic (Heckathorn 2007).

Functional Assumptions

Three functional assumptions must be met during RDS recruitment. Each of these assumptions should be reviewed before RDS is considered. If these assumptions are not met, a number of biases may result, including failure to accumulate a large enough number of respondents.

1. Respondents within the target population hold interpersonal ties. RDS is based on the assumption that group members can most effectively recruit other members of their own group (Heckathorn and Rosenstein 2002). Essentially, peer-to-peer recruitment is believed to increase credibility and encourage participation, especially among populations that prefer to be hidden and that are hard to reach. In order to ensure that RDS is applicable to a certain target population, it is important to understand whether or not members of the target population are linked by preexisting contact patterns and reciprocal relationships.

The combination of recruitment quotas (a set number of recruitment coupons for each respondent) and provision of a secondary incentive for successful recruitment increases the likelihood that respondents will try to recruit from members of the target population with whom they already have a relationship rather than approaching strangers. Previous successful applications of RDS demonstrate that recruiters and recruits had some form of ongoing personal relationship in approximately 98% of cases (Gile et al. in press).

2. Interpersonal ties within the target population residing in a defined geographical area are dense. The interpersonal ties within the target population must be dense enough to sustain recruitment. In other words, there must be multiple preexisting links between members of the target population and members must be accessible to each other (e.g., not so geographically dispersed that distance would prevent them from contacting each other and passing on recruitment coupons). While respondents may know many potential recruits who meet the eligibility criteria for a survey, if they cannot contact them easily, recruitment will likely not be sustained. To ensure numerous network connections, respondents should be allowed to recruit those with whom they have "weak links," such as acquaintances, as well as those with whom they have "strong links," such as friends and family members.

3. RDS sample is a small fraction of the target population. Sampling with replacement is one of the statistical requirements for many of the RDS estimators to be valid. Theoretically, sampling with replacement means that all members of the population have multiple chances to participate. Most surveys do not allow respondents to participate more than once, as a very small number of respondents may be likely to overwhelm the sample. Instead of allowing respondents to participate more than once, RDS assumes that the sampling fraction (the number of individuals in the sample divided by the total number of individuals in the target population) be small. There is debate about whether RDS is a sampling with replacement method. On the surface it is not since a respondent is allowed to enroll only once (Gile and Handcock 2010; Gile et al. in press); however, the assumption is viewed more loosely if the sample size is small relative to the population size (Volz and Heckathorn 2008).

Analytic Assumptions

Analytic assumptions must be assessed to measure the level of bias in the final estimates. Not all assumptions can be proven and some assumptions may not be completely met (Gile et al. in press).

1. *Self-reported personal social network size accurately reflects the true network size of respondents.* The personal social network size is defined as the number of relatives, friends, and acquaintances that the respondent knows and who know the respondent, who are part of the target population. Because respondents recruit each other, it is important to know how many individuals a respondent could potentially recruit. There are multiple paths to each respondent: those with larger social networks are more likely to be recruited than those with smaller social networks. Those respondents with small social networks are given a larger weight in the analysis because there are fewer recruitment paths that lead to them.

The social network size question should reflect the pool of individuals that the respondent could recruit from the target population. The measurement (as accurate as possible) of social network sizes depends on many factors, including how the question is structured, how well the interviewers are trained to probe for accurate responses to this question, and the impact of recall bias. (See examples of questions for determining social network size, below; also see Johnston 2013a; Johnston et al. 2014.)

2. *Peer recruitment is a random selection from the recruiter's network.* The assumption of random recruitment is difficult to assess (Gile et al. in press). There are three occasions when respondent behavior may affect recruitment: (1) random coupon distribution (respondents do not distribute their coupons among different subgroups within their social network); (2) coupon acceptance (those approached do not accept coupons); and (3) coupon redemption (those who accept a coupon do not enroll in the survey).

Nonrandom coupon distribution is more likely when seeds are homogenous in terms of an important variable (e.g., migrant population seeds are identified through an active migrant outreach organization and therefore recruit only from among their own subgroup [e.g., politically active migrants], without reaching into other important subgroups such as nonpolitically active migrants). Nonrandom coupon acceptance occurs when members of one subgroup (e.g., employed

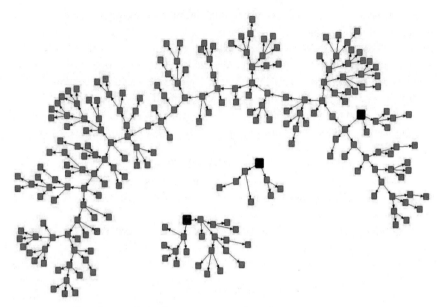

FIGURE 7.2. Recruitment chains from a survey conducted among 230 undocumented Central American Women, conducted in Houston, Texas, 2010. (Appreciation to Jane Richards Montealegre for sharing this graphic.)

migrants) are more reluctant to accept a coupon than members of another subgroup (e.g., unemployed migrants).

The random recruitment assumption is plausible only if members of the target population have reasonably easy and comfortable access to the interview site, an appropriate time frame is used for the network size question, and appropriate incentives are employed (Heckathorn 2002). However, nonrandom recruitment, if it occurs, will not necessarily bias the RDS estimator as long as recruitment is not correlated with any variable important for estimation (Volz and Heckathorn 2008).

3. *Each respondent recruits a single peer.* RDS relies on peers recruiting peers. Most RDS surveys begin with multiple recruitments, with seeds receiving more than one coupon, because recruitment tends to die out quickly when only a single recruitment per seed is allowed at the beginning of a survey.

HOW TO END THE RDS RECRUITMENT PROCESS

The maximum number of waves in an RDS sample is based on the longest chain produced by any single seed in that sample. For example, in fig. 7.2., the seed (larger square) in the upper right corner has produced the longest wave (26 waves).

It is fairly common that one seed becomes a "super" recruiter, producing more waves in the chain than any other seed in the sample. Indeed, it is not uncommon for a "super seed" to produce a very long chain that comprises one third of the entire sample, whereas other seeds may produce only two, three, or four waves, and some seeds may not recruit anyone.

Fig. 7.2 shows recruitment chains from three seeds who recruited a sample of 230 migrants for an RDS survey conducted in Houston, Texas, in 2010 among undocumented Central American women.

ADVANTAGES AND DISADVANTAGES OF RDS
Advantages

When deciding about which sampling method to use for surveying migrant populations, researchers should take into consideration the advantages of RDS. Specifically, RDS methods

- involve a statistical and theoretical basis that, when the method is done correctly, enables RDS to produce representative estimates for network characteristics of the population sampled;
- have relatively easy field operations once the survey is under way;
- use peer-to-peer recruitment that is based on trust and that allows for anonymity (an important factor for migrants to participate in surveys);
- require no mapping and relatively limited formative research (however, formative research is essential to understand the underlying network structure of the populations);[5]
- can rapidly reach the calculated sample size through peer-to-peer recruitment in socially networked populations;
- reach less visible segments of the sampled population when recruitment chains are long;
- require a minimal number of additional questions to ensure proper statistical analysis;
- may be the most cost-effective and only practical and available method to obtain a representative sample of migrants; and
- have been conducted successfully in many countries among numerous hard-to-reach populations around the world, although mostly among groups at high risk for HIV.

In addition:

- Most of the templates for implementation materials (e.g., implementation manual, monitoring forms, protocols, survey steps, etc.) have already been developed and are freely accessible (Johnston 2013a, also see http://global healthsciences.ucsf.edu/pphg/gsi/epidemiologic-surveillance/ibbs-toolbox).

- Two open-source computer software programs, RDS Analyst (www.hpmrg. org) and Respondent-Driven Sampling Analysis Tool (RDSAT) (www. respondentdrivensampling.org), have been specifically designed to analyze RDS data.

Disadvantages

Several issues may limit the wide use or applicability of RDS, including the following:

- Because screening for eligibility relies on self-reported data, it can be difficult to verify respondents' group membership (i.e., how can we verify whether a migrant is really a migrant and still maintain anonymity?). Using target population members as screeners may mitigate this disadvantage since migrants can easily evaluate whether somebody is from the same country of origin and speaks the language of the country of origin, and can screen respondents by asking them to describe aspects of their country's history or culture, type of visa or immigration status, migration history and process, and so on.[6]
- Mobility of migrants can complicate planning and fieldwork for RDS.
- RDS requires strict adherence to theory and assumptions (e.g., the necessity of tracking links between recruiters and recruiting through coupon management assumes limited in- and out-migration during sampling).
- The use of incentives is not universally accepted by some investigators (Semaan et al. 2008).[7]
- Data analysis can be challenging, and the use of the available analysis tools (RDS Analyst or RDSAT) usually requires special training.[8]
- Analysis of RDS data is still being developed, and the best practices on how to do multivariate analysis are under debate.
- Migrants may have transportation barriers, making it difficult for them to go to a central place for interviews.
- It is difficult to deal with selective nonresponse bias due to lack of direct access to those who refuse to accept coupons from recruiters or do not use the coupon to participate.

USEFUL RDS MATERIALS

Survey implementers should prepare several essential documents for conducting an RDS survey. These documents include the following:[9]

- survey protocol
- field operations manual

- survey management forms
- survey questionnaire (including questions that assess network size and the relationships between recruiters and potential recruits)

Survey Protocol

The survey protocol, which is usually submitted as part of the ethical review process, describes every step of a survey and is an essential tool to have while preparing for and conducting any survey. A description of the recruitment process is a key part of the survey protocol; examples are provided here.

Recruitment Process.   Figs. 7.3 and 7.4 provide examples of the first and second recruitment visits to an RDS survey site. These examples are intended to provide guidance and will vary based on the number and type of staffing and the steps in the survey process (e.g., some surveys collect biological specimens). The examples also mention management forms that can be used during the first and second visits. These forms are explained in more detail below.

These examples assume four staff members participating in the recruitment process:

- The *screener* (also called a receptionist in some surveys) greets respondents, screens for eligibility, completes consent, and asks the social network size question.
- The *interviewer* completes the interview (this assumes face-to-face interviewers, but many RDS surveys use computer-assisted survey instruments). Depending on the sample size, surveys often have more than one interviewer.
- The *coupon manager* explains the coupon recruitment process, gives out the recruitment coupons, and pays out the primary (first visit) and secondary (second visit) incentives.
- The *site supervisor* ensures that staff has all the materials it needs, deals with challenging situations when they arise, helps out staff when the survey site gets too busy, manages paperwork, and ensures quality throughout the survey process.

Staff should be knowledgeable about the customs and culture and speak the language(s) of the population being sampled.

Coupons.   Coupons must be easy to track and contain a unique RDS identification code, so that recruiters can be linked to recruits without using any personal identifying information about the respondents. Coupons should be easy to read, provide useful information (e.g., hours of operation, location of interview site, expiration dates, etc.), and have a pleasant appearance so that survey

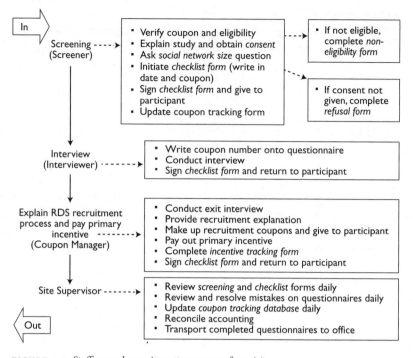

FIGURE 7.3. Staffing and recruitment process at first visit.

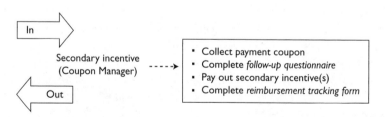

FIGURE 7.4. Staffing and recruitment process at second visit.

respondents realize that the coupons have value. Examples of coupons are given in Figs. 7.5 and 7.6.

Sample Size Calculation.   Calculating the sample size is a key part of the survey protocol that must be completed before you start the survey. The practical objective of a sample size calculation is to better plan for the survey based on the number of respondents (i.e., funding, staff support, etc.). The scientific objective of a sample size calculation is to determine the number of respondents needed to estimate prevalence of key indicators (i.e., unemployment, access to health care, illiteracy, etc.) or change in the proportion of an indicator from one survey round to the next. Here, we have provided a formula for one survey round.

The formula for the needed sample size *(n)* to detect a point prevalence of a certain indicator using RDS is as follows:

$$n = D * \frac{[Z_{1-\alpha}]^2 * P^* (1 - P)}{E^2}$$

Where:

n: Sample size required per survey[10]

Z1 - α: The $Z_{1-\alpha}$ score is a statistic that corresponds to the level of significance desired. Usually a significance level of 0.05 (or, equivalently, a 95% confidence level) is selected and corresponds to a value of 1.96. The smaller the significance level (that is, higher confidence level), the larger the sample size you will need.

P is the estimated proportion of the indicator of interest. For example, you wish to show that access to health care for migrant population was 20% in 2007, so P is equal to 0.2. The closer P is to 50%, the larger the sample size you will need.

E is the margin of error, which is defined as the radius of a confidence interval for the estimated proportion. For example, if the margin of error is 5%, you wish to show that the estimated access to health care proportion (in this case 20%) falls within +5% of 20% (15%–25%). The smaller the margin of error, the larger sample size you will need.

D, the design effect, accounts for the similarities individuals have when they are sampled within the same cluster. For example, migrants within a particular cluster may be similar with respect to employment because they are living in areas where employers are willing to hire migrants. The design effect can be thought of as a correction factor for how much an RDS sample differs from a simple random sample. Effectively, the design effect multiplies the sample size by the factor of D. The bigger the D, the larger the sample size needed. Preferably, design effect for RDS survey should be calculated based on prior survey data. Design effects of 2 are standard for most RDS surveys; however, a design effect closer to 3 or 4 may be more appropriate (Johnston, Chen, et al. 2013; Wejnert et al. 2012).

Ipsos MORI
University of Essex

Being in Britain

Take part in important research and earn up to £40 in High Street Vouchers

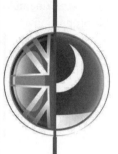

Are you…

✓ Of Pakistani nationality?

✓ Have you moved to Britain from Pakistan in the last 18 months?

✓ Are you aged between 18-60 years old?

✓ Do you live in London?

If the answer to all of these questions is YES…

You can earn up to **£40 in High Street Vouchers** by taking part in an interview about your experiences of life in Britain.

Please contact:
Jonathan Wooddin
Email: BeinginBritain@ipsos-mori.com
Tel : 0808 238 5424
Ipsos MORI, 79-81 Borough Road, London, SE1 1FY

We will ask for your reference numbers.
(1) YOUR NUMBER IS:

(2) YOU WERE RECOMMENDED BY NUMBER:

THIS LEAFLET IS ONLY VALID UNTIL

برطانیہ میں موجودگی

اہم تحقیق میں حصہ لیں اور ہائی اسٹریٹ واؤچر کی صورت میں £40 تک کمائیں

کیا آپ…

✓ پاکستانی شہریت رکھتے ہیں؟

✓ گزشتہ 18 مہینوں میں پاکستان سے برطانیہ میں منتقل ہوئے ہیں؟

✓ عمر 18-60 سال کے درمیان ہے؟

✓ کیا آپ لندن میں رہتے ہیں؟

اگر ان تمام سوالات کا جواب ہاں ہے…

آپ ان کی زندگی کے بارے میں ایک انٹرویو میں شرکت کر کے £40 تک کما سکتے ہیں

یہ رابطہ کریں
Jonathan Wooddin
Email: BeinginBritain@ipsos-mori.com
Tel : 0808 238 5427
Ipsos MORI, 79-81 Borough Road, London, SE1 1FY

(1)

(2) آپ کی نشانی نمبر

یہ لیفلٹ صرف اس تاریخ تک کارآمد ہے

برطانیہ وچ پوند

سرشت واؤچر دی صورت وچ £40 تیک کماؤ

کیہ تسیں

✓ پاکستانی قومیت دے ہو؟

✓ کیہ تسیں پاکستان توں برطانیہ پچھلے 18 مہینیاں دے وچ آئے ہو؟

✓ کیہ تہاڈی عمر 18-60 ورہے ہے؟

✓ کیہ تسیں لندن وچ رہندے ہو؟

جے ایہناں سارے سوالاں دا جواب ہاں ہے

Jonathan Wooddin
Email: BeinginBritain@ipsos-mori.com
Tel : 0808 238 5426
Ipsos MORI, 79-81 Borough Road, London, SE1 1FY

(1)

(2) تہاڈا نمبر ایہہ ہے

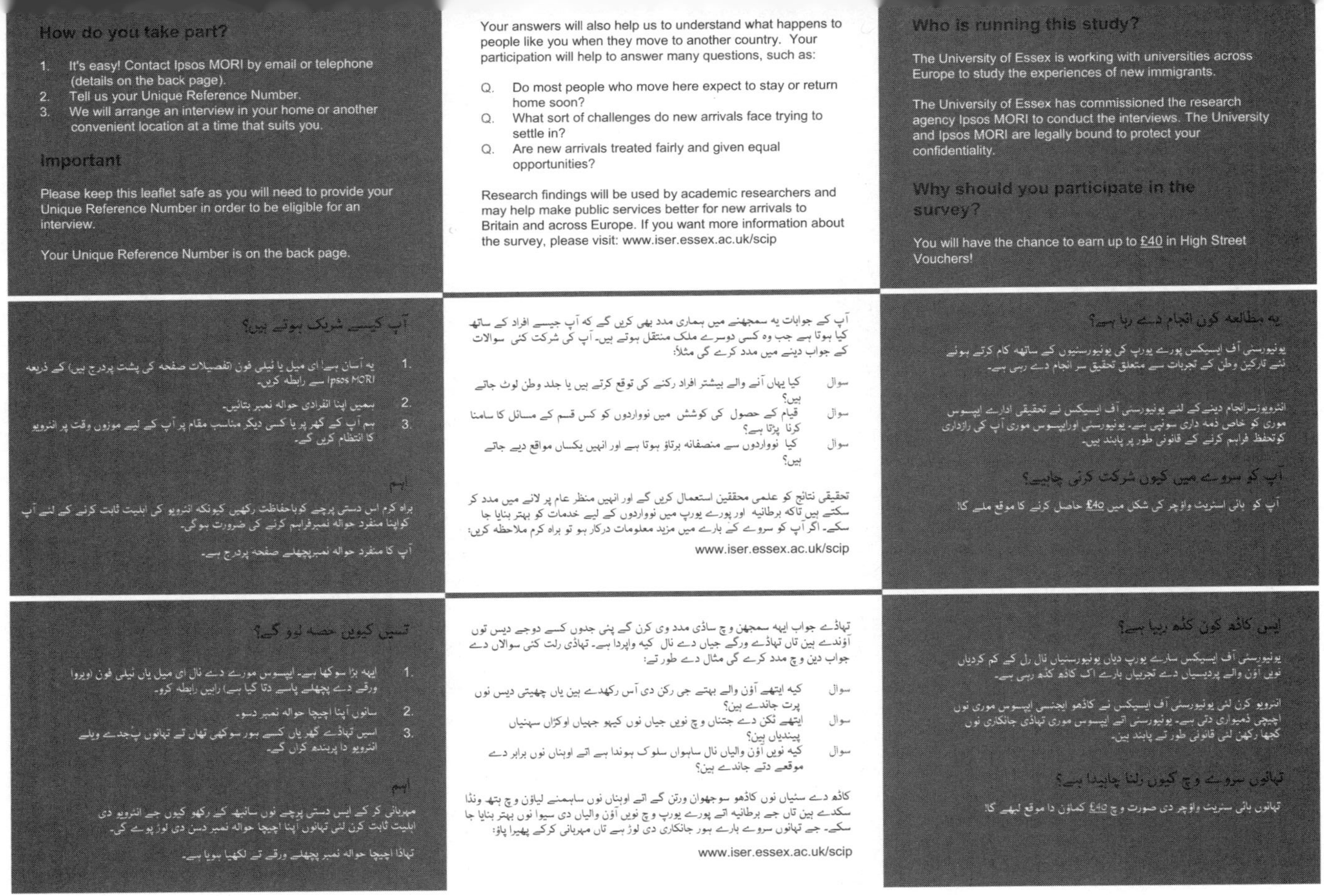

Who is running this study?

The University of Essex is working with universities across Europe to study the experiences of new immigrants.

The University of Essex has commissioned the research agency Ipsos MORI to conduct the interviews. The University and Ipsos MORI are legally bound to protect your confidentiality.

Why should you participate in the survey?

You will have the chance to earn up to £40 in High Street Vouchers!

Your answers will also help us to understand what happens to people like you when they move to another country. Your participation will help to answer many questions, such as:

Q. Do most people who move here expect to stay or return home soon?

Q. What sort of challenges do new arrivals face trying to settle in?

Q. Are new arrivals treated fairly and given equal opportunities?

Research findings will be used by academic researchers and may help make public services better for new arrivals to Britain and across Europe. If you want more information about the survey, please visit: www.iser.essex.ac.uk/scip

---

How do you take part?

It's easy! Contact Ipsos MORI by email or telephone (details on the back page).

1. Tell us your Unique Reference Number.
2. We will arrange an interview in your home or another convenient location at a time that suits you.

Important

Please keep this leaflet safe as you will need to provide your Unique Reference Number in order to be eligible for an interview.

Your Unique Reference Number is on the back page.

یہ مطالعہ کون چلا رہا ہے؟

آپ کو اس سروے میں کیوں شرکت کرنی چاہیے؟

اس کارڈ کو کیسے استعمال کیا جائے؟

تلاش کیونکر حصہ لیں گے؟

آپ کیسے شریک ہوتے ہیں؟

www.iser.essex.ac.uk/scip

www.iser.essex.ac.uk/scip

FIGURE 7.5. Coupon used in a survey of Pakistani migrants in Britain, 2010. (Appreciation to Renee Luthra, Lucinda Platt, and Ipsos Mori for sharing this coupon.)

CUPON DE INVITACION PARA PARTICIPAR

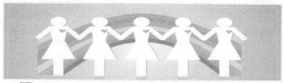

Proyecto Enlances

La Escuela de Salud Pública de la Universidad de Tejas

Encuesta sobre la salud de las mujeres centroamericanas en Houston

____/____/____
Fecha de emisión

____/____/____
Fecha de vencimiento

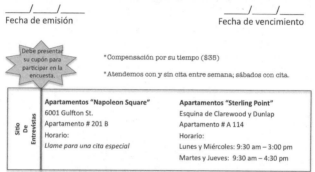

Debe presentar su cupón para participar en la encuesta.

* Compensación por su tiempo ($35)

* Atendemos con y sin cita entre semana; sábados con cita.

Sitio De Entrevistas	Apartamentos "Napoleon Square"	Apartamentos "Sterling Point"
	6001 Gulfton St.	Esquina de Clarewood y Dunlap
	Apartamento # 201 B	Apartamento # A 114
	Horario:	Horario:
	Llame para una cita especial	Lunes y Miércoles: 9:30 am – 3:00 pm
		Martes y Jueves: 9:30 am – 4:30 pm

¿Preguntas? O para hacer una cita, llame al
713-992-9502 ó al 504-920-5567

DIRECCIONES

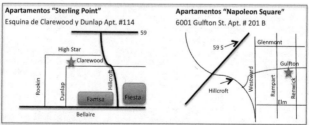

Apartamentos "Sterling Point"
Esquina de Clarewood y Dunlap Apt. #114

Apartamentos "Napoleon Square"
6001 Gulfton St. Apt. # 201 B

TEL: 713-992-9502 ó 504-920-5567

FIGURE 7.6. Coupon (front, back and attachment) used in a survey of Central American female migrants in Houston, Texas, US, 2009. (Appreciation to Jane Richards Montealegre for sharing this coupon.)

Field Operations Manual

A field operations manual describes the procedures that must be followed during an RDS survey. A good field operations manual anticipates problematic situations and includes contingency plans for these situations.

Survey Management Forms

Think about the steps involved in conducting your RDS survey and prepare the forms that will be needed to ensure quality collection of data.[11]

Survey Questionnaire

The questionnaire will need to be developed and piloted during the preparation stage of an RDS survey. A measurement of social network size of each respondent is a critical part of the RDS survey and will need to be added to either the questionnaire or a screening form.

PERSONAL NETWORK SIZE QUESTIONS

The personal network size question is developed from the eligibility criteria used in the survey with the addition of some reasonable period of time in which the respondent saw or met with individuals in their social network. For most surveys conducted through the direct passing of coupons, the inclusion of someone having been in contact with a peer is an indication that he or she would be able to pass a coupon to that person. For instance, in a survey with the eligibility criteria of female, originally from Turkey, eighteen years and above, living in Amsterdam, the network size question would be as follows:

> How many women of Turkish origin do you know (and they know you, you know their name and they know yours) who are at least eighteen years of age, live in Amsterdam, that you have seen in the past thirty days?

To gather data about social networks, we often ask questions using the phrase "*knowing* someone," which may have different meanings in different languages and cultures. In some languages, there are two words used to *know* someone. One word of *know* may be that the person knows the other person well, that is, know the person's phone number, address, first and last name, and so on. These are persons with strong ties. The other word of *know* may include these strong ties but also weaker ties. It is better to use the word for *know* that includes weak and strong ties. In addition to knowing someone, the question should also convey the meaning that the person has reciprocal relationships (i.e., you know the person and the person knows you). We often include the phrase "you know their name and they know yours" to ensure that all respondents have the correct understanding of what it means to *know* someone.

MULTIPLIER QUESTIONS TO ESTIMATE THE
POPULATION SIZE

RDS is a useful tool for measuring population size. We only briefly discuss the concept here, as there are resources available that cover this in depth (WHO/ UNAIDS 2010).

The multiplier method is one of the more commonly used methods for population size estimates of hard-to-reach populations (Johnston, Prybylski, et al. 2013). To employ this method, you need to have information from two sources. The first source is usually an institution or service-based site, such as a governmental or nongovernmental migrant assistance program with which the target group members are in contact. The second source is a survey using a probability-based sampling method (in this case, RDS) that has questions about the usage of these specific services. These two data sources should correspond to each other in respect to the geographical area, time frames of visits, and definitions of the sampled population.

For example, in an RDS survey of francophone sub-Saharan African migrants living in Rabat, Morocco, respondents were asked whether they received services from a local nongovernmental health organization during a specific time period prior to the survey. An adjusted analysis with RDS Analyst indicated that 22.1% of respondents reported that they received services from the organization. This organization reported that 916 francophone sub-Saharan African migrants received services in the survey catchment area during the same time period used in the survey. The calculation of 916/.221 revealed that there were 4,427 francophone sub-Saharan African migrants residing in Rabat (Johnston 2013b). Some disadvantages to this method are that service-based data may be biased and contain an unknown number of duplicates, as well as lack of independence between the survey and the service (WHO/UNAIDS 2010; Johnston, Prybylski, et al. 2013).

SUMMARY

Migrant populations are considered hard-to-reach for research purposes due to various reasons, including not being registered on any list or being affiliated with any institutions, being geographically dispersed, being subject to stigma and discrimination in the host country, or having an illegal immigration status and language barriers. Conventional probability sampling methods that require a sampling frame are not feasible for such populations.

RDS, a network-based sampling method, has been shown to be an effective tool for accessing and recruiting hard-to-reach populations across the globe, including migrants. RDS comprises two parts: a recruitment strategy and a statistical adjustment analysis component. Each is required in order to ensure unbiased estimates that represent the network of the population sampled. In order to make statistical adjustments, it is critical to carefully collect two pieces of data from respondents: (1) information about the personal network size and (2) who recruited whom. Without the necessary analytical adjustments, RDS-generated estimates may not be differentiated from those generated by "convenient" chain referral samples.

Migrants tend to form strong social ties in host countries for reasons such as being from the same country of origin, sharing similar cultural backgrounds and languages, and relying on one another to find jobs, schooling, and housing. These factors provide an opportunity for the application of social network–based sampling methods among migrants.

A preparatory formative assessment helps to determine whether or not RDS is appropriate for the target population and to plan for logistical and implementation considerations (e.g., identifying survey location, determining appropriate incentives, and identifying seeds and culturally competent staff). As in all survey methods, RDS has several advantages and challenges that should be considered prior to its use.

NOTES

1. For more information on the specific steps involved in RDS see *Introduction to Respondent Driven Sampling* (Johnston 2013a).

2. This example assumes that 100% of coupons are being redeemed. However, it is often impossible to predict the number of coupons that will be passed by each respondent during the course of a survey. In general you cannot expect to ever achieve 100% passing /redemption of coupons distributed. In most situations, approximately 30% of coupons are redeemed.

3. For instructions on how to develop the social network size question see Johnston 2013a; Johnston et al. 2014.

4. For instructions on coupon numbering see Johnston 2013a.

5. For instructions on formative research in RDS surveys see Johnston 2013a; Montealegre et al. 2014; Friberg and Horst 2014.

6. For instructions on screening respondents in RDS surveys see Johnston 2013a; Montealegre et al. 2014.

7. For instructions on incentives in RDS surveys see Johnston 2013a; Tyldum et al. 2014.

8. For more on RDS analysis see Johnston 2013a; Johnston and Luthra 2014; Montealegre et al. 2014.

9. For examples of documents used in RDS surveys see Johnston 2013a.

10. The size of the target population has a negligible effect on the size of the required sample if the sample size is relatively small compared to the size of the target population. Also, if all other factors remain constant, the size of the required sample increases, as the estimated point prevalence increases up to 50%. Note that the maximum required sample size is at the 50% prevalence estimate. Because of the characteristics of the sample size formula, the required sample size reduces for prevalence estimates above 50%.

11. Examples of RDS survey management forms are available in the manual (Johnston 2013a).

REFERENCES

Atkinson, R., and J. Flint. 2001. "Accessing Hidden and Hard-to-Reach Populations: Snowball Research Strategies." *Social Research Update* 33(1):1–4.

Bernhardt, A., R. Milkman, N. Theodore, D. Heckathorn, M. Auer, J. DeFilippis, A. Luz González, V. Narro, J. Perelshteyn, D. Polson, and M. Spiller. 2009. *Broken Laws, Unprotected Workers*. New York: National Employment Law Project.

Biernacki, P., and D. Waldorf. 1981. "Snowball Sampling: Problems and Techniques of Chain Referral Sampling." *Sociological Methods and Research* 10(2):141–63.

Erickson, B. H. 1979. "Some Problems of Inference from Chain Data." *Sociological Methodology* 10(1):276–302.

Friberg, J. H., and Eldring, L., eds. 2013. *Labour Migrants from Central and Eastern Europe in the Nordic Countries: Patterns of Migration, Working Conditions and Recruitment Practices*. Copenhagen: Norden.

Friberg, J. H., and C. Horst. 2014. "RDS and the Structure of Migrant Populations." G. Tyldum and L. G. Johnston (Eds.), *Applying Respondent Driven Sampling to Migrant Populations: Lessons from the Field*. London: Palgrave.

Friberg, J. H., and G. Tyldum. 2007. *Polonia i Oslo: En studie av arbeids- og levekår blant polakker i hovedstadsområdet*. Fafo-report 2007-27. Oslo: Fafo.

Gile, K. J., and M. S. Handcock. 2010. "Respondent-Driven Sampling: An Assessment of Current Methodology." *Sociological Methodology*, 40:285–327.

Gile K. J., L. G. Johnston, and M. J. Salganik. in press. "Diagnostics for Respondent-Driven Sampling." *Journal of the Royal Statistical Society*. http://arxiv.org/abs/1209.6254.

Hansen, J. A., and N. W. Hansen. 2009. "Polonia i København: Et studie af polske arbejdsmigranters løn-, arbejds- og levevilkår i Storkøbenhavn." *LO-dokumentation* 1.

Heckathorn, D. 1997. "Respondent Driven Sampling: A New Approach to the Study of Hidden Populations." *Social Problems* 44(2):174–99.

Heckathorn D. 2002. "Respondent Driven Sampling II: Deriving Valid Population Estimates from Chain-Referral Samples of Hidden Populations." *Sociological Problems* 49 (Suppl 1):11–34.

Heckathorn, D. 2007. "Extensions of Respondent Driven Sampling: Analysing Continuous Variables and Controlling for Differential Recruitment." *Social Methodology* 37(1):151–207.

Heckathorn, D., and J. E. Rosenstein. 2002. "Group Solidarity as the Product of Collective Action: Creation of Solidarity in a Population of Injection Drug Users." S. R. Thye and E. Lawler (Eds.), *Advances in Group Processes*. Vol. 19. London: Emerald Group. 37–66.

Johnston, L. G. 2013a. *Introduction to Respondent Driven Sampling*. Geneva: WHO. http://applications.emro.who.int/dsaf/EMRPUB_2013_EN_1539.pdf.

Johnston, L. G. 2013b. *HIV Integrated Behavioral and Biological Surveillance Surveys—Morocco 2013: Sub-Saharan Migrants in an Irregular Administrative Situation in Morocco*. Rabat, Morocco: UNAIDS. www.lisagjohnston.com.

Johnston, L. G., Y. H. Chen, A. Silva-Santisteban, and A. H. Raymond. 2013. "An Empirical Examination of Respondent Driven Sampling Design Effects among HIV Risk Groups from Studies Conducted around the World." *AIDS and Behavior* 17(6):2202–10.

Johnston L. G., and R. Luthra. 2014. "Analyzing data in RDS." G. Tyldum and L. G. Johnston (Eds.), *Applying Respondent Driven Sampling to Migrant Populations: Lessons from the Field.* London: Palgrave.

Johnston, L. G., M. Malekinejad, C. Kendall, I. M. Iuppa, and G. W. Rutherford. 2008. "Implementation Challenges to Using Respondent-Driven Sampling Methodology for HIV Biological and Behavioral Surveillance: Field Experiences in International Settings." *AIDS and Behavior* 12(4 Suppl):S131–41.

Johnston, L. G., D. Prybylski, H. F. Raymond, A. Mirzazadeh, C. Manopaiboon, and W. McFarland. 2013. "Incorporating the Service Multiplier Method in Respondent Driven Sampling Surveys to Estimate the Size of Hidden and Hard-to-Reach Populations: Case Studies from around the World." *Sexually Transmitted Diseases* 40(4):304–10.

Johnston L. G., L. Rodriguez, J., and Napierala. 2014. "Measuring Personal Network Size in RDS." G. Tyldum and L. G. Johnston (Eds.), *Applying Respondent Driven Sampling to Migrant Populations: Lessons from the Field.* London: Palgrave.

Johnston, L. G., T. R. Thurman, N. Mock, L. Nano, and V. Carcani. 2010. "Respondent-Driven Sampling: A New Method for Studying Street Children with Findings from Albania." *Vulnerable Children and Youth Studies* 5(1):1–11.

Johnston, L. G., S. Whitehead, M. Simic-Lawson, and C. Kendall. 2010. "Formative Research to Optimize Respondent-Driven Sampling Surveys among Hard-to-reach Populations in HIV Behavioral and Biological Surveillance: Lessons Learned from Four Case Studies." *AIDS Care* 22(6):784–92.

Khamsiriwatchara, A., P. Wangroongsarb, J. Thwing, J. Eliades, W. Satimai, C. Delacollette, and J. Kaewkungwal. 2011. "Respondent-Driven Sampling on the Thailand-Cambodia Border. I. Can Malaria Cases Be Contained in Mobile Migrant Workers?" *Malaria Journal* 10:120.

Kubal, A., I. Shvab, and A. Wojtynska. 2014. "Initiation of the RDS Recruitment Process: Seed Selection and Role." G. Tyldum and L. G. Johnston (Eds.), *Applying Respondent Driven Sampling to Migrant Populations: Lessons from the Field.* London: Palgrave.

Malekinejad, M., L. G. Johnston, C. Kendall, L. R. Kerr, M. R. Rifkin, and G. W. Rutherford. 2008. "Using Respondent-Driven Sampling Methodology for HIV Biological and Behavioral Surveillance in International Settings: A Systematic Review." *AIDS and Behavior* 12(4 Suppl):S105–30.

Montealegre, J. R., L. G. Johnston, C. Murrill, and E. Monterroso. 2013. "Respondent Driven Sampling for HIV Biological and Behavioral Surveillance in Latin America and the Caribbean." *AIDS and Behavior* 17(7); 2313–40.

Montealegre, J. R, L. G. Johnston, and K. Sabin 2011. "Letter to the Editor: Snowball Is not the Only Method for Sampling Refugees and Similar Populations." *BMC International Health and Human Rights* 11(2).

Montealegre J. R., J. M. Risser, and B. J. Selwyn. 2012. "Prevalence of HIV Risk Behaviors among Undocumented Central American Women in Houston, Texas." *AIDS and Behavior* 16(6):1641–48.

Montealegre, J. R., J. M. Risser, B. J. Selwyn, K. Sabin, and S. A. McCurdy. 2011. "HIV Testing Behaviors among Undocumented Central American Women in Houston, Texas." *Journal of Immigrant and Minority Health* 14(1):116–23.

Montealegre, J. R., A. Röder, and R. Ezzati. 2014. "Formative Assessment, Data Collection and Parallel Monitoring for RDS Fieldwork." G. Tyldum and L. G. Johnston (Eds.), *Applying Respondent Driven Sampling to Migrant Populations: Lessons from the Field.* London: Palgrave.

Mühlau, P., M. Kaliszewska, and A. Röder. (2011). *Polonia in Dublin: Preliminary Report of Survey Findings—Demographic Overview.* Dublin: Employment Research Centre.

Ramirez-Valles, J., D. D. Heckathorn, R. Vázquez, R. M. Diaz, and R. T. Campbell. 2005. "From Networks to Populations: The Development and Application of Respondent-Driven Sampling among IDUs and Latino Gay Men." *AIDS and Behavior* 9(4):387–402.

Rodriguez, L. 2009. "Economic Adaptation and the Self-Employment Experience of Nigerian Immigrants in New York City." PhD diss., Pennsylvania State University.

Salganik, M. J., and D. Heckathorn. 2004. "Sampling and Estimation in Hidden Populations Using Respondent-Driven Sampling." *Sociological Methodology* 34:193–240.

Semaan, S., S. Santibanez, R. S. Garfein, D. D. Heckathorn, and D. C. Des Jarlais. 2008. "Ethical and Regulatory Considerations in HIV Prevention Studies Employing Respondent-Driven Sampling." *International Journal of Drug Policy* 20(1):14–27.

Sudman, S., and G. Kalton. 1986. "New Developments in the Sampling of Special Populations." *Annual Review of Sociology* 12:401–29.

Sudman, S., M. G. Sirken, and C. D. Cowan. 1988. "Sampling Rare and Elusive Populations." *Science* 240(4855):991–96.

Þórarinsdóttir, H., and A. Wojtyńska. 2011. *Polonia Reykjavik 2010: Preliminary Report.* Reykjavik: MIRRA.

Tyldum, G., and L. G. Johnston, eds. 2014. *Applying Respondent Driven Sampling to Migrant Populations: Lessons from the Field.* London: Palgrave.

Tyldum G., L. Rodriguez, I. Bjørkhaug, and A. Wojtynska. 2014. "Deciding on and Distributing Incentives in RDS." G. Tyldum and L. G. Johnston (Eds.), *Applying Respondent Driven Sampling to Migrant Populations: Lessons from the Field.* London: Palgrave.

Volz, E., and D. D. Heckathorn. 2008. "Probability Based Estimation Theory for Respondent Driven Sampling." *Journal of Official Statistics* 24(1):79–97.

Wejnert, C., H. Pham, N. Krishna, B. Le, and E. DiNenno. 2012. "Estimating Design Effect and Calculating Sample Size for Respondent-Driven Sampling Studies of Injection Drug Users in the United States." *AIDS and Behavior* 16(4):797–806.

WHO/UNAIDS. 2010. Estimating the Size of Populations Most at Risk for HIV Infection. Geneva: WHO/UNAIDS. http://www.who.int/hiv/pub/surveillance/estimating_populations_HIV_risk/en/index.html.

Zhang, S. X. (2012). *Trafficking of Migrant Laborers in San Diego County: Looking for a Hidden Population.* San Diego: San Diego State University.

The findings and conclusions in this chapter are those of the authors and do not necessarily represent the views of the Centers for Disease Control and Prevention.

8

Time-Space Sampling of Migrant
Populations

Salaam Semaan
Elizabeth DiNenno

INTRODUCTION

Time-space sampling (TSS), also known as time-location sampling, through use of venue-based sampling, is a probability-based sampling method useful for investigating well-defined populations that congregate at specific locations and times. Since the early 1990s, researchers have gained extensive experience with implementing TSS of hard-to-reach populations. TSS has been especially useful in sampling persons at risk for HIV infection, a hard-to-reach population in the United States (Mackellar et al. 2007; Marpsat and Razafindratsima 2010; Semaan et al. 2002; Semaan 2010). This extensive experience with TSS in HIV-related projects can be leveraged and tailored for sampling migrant populations, which are also often hard-to-reach from a sampling perspective. TSS can serve as an effective approach that takes advantage of congregation patterns of migrant populations.

We consider the challenges in surveying migrant populations statistically and sociologically (Kish 1991). Statistically, traditional sampling frames that list individual members of migrant populations are not usually available because it is difficult to construct these frames for those populations (Lepkowski 1991; Sudman et al. 1988). From a sociological perspective, migrant populations can be linked by nationality, race or ethnicity, socioeconomic conditions, societal structures, cultural bonds, or common experiences and behaviors (see chapter 1 by Schenker, and chapter 2, by Rodriguez-Lainz and Castañeda, in this volume). Migrant populations may refrain from moderate or heavy involvement in majority social institutions for social reasons (e.g., stigma, discrimination, culture) or legal reasons (e.g., illegal status or behaviors).

Simple or stratified random sampling or multistage cluster sampling, used when it is possible to construct complete sampling frames that list individual members of the target population, are typically used with door-to-door household surveys, telephone surveys, or facility-based surveys (Lepkowski 1991). Effective adaptations of household and telephone surveys of migrant populations can overcome certain cost and implementation concerns of probability sampling of migrant populations (Levy and Lemshow 1991; also see chapter 10, by Grant et al., and chapter 6, by Marcelli, in this volume). Nonetheless, considerable costs and resources of household or facility-based surveys can encourage public health and other professionals to use TSS with migrant populations (Wasserman 2005).

The purpose of this chapter is to explore the purpose, procedures, advantages, and disadvantages of using TSS with migrant populations. We highlight important factors for the successful application of TSS, including relevant factors in different sampling phases (presampling, during sampling, and postsampling). We also discuss specific considerations (e.g., logistical, regulatory, legal, and ethical) that can enhance TSS of migrant populations and lead to the production of representative samples and generalizable results.

PURPOSE OF TIME-SPACE SAMPLING

TSS is intended to produce estimates of populations when sampling frames (i.e., lists) of individual members of those populations do not exist or are difficult to construct. Venue-day-time units (VDTs) (e.g., a given location, such as an ethnic grocery store, Tuesday, 9 A.M. to 12 P.M.), representing the universe of venues (i.e., locations), days, and times of congregation of defined populations form the sampling frame. In TSS, the probability of sampling depends on the frequency with which participants attend a specific venue. In probability sampling methods (e.g., simple random sampling) or in probability-household or facility-based surveys, the probability of sampling depends on the population from which the sample is drawn.

TSS differs from two other sampling methods that use locations as the basis for sampling and recruiting participants (Levy and Lemshow 1991). In facility-based probability sampling, investigators use a sampling frame of individual members in each facility. The list already exists or can be easily constructed to select participants randomly. In convenience sampling carried out in a facility, participants are selected because they are readily distinguished, identified, or available in that facility.

PROCEDURES OF TIME-SPACE SAMPLING

TSS proceeds in four main phases: (1) the formative phase, (2) the preparatory phase, (3) the sampling phase, and (4) the analytic phase (Mackellar et al. 2007; Muhib et al. 2001; Semaan 2010).

Formative Phase

The goal of the formative phase is to collect information on the target population and its demographics, including information on how best to interact with the population and communicate study goals to stakeholders. This phase focuses on conducting formative research, including collection of ethnographic data, interviews with key informants, and analysis of indicator data (i.e., proxy variables) that describe population characteristics. Indicator data on the target population can include sociodemographic characteristics (e.g., racial and ethnic composition, age and gender distribution, country of origin, migration patterns, and language and culture of the population), access challenges to the target population at public venues, and anticipated responses of the target population to recruitment intercepts in public venues.

The formative phase enhances tailoring TSS procedures to address the contextual and diverse factors that characterize migrant populations. This phase provides information that defines the population of interest, information on ways to access the population, and information on specific attributes related to project goals (e.g., the public health topic of interest). Relevant information includes socioeconomic strata and sociodemographic characteristics of the population, geographic areas and identifiable venues where the target population congregates, the level of stigma experienced by the population and its migration and legal status and health needs, and the communities where the population lives, works, and socializes.

Preparatory Phase

During the preparatory phase, staff members identify all the venues where the target migrant populations congregate. Typically, venues include community-based organizations, places of worship, social and cultural organizations, street locations, markets, stores, bars, cafes, restaurants, dance clubs, brothels, beaches, parks, farms, and other sites where a specific population congregates. Ensuring that all venues or a high proportion of venues attended by the target population are included in the sampling frame increases the likelihood of obtaining a heterogeneous and representative sample of the target population, and adds sampling rigor. It is worth noting that not all venues are equal from a sampling perspective. The goal of TSS is to ensure that all members of the population who go to venues could be sampled in the forthcoming sampling phase. Thus, getting access to a hard-to-reach venue whose users are similar to those of a venue that has already been included may not be worth the effort. However, if the users of that venue have unique characteristics and do not visit other venues included in the sampling frame, an extra effort to get access to that venue can be worthwhile. Once a venue is identified, the appropriate day and time (day-time) periods are investigated to determine the most advantageous blocks of time (e.g., 4 hours or 2 hours) to recruit individuals into the study. A four-hour time period is often used as a standard period because it can maximize yield of participants (i.e., number of surveys completed) without overburdening staff. A two-hour time frame can be used in heavily attended venues to ensure that staff members are not overburdened by recruitment for a longer duration, such as four hours.

During the preparatory phase, staff members canvass all the venues that were enumerated during this phase to assess (typically by using a hand tally counter, such as a clicker) the number of persons who seem to belong to the target population and can potentially be recruited during specific day-time periods. The "primary enumeration" assessment allows staff members to determine whether the venues identified through the formative phase are indeed attended by the migrant population. This first assessment is generally sufficient to ensure that the proper day-time periods are chosen for venues that are known to have large numbers of the target population. However, for new venues or for those where the number and frequency of attendees are unknown, staff members may conduct brief screening interviews to estimate, for each VDT period, the number and proportion of persons who meet eligibility criteria. In this assessment, staff members attempt to interview all persons whom they intercept during a shorter time period (e.g., 1 hour) in a given venue, through brief "street intercepts." During these intercepts and brief interviews, staff members ask a very limited number of questions to ascertain whether there are enough potentially eligible persons attending the venue to characterize it as an efficient venue for recruiting the target population during the forthcoming sampling phase. The brief street intercepts, which are subsequent to participants' informed consent, allow for collecting relevant data such as the number of migrant persons who attend the venues and their country of birth; occupation, gender, racial, ethnic, and age distribution; and other characteristics (e.g., migrant status) that are not visible by observation or known to key informants. This assessment (sometimes referred to as "secondary enumeration") is useful for estimating the effective yield, defined as the potential number of interviews a VDT can generate during a forthcoming sampling event (e.g., a 4-hour period).

The preparatory phase allows staff members to determine whether TSS is logistically feasible by identifying enough viable and safe venues to approach the target population. During this phase, staff members can learn about logistical needs or challenges that can be encountered during forthcoming sampling events (e.g., safety, privacy, traffic patterns, and other concurrent activities that can support or impede sampling and data collection) and can plan for how best to address such needs or challenges. The preparatory phase, which facilitates assessment of attendance habits of the target population at the listed venues, also facilitates determination of whether exclusion of venues with low attendance or inaccessible venues would create selection bias, and the staff decision about whether a higher budget (e.g., more staff, more time) is needed.

Sampling Phase

During the sampling phase, staff members may use a two-stage process. This process involves constructing a monthly sampling frame of sampling events and VDTs and recruiting participants to attain the a priori–determined sample size desired for the project. Staff members decide how many VDTs can be scheduled in a given month, based on staff availability and schedules. First, venues are sampled at random (Finlayson et al. 2011) or by using a probability proportional to the potential number of eligible persons at each listed venue (Karon and Wejnert 2012). Random selection of venues reduces selection bias (e.g., by including both easily and not-so-easily accessible venues). A stratified sample of venues can also be used by sampling within venue strata or types (e.g., social or clinical venues; geographically defined venues; small or large venues). Next, staff members randomly select day-time periods from the list of all possible day-time periods for each venue (table 8.1). The day-time periods, identified during the preparatory phase, refer to those periods when venue attendance is expected to be reasonably high, adequate, representative of the population, and can provide optimal participation in data collection.

Following these steps, staff members engage in sampling and data collection at each selected VDT through random or systematic sampling of participants. Staff members may count and consecutively intercept every person or every Kth person entering an intercept zone. A recruitment zone is an intercept zone, characterized by an imaginary line or as a geographically defined area, through which the target population passes, and can be counted and subsequently approached by study staff.

Following informed consent, staff members screen prospective participants, invite eligible participants to learn more about the project, carry out the data collection process, and collect relevant data on those who refuse or withdraw from participation. Participants who refuse to participate in data collection (e.g., responses, "I do not have time," "I am not interested," "I do not want to leave my friends") can differ in their characteristics from those who agree to participate. Selective participation can be associated with selection bias. Although it may be difficult to collect data on the number of those who refused to participate in data collection and on their reasons, project staff should attempt to gather and record this data. Persons who indicate to staff members their willingness and agreement to learn more about the project are taken to a secure private area inside the venue or to a van used for the study and are presented with information about the study and with the consent forms.

Different terms are used to describe the sampling phase. "Enumeration" refers to counting all persons who cross into a recruitment zone; "intercept" refers to approaching and speaking with randomly or systematically selected persons; "determining eligibility" through a "screener" refers to asking questions to assess

TABLE 8.1 Venue and VDT Identification Samples

Venue ID	Venue Name[a]	Address[a]	Contact[a]	Phone number/email	Observations					Enumerations					Interviews with stakeholder	
					Age distribution	Gender distribution	Safety issues	Venue owner approval	Barriers to interviewing/viewing/recruiting	Primary or secondary	Date/time of enumeration	Count during enumeration period	% ineligible (nonmigrant)[b]	VDT produces ≥8 eligible persons?	Suitable, safe venue?	VDTs with high attendance
B001	Woody's Barbershop	1234 Walnut St.	Bryan (manager)	xxx-xxxx	All ages	Mostly male	N	Y	Crowded recruiting	1	2/22/08, 2:00–2:30 P.M.	30	N/A	Y	Y	Thurs.–Sat., 12:00 P.M.–5:00 A.M.
C028	Esposito's Resturant	123 St 4th st.	Robert (owner)	xxx-xxxx	Old	50/50	N	Y	None	1	2/28/08, 5:00–5:30 P.M.	16	N/A	Y	Y	Tues.–Sat., 5:00 P.M.–9 P.M.
P001	Memorial Park	34 W. 123th St.	N/A	N/A	Mixed	Mostly male	Y	N/A	HIV testing difficult	1	2/15/2008, 12:30–1:30 P.M.	4	N/A	N	N	N/A
P001	Memorial Park	34 W. 123th St.	N/A	N/A	Young	50/50	Y	N/A	Requires mobile unit	2	2/16/08, 10:00–11:00 P.M.	88	12%	Y	Y	Sat., 10 P.M.–2 A.M.
D002	Rita's Beauty Shop	123 E. 4th	Leslie	xxx-xxxx	Young	Female	N	Y	Very large space	None	N/A	N/A	N/A	Y	Y	Wed.–Fri., 10 A.M.–2 P.M.
X001	Corner of 14th and Callowhill	14th and Callowhill	3rd ward police dept.	xxx-xxxx	Mixed	50/50	Y	N/A	Dark	2	2/18/08, 9:00–10:00 P.M.	32	21%	Y	Y	Wed.–Sun., 8–12 P.M.
C94	Garden Shoppe	123 Meridian	Clarke Smith	xxx-xxxx	Mixed	Mostly female	N	Y	Small space; HIV testing difficult	2	3/1/2008, 4:00–4:30 P.M.	16	30%	Y	N	N/A
O001	The Club	22nd and Front	Kim	xxx-xxxx	Mixed	50/50	N	Y	None	2	3/20/2008, 2:00–2:30 P.M.	8	0%	Y	Y	Mon.–Sat., 2–6 P.M.

NOTE: N/A means not applicable.
[a] All names of persons and places are fictional.

whether the intercepted persons meet participation criteria; "enrollment" refers to asking persons to participate in the study following their consent; and "completion of the survey" refers to the participant's provision of data for the survey.

Analytic Phase

TSS can produce a probability-based sample of the target population when each venue has a known chance of inclusion, when members of the target population do indeed attend the venues during the day-time periods listed in the sampling frame, and when eligible participants are enrolled in the survey and provide data, with no bias in selection of VDTs or in selection of participants.

Staff members can consider relevant factors in evaluating the success of TSS. These factors include extent of coverage of the target population, range (e.g., strata, type) of venues covered, extent of recruitment during the sampling events, number of completed interviews or surveys by type of venues, and characteristics of the sample (Pollack et al. 2005). Other examples for the process evaluation of TSS include the number of sampling events needed to achieve the sample size given staff availability and workload, effect of weather conditions on recruitment and on duration of the fieldwork (including the sampling phase), number of participants at each VDT (which can be used for producing weights for relevant variables), number and percentage of intercepts attempted (based on random or systematic sampling), number of intercepts completed, number and reasons for refusing to participate, number of eligible respondents who were enrolled, and number of completed interviews. A cutoff point of 80% or higher for intercepts is often used as a good target—to minimize participation bias and selection bias. A cutoff point of 70% or higher of the eligible target population who participated in data collection can be a good target—to reduce participation bias. A reasonably large percentage (50% or more) of venues listed in the sampling frame is also a good target for the sampling phase.

Other performance-evaluation criteria may include the duration of data collection (e.g., 6 to 12 months), the number of completed sampling events per month (e.g., at least 14 sampling events per month), the minimum number of completed interviews per sampling event (e.g., 4), the completion of all (100%) sampling events, and the achievement of the required sample size based on a priori sample size calculations (Finlayson et al. 2011).

In analyzing selection biases, staff members need to examine the data collected during the screening and core (sampling phase) surveys. For example, it is important to compute overall attendance rates and participation rates by different strata, or types of venues, and to compare (e.g., by venue type) a priori selected characteristics of participants, especially those characteristics that are associated with project outcomes. Staff members can assess extent of participation in the screening and core interviews and reasons for refusal or withdrawal for each venue stratum or "type" (e.g., participation at bars or clubs vs. religious events). Determining whether number and characteristics of those who refused participation produce selection bias and assessing representativeness of the selected sample by comparing data collected through TSS with other datasets (e.g., a similar sampling strategy in a different setting or a different sampling strategy in a similar setting, information gathered during the formative phase) can assist project staff in detecting selection bias and the extent of generalizability of results (Kendall et al. 2008; Kral et al. 2010; Lavange et al. 2010; McKenzie 2007; McKenzie and Mistiaen 2009; Platt et al. 2006; Quaglia and Vivier 2010; Robinson et al. 2006).

Additionally, in analyzing selection bias, staff members can use data collected through the screening and core surveys. The questionnaire(s) should, therefore, include questions on mobility patterns of respondents (attendance patterns affect probability of selection) because participants can potentially attend several venues and have unequal venue attendance patterns (resulting in frequent attendees being more likely to be intercepted at a certain venue than others). These selection probabilities greatly influence the precision of estimates of outcomes and accordingly may need to be incorporated statistically in the analysis. Respondents can be queried about their frequency of attendance, not only of the venue at which they were recruited but also of all other venues listed in the sampling frame (Karon and Wejnert 2012). Questions can also address whether some participants (e.g., women) or other groups (e.g., certain racial or ethnic groups) are less likely to agree to an interview because they have less time to take a survey or are less willing to participate in a survey. Different methods for producing weights and for statistical adjustment can be used when study outcomes are associated with attendance of venues and when VDTs have heterogeneous attendance patterns (Kalton 2009; Karon and Wejnert 2012; MacKellar et al. 1996, 2007; Muhib et al. 2001; van Griensven et al. 2005).

To treat the visitor as the unit of analysis, data on unequal selection probabilities must be collected and analyzed (Mackellar et al. 2007). This analysis is relevant because during each monthly sampling event, many members of the defined population may revisit the venues, providing for multiple chances of selection, while others may rarely visit the venues listed in the sampling frame. Accordingly, a weighted analysis can be used, where the weight represents the inverse of the participant's selection probability as determined by attendance data of VDTs (Karon and Wejnert 2012; Mackellar et al. 2007). Differences in attendance patterns of VDTs can introduce different sampling probabilities and clustering of participants as defined by participant characteristics and behaviors. Thus during the last phase, the analytic phase, sampling-related variables and data are assessed and analyzed using relevant weights on the basis of data collected during the sampling phase.

Staff members need to examine whether it is necessary to statistically adjust the data obtained in studies that use TSS to enhance the validity of the data obtained and analyzed and the results of the study (Jenness et al. 2011). In general, TSS produces many small clusters of participants rather than a few large homogenous clusters, which tends to minimize design effects and changes between crude and adjusted estimates of outcomes of interest. Staff members need to assess the need to use statistical programs that incorporate intraclass correlations (representing the effect of clustering), which arise when persons at VDTs have homogenous characteristics. Because responses from homogenous groups have a propensity to provide data that are correlated (referred to as "intraclass correlation"), the variance of estimates could be underestimated if this correlation is ignored in statistical analyses (Levy and Lemshow 1991). As a result, the apparent precision of information can be overestimated. Thus, considering the magnitude and effect of clustering and of unequal probability of selection on statistical results is important (Karon and Wejnert 2012).

Thus, in sum, important steps in the successful implementation of TSS include (1) operational procedures (e.g., defining eligibility criteria, using appropriate incentives), (2) design procedures (e.g., characterizing extent and nature of VDTs), and (3) analytic procedures (e.g., using weights to adjust for unequal probability of selection).

ADVANTAGES AND DISADVANTAGES OF TIME-SPACE SAMPLING

TSS offers several advantages for sampling migrant populations. TSS allows investigators to identify venues where the target migrant population congregates, obtain a large, diverse sample, and generalize the results from the survey to the migrant population of interest who attend those venues. TSS also allows for identifying venues where migrant populations can receive services, if service delivery is a project goal (E. Negro-Calduch et al. 2008). In addition, TSS can be used to collect biologic samples from participants; mobile units located at or close to the venues are particularly useful for this purpose. Furthermore, TSS can be reproducible in many areas and over time, an important consideration in multicity or multiyear projects (Semaan et al. 2002). The sampling design can be repeated during the project period in multiyear projects, thus enhancing internal validity and providing an opportunity for including participants in relevant interventions.

When it is not possible to construct sampling frames for probability sampling of participants (e.g., simple, stratified, or cluster sampling) or network-based sampling (Semaan et al. 2010; Spreen and Swaagstra 1994), TSS can serve as a viable strategy for sampling migrant populations. Formative research and ethnographic surveys can shed light on the assimilation patterns of the migrant population and its congregation habits and on the feasibility of TSS by identifying the venues where the migrant population congregates (Mills et al. 2004). Staff members can examine the congregation and assimilation patterns based on data collected during the formative and preparatory phases to assess the utility of TSS as a sampling strategy.

Venue identification provides information on the geographic and spatial distribution of the migrant population and on the characteristics, behaviors, and needs of venue users. TSS can be the method of choice when migrant populations congregate in accessible and identifiable VDTs, when it is feasible to create a list of all venues and their related day-time periods, when it is feasible to access the eligible population at these VDTs, and when it is possible to collect data on sampling-related variables for calculating weights to produce outcome estimates for the target population. The presence of institutions that support migrant populations (e.g., ethnic- or nationality-based institutions such as consulates, hometown organizations, community groups, ethnic grocery stores, places of worship, social sites) can greatly facilitate implementation of TSS. Staff members should work with these institutions to get their support to conduct TSS. For migrant populations with low congregation patterns (e.g., few and geographically disparate venues), TSS may not be appropriate (e.g., migrant populations living in rural areas, racial or ethnic minority migrant populations).

Migrant populations should not be considered as one entity for sampling purposes. Because migrant populations are not a homogenous group and are linguistically and culturally diverse, there are differences among subgroups of migrant populations in their association patterns with other each other and with other populations. Some migrant populations may associate only with immediate family members or business groups and may avoid migrants from their country of origin. Other migrant populations may associate only with migrants from their country of origin and avoid those from other countries.

Several factors can enhance the success and rigor of TSS, including whether all venues were included in the sampling frame and whether the number of the migrant population attending or congregating at each venue during the designated day-time period could be estimated. Staff members can determine the proportional allocation of the selected sample between different types of venues (e.g., business strata, recreational strata, clinical strata). A multisite study showed the importance of understanding key differences in the types of venues preferred by young males and females; for example, female-preferred venues were closer to their homes (Chutuape et al. 2008).

Given potentially changing circumstances that can affect the sampling process (e.g., changes in attendance patterns influenced by weather or by social, economic, or legal factors), there is often a need to continually identify new VDTs and to evaluate the potential yield of VDTs already listed in the sampling frame (Thompson & Collins 2002). Sampling projects conducted over a period of several months often require monthly reconstruction of the sampling frame of VDTs and development of sampling-event calendars to organize deployment of staff members (Mackellar et al. 2007).

In terms of rigor, TSS can approximate probability sampling, especially when weights are used to overcome selection biases, because venues serve as proxy settings for randomly selecting participants and because TSS can allow for inferences to be made about the target population. TSS can resemble a multistage cluster sample when people in the cluster (e.g., those attending randomly selected VDTs) have a known chance of being sampled randomly at each sampling event and when staff members can use weights to estimate outcomes of interest (e.g., prevalence of disease or risk behaviors in that population).

TSS allows for sampling migrant populations in circumstances where exhaustive sampling frames of individual members of the migrant population do not exist, without unduly delaying data collection or incurring inordinately high costs. Because TSS takes advantage of the attendance patterns of migrant populations in a universe of venues at identifiable and specific days and times, random or stratified selection of VDTs and random or systematic sampling of the target population (e.g., by using selection rules for potential respondents that are feasible in the field) at the selected VDTs adds sampling rigor.

Similar to other sampling methods, TSS can be used to estimate the size (e.g., total number of individuals) of a migrant population. Capture-recapture methods use two or more independent samples, or data sources, of the target population, with one sample being representative of that population (Heimer and White 2010; International Working Group for Disease Monitoring and Forecasting 1995). Independent samples, or data sources, are especially useful when estimates from one source fail to include all individuals of the target population.

There are, however, disadvantages of TSS. Because implementing TSS requires developing a complete list of venues, TSS advantages can also be labeled as disadvantages. It is very likely that some members of the target population will never or rarely attend the venues listed in the sampling frame, and, therefore, can be excluded from the sample. Including only venues that are easily accessible to the target population can produce selection bias, especially if characteristics of persons who attend venues differ substantially (e.g., by race, gender, or other variables associated with outcomes of interest) from those of persons who do not attend venues or from those of persons who are not easily identifiable or approachable at the venues and were, therefore, excluded from project participation. In such cases, results need to be interpreted as limited to the venues or to the population who attended the venues listed in the sampling frame, unless data were collected and weights were developed to estimate probability of attendance across the universe of venues and the intended target population.

TSS cannot capture people who do not attend any venue, for example, homeless persons who are migrants and who do not use outreach services or shelter accommodations. Accounting for their characteristics and how such characteristics might influence study results is important. Varied attendance at venues by members of the target population can affect selection bias, especially in multiyear studies. Thus, a potential TSS limitation includes having results that are limited or generalizable only to accessible venues, venue attendees, and to more visible or active members of the target population. Lack of access to a substantial percentage of venues can provide biased results. For this reason, obtaining permission from proprietors and venue owners to access as many venues as possible can increase their acceptance to conduct data collection at selected VDTs. Increasing cooperation of venue managers can be enhanced by conducting activities that build trust and relationships, such as sponsoring relevant events at the venues, providing healthful materials, and assisting with community needs (e.g., referrals to health services). Because of the new relationships that staff members or migrant populations need to develop with each other or with research institutions and activities, presence of staff members at venues, including during selected day-time periods, might increase migrant populations' trust of staff members and of their professional disciplines, domains, and research, including public health.

Collecting data (e.g., questions on venue attendance, particularly the frequency with which a person attends each type of venue listed in the sampling frame) can be instrumental in assessing the impact of attendance patterns on the validity of the data collected (Karon and Wejnert 2012). Development of TSS sampling plans requires sufficient knowledge of the target migrant population and communities, intense fieldwork for enumeration of venues, training bilingual and culturally sensitive interviewers, and thorough supervision of the sampling process and procedures. Formative research can help in understanding the level of remuneration that would be appropriate, but not coercive, to motivate project participation of both economically disadvantaged and well-off migrant populations.

Disadvantages of TSS include logistical challenges, particularly enumeration of all venues and their associated day-time periods through extensive initial formative and ethnographic research and fieldwork. Nevertheless, once information on VDTs or mapping of VDTs is completed, TSS can be used in subsequent studies that can include periodic updates of VDTs, as necessary, especially when certain venues or VDTs become less popular or when new venues or VDTs emerge. The research goals and data collection activities may be incompatible with the purpose of activities occurring naturally at the venues, which may yield low participation rates or pose security threats to project staff (e.g., late-night VDTs). Racial-ethnic minority-focused venues or venues for young racial-ethnic migrant populations can be rare, or located in remote or dispersed locations, which can reduce the efficiency of data collection, especially if most venues in the sampling frame are only available at the same day-time periods of the week. TSS may not be appropriate for sizeable migrant populations with very complex congregation and mobility patterns; for example,

Mexican-born residents in Los Angeles County. However, even in such instances, TSS can be used to complement other sampling methods, or it can be used in specific venues (e.g., consulates). The type of venues and their related activities may impact decisions on the length of the questionnaire used in data collection and on the time available for interviewing and data collection. For example, in venues where participants are entering and exiting rapidly, a long questionnaire may not be viable.

In sum, recognizing the potential logistical needs of TSS and making plans to address them before TSS implementation can enhance the generalizability of results. Critical resources such as expertise in the content and topical areas of the project, characteristics of the target population, theoretical and practical aspects of sampling, and in logistical, regulatory, legal, and ethical aspects of sampling can enhance success of TSS of migrant populations.

STUDIES OF TIME-SPACE SAMPLING OF MIGRANT POPULATIONS

The success of TSS projects with migrant populations can be enhanced through relevant planning, execution, and evaluation. TSS can be used in sampling various groups of migrant populations, including immigrants, refugees, deportees, temporary workers, mobile populations, and displaced people (e.g., through war, famine, political or social upheaval, and natural disasters). Data collected through TSS of migrant populations in different research studies (e.g., injury prevention, environmental health, mental health) can be used to develop interventions to enhance the health and well-being of migrant populations. In such projects, venues for farmworkers, for example, can include farms where migrants work and migrant camps where migrants live. Venues for day laborers can include street corners, construction sites, or home improvement stores. Venues for international migrant border crossers can include congregation sites at ports of entry. Venues for migrant truck drivers can include bus stops and truck stops. Staff members should also consider cultural festivals, places of worship, and ethnic stores for recruiting migrant populations with diverse backgrounds.

TSS can be used in HIV-related research with migrant populations such as migrant males who have sex with men, migrant sex workers, and migrant populations who use or inject drugs or engage in other high-risk behaviors. Different studies of migrant populations, including those that have not used TSS, highlight practical considerations and relevant sampling venues (Deren et al. 2003, 2005; Hernandez et al. 2009; Rangel et al. 2006).

Three studies have used TSS with migrant populations in states with substantial migrant populations (Fernandez et al. 2005; Kissinger et al. 2008; Valenzuela 2002). The samples ranged in size from 180 to almost 500, and venues ranged substantially in number, between 3 and 87. Valenzuela (2002) conducted a face-to-face survey with 481 day laborers in 87 venues in Los Angeles and Orange Counties in California. Fernández et al. (2005) recruited 244 male and female Hispanic migrant-seasonal farmworkers in southern Miami-Dade County, Florida. Kissinger et al. (2008) recruited a sample of 180 Latino migrant workers on weekends during August and September 2006 in New Orleans. The studies used a wide range of venues (e.g., labor pickup sites, home improvement stores, churches, soccer stadiums, work sites, camps, fields, parks, and markets) and followed TSS methods. However, each study treated the sample as a simple random sample (e.g., did not use weights to account for unequal probability of participants' attendance of venues). It is unclear from the articles if the authors collected sampling data that would have allowed for calculating and using weights in data analysis.

CONTEXTUAL FACTORS AFFECTING TSS OF MIGRANT POPULATIONS

Conducting health-related TSS projects with migrant population is important for the development of interventions intended to protect and promote the health of migrant populations and to increase their access to health care (Arcury and Quandt 2007). Early detection and treatment of infectious and chronic diseases and better access to prevention and care provide enormous clinical and public health benefits to migrant populations (Cashman et al. 2011; Louther et al. 2011; Magis-Rodriguez et al. 2009; Rabito et al. 2011). Public health prevention and treatment programs for migrant populations are based on both human rights and public health principles (e.g., enabling people to remain socially and economically active and healthy).

As with any other population, different factors affect the lives and well-being of migrant populations (Campbell et al. 2011; Ramo et al. 2010; Wasserman 2005). Understanding the circumstances and heterogeneity of migrant populations can lead to better TSS experiences and outcomes, especially in public health projects. Some migrant populations may fear speaking with public health staff conducting surveys, mistaking them for immigration agents and fearing immigration authorities and deportation (Hardy et al. 2012). As a result of vulnerable economic status, some migrant populations experience mental distress, a great sense of vulnerability and anonymity, and physical, social, or cultural isolation (Das-Munshi et al. 2012). These experiences, along with environmental conditions (e.g., loss of familiar social environments, long working hours, changes in social networks), can sometimes lead people to engage in high-risk behaviors (influencing exposure to infectious diseases) and in lifestyle risk factors (influencing risk for chronic diseases) (Kissinger et al. 2012; Parrado et al. 2004; Rabito et al. 2011; Ramo et al. 2010). However, risk for infectious and chronic diseases varies by type and reason for migration, gender, and age, as well as by other social and economic factors

(Rachlis et al. 2007; Stauffer et al. 2012). Female migrants, for example, may experience different social and economic factors than migrant males. Some women may migrate due to discrimination and lack of opportunities in their countries or regions of origin. Male and female migrants who work in low-skilled jobs or illegally, particularly in unregulated sectors such as domestic employment, may be at risk for violence, poor working conditions, sexual exploitation, and poor health.

Staff members need to understand contextual factors that affect TSS sampling of migrant populations, including the vulnerable legal and economic status of migrant populations. This understanding can improve the willingness of migrant populations to participate in research projects and enhance the validity of the collected data. Migrant populations, particularly illegal migrants, may experience stigma and discrimination, which can reduce project participation. Additionally, the great variations in self-perceived health and in utilization of health services may affect project participation. These contextual factors can be magnified by taboos regarding certain behaviors or health conditions and can influence the validity of the data.

TIME-SPACE SAMPLING OF NONMIGRANT POPULATIONS

TSS has been used in the United States in HIV-related projects with hard-to-reach populations since the early 1990s. TSS was used to recruit men who have sex with men (MSM) in an HIV behavioral intervention research study of young MSM in five cities in the United States (Mackellar et al. 1996). Shortly thereafter, TSS was used in sampling young MSM in survey research (Muhib et al. 2001). TSS was subsequently used to sample MSM for a US national behavioral surveillance project in seventeen to twenty-three metropolitan areas in the United States (Mackellar et al. 2007). TSS continues to be used in the National HIV Behavioral System with MSM (Finlayson et al. 2011; Oster et al. 2011). TSS was used to sample other populations, including Latino MSM (Stueve et al. 2001), young (13–24) lesbian, gay, bisexual, transgender, and heterosexual youth in a study of tobacco use, and heterosexual persons at high risk for HIV infection (Remafedi et al. 2008, DiNenno et al. 2012). Internationally, TSS was used with diverse hard-to-reach populations; for example, sex workers in Congo (Kayembe et al. 2008) and Kenya (Geibel et al. 2008) and truck drivers in northeast Brazil (Ferreira et al. 2008). TSS experiences with diverse populations highlight the importance of practical considerations for planning and implementing TSS of migrant populations.

PRACTICAL CONSIDERATIONS OF TIME-SPACE SAMPLING OF MIGRANT POPULATIONS

Similar to other sampling methods, TSS has important, often coexisting, logistical, regulatory, legal, and ethical considerations that influence sampling of migrant populations (Semaan et al. 2010). Each consideration needs relevant safeguards that are specific to five dimensions: (1) the defined population of interest, especially when it is a hard-to-reach population; (2) the particular topic of the project, especially sensitive, private, or potentially stigmatizing topics (e.g., illegal status, illegal use of drugs, intimate and personal behaviors); (3) the study procedures, particularly those that carry social stigma (e.g., testing for a particular infection or disease, questions about domestic violence); (4) the regulatory nature of the project (e.g., research or surveillance), often subject to regulatory requirements, ethical principles, policies, procedures, and scientific standards; and (5) several considerations of sampling or of TSS (e.g., eligibility criteria, remuneration levels). Reports on each of these five dimensions as they relate to a particular topic and target population (e.g., data from sex workers who are migrants of a certain region or country on use of condoms) have appeared in the scientific literature and can be useful in highlighting relevant procedures and safeguards for TSS.

Regarding logistical procedures, safeguards include extensive field experience of staff with migrant populations and attention to local and cultural factors that influence fieldwork. Staff members need to be sensitive to norms governing interactions and discussions of high-risk behaviors or health conditions. The diversity of migrant populations should be reflected in hiring and training project staff. Partnerships with local community-based organizations and public health systems, and use of linguistically and culturally appropriate data collection instruments and mechanisms can help in increasing success of TSS. Equally important is the need to train project staff in the sampling strategy and procedures, and to consider and implement strategies to boost participation in the screening and core interviews (e.g., remuneration, incentives, appointments for interviews, privacy of data collection). Well-trained and experienced sampling managers are instrumental for supervising the sampling process and for carrying out the sampling process efficiently and effectively, including implementing corrective measures, as needed (Barnhart et al. 2010).

Sample size for TSS studies can affect logistical considerations. Sample size needs to be determined statistically to ensure sufficient statistical power for key outcomes. The design effect in studies that use TSS is often large enough that project managers must double or triple the sample size in projects that use TSS as compared to the sample size in projects that use a simple random sample (Karon and Wejnert 2012). Sample size is also influenced by the time and funds available for the study, and by a power calculation determined a priori to be adequate for the study and its goals and outcomes. The determination for the sample size and duration of sampling (e.g., completing 500 interviews in six months) should be made at the beginning of the study and can be used to monitor the sampling process (e.g., 9 months of sampling, 14 sampling events per month, and a minimum of 4 participants per event produces 504 interviews).

In terms of regulatory considerations, it is important to train project staff in procedures intended to protect the rights and welfare of participants and project integrity (Emanuel et al. 2011). Staff members need to be knowledgeable of guidelines and regulations for protecting project participants and skilled in their application of this information in their projects. Federal regulations for protection of persons enrolled in the project (e.g., informed consent) should be afforded to all key informants, "street intercept" participants, and survey participants.

Staff members need to discuss with potential participants the consent process and form and ensure that participants do not feel pressured to participate in the project. Oversight of institutional boards, review committees, and community advisory boards, and, as necessary, logistical procedures such as pilot testing of relevant procedures (e.g., remuneration amount) are necessary to avoid or minimize mid-project corrections. Equally important is to inform potential participants through the informed consent process and forms that remuneration is intended as reimbursement for time and effort in project participation. Government research institutions in several countries may have laws or other prohibitions against some or all project-related monetary remuneration. In these situations, nonmonetary remunerations can be an option. Remuneration or compensation for time and effort in projects that use TSS is an important element because although altruism is necessary for voluntary participation, it may not be sufficient (Semaan et al. 2009). Arguments against monetary remuneration include the potential use of remuneration payments for harmful behaviors and subversion of altruistic motivations for project participation. However, remuneration payments show respect for participants' judgment to use the remuneration to meet personal needs (Semaan et al. 2009).

A checklist of remuneration-related variables for systematic data collection and reporting, as feasible, in studies that use TSS can be helpful in monitoring and evaluating TSS implementation. The variables can include (1) motivation for project participation, (2) the extent of any coercion or undue influence, (3) the amount of remuneration for study participation, (4) the methods used to determine remuneration amounts, and (5) the effects of monetary and nonmonetary remuneration.

Regulatory considerations should be built into the review and approval process of projects before project initiation. All involved parties, including project staff members, have a responsibility to discuss and address warning signs of factors that affect the rights and welfare of study participants and integrity of projects as soon as project staff members recognize such signs (e.g., risk to privacy or coercion). Project directors also need to take into consideration the heterogeneity in social and cultural characteristics and the barriers and obstacles that may affect project participation (Arcury and Quandt 2007). Migrant populations who have limited ability to speak English should be interviewed in their native language. Project directors should also consider the literacy level of the population as well as the primary or only language of the population and develop project-related materials (e.g., consent form) in relevant languages or dialects that also reflect the cultural norms of the population.

There are general procedures and safeguards that can be used in projects irrespective of the sampling strategy used. Relevant procedures include using audio computer-assisted self-interviewing (ACASI) to enhance the reliability and validity of self-reported data, particularly for sensitive and personal data (Gorbach et al. 2013; Yan et al. 2012). When deemed necessary, describing relevant concerns or failures of TSS projects needs to be based on project data and experiences to avoid creating inaccurate impressions that the planning process for TSS and the safeguards used were inadequate or that harms were actualized. Equally important is the need to share information about the process and results of TSS projects with representatives of migrant populations for implementing relevant individual- and community-level interventions to enhance the well-being of migrant populations.

In terms of legal considerations, as relevant and feasible, health jurisdictions can consider developing collaborative agreements with bordering countries (e.g., Canada and Mexico) to assist in understanding and meeting the needs of migrant populations (WHO 2010). Staff members need to be aware of federal, state, and local laws and regulations that might affect data collection of undocumented migrants, especially when they are less likely to participate in projects for fear of legal consequences. The right to health, regardless of the legal status of individuals, is recognized widely in different international and national legislative frameworks. Many related conventions on immigration and health matters have been ratified by most countries in the world (WHO 2010). The conventions include the WHO Constitution, the Universal Declaration on Human Rights, the International Labor Organization Conventions, the Declaration on the Human Rights of individuals who are not nationals of the country in which they live, the Convention on the Status of Refugees, and the principles on internal displacement (GAUN 1948, 1951, 1985, 1990; ILO 1949, 1975; WHO 1946; UNHRC 1998).

In terms of ethical considerations, procedures for protecting participants have become highly refined. These procedures specify how sensitive information must be guarded and how remuneration for time and effort in project participation must be balanced to preclude undue inducement or coercion and to provide an opportunity to choose, refuse, or withdraw from project participation. In working with migrant populations, it is important that potential participants do not feel coerced or pressured to participate and that staff members protect against such pressure. Participants need to know that participation is voluntary and that there is no penalty should they decline participation or withdraw from participation.

Relevant guidelines and regulations are important for protecting the integrity of projects with migrant populations (National Commission for the Protection of Human Subjects of Biomedical and Behavioral Research 1978; Centers for Disease Control and Prevention 1999). For example, US federal regulations require all US federally funded research to be reviewed by an institutional review board or approved by designated officials for protection of participants in projects (USD-HHS 1981). When US federally funded research is conducted outside the United States, the regulations require that the project protocols be reviewed in both the United States and the host country (USDHHS 1981). Projects conducted outside the United States need to follow the regulations and codes of the host country and relevant literature (WHO 2000, 2009). To ensure the rights and well-being of participants and integrity of projects, staff members need to develop clear protocols that meet regulatory requirements and receive approval by regulatory and ethical review bodies and offices before initiation of data collection. Typically, such protocols need to outline the purpose of the project, project development and design methods, data collection procedures, intended use of the collected data, and data security procedures. Standardized protocols—including information on formative research, sampling and recruitment methods, data collection instruments, informed consent procedures and forms, collection of self-report or biologic data, data management procedures, plans for data analysis and for dissemination of results, data security and confidentiality procedures, and procedures for protecting participants as human subjects—are also useful for ensuring comparability of procedures in multisite studies. In multisite studies, protocols might need to be submitted to one or more local institutional review boards or bodies, as deemed required by the institutions supporting the projects.

Because migrants can be exposed to stigma and ostracism, screening of migrants for infectious diseases or chronic conditions should always be voluntary. Different government and nongovernmental agencies often provide health care services for migrants and often highlight the vulnerability of migrant populations (Arcury and Quandt 2007; European CDC 2009). Reaching out to migrant populations to engage them in the development of TSS projects is crucial to building community trust and capacity, as for example in training and engaging community health workers in the prevention of HIV among Latino migrant workers in South Florida (Sanchez et al. 2012).

Ethical considerations in using TSS include issues related to disclosure of information relevant to the health and well-being of others, especially as staff members become aware of health-related information through the data collection process (Semaan et al. 2009). For example, the ethical principle of respect for participants highlights obligations of staff members to the public health of networks and communities and calls for informing participants, through institutionally approved project protocols and informed consent, whether staff members are going to share with authorities or population databases information that has a bearing on the health of others (e.g., domestic violence, child abuse, an infectious health condition, a genetic marker). The principle of respect also requires that investigators protect the privacy of participants, confidentiality of data, and participants' choices. This information should be clearly indicated in project-approved protocols and discussed with potential participants during the informed consent process. TSS projects can use a checklist for describing procedures related to disclosure of sensitive information. The checklist can include information on (1) procedures used to protect the privacy of participants and confidentiality of personal information, (2) disclosure options offered to participants, (3) procedures used to protect relationships in projects involving collection or disclosure of sensitive information, and (4) beliefs and behaviors of participants regarding their responsibility to adopt safer behaviors and their responsibility to disclose sensitive information to protect the health of others in their networks and communities. Staff members need to know the ethical literature because it influences success of TSS projects (Lee et al. 2013).

The five dimensions of sampling (i.e., logistical, regulatory, legal, ethical, and scientific) often interact in a complex manner, especially in TSS projects of migrant populations that collect data on socially sensitive topics (Semaan 2010). Clarity on the separate, combined, and synergistic role of logistical, regulatory, legal, and ethical requirements and implementation of relevant safeguards in TSS projects are important. Thus, staff members need to be aware of the influence and interactions of the five dimensions and of the relevant safeguards for logistical, regulatory, legal, and ethical considerations in their projects. Addressing these considerations in TSS projects is important to ensure that projects that use TSS are feasible, provide statistically and scientifically valid data, and are ethically sound.

CONCLUSION

The collective experience gained since the 1990s in using TSS with hard-to-reach or hidden populations at risk for HIV infection can be useful for employing TSS with migrant populations (Barbosa et al. 2011). TSS can be used in sampling migrant populations with appropriate planning and monitoring, and with application of relevant theoretical and practical knowledge distilled from prior experience in implementing this approach.

Several factors influence the successful TSS of migrant populations, including having a clear and complete institutionally approved protocol (e.g., by an institutional review board or an ethics review committee), adequate formative research, pilot studies, articulation of eligibility criteria, sampling goals, and evaluation of the sampling process and outcomes (Semaan et al. 2002). TSS requires adequate formative research to acquire relevant information about migrant populations and to provide the basis and rationale for choosing TSS. The formative phase is important to ensure the successful implementation and outcomes of TSS. Pilot testing relevant procedures, training staff members, implementing quality control procedures, monitoring the sampling process, establishing criteria to define successful implementation of TSS, and hiring an interdisciplinary (e.g., ranging from anthropology to statistics) and culturally competent staff are important steps to ensure the success of TSS. A rigorous TSS strategy can result in data that can be effectively used to ensure that local resources are appropriately used and that communities can adapt programs to fit their particular population needs and characteristics. Development of timely and responsive interventions, programs, and policies to enhance the health and well-being of migrant populations does not need to be hindered by lack of scientifically valid data. Knowledge and experience working with guidelines and regulations for the protection of participants can enhance the implementation of TSS. Project directors may obtain input from community advisory boards for protecting participants and from project staff to assess project implementation and the need for relevant corrections. Attention to sampling procedures, regulations, and ethical considerations, including dialogue among all stakeholders and attention to lessons learned, can enhance the successful implementation of TSS with migrant populations.

REFERENCES

Arcury, T., and S. Quandt. 2007. "Delivery of health services to migrant and seasonal farmworkers." *Annual Review of Public Health* 28: 345–63.

Barbosa Júnior, Aristides, Pati Roberta Ana Pascom, Celia Szwarcwald Landman, Carl Kendall, and W. McFarland. 2011. "Transfer of sampling methods for studies on most-at-risk populations (MARPs) in Brazil." *Cadernos de Saúde Pública* 27 (Supplement 1): S36–S44.

Barnhart, J., K. Liu, A. Giachello, D. Lee, J. Ryan, M. H. Criqui, and J. P. Elder. 2010. "Sample design and cohort selection in the Hispanic community health study/Study of Latinos." *Annals of Epidemiology* 20: 642–49.

Calduch Negro, E., A. Diaz, and M. Diez. 2008. "Ethical and legal issues related to health access for migrant populations in the Euro-Mediterranean area." *Eurosurveillance* 13(50): Pii 19061.

Campbell, Eugene K., and Kandala Ngianga-Bakwin. 2011. "Remittances from internal migration and poverty in Botswana." *Sociology Mind* 1(3): 130–37.

Cashman, Rebecca, Eugenia Eng, Florence Siman, and Scott D. Rhodes. 2011. "Exploring the sexual health priorities and needs of immigrant Latinas in the southeastern United States: A community-based participatory research approach." *AIDS Education and Prevention* 23(3): 236–48.

Centers for Disease Control and Prevention. 1999. "Guidelines for defining public health research and public health non-research." Accessed October 2, 2012. http://aops-mas-iis .cdc.gov/Policy/Doc/policy557.pdf.

Chutuape, K. S., M. Ziff, C. Auerswald, M. Castillo, A. McFadden, J. Ellen, et al. 2008. "Examining differences in types and location of recruitment venues for young males and females from urban neighborhoods: Findings from a multi-site HIV prevention study." *Journal of Urban Health* 86(1): 31–42.

Das-Munshi, J., G. Leavey, S. A. Stansfel, and M. J. Prince. 2012. "Migration, social mobility and common mental disorders: Critical review of the literaturè and meta-analysis." *Ethnicity and Health* 17(1–2): 17–53.

Deren, S., S. Y. Kang, H. M. Colon, J. F. Andia, R. R. Robles, D. Oliver-Velez, and A. Finlinson. 2003. "Migration and HIV risk behaviors: Puerto Rican drug injectors in New York City and Puerto Rico." *American Journal of Public Health* 93(5): 812–16.

Deren, S., M. Shedlin, C. U. Decena, and M. Mino. 2005. "Research challenges to the study of HIV/AIDS among migrant and immigrant Hispanic populations in the United States." *Journal of Urban Health* 82(2 Supplement 3): iii13–iii25.

DiNenno, E. A., A. M. Oster, C. Sionean, P. Denning, and A. Lansky. 2012. "Piloting a system for behavioral surveillance among heterosexuals at increased risk of HIV in the United States." *The Open AIDS Journal* 6 (Supplement 1: M15): 169–76.

Emanuel, E. J., and J. Menikoff. 2011. "Reforming the regulations governing research with human subjects." *New England Journal of Medicine* 365(12): 1145–50.

European Centre for Disease Prevention and Control. 2009. "Migrant health: Epidemiology of HIV and AIDS in migrant communities and ethnic minorities in EU/EEA countries." Technical report.

Fernández, M. I., J. B. Collazo, G. S. Bowen, L. M. Varga, N. Hernandez, and T. Perrino. 2005. "Predictors of HIV testing and intention to test among Hispanic farmworkers in South Florida." *Journal of Rural Health* 21(1): 56–64.

Ferreira, L. O. C., E. S. de Oliveira, H. F. Raymond, S. Y. Chen, and W. McFarland. 2008. "Use of time-location sampling for systematic behavioral surveillance of truck drivers in Brazil." *AIDS and Behavior* 12: S32–S38.

Finlayson T. J., B. Le, A. Smith, K. Bowles, M. Cribbin, I. Miles, A. M. Oster, T. Martin, A. Edwards, and E. DiNenno. 2011. "HIV risk, prevention, and testing behaviors among men who have sex with men: National HIV behavioral surveillance system, 21 U.S. Cities, United States, 2008." MMWR Surveillance Summaries 60(SS14): 1–34.

Geibel, S., S. Luchters, N. King'Ola, E. Esu-Williams, A. Rinyiru, and W. Tun. 2008. "Factors associated with self-reported unprotected anal sex among male sex workers in Mombasa, Kenya." *Sexually Transmitted Diseases* 35: 746–52.

General Assembly of the United Nations (GAUN). 1948. The universal declaration of human rights. http://www.un.org/Overview/rights.html.

General Assembly of the United Nations (GAUN). 1951. Convention relating to the status of refugees. Geneva. The Office of the High Commissioner for Human Rights. http://www.unhchr.ch/html/menu3/b/o_c_ref.htm.

General Assembly of the United Nations (GAUN). 1985. Declaration on the human rights of individuals who are not nationals of the country in which they live. Geneva: The Office of the High Commissioner for Human Rights. http://www.unhchr.ch/html/menu3/b/o_nonat.htm.

General Assembly of the United Nations (GAUN). 1990. The international convention on the protection of the rights of all migrant workers and members of their families. http://www.unhchr.ch/html/menu3/b/m_mwctoc.htm.

Gorbach, P. M., B. S. Mensch, M. Husnik, A. Coly, B. Masse, B. Makanani, et al. 2013. "Effect of computer-assisted interviewing on self-reported sexual behavior data in a microbicide clinical trial." *AIDS and Behavior* 17: 790–800.

Hardy, L. J., C. M. Getrich, J. C. Quezada, A. Guay, R. J. Michalowski, and E. Henley. 2012. "A call for further research on the impact of state-level immigration policies on public health." *American Journal of Public Health* 102: 1250–54.

Heimer, R., and E. White. 2010. "Estimation of the number of injection drug users in St. Petersburg, Russia." *Drug and Alcohol Dependence* 109: 79–83.

Hernandez, M. A., M. A. Sanchez, L. Ayala, C. Magis-Rodriguez, J. D. Ruiz, M. C. Samuel, B. K. Aoki, A. H. Garza, and G. F. Lemp. 2009. "Methamphetamine and cocaine use among Mexican migrants in California: The California-Mexico epidemiological surveillance pilot." *AIDS Education and Prevention* 21 (Supplement B): 34–44.

Hickman, M., V. Hope, B. Coleman, J. Parry, M. Telfar, J. Twigger, et al. 2009. "Assessing IDU prevalence and health consequences (HCV, overdose, and drug-related mortality) in a primary care trust: Implications for public health action." *Journal of Public Health* 31: 374–82.

International Labour Organization (ILO). 1949. Convention 97. http://www.ilo.org/ilolex/english/convdisp1.htm.

International Labour Organization (ILO). 1975. Convention 143. http://www.ilo.org/ilolex/english/convdisp1.htm.

International Working Group for Disease Monitoring and Forecasting. 1995. "Capture-recapture and multiple-record systems estimation I: History and theoretical development." *American Journal of Epidemiology* 142: 1047–58.

Jenness, S. M., A. Neaigus, C. S. Murrill, C. Gelpi-Acosta, T. Wendel, and H. Hagan. 2011. "Recruitment-adjusted estimates of HIV prevalence and risk among men who have sex with men: Effects of weighting venue-based sampling data." *Public Health Reports* 126: 635–42.

Kalton, G. 2009. "Methods for oversampling rare subpopulations in social surveys." *Survey Methodology* 35(2): 125–41.

Karon, J. M., and C. Wejnert. 2012. "Statistical methods for the analysis of time-location sampling." *Journal of Urban Health* 89(3): 565–86.

Kayembe, P. K., M. A. Mapatano, A. F. Busangu, J. K. Nyandwe, G. M. Musema, J. P. Kibungu, et al. 2008. "Determinants of consistent condom use among female sex workers in the Democratic Republic of Congo: Implications for interventions." *Sexually Transmitted Infection* 84: 202–6.

Kendall, C., L. R. Kerr, R. C. Gondim, G. L. Werneck, R. H. Macena, M. K. Pontes, et al. 2008. "An empirical comparison of respondent-driven sampling, time-location sampling, and snowball sampling for behavioral surveillance in men who have sex with men, Fortaleza, Brazil." *AIDS and Behavior* 12: S97–S104.

Kish, L. 1991. "Taxonomy of elusive populations." *Journal of Official Statistics* 7: 340–47.

Kissinger, P., S. Kovacs, C. Anderson-Smits, N. Schmidt, O. Salinas, J. Hembling, A. Beaulieu, L. Longfellow, N. Liddon, J. Rice, and M. Shedlin. 2012. *AIDS and Behavior* 16: 199–213.

Kissinger, P., N. Liddon, N. Schmidt, E. Curtin, O. Salinas, and A. Narvaez. 2008. "HIV/STI risk behaviors among Latino migrant workers in New Orleans Post–Hurricane Katrina Disaster." *Sexually Transmitted Diseases* 35(33): 924–29.

Kral, A. H., M. Malekinejad, J. Vaudrey, N. Martinez Alexis, J. Lorvick, W. McFarland, and H. Raymond Fisher. 2010. "Comparing respondent-driven sampling and targeted sampling methods of recruiting injection drug users in San Francisco." *Journal of Urban Health* 87(5): 839–50.

Lavange, L. M., W. D. Kalsbeek, P. D. Sorlie, Aviles-Santa, M. Lariisa, R. C. Kaplan, J. Barnhart, K. Liu, A. Giachello, D. J. Lee, J. Ryan, M. H. Criqui, and J. P. Elder. 2010. "Sample design and cohort selection in the Hispanic community health study/Study of Latinos." *Annals of Epidemiology* 20(8): 642–49.

Lee, L. M., B. Wright, and S. Semaan. 2013. "Expected ethical competencies of public health professionals and graduate curricula in accredited schools of public health in North America." *American Journal of Public Health* 103: 938–42.

Lepkowski, J. 1991. "Sampling the difficult to sample." *Journal of Nutrition* 121: 416–23.

Levy, P., and S. Lemshow. 1991. Sampling of populations: *Methods and applications.* 3rd ed. New York: Wiley.

Lowther, Sara A., Roque Miramontes, Barbara Navara, Nadya Sabuwala, Milyana Brueshaber, Sarah Solarz, Maryam Haddad, Deborah, Sodt, and Ruth Lynfield. 2011. "Outbreak of tuberculosis among Guatemalan immigrants in rural Minnesota, 2008." *Public Health Reports* 126: 726–32.

Mackellar, D. A., K. M. Gallagher, T. Finlayson, T. Sanchez, A. Lansky, and P. S. Sullivan. 2007. "Surveillance of HIV risk and prevention behaviors of men who have sex with men—A national application of venue-based, time-space sampling." *Public Health Reports* 122: 39–47.

Mackellar, D. A., L. Valleroy, G. Karon, G. Lemp, and R. Janssen. 1996. "The Young Men's Survey: Methods for estimating HIV seroprevalence and risk factors among young men who have sex with men." *Public Health Reports* 111: 138–44.

Magis-Rodriguez, C., G. Lemp, M. Hernandez, M. Sanchez, F. Estrada, and E. Bravo-Garcia. 2009. "Going north: Mexican migrants and their vulnerability to HIV." *Journal of Acquired Immune Deficiency Syndromes* 51: S21–S25.

Marpsat, M., and N. Razafindratsima. 2010. "Survey methods for hard-to-reach populations: Introduction to the special issue." *Methodological Innovations Online* 5(2): 3–16.

McKenzie, D. J. 2007. "Surveying migrant households: A comparison of census-based, snowball, and intercept point surveys." The World Bank, Policy Research Working Paper 4419: 1–41.

McKenzie, D. J., and J. Mistiaen. 2009. "Surveying migrant households: A comparison of census-based, snowball, and intercept point surveys." *Journal of the Royal Statistical Society Series A* 172(2): 339–60.

Mills, S., T. Saidel, R. Magnani, and T. Brown. 2004. "Surveillance and modeling of HIV, STI, and risk behaviours in concentrated HIV epidemics." *Sexually Transmitted Infection* 80: ii57–ii62.

Muhib, F. B., L. S. Lin, A. Stueve, R. L. Miller, W. L. Ford, W. D. Johnson, et al. 2001. "A venue-based method for sampling migrant populations." *Public Health Reports* 116: 216–22.

National Commission for the Protection of Human Subjects of Biomedical and Behavioral Research. 1978. "The Belmont Report: Ethical principles and guidelines for the protection of human subjects of research." Accessed October 2, 2012. http://www.hhs.gov /ohrp/humansubjects/guidance/belmont.html.

Oster, A., et al. 2011. "HIV testing among men who have sex with men—21 cities, United States, 2008." *Mortality and Morbidity Weekly Report* 60(21): 694–99.

Parrado, E., C. Flippen, and C. McQuiston. 2004. "Use of commercial sex workers among Hispanic migrants in North Carolina: Implications for spread of HIV." *Perspectives on Sexual and Reproductive Health* 36: 15–156.

Platt, L., M. Wall, T. Rhodes, A. Judd, M. Hickman, L. Johnston, et al. 2006. "Methods to recruit migrant groups: Comparing two chain referral sampling methods of recruiting injecting drug users across nine studies in Russia and Estonia." *Journal of Urban Health* 83: 39–53.

Pollack, L. M., D. H. Osmond, J. P. Paul, and J. Catania. 2005. "Evaluation of the Centers for Disease Control and Prevention's HIV behavioral surveillance of men who have sex with men: Sampling issues." *Sexually Transmitted Diseases* 32: 581–89.

Quaglia, M., and G. Vivier 2010. "Construction and field application of an indirect sampling method (time-location sampling): An example of surveys carried out in homeless persons and drug users in France." *Methodological Innovations Online* 5(2): 17–25.

Rabito, F. A., S. Perry, O. Salinas, J. Hembling, N. Schmidt, P. J. Parsons, and P. A. Kissinger. 2011. "Longitudinal assessment of occupation, respiratory symptoms, and blood lead levels among Latino day laborers in a non-agricultural setting." *American Journal of Industrial Medicine* 54(5): 366–74.

Rachlis, B., K. C. Brouwer, E. J. Mills, M. Hayes, T. Kerr, and R. S. Hogg. 2007. "Migration and transmission of blood-borne infections among injection drug users: Understanding the epidemiologic bridge." *Drug and Alcohol Dependence* 90: 107–19.

Ramo, Danielle E., Christian Grov, Kevin Delucchi, Brian C. Kelly, and Jeffrey T. Parsons. 2010. "Typology of club drug use among young adults recruited using time-space sampling." *Drug and Alcohol Dependence* 107: 119–27.

Rangel, Gudelia M., A. P. Martinez-Donate, M. F. Hovell, J. Santibanez, C. L. Sipan, and J. A. Izazola-Licea 2006. "Prevalence of risk factors for HIV infection among Mexican migrants and immigrants: Probability survey in the North border of Mexico." *Salud Pública de México* 48(1): 3–12.

Remafedi, G., A. M. Jurek, and J. M. Oakes. 2008. "Sexual identity and tobacco use in a venue-based sample of adolescents and young adults." *American Journal of Preventive Medicine* 35: S463–S470.

Robinson, W., J. Risser, S. McGoy, A. Becker, M. Rehman, M. Jefferson, et al. 2006. "Recruiting injection drug users: A three-site comparison of results and experiences with respondent-driven and targeted sampling procedures." *Journal of Urban Health* 83: 29–38.

Sanchez, J., G. Silva-Suarez, C. A. Serna, and M. De La Rosa. 2012. "The Latino migrant worker HIV prevention program: Building a community partnership through a community health worker training program." *Family and Community Health* 35(2): 139–46.

Semaan, S. 2010. "Time-space sampling and respondent-driven sampling with hard-to-reach populations." *Methodological Innovations Online* 5(2): 60–73.

Semaan, S., D. D. Heckathorn, D. C. Des Jarlais, and R. S. Garfein. 2010. "Ethical considerations in surveys employing respondent-driven sampling." *American Journal of Public Health* 100(4): 582–83.

Semaan, S., J. Lauby, and J. Liebman. 2002. "Street and network sampling in evaluation studies of HIV risk-reduction interventions." *AIDS Review* 4: 213–23.

Semaan, S., S. Santibanez, R. S. Garfein, D. Heckathorn, and D. C. Des Jarlais. 2009. "Ethical and regulatory considerations in HIV prevention studies employing respondent-driven sampling." *International Journal of Drug Policy* 20: 14–27.

Spreen, M., and R. Swaagstra. 1994. "Personal network sampling, outdegree analysis, and multilevel analysis: Introducing the network concept in studies of hidden populations." *International Sociology* 9: 475–91.

Stauffer, W. M., J. Painter, B. Mamo, R. Kaiser, M. Weinberg, and S. Berman. 2012. "Sexually transmitted infections in newly arrived refugees: Is routine screening for Neisseria gonorrheae and Chlamydia trachomatis infection indicated?" *American Journal of Tropical Medicine and Hygiene* 86(2): 292–95.

Stueve, A., L. N. O'Donnell, R. Duran, A. San Doval, and J. Blome. 2001. "Time-space sampling in minority communities: Results with young Latino men who have sex with men." *American Journal of Public Health* 91: 922–26.

Sudman, S., M. Sirken, and C. Cowan. 1988. "Sampling rare and elusive populations." *Science* 240: 991–96.

Thompson, S. K., and L. M. Collins. 2002. "Adaptive sampling in research on risk related behaviors." *Drug and Alcohol Dependence* 68: S57–S67.

United Nations Human Rights Commission (UNHRC). 1998. *Guiding principles on internal displacement.* Geneva: The Office of the High Commissioner for Human Rights. http://www.unhchr.ch/html/menu2/7/b/principles.htm.

United States Department of Health and Human Services (USDHHS). 1981. *Code of Federal Regulations, Title 45, Part 46. Protection of human subjects* (aka "The Common Rule"). Accessed January 11, 2013. http://www.hhs.gov/ohrp/humansubjects/guidance/45cfr46.html.

Valenzuela, A., Jr. 2002. "Working on the margins in metropolitan Los Angeles: immigrants in day-labor work." *Migraciones Internacionales* 1(2): 6–28.

van Griensven F., S. Thanprasertsuk, R. Jommaroeng, G. Mansergh, S. Naorat, R. A. Jenkins, K. Ungchusak, P. Phanuphak, J. W. Tappero, and the Bangkok MSM Study Group. 2005. "Evidence of a previously undocumented epidemic of HIV infection among men who have sex with men in Bangkok, Thailand." *AIDS* 19: 525–26.

Wasserman, M. R. 2005. "A church-based sampling design for research with Latina immigrant women." *Population Research and Policy Review* 24: 647–71.

World Health Organization (WHO). 1946. *Constitution of the World Health Organization.* New York. http://www.who.int/governance/eb/who_constitution_en.pdf.

World Health Organization (WHO). 2000. "Declaration of Helsinki: Ethical principles for medical research involving human subjects." Geneva: World Health Organization.

Accessed January 11, 2013. http://www.wma.net/en/30publications/10policies/b3/index .html.

World Health Organization (WHO). 2009. "Research ethics committees: Basic concepts for capacity building." Geneva: World Health Organization. Accessed January 11, 2013. http://www.who.int/ethics/Ethics_basic_concepts_ENG.pdf.

World Health Organization (WHO). 2010. "Health of Migrants—The Way forward: Report of a global consultation 2010. Accessed January 11, 2013. http://www.who.int/hac/events /consultation_report_health_migrants_colour_web.pdf.

Yan, T., F. Kreuter, and R. Tourangeau. 2012. "Latent class analysis of response inconsistencies across modes of data collection." *Social Science Research* 41: 1017–27.

The findings and conclusions in this chapter are those of the author and do not necessarily represent the views of the Centers for Disease Control and Prevention.

9

Prior Enumeration

A Method for Enhanced Sampling with Migrant Surveys

Richard Mines
Coburn C. Ward
Marc B. Schenker

INTRODUCTION

One challenge in conducting research with hard-to-reach migrant populations, including farmworkers, is defining a population sampling frame in order to obtain an unbiased sample. Several innovative approaches have been used in the sampling of farmworkers in the United States, and these approaches can be useful for working with other migrant populations. Although these customized approaches are an improvement over noncustomized schemes, they still likely fail to capture the poorest, least educated, and most socially displaced migrant workers. Prior enumeration (PE) is a sampling strategy that can minimize this problem. Prior enumeration is a two-stage process of creating a cluster sample in the first stage and then drawing a stratified sample within each of the clusters in the second stage. The advantages of PE include reducing nonsampling errors, improving assessment of underrepresentation of subgroups, and providing a sample from which generalized inferences can be made. This approach may be useful for migrant health researchers, service providers, and policy makers who work with migrant populations to better understand their unique needs and develop and implement appropriate programs.

The majority of farmworkers in the United States are immigrants, and in California this number is over 85%. Survey work with farmworker populations in the United States has begun to be carried out in recent years. Progress has been made in collecting probability samples that can inform policies and programs for farmworkers. However, an inherent bias of underrepresentation of the most underprivileged farmworkers has not been removed (Kamel et al. 2001; Zahm and Blair

2001). These particularly disadvantaged individuals and their households face uniquely prevalent problems, including tuberculosis, mental illness, child labor practices, minimum wage violations, and illegal charges for rides and equipment. Such challenges are common in research involving migrant populations and require distinct solutions, such as survey techniques that are honed to reduce bias to an absolute minimum. The aim of this chapter is to present prior enumeration (PE), an enhanced sampling approach adapted for farmworkers, that can also be used with other migrant populations. This chapter reviews common sampling methodologies and provides examples of their use in farmworker populations. Details on implementation of PE are provided. Finally, we highlight advantages and strengths of PE that argue for this approach in obtaining unbiased information on hard-to-reach migrant populations.

As with other hard-to-reach migrant populations, it is difficult to define the population sampling frame of farmworkers and, therefore, obtain a complete and unbiased sample of the community. This is because there is often no preexisting list of farmworkers from which to sample (Sudman et al. 1988; Zahm and Blair 2001). This situation is also true of many other migrant populations, making it difficult to obtain reliable information that could improve the lives of farmworker subgroups. Useful information can be collected with nonrandom approaches, such as ethnographic research based on snowball sampling techniques. However, probability-based sampling is crucial to the work of program designers, policy makers, and advocates. Probability-based sampling has a built-in estimation procedure, forces better control of non-sampling problems, and allows for a random infrastructure for ancillary work done using nonrandom selection methods (Sudman et al. 1988).

CUSTOMIZED SAMPLING APPROACHES FOR FARMWORKERS

There have been several attempts in recent years to correct the bias in official farmworker data through variation in sampling design, and three approaches are described below. The Binational Farmworker Health Survey (BFHS) utilized a network approach, the National Agricultural Workers Survey (NAWS) used an employment-based method, and the California Agricultural Workers Health Survey (CAWHS) used a household sampling method. All three surveys used in-person interviews with trained bilingual interviewers who were familiar with the respondent population and skilled at obtaining the confidence of the respondents.

Binational Farmworker Health Survey (BFHS)

The BFHS was conducted in 1999–2000 in Mexico and the United States (Mines et al. 2001). The staff traveled to the southern state of Zacatecas, Mexico, and identified ten villages that had heavy participation in US farmwork. Based on information collected from village elders, a universe list was created of every living person who had done US farmwork and was raised in the villages. These lists were crosschecked by other informants in the community. At the time of the survey, some of the individuals were in the home villages while others could be found in settlement communities in the United States. A random selection was taken from the universe list for each village. The survey began in Mexico and, after approximately 300 interviews were done in the villages, the survey team moved to the United States, where another 150 interviews were done with village members living in settlement communities there. During the survey period in the villages, the addresses and phone numbers of the randomly selected members of the village community in the United States were collected from relatives and friends in Mexico. Since there was a high degree of concentration of emigrants in just a few settlement areas from each village, it was possible to obtain a very high completion rate of the randomly selected individuals on both sides of the border at a reasonable cost. With this network selection approach, the interviewers became known to each village network because they spent several months interviewing people in each community. The refusal rate was extremely low since most respondents were familiar with the survey and its objectives before an interviewer approached them. Also, because the interviewers spent time in the home village, rapport with respondents was easy to establish, rendering the collected information more accurate.

A primary advantage of the BFHS was that the survey included ex-farmworkers and people living on both sides of the border. By collecting information about ex-farmworkers, the reasons for their leaving farmwork and the long-term impacts of their work could be investigated, thus reducing the potential for the healthy worker effect, a bias that can result when sick or injured farmworkers are selectively excluded from research. Additionally, the transnational context of the BFHS improves the completion and accuracy of data collection over competing survey approaches. Difficult-to-reach farmworkers give more reliable information in the confines of their home village, where family and friends surround them. Equally important, the sample is more inclusive if some interviews are done south of the border because individuals unlikely to cooperate north of the border are included. Furthermore, individuals that are residing outside of the United States at the time of the survey that would ordinarily be excluded from the sample have a greater probability of being included as other eligible respondents.

The biggest disadvantage of the BFHS approach is the inability to generalize the results to a larger population. Although the selection within the villages was random, the choice of the villages was not representative of all parts of Mexico. Therefore, a large sample with many points of origin from many places in Mexico would be required to assure that the data could be generalized to larger populations of farmworkers. In addition, whole families who have migrated from the study areas and emigrants in the US who have lost contact with their communities will not be included in the survey.

National Agricultural Workers Survey (NAWS)

The NAWS is a survey of farmworkers conducted by the US Department of Labor since October 1988 (US Department of Labor 2011). Each year, interviews are done in three cycles (February, June, and October) to account for the seasonal nature of farmworker employment. Because over 50,000 farmworkers have been interviewed since the NAWS inception, it is indisputably the best national sample of farmworker data ever collected. The NAWS employs a multistage technique in which counties are chosen using a probability proportional to size approach based on payroll spent on farmworkers by county. Within the counties, grower lists are constructed from Bureau of Labor Statistics and Department of Agriculture employer inventories. The interviewers follow a rigorous and systematic procedure in choosing the growers and then another procedure to select the workers employed by those growers in the chosen counties. The technique is similar to venue-based sampling, in which respondents are chosen at a common venue (Muhib et al. 2001; see also chapter 8, by Semaan and DiNenno, in this volume); theoretically, all employed farmworkers have an equal chance of being included in the sample.

The advantages of NAWS are its large size, the fact that it is a long-term time series data collection effort, and the potential completeness of the sample. The data from the survey show that poor, undocumented, and solo males (unaccompanied by their nuclear family) are well represented in the survey. Another important advantage is the seasonal timing of the sampling, which increases the likelihood that workers engaged in only one season will be included.

The disadvantages of NAWS derive from the unwillingness of some employers to collaborate. Since sampling is done after communication with the employer who identifies where the workers can be located, uncooperative growers may bias the results. Another continuing challenge for the NAWS is to provide its interviewers with complete and accurate grower lists. The lists tend to be inaccurate and duplicative unless constantly updated and improved—an expensive process.

California Agricultural Workers Health Survey (CAWHS)

The CAWHS was a community-based household survey that used a multistage sampling strategy focused on small farmworker towns (Villarejo et al. 2000; Villarejo and McCurdy 2008). One community was chosen randomly from each of the six major farm areas in California. An additional site was added in the San Joaquin valley to oversample this region, where most California farmworkers live. Research teams mapped all the dwelling units located within each community. This prior screening of the sampled dwellings, like the prior enumeration described in this chapter, involved walking through the entire randomly selected geographic unit and visually locating every dwelling unit. Then, dwelling units were randomly selected for enumeration and visited by an interviewer. If at least one eligible farmworker was present, then all the eligible farmworkers were enumerated at that time. One worker was chosen randomly from the dwelling for an interview.

Sampling advantages of the CAWHS approach were derived from the partial prior enumeration of the dwellings, which allowed for the inclusion of informal dwellings that are often overlooked in other sampling designs. Bias against the most disadvantaged population was greatly reduced in the CAWHS compared to more conventional surveys. Although the partial enumeration in the CAWHS was crucial, the individuals associated with the household addresses were not enumerated with a separate visit prior to the interview phase of the survey. In the CAWHS, both enumeration and the survey interview occurred during the same visit. Another strength of the CAWHS is that it conducted physiological measurements (e.g., height, weight, and blood pressure) and collected biological specimens for laboratory testing.

The disadvantages of this approach are that the sample is drawn at the time of the enumeration without an analysis of the population and without a careful sampling from this universe provided by a full prior enumeration. It is easier to obtain the full array of individuals associated with an address when that is the focus of the visit rather than when the interviewer is pressured to complete an interview simultaneously with the household enumeration. The persistent bias of underrepresenting the most disadvantaged (due to the timidity of this population) was likely present during the CAWHS implementation. Additionally, CAWHS was limited to a few small farmworker communities. Many, if not most, farmworkers live in farmworker neighborhoods of mid-sized towns and even cities in agricultural areas. By focusing on just a few towns, the efficiency for interviewers of finding farmworkers was increased, but many farmworkers living in larger towns were excluded.

DEMONSTRATION OF REDUCTION OF BIAS IN FARMWORKER-CUSTOMIZED SURVEYS

Although none of the above-described farmworker-customized surveys remove bias completely, they do minimize it compared to mainstream or general population surveys (e.g., Current Population Survey). The bias manifests itself in an overrepresentation of the better-off, more established farmworkers and in undersampling among the less assimilated and more disenfranchised individuals, which is what the customized surveys strive to minimize. Unfortunately, data from the respondents in mainstream surveys are often misleadingly used to design programs or create policies for farmworkers that result in inappropriate programmatic and policy changes.

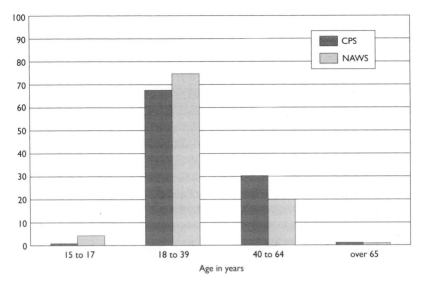

FIGURE 9.1. Proportion by age group, CPS 2004, NAWS 2000.

To demonstrate the reduction of bias in customized surveys versus mainstream surveys, we compared the 2000 NAWS (US Department of Labor 2011) with the Current Population Survey (CPS) annual summary of March 2004 (Bureau of Labor Statistics; http://www.census.gov/cps/). Because of the limited availability of detailed occupational codes in the CPS, comparisons were made between two comparable foreign-born groups in the two surveys. All foreign-born in the CPS 2004 who worked in crop, livestock, or agricultural services were selected with the assumption that almost all would be farmworkers. In the NAWS, only the foreign-born were chosen since one must be a farmworker to be eligible for the NAWS.

While NAWS and CPS respondents were not significantly different by age, NAWS respondents included individuals under age eighteen years (figure 9.1). NAWS respondents were less educated and earned significantly less than CPS respondents. There was a smaller proportion of workers with a high school diploma or more schooling in the NAWS compared to the CPS group ($p < 0.004$) (figure 9.2). Comparisons of annual income showed 57% of NAWS respondents and 39% of CPS respondents earned less than $12,500 per year, while only 14% of NAWS respondents and 41% of the CPS respondents earned over $17,500 ($p < 0.0001$) (figure 9.3). Estimated median annual income was $11,800 for NAWS respondents and $15,600 for CPS respondents.

Noting that the CPS and NAWS comparison was limited by the aggregated nature of the CPS data available to the public, we then compared the 2001 California

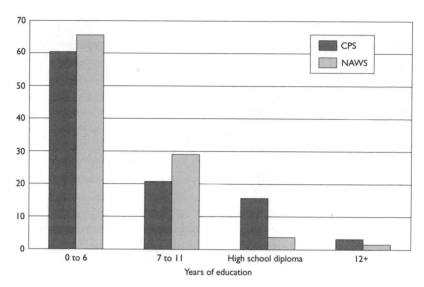

FIGURE 9.2. Years of education, CPS 2004, NAWS 2000.

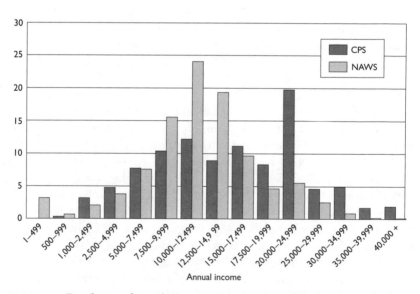

FIGURE 9.3. Distribution of annual income, CPS 2004, NAWS 2000.

TABLE 9.1 Demographic Characteristics of California Health Interview Survey (CHIS) 2001 Adult Respondents and California Agricultural Workers Health Survey (CAWHS) 2000 Adult Respondents

	CHIS	CAWHS	p value
Education			
Less than 6th grade	47%	65%	<0.001
7th–11th grade	22%	25%	
High school graduate or higher	31%	10%	
Annual household income			
Less than $10,000	16%	36%	<0.001
$10,000–$19,999	40.5%	38%	
$20,000+	43.5%	22%	
English language proficiency			
Well/very well	15%	6%	0.04
Not well/not at all	85%	94%	
Health insurance			
Uninsured	41%	76%	<0.0001
Insured	59%	24%	
Doctor visits			
Never	2%	25%	<0.0001
More than 5 years ago	9%	6%	
1–5 years ago	26%	26%	
Within the last 12 months	63%	43%	
Dental Visits			
Never	9%	50%	<0.0001
More than 5 years ago	14%	8%	
1–5 years ago	28%	25%	
Within the last 12 months	48%	17%	

Health Interview Survey (CHIS) to the CAWHS, which more precisely highlights the potential bias. The CHIS is a random selection of the entire California population and is done by telephone (CHIS 2001). Farmworkers in the CHIS were selected as a comparable group to the CAWHS. Both the CHIS and CAWHS are household-based health surveys that ask similar questions of respondents.

The CHIS-sampled individuals appeared well connected and more assimilated than the CAWHS respondents, and in fact the CHIS sample seemed to greatly overrepresent those of higher socioeconomic status (SES) while underrepresenting the less well off (table 9.1). The CAWHS sample, in contrast, had a small proportion of higher SES workers, consistent with data from the NAWS. Ten percent of the CAWHS respondents achieved high school or greater education while 31% in the CHIS sample did so ($p < 0.001$). Additionally, 22% of CAWHS participants reported annual incomes over $20,000 compared to 44% of the CHIS sample

($p < 0.001$). English proficiency also differed significantly between the two groups, with 6% of CAWHS reporting that they spoke English well or very well and 15% in the CHIS.

Examination of health care access and utilization showed similar differences between CHIS and CAWHS participants. Seventy-six percent of CAWHS and 41% of CHIS participants reported that they had no health insurance coverage ($p < 0.0001$). Additionally, 25% of CAWHS respondents reported they had never been to the doctor compared to 2% among CHIS respondents ($p < 0.0001$). Among the CAWHS sample, only 17% of adults reported dental visits in the last year, whereas in the CHIS sample, 48% had visited a dentist in the year prior to the survey. These data suggest that the CHIS sample is a group much more able to access services and institutions.

PRIOR ENUMERATION IN FARMWORKER HOUSEHOLD SURVEYS

The customized farmworker survey approaches described above contributed to the goal of gathering better farmworker data and appear to reduce bias that is present in mainstream surveys. However, each customized approach has its limitations by not verifying the data against a full or partial universe or sampling list. Even the NAWS, with its large sample size and continuous data collection, can be checked only against employment estimates. We propose prior enumeration (PE) as an approach to overcome existing limitations to obtain a more representative sample for working with migrant populations.

SAMPLING SCHEME FOR PE

Prior to beginning PE, the staff must advertise in the community that the survey will occur so that people are not surprised by the appearance of interviewers. The proposed sampling scheme consists of two stages, with the PE occurring between them. The first stage is a cluster sampling with clusters being, for example, the census blocks in the geographic area under study. The census block is a convenient unit for which the census bureau can estimate the number of farmworkers or other immigrant workers. The second stage is accomplished with a stratified sample drawn within each of the chosen clusters.

In the first stage, for cost efficiency, it is suggested that the possible selections be limited to only those blocks with a minimum number of farmworkers. Due to the concentrated nature of farmworker populations, this process will eliminate the vast majority of census blocks except in neighborhoods with a high density of farmworker households. This resource-efficient limitation will introduce a degree of invalidity whenever conclusions are drawn about a whole group of farmworkers that covers those in the census block that were excluded a priori. However, the error is small if the procedure excludes only a small proportion of farmworkers. The error will also be small if there is no strong statistical association between variables of the study and the number of farmworkers in a given census block. Among the N eligible clusters (i.e., census blocks), n of them are chosen by a probability proportional to size (with replacement) sampling scheme. This scheme allows an individual cluster to be chosen more than once; if an individual cluster is chosen more than one time (t 1), the second stage sampling is done t independent times within that cluster.

The first step of PE is to map, by walking through the neighborhoods, every address in the selected blocks and identify all possible dwelling places and their associated addresses. Informal dwellings (without an official address) such as garages, trailers, sheds, and cars are included in this step. Once all potential dwelling places have been identified, interviewers go to the addresses and determine if there are any farmworkers living at or associated with the addresses. Only addresses with at least one member of the target population are eligible for the survey. At each eligible address, interviewers ask a series of simple questions about each person associated with the dwelling. The questions asked are limited and no names are taken so as to maintain maximum trust. Questions vary depending on the goals of the survey. Once the PE is complete, the information obtained serves as the sampling frame, and survey staff select the sample according to sampling procedures (e.g., stratification on predetermined characteristics, if appropriate). The implementation stage commences with preselected individuals (identified by characteristics such as age, gender, and nationality), with predetermined backups for each address.

The second stage of the sampling scheme involves stratified sampling within each chosen census block using the sampling frame created with the PE and precise information about possible strata and their relative sizes. It is possible to choose the sample size of strata in the second stage.

PE is best explained with an example. In the summer of 2005, a PE was conducted in Mendota, California, for a health survey of farmworkers (Stoecklin-Marois et al. 2011). Initially, a random selection of census blocks within each census tract in Mendota was taken. Each address and some vacant lots with inhabitants within these selected blocks were mapped for possible dwellings and then visited by enumerators to compile the database. Next, each address was visited and a series of questions were asked about each farmworker associated with the address. First, the relationship of each adult in the household (head of household, spouse, sibling, other relative, roomer) was determined. Additional questions attempted to establish the age, gender, place of birth, years residing in Mendota, and whether the person had done two or more weeks of US farmwork in the prior year. Finally, the number of minors less than eighteen years of age associated with the address

TABLE 9.2 Distribution of Addresses by Married Couple or Solo Male: Mendota
Farmworkers, July 2005

	Addresses *(n)*	Adults *(n)*	Children <18 *(n)*	Total individuals
Solo male	175	619	73	692
Married couple	554	1821	994	2815
Total	729	2440	1067	3507

TABLE 9.3 Demographic Characteristics by Married Couple and Solo Male Addresses:
Mendota Farmworkers, July 2005

Characteristic	Married couple address	Solo male address
Male > 18 years	61%	80%
Central American	29%	50%
Mean years Mendota resident	10 years	5 years
Mean age	33 years	30 years
Children <18 years	35.30%	10.50%

was ascertained. These data, though very limited in scope and without names, allowed for a careful review of the population for sampling purposes. Also, this step provided sufficient information for verifying the representativeness of the sample against the total enumerated population.

Preliminary analysis of these data provided information on farmworker community traits that were useful for selecting strata to sample. For example, by manipulating the data points that were acquired, the distribution of solo male and married, couple-based households was determined (table 9.2). In addition, we could identify the relationship of solo males living in married-couple households—often they were siblings, cousins, or other relatives. Addresses could be analyzed in many other ways that help in stratifying and weighting the sample after the data is collected. Table 9.3 presents characteristics of the population in terms of age, gender, country of birth, average length of residence in Mendota, and the number of minor children by the type of address (solo male or married couple). This kind of analysis of the population prior to sampling is crucial for verifying the representativeness of the sample obtained from PE.

DISCUSSION

One challenge in conducting research with farmworker and other migrant populations is defining a population sampling frame in order to obtain an unbiased sample. Several sampling customized approaches, such as network sampling, employment-based methods, and household sampling with partial prior enumeration, provide improvements over using data from mainstream surveys. Comparisons between CPS and NAWS data and CHIS and CAWHS data demonstrate that use of these mainstream surveys may not capture the poorest and most socially displaced workers. The methods used to create a sampling frame by mainstream surveys are often inadequate to accurately reach farmworker and other migrant populations. For example, census data do not accurately count all farmworkers, not all households or families maintain telephones, and inclusion of persons in the US without documentation precludes the use of immigration records. Also, potential participants may not be included in other population lists, such as those created by census records or assistance programs, due to participants' lack of familiarity with these types of agencies, language and cultural barriers, immigration status, informal living arrangements, or apprehension about government agencies (Kamel et al 2001; Garcia and Marinez 2005).

One crucial advantage of PE is that it allows for the reduction of nonsampling errors. PE allows for the careful choice of whom to sample, including the use of stratified sampling. It also allows for ex-post weighting of the sample using the total enumerated population as a universe of all farmworkers in the census tracts chosen for study. The interviewers' prior visit to the addresses, which establishes the composition of the members of the households living at the address, allows for sampling prior to the survey implementation stage. The interviewer can enter the premises and request to speak to the proper respondent without having to go through the cumbersome and distracting process of choosing a respondent after arriving. Also, familiarity with the nationality, age, and relationships of residents at the address allows for better rapport between the interviewer and the members of the household (see F. Floyd in Biemer et al. 1991, p. 259). Another nonsampling advantage of PE is that the questions included in the questionnaire can be predesigned for the demographic traits of the persons to be interviewed. This allows for the avoidance of skip patterns and the expansion of questions customized for one stratum of workers. Also, prior knowledge of the characteristics of the interviewees can be utilized during the training of interviewers. Interviewers can be trained to specialize in certain types of respondents and given special lessons on how to gather information from these individuals. For example, backup prompts that are designed to elicit responses for questions that interviewees may not comprehend can be tailored for the different demographic groups without jeopardizing the standardization of possible responses. Since the type of respondent at each address is known prior to the survey, the interviewers can be assigned to interview predominantly respondents for whom they have received customized training (see Fowler in Biemer et al. 1991).

There are advantages also in reducing sampling errors by using the PE approach with farmworkers and other migrant populations. In general population surveys, for example, underrepresentation is typically associated with homelessness and street people (Cox and Cohen 1985), but among migrant populations, overcrowded and ancillary dwelling units can cause the same problems. The PE approach allows for sampling among the most disadvantaged groups, which usually are greatly undercovered by traditional population surveys. The PE approach allows for the identification and selection of difficult-to-reach individuals without eliciting names, allowing them to be sampled and found. Further, prior knowledge of the probability of selection of (almost all) the universe elements in the chosen census blocks can lead to accurate measurement of undercoverage of subgroups. The nonresponse to certain questions can also be monitored by subgroup more carefully. For example, Hispanics are known to avoid answering questions about social relations (Owens et al. 1999).

PE improves the ability to correctly stratify a sample. The near complete coverage of certain limited demographic traits of the universe reduces any misclassification and improper assignment of individuals to strata. PE can also integrate "insider information" gathered informally in a community to probe for missing individuals to achieve as complete an enumeration as possible. PE allows for the oversampling of certain small or hard-to-reach strata and the use of postsurvey weights to adjust the results. It also allows for weighting of undercovered strata or subgroups. Survey results can be best analyzed if they can be checked so that estimates agree with existing parameters (Cox and Cohen 1985, chapter 2). However, without a PE sampling frame, there are no reliable benchmarks for farmworkers.

With PE, a random sample infrastructure can be established that can be utilized in interpreting and situating the work of complementary nonrandom network-based interviewee selection projects. Further ethnographic work can be done pursuing questions irresolvable by quantitative surveys among certain subgroups of the population. The significance of the findings of this nonrandom work can then be put into perspective by situating the group analyzed in the total universe of farmworkers or another specific migrant population. For example, problem networks like affinity groups with high rates of diabetes can be studied, and then the importance of the findings can be quantified by reference to the universe of farmworkers gathered by the PE database. Finally, PE allows for the analysis of the data by various units of inquiry depending on the goals of the research; the individual, nuclear family, household, and residents of a given address can all be chosen as units of analysis with access to the PE sampling frame. The main disadvantage of PE is the additional cost and time needed to map and collect basic information on all dwellings and residents in the selected clusters.

The PE approach offers unique advantages for the investigation of farmworker and other migrant populations that are often misrepresented in mainstream surveys.

ACKNOWLEDGMENTS

This research was supported by the National Institute for Occupational Safety and Health through the Western Center for Agricultural Health and Safety (Cooperative Agreement #2U50OH007–550) and the California Endowment, Grant 20043221.

REFERENCES

Biemer, P., R. Groves, et al. 1991. *Measurement Errors in Surveys.* Wiley: New York.

California Health Interview Survey (CHIS). 2001. Accessed March 20, 2013. http://health-policy.ucla.edu/chis/data/Pages/public-use-data.aspx.

Cox, B., and S. Cohen. 1985. *Methodological Issues for Health Care Surveys.* New York: Marcel Drekker.

Garcia, V., and J. Marinez. 2005. "Exploring Agricultural Census Undercounts among Immigrant Hispanic/Latino Farmers with an Alternative Enumeration Project." *Journal of Extension* 43(5). Accessed March 20, 2013. http://www.joe.org/joe/2005october/a2.php.

Kamel, F., T. Moreno, et al. 2001. "Recruiting a Community Sample in Collaboration with Farmworkers." *Environmental Health Perspectives* 109 (Suppl. 3): 457–59.

Mines, R., N. Mullenax, and L. Saca. 2001. *The Binational Farmworker Health Survey.* California Institute for Rural Studies, Davis. Accessed March 20, 2013. http://www.cirsinc.org/index.php/component/search/?searchword = binational+farmwork&ordering = newest&searchphrase = all.

Muhib, F., L. S. Lin, A. Stueve, R. L. Miller, W. L. Ford, W. D. Johnson, and P. J. Smith. 2001. "A Venue-based Method of Sampling Hard-to-reach Populations. *Public Health Reports* 116(1) Suppl.: 216–22.

Owens, L., T. P. Johnson, et al. 1999. "Culture and Item Nonresponse in Health Surveys." Seventh Conference on Health Survey Research Methods, Hyattsville, Maryland, Department of Health and Human Services, Centers for Disease Control and Prevention, National Center for Health Statistics.

Stoecklin-Marois, M.T., T. E. Hennessey-Burt, and M. B. Schenker. 2011. "Engaging a Hard-to-reach Population in Research: Sampling and Recruitment of Hired Farm Workers in the MICASA Study. *Journal of Agricultural Safety and Health* 1714(4): 291–302.

Sudman, S., M. G. Sirken, et al. 1988. "Sampling Rare and Elusive Populations." *Science* 240(4855): 991–96.

US Department of Labor. 2011. *Statistical Methods of the National Agricultural Workers Survey.* http://www.doleta.gov/agworker/statmethods.cfm.

Villarejo D., D. Lighthall, D. Williams, A. Souter, R. Mines, B. Bade, S. J. Samuels, and S. A. McCurdy. 2000. "Suffering in Silence: A Report on the Health of California's Agricultural Workers." California Institute for Rural Studies, Davis.

Villarejo D., and S. A. McCurdy. 2008. "The California Agricultural Workers Health Survey." *Journal of Agricultural Safety and Health* 14(2): 135–46.

Zahm, S. H., and A. Blair. 2001. "Assessing the Feasibility of Epidemiologic Research on Migrant and Seasonal Farmworkers: An Overview." *American Journal of Industrial Medicine* 40(5): 487–89.

10

Telephone-Based Surveys

David Grant
Royce J. Park
Yu-chieh Lin

INTRODUCTION

Telephone surveys are a popular and cost-effective data collection methodology. They have been widely used for general population surveys and also in some migration studies and research (National Public Radio et al. 2004; Pew Hispanic Center 2006; Statistics New Zealand 2007). Since the advent of random-digit dialing (RDD) sampling methods in the 1980s, RDD telephone surveys have become perhaps the most common method of fielding a survey. And while RDD telephone surveys remain popular, declining response rates and the growth of cell-phone-only households present significant challenges to the dominance of this method.

Following the introduction, we describe telephone surveys, telephone survey sampling, and the unique characteristics of this data collection method generally as well as within the context of migration studies. We then discuss the utility of using telephone surveys for studying migrant populations based primarily on a decade of experience with the California Health Interview Survey (CHIS), a large, population-based telephone survey. Examples are provided of how telephone surveys have been used for studying immigrant health, drawing largely on the CHIS experience. The chapter concludes with consideration of the strengths and limitations of telephone surveys.

TELEPHONE SURVEYS

What distinguishes telephone surveys from other data collection methods is the simple fact that a survey interview is conducted using the telephone. It is, thus, the mode that makes telephone surveys distinct from other types of surveys. Telephone surveys share many characteristics with other research methods and surveys, such as a sample universe, sampling frame, survey instruments, and so forth. Telephone surveys share many characteristics with other survey methods and are often supplemented by other contact modes (such as a mailed advance letter) or combined with other methods such as mail surveys and/or web surveys, resulting in mixed or multimodal surveys. The Gallup World Poll, for example, implements a mixed-mode design in which the telephone is used in countries where 80% or more of the target population is covered, and face-to-face interviewing is used in countries with lower telephone coverage (Gallup Inc. 2007).

Since telephone surveys depend on telephones for data collection, they may have limited application depending on the research purpose, study location and population, and sample frame. For example, a general household health survey would be out of the question if the majority of households in a location did not have telephone service, while a telephone survey of hospitals in the same country may be appropriate. Surveys have always tracked communication technology, and technology continues to drive the possibilities of data collection methods. The development of cellular telephones, for example, may facilitate some aspects of telephone surveys for studies that include migrant populations (more on this below).

TELEPHONE SURVEY SAMPLING

To conduct a telephone survey, telephone numbers are sampled from an appropriate sampling frame—a comprehensive list of available telephone numbers that represents the population of interest. This list may come from an organization of members, purchased through a survey sampling firm to meet specific study parameters, or from some other source. For general population surveys, the most common type of telephone sampling is random-digit dialing. RDD sampling is relatively inexpensive and able to produce representative samples with known sampling probabilities, making it very useful for general population surveys of areas with high telephone coverage. RDD sampling is often "list assisted" in that a seed number is generated from a random draw of a published phone number and the next 100 telephone numbers (sequentially) are generated as the sample with additional blocks of 100 (or 1,000) telephone numbers drawn to reach the desired sample. Traditionally, RDD methodology targeted landline telephones only. As cell-phone-only households have become more common, RDD surveys increasingly use "dual-frame" sampling to include both landline and cell-phone telephone numbers, thereby reducing the potential for noncoverage bias. Cell-phone surveys and noncoverage bias are further discussed toward the end of this chapter.

The inclusion of cell-phone samples in surveys of migrants or immigrants is particularly important. Estimates from the National Health Interview Survey (NHIS), for example, indicate that in the last six months of 2011, 34% of adults nationally lived in households with cell-phone-only service. Latinos (43.3%) were more likely to live in cell-phone-only households than either whites (29.0%) or African Americans (36.8%) (Blumberg and Luke 2012). Adults living in poverty (51.4%) and adults living with unrelated roommates (77.5%) had high rates of residing in households that were cell-phone only—demographic factors that may be important for studies about, or that include, migrants.

Overall, most adults in the US live in homes with telephone access, about 98% according to the most recent estimates from the NHIS. The US Census Bureau's American Community Survey shows a slightly higher proportion of adults living in households without telephone service (2.5% in 2010) and that these proportions are nearly identical among native-born and foreign-born adults; this suggests that telephone coverage of immigrants in the US is high and a viable option for immigrant health data collection methods. Since cell phones are mobile and not tied to a household, the growth, availability, and affordability of cellular telephones has likely increased telephone coverage of certain populations, including migrants and those living in transitory housing such as migrant farmworkers.

SAMPLING WITHIN HOUSEHOLDS

For landline telephones, telephone numbers are generally shared among household members (this may be true for cell phones as well, particularly among low-income persons or families). Therefore, in addition to sampling telephone numbers, the sampling of individuals within a household must also be considered. Depending on the purpose of the survey, any household adult who is available may be appropriate for interview. For health surveys that attempt to represent the population of household dwelling adults, randomization of eligible household members is essential; otherwise the data will not represent the general population, but the population subset that tends to be at home and answer the telephone.

TELEPHONE QUESTIONNAIRE ADMINISTRATION

Administering a questionnaire over the telephone has both benefits and drawbacks. Among the principal benefits of telephone administration is the use of computer-assisted telephone interviewing (CATI), which allows survey interviewers to move quickly and seamlessly through standardized, long, and complicated survey instruments where the next appropriate question depends on information gathered previously; long surveys with difficult skip patterns may not, for example, be feasible for paper-based surveys. Using CATI, interviewers read the questions from a computer screen to the respondent and enter the response into the computer, which then displays the next appropriate question. Telephone surveys allow for administration in multiple languages and are useful with populations where low literacy rates may be a concern (such as migrants)—factors that are problematic for self-administered paper- or web-based surveys. The use of CATI also simplifies data capture and reduces error relative to methods in which results must be transferred from one format to another (e.g., paper to computer). Finally, telephone administration can efficiently and cost-effectively cover large geographic areas such as states or nations where using other methods (e.g., face-to-face interviews) might be cost prohibitive.

However, while survey response rates have generally been declining among all modes, declines have been most precipitous among telephone surveys, likely due to the combination of commercial telemarketing and telephone screening devices. The decline in telephone survey response rates increases the potential for nonresponse bias and may raise concerns about data quality and representativeness among survey sponsors and data consumers (Curtin et al. 2005). Telephone surveys also do not generally permit the collection of paradata[1] that might be gathered using other survey modes such as face-to-face surveys.

CONTENT FOR TELEPHONE ADMINISTRATION

Questions used in telephone surveys should be short, simple, easy to understand, unambiguous, and easy to respond to. There is a science and art to writing good questionnaires and as a general rule, the best first option is to find questions that have been carefully developed and successfully used on other surveys, such as the National Latino and Asian American Study or the Behavioral Risk Factors Surveillance System. Many federal surveys are in the public domain and their content is generally of high quality, developed with extensive testing and validation.

When adapting content from other surveys, the researcher must consider the mode, purpose, and sample of the survey source. Questions used in face-to-face surveys, for example, may be more complex and use visual aids during administration that cannot be readily and successfully administered by telephone. Some survey questions are developed for special populations such as veterans or doctors and may be inappropriate for use with a general population. Determining survey content may depend not only on the sample but also on the interviewers who administer the questions. For example, questions to assess compliance with a medical treatment plan may require specially trained nurses rather than lay interviewers.

For survey data to adequately represent the sample population for studies of migrant populations, survey instruments must be available in the languages spoken by the sample population. Translation and cultural adaptation of materials is an essential part of this process, and there is a broad literature on best practices for translation procedures and cross-cultural interviewing guidelines (including chapter 24 in this volume, by Gany et al.).

The Survey Research Center (2010) at the University of Michigan has developed an extensive and comprehensive resource, *Guidelines for Best Practice in Cross-Cultural Surveys*, which includes chapters on questionnaire design, adaptation, translation, and sample design. This publicly available online resource provides a wealth of information about conducting surveys, including telephone surveys, that is applicable to studies of migrant health.

CASE STUDY: CALIFORNIA HEALTH INTERVIEW SURVEY (CHIS)

The California Health Interview Survey (CHIS) is a population-based telephone survey of California's general population conducted every other year since 2001 and on a continuous basis since 2011. CHIS is the largest health survey conducted in any state and one of the largest health surveys in the nation. CHIS is based at the UCLA Center for Health Policy Research and is sponsored by federal and state agencies and philanthropic organizations. Much more information about CHIS is available at www.chis.ucla.edu.

CHIS collects extensive information for three age groups on health status, health conditions, health-related behaviors, health insurance coverage, access to health care services, and other health and health-related issues. The sample is designed to meet and optimize two objectives: (1) provide estimates for large- and medium-sized counties in the state, and for groups of the smallest counties (based on population size), and (2) provide statewide estimates for California's overall population, its major racial and ethnic groups, and its Asian and Latino ethnic subgroups. To help compensate for the increasing number of households without landline telephone service, a separate RDD sample of telephone numbers assigned to cellular service was first pilot-tested in CHIS 2005 and then included as a growing part of the CHIS sample in every cycle since 2007 (CHIS 2008).

To capture the rich diversity of the California population, interviews are conducted in five languages: English, Spanish, Chinese (Mandarin and Cantonese dialects), Vietnamese, and Korean. These languages were originally chosen based on analysis of 2000 census data to identify the languages that would cover the largest number of Californians in the CHIS sample that either did not speak English or did not speak English well enough to otherwise participate. The development of CHIS questionnaire items for administration in languages other than English undergoes an extensive process of English simplification, cultural adaptation, multiple forward translations with review, and a final group reconciliation process (Ponce et al. 2004).

CHIS interviews one randomly selected adult in each sampled household. In those households where the selected adult respondent is the parent or legal guardian of one or more adolescents between the ages of twelve and seventeen, one is chosen at random and interviewed directly after receiving the parent's permission. And if the adult respondent is the parent of one or more children under the age of twelve, one is selected at random and is the subject of an interview conducted with the adult most knowledgeable about the child's health. Each participating CHIS household may produce up to three interviews for these different age groups.

CHIS interviews capture demographic information on racial and ethnic identification, ancestry or ethnic group, tribal affiliation, country of birth, parent's place of birth, years lived in the US, languages spoken at home, English language ability, citizenship, and green card status. In addition, CHIS collects a broad range of other demographic information and content on health conditions, health behaviors, access to and utilization of health care services, health insurance coverage, mental health, neighborhoods, and other topics depending on the CHIS cycle.[2] Prior to some questions on sensitive content, such as the legal residency status of persons born outside of the US, respondents are reminded that their information is confidential. To further protect participants, CHIS obtained a Certificate of Confidentiality from the National Institutes of Health. This certificate protects CHIS against forced disclosure, such as legal subpoena, of confidential information obtained from CHIS respondents.

While CHIS was not conceptualized as a migrant health study, it was designed as an omnibus public health survey able to capture the rich demographic diversity of California. Given the large CHIS sample size (roughly 40,000 to 50,000 households per two-year cycle) and the fact that in 2010 more than 10 million Californians (27%) had been born outside of the US,[3] CHIS is a fertile data source for studies of migrant population health. The diverse California population, large CHIS sample, and the multilingual administration generate relatively large samples of groups that are inadequately represented in many other data sources. Rather than combining many distinct groups under the banner of "Asian," for example, the CHIS sample permits separate analyses of many Asian ethnic groups including Chinese, Filipino, Japanese, Korean, South Asian, Vietnamese, and other Southeast Asian (table 10.1).

The ability to disaggregate health-related indicators for multiple Asian and Latino ethnic groups has led to CHIS being accepted as the only state-level data reported in the congressionally mandated National Health Disparities Report produced by the Agency for Healthcare Research and Quality (AHRQ). Since CHIS

TABLE 10.1   California Health Information Survey (CHIS) 2009 Adult Sample Size: Race and Asian and Latino Ethnic Groups by Place of Birth

	Place of Birth		
	US	Other	Total
Race (census)			
Pacific Islander	64	26	90
American Indian/Alaska native	535	72	607
Asian	908	4,001	4,909
African American	1,734	173	1,907
White	30,128	4,077	34,205
Other single race	1,727	3,058	4,785
More Than One Race	1,037	74	1,111
Total	36,133	11,481	47,614
	(75.9%)	(24.1%)	(100.0%)
Asian ethnic groups			
Chinese	260	805	1,065
Japanese	326	102	428
Korean	97	861	958
Filipino	154	353	507
South Asian	36	384	420
Vietnamese	85	1,338	1,423
Other Southeast Asian	29	60	89
Other Asian/two or more Asian types	80	134	214
Total	1,067	4,037	5,104
	(20.9%)	(79.1%)	(100.0%)
Latino ethnic groups			
Mexican	2,742	3,752	6,494
Salvadoran	45	353	398
Guatemalan	21	165	186
Central American	27	122	149
Puerto Rican	111	1	112
Latino European	251	40	291
South American	58	208	266
Other Latino	84	44	128
Two or more Latino types	244	39	283
Total	3,583	4,724	8,307
	(43.1%)	(56.9%)	(100.0%)

data became available for research in 2003, more than 240 peer-reviewed journal articles have been published, and about one-third of these publications used place of birth and/or other measures of "acculturation" in their analyses. Publications based on CHIS data address a wide variety of immigrant health issues, such as cancer screening rates among Latino and Asian ethnic groups, risk factors for other chronic illnesses, physical activity levels, risk factors for overweight teens, and many other topics.[4]

STRENGTHS AND LIMITATIONS OF TELEPHONE SURVEYS

Compared to face-to-face, Internet, or other self-administered questionnaires, telephone surveys are cost-effective, approach the maximum number of potential respondents in the shortest period of time, and provide representative samples with the ability to cover multiple geographical designations (Gwartney 2007). Interviewers working from a centralized location can speak with respondents living in a variety of different locations. Calling from the centralized location allows interviewers to obtain on-the-spot guidance and assistance from supervisors as needed, and supervisors can readily monitor interviews for accuracy, completeness, and comparability. Many respondents are more comfortable discussing sensitive topics on the telephone with an interviewer than doing so face to face with a stranger. Moreover, computer-assisted telephone interviewing (CATI) can handle complex or multilanguage instruments easily, providing a flexible tool for interviewers.

However, telephone surveys tend to be short, with simpler questions, fewer questions, and fewer answer categories than other types of surveys. Most telephone interviews are less than fifteen minutes in length, while face-to-face interviews often last thirty minutes or more. Telephone interviewers also cannot use visual aids to help respondents understand a complex concept or assist with accurate measurements. Although telephone interviewers may be able to read a respondent's tone of voice for impatience or misunderstanding, they cannot see that respondent's body language for additional nonverbal cues, like an in-person interviewer can.

Telephone surveys may not reach all individuals or households of interest. The growth of cell-phone-only households, especially among young adults and migrants, is potentially problematic for telephone surveys because landline RDD samples exclude cell-phone numbers. Telephone surveys also tend to exclude households whose residents are rarely home, homeless persons, and households without telephones. Sample frames that inadequately cover the sample population may lead to noncoverage bias. Response rates for surveys in general and telephone surveys in particular have declined substantially over the past several decades. The decline in telephone survey response rates increases the potential for nonresponse bias. Together, noncoverage and nonresponse bias have generated concern about the data quality and representativeness of telephone surveys, particularly RDD sample surveys. To explore these issues further, we again turn to CHIS as a case study to examine how noncoverage and nonresponse may bias data estimates.

NONCOVERAGE AND NONCOVERAGE BIAS

Noncoverage bias occurs when the sample frame does not adequately cover the target population, and those excluded from the frame differ from those included along some dimension of interest. In practice, sample frames rarely cover the sample universe perfectly; the issue is whether or not noncoverage results in biased estimates. For example, CHIS attempts to cover all persons living in households in California. For RDD telephone surveys like CHIS, noncoverage bias could result from the exclusion of households without any telephone service as well as households that have cell-phone service only. As noted above, studies using data from the NHIS suggest that nontelephone households pose little threat of noncoverage bias because the proportion of such households is low and stable. Cell-phone-only households, by contrast, have grown dramatically in recent years, leading to the now common practice of dual-frame sampling to include landline and cellular telephones.

NONRESPONSE BIAS

Nonresponse bias occurs when nonresponders systematically differ from responders in relation to some measure of interest (Groves 2006). For example, if nonresponders tend to smoke more than responders, nonresponse bias would result in smoking prevalence estimates that were lower than the prevalence of the true population. CHIS has conducted several studies to test strategies to avoid refusals, improve contact rates, and assess potential nonresponse bias; more information about these studies and results are available in the CHIS methodology reports and on the data quality section of the CHIS website (see www.chis.ucla.edu).

TESTING FOR NONCOVERAGE AND
NONRESPONSE BIAS

Survey methodologists use a variety of methods to assess data quality and sources of potential bias. Over the years, CHIS has conducted a number of studies to assess data quality, including benchmarking CHIS estimates against the California samples of federal surveys that were conducted in person and had high response rates (such as NHIS and the National Survey of Drug Use and Health), and benchmarking CHIS estimates against other California-based telephone surveys (such as the Behavioral Risk Factors Surveillance System). In most cases, CHIS estimates are similar to those from other surveys, and when differences are detected, they are small and do not demonstrate a pattern that suggests systemic bias.[5]

It is difficult to assess whether response rates differ among native and foreign-born adults since we are unable to collect information about nativity from households that do not participate in the survey. By comparing neighborhood characteristics of responders and nonresponders based on addresses matched to phone numbers, however, Lee et al. (2009) found few differences in response propensity across census tracts in California. Although the differences were small, this study found lower average response rates in tracts with higher concentrations of Latinos, Asians, and linguistically isolated households, indicating the potential for nonresponse bias among key populations of interest to immigrant health researchers. Nonresponse adjustments made to the sampling weights are effective in reducing nonresponse bias in CHIS-based estimates.

As part of CHIS 2007, an area probability sample of addresses was selected within Los Angeles County, the California county with the lowest response rate in CHIS 2005, in order to test for noncoverage and nonresponse bias. An attempt was made to match each sampled address to a telephone number, and if the match was successful, a standard CHIS interview was attempted. For households that could not be matched to a telephone number, as well as matched households that did not respond to the telephone interview, survey recruiters were sent door-to-door to actively invite sampled household members to participate in CHIS. Respondents were asked about the status of telephone usage in their household so that households with landline service could be compared to the "complete" sampling frame that included both landline and cell-phone-only households. This strategy allowed comparison of estimates based on initial responders only to data that included both initial responders and those more intensely recruited with in-person contact to test estimates for nonresponse bias.

Analyses conducted with the CHIS 2007 area probability sample compared more than forty CHIS estimates from a variety of topical areas (including health conditions, health behaviors, and access to health services), and after sample weights were applied, very little evidence of noncoverage or nonresponse bias was detected. These results, in addition to the benchmarking and neighborhood-level comparison of responders and nonresponders mentioned above, provide assurance that the CHIS data accurately represents the population residing in California households.

As cell phones and declining response rates complicate the telephone survey landscape, survey methods and statistics have become increasingly sophisticated and an important part of data quality. It is imperative that the sample weights applied to the collected data during the analysis phase are carefully crafted to adjust for noncoverage and differential nonresponse. Calculating appropriate weights is complicated by the now common practice of fielding overlapping landline and cell-phone samples. CHIS has been at the fore of these efforts and has carefully documented its weighting procedures, including methods for combining landline and cell samples (see Brick et al. 2007; CHIS 2011).

LESSONS LEARNED

Telephone surveys are a popular, cost-effective method for collecting data that have broad application for migrant health surveys. Whether or not a telephone survey is an appropriate survey method depends on the particulars of a given study and the ability of the telephone as a communication medium to adequately cover the population of interest. Survey instruments must be simplified and appropriate for telephone administration, and carefully translated to the languages spoken by respondents as needed, and interviewers must be carefully trained to administer the questionnaire in a value-neutral, culturally appropriate manner. Increasingly, telephone survey methods are complicated by rapid changes in communication technology, but also create new opportunities as, for example, less expensive cell phones become available to an increasing proportion of the population. As the CHIS experience demonstrates, migrant health studies based on telephone survey data can inform a wide variety of public health and health policy issues from the use of emergency room visits among undocumented populations to differences in cancer screening behaviors based on ethnicity and country of birth. Despite a number of challenges, telephone surveys remain a viable and important method for collecting information about the health of migrants and their host communities.

NOTES

1. Paradata is information that is systematically collected about the survey process, such as number of contact attempts, language problems, etc. (see Taylor 2008).

2. Previously administered CHIS questionnaires are available online at http://www.chis.ucla.edu/questionnaires.html.

3. American Community Survey, 2010 one-year estimate. US Census Bureau (http://factfinder2.census.gov/faces/tableservices/jsf/pages/productview.xhtml?pid=ACS_10_1YR_DP04&prodType=table).

4. A list of peer-reviewed CHIS-based publications is available at http://www.chis.ucla.edu/peerpubs/.

5. More information on the CHIS benchmarking studies is available in the data quality section of the CHIS website.

REFERENCES

Blumberg, S. J., and J. V. Luke. 2012. "Wireless Substitution: State-level Estimates from the National Health Interview Survey, July–December 2011. Accessed August 07, 2012. http://www.cdc.gov/nchs/data/nhis/earlyrelease/wireless201206.pdf.

Brick, J. M., W. S. Edwards, and S. Lee. 2007. "Sampling Telephone Numbers and Adults, Interview Length, and Weighting in the California Health Interview Survey Cell Phone Pilot Study." *Public Opinion Quarterly* 71: 793–813.

California Health Interview Survey. 2008. "CHIS 2007 Cell-Phone Only Sample to Assess Noncoverage Bias." CHIS Working Paper Series. Los Angeles: UCLA Center for Health Policy Research.

California Health Interview Survey. 2011. "CHIS 2009 Methodology Series: Report 5— Weighting and Variance Estimation." Los Angeles: UCLA Center for Health Policy Research.

Curtin, R., S. Presser, and E. Singer. 2005. "Changes in Telephone Survey Nonresponse over the Past Quarter Century." *Public Opinion Quarterly* 69(1): 87–98.

Gallup, Inc. 2007. "Gallup World Poll Research Design." Accessed April 27, 2007. http://media.gallup.com/WorldPoll/PDF/WPResearchDesign091007bleeds.pdf.

Groves, R. M. 2006. "Nonresponse Rates and Nonresponse Bias in Household Surveys. *Public Opinion Quarterly* 70(5): 646–75.

Gwartney, P. A. 2007. *The Telephone Interviewer's Handbook: How to Conduct Standardized Conversations.* San Francisco: Jossey-Bass.

Lee S., E. R., Brown, D. Grant, T. R. Belin, and J. M. Brick. 2009. "Exploring Nonresponse Bias in a Health Survey Using Neighborhood Characteristics." *American Journal of Public Health* 99: 1811–17.

National Public Radio, the Henry J. Kaiser Family Foundation, and Harvard University John F. Kennedy School of Government. 2004. Immigration in America: Survey Overview. Retrieved October 10, 2011. http://www.npr.org/templates/story/story.php?storyId = 4062605.

Pew Hispanic Center. 2006. National Survey of Latinos: The Immigration Debate. Retrieved October 10, 2011. http://pewhispanic.org/files/reports/68.pdf.

Ponce, N., S. A. Lavarreda, W. Yen, E. R. Brown, C. DiSogra, and D. Satter. 2004. The California Health Interview Survey 2001: Translation of a Major Survey for California's Multiethnic Population. *Public Health Reports* 119(4): 388–95.

Statistics New Zealand. 2007. "Survey of Dynamics and Motivations for Migration (DMM)." Accessed October 10, 2011. http://www.stats.govt.nz/browse_for_stats/population /Migration.aspx.

Survey Research Center. 2010. *Guidelines for Best Practice in Cross-Cultural Surveys.* Ann Arbor: Survey Research Center, Institute for Social Research, University of Michigan. Accessed July 18, 2012. http://www.ccsg.isr.umich.edu/.

Taylor, Beth L. 2008. "The 2006 National Health Interview Survey (NHIS) Paradata File: Overview and Applications." Proceedings of the Section on Survey Research Methods of the American Statistical Association. Joint Statistical Meetings. 1909–13.

11

Case-Control Studies

Clelia Pezzi
Philip H. Kass

WHAT IS A CASE-CONTROL STUDY?

The case-control study is an efficient approach to assessing the association between exposures and disease or health outcomes. In a case-control study, the exposure histories of cases, individuals with a disease or other health outcome, are compared to the exposure histories of controls, those at risk of the outcome (i.e., without the disease of interest), to identify potentially causal associations. For example, this method could be used to study the effects of exposure to different pesticides and cancer risk among farmworkers. Unlike cohort studies, study subjects are selected based on disease status, and controls are a sample (rather than a census) of the disease-free population of interest. Investigators collect information on exposures in cases and controls, contrasting the odds of exposure between the two groups to measure their association with disease (Figure 11.1). Numerous applications of the case-control approach exist for the study of migrant populations and evaluation of the role of migration-related exposures or factors in health outcomes.

There are a number of benefits to using case-control studies compared to other study designs, and the case-control design lends itself particularly well to studies of migrant or mobile populations. Because case-control studies sample study individuals based on the outcome of interest and use data on exposures prior to outcome occurrence, they are well suited for the study of rare diseases and diseases with long latent periods (e.g., cancer, when an exposure can take place many years or decades before disease onset). In the prospective study of diseases with long latent periods in mobile populations, a significant proportion of study subjects

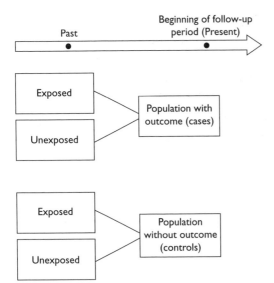

FIGURE 11.1. Diagram of the case-control study design.

may be lost to follow-up, a problem that can be avoided with a case-control study design as long as mobility is unassociated with exposure(s).

This study method is typically less resource intensive because it does not require a sample size as large as those required for cross-sectional or longitudinal designs of rare diseases; its outcome-based sampling makes it statistically and financially more efficient. Case-control studies can use data extracted from existing data sources, or researchers can collect their own data directly from the study population. Instead of including the exposure experience of the entire source population in the analysis, only a sample (controls) is chosen for comparison. The smaller size and often shorter period required to gather exposure information usually results in studies that are less costly and faster to develop and conduct, which is beneficial for working in resource-limited environments or with mobile populations that make follow-up challenging. Finally, case-control studies permit the simultaneous examination of multiple exposures or factors in terms of their association with a single health outcome, making them a strong tool for exploratory studies and outbreak investigations.

There are some limitations associated with the case-control methodology. Similar to other observational studies, investigators lack control over the environments of study subjects they would normally have with an experimental design. Also, the absence of randomization and potential for uncontrolled confounding prevents researchers from confirming cause-and-effect relationships between exposures and outcomes. The study is based on outcome sampling, meaning that investigators select subjects based on their case status and then ascertain past exposures. This feature of case-control studies can lead to differential recall bias, where the accuracy of recall is systematically different between cases and controls. One reason this can happen is that a subject's outcome status can influence his or her memories of potential exposures. For example, people diagnosed with a particular outcome may have more motivation to remember potential exposures; conversely, their memories may have been adversely affected by disease progression (e.g., when the disease affects their memory or cognitive capacity). It can be difficult, if not impossible, to validate exposure information on the basis of self-reported data. Also, identifying appropriate controls that represent the true distribution of exposure(s) in the source population can be challenging. However, while case-control studies are not appropriate for all circumstances, the study method may be the only realistic approach to investigating potential causal relationships in many contexts where alternative designs are either infeasible or unethical. For example, it would be unethical to deliberately expose a population to a potentially carcinogenic substance to determine if the population later develops cancer at increased rates when compared with an unexposed control group.

Health issues related to migration can be effectively addressed by case-control studies in a number of ways. First, a study can be conducted on a specific migrant population. For example, a case-control study examining the relationship between lifelong vegetarianism and breast cancer risk in England focused exclusively on a population of South Indian migrant women born outside of England (Dos Santos Silva et al. 2002). In another instance, a number of nested case-control studies were conducted using a database for migrant farmworkers and the California Cancer Registry to examine the relationship between pesticide exposures and cancer incidence (Mills and Yang 2003, 2005, 2007; Mills et al. 2005).

Another approach is to stratify a study population according to country of birth to compare the unique exposures or experiences of the foreign-born (or individuals from specific birth countries) to those of native populations. For example, a study from Turin, Italy, explored the increased risk of diabetes in Sardinian migrants, using birthplace of parents and social class as exposures of interest (Bruno et al. 2000). In addition, migration-associated variables, including the timing and duration of migration, can be considered exposures of interest. In a study of migration, acculturation, and breast cancer risk in Hispanic women living in the United States, age of migration, duration of residence in the United States, and type of residence (urban vs. rural) were captured for the foreign-born women. Acculturation was assessed by way of variables based on language usage and generational status (John et al. 2005). Case-control studies have also been used to identify potential sources of disease outbreaks in migrant communities, such as a listeriosis outbreak in Hispanic farmworkers in the US, typhoid in rural-to-urban migrants in squatter settlements in Pakistan, and cholera in refugees in a Kenyan refugee camp (MacDonald et al. 2005; Siddiqui et al. 2008; Shultz et al. 2009).

DESIGN OF THE CASE-CONTROL STUDY

Research Question

The first step in designing a case-control study is the development of a clearly defined research question based on existing information. An initial research interest should be broken down into the various hypotheses about the relationship between dependent (outcome) and independent (exposure) variables being studied. Investigators should take all hypotheses into account when designing the study to ensure that the necessary sample size and information are obtained, including information on potential confounding variables. Confounding occurs when some extraneous factor such as age, vitamin usage, or exercise habits is associated with both the study exposure and with the outcome of interest and is not evenly distributed among the groups being compared (e.g., the cases and controls). Confounding can lead to a distortion of the effect measure estimate between the exposure and disease. For example, maternal age is a confounder in the relationship between birth order and Down's syndrome; maternal age is related to both the exposure and birth order (mothers are older at the birth of each subsequent child), and is also independently associated with Down's syndrome. Failing to account for maternal age as a confounder could result in the incorrect interpretation of the effect of birth order on Down's syndrome risk.

The following scenario is an example that will be used throughout this discussion to illustrate the case-control method. Research has shown that breast cancer risk increases for women who move from countries with low breast cancer incidence to countries with high incidence. In order to ascertain the potential causes for this pattern, researchers might be interested in studying the risk factors or exposures of immigrant women from country Y, a low-incidence country, after they move to city Z in country X, a high-incidence country. The researchers might hypothesize that women from country Y experience higher breast cancer risk the younger they migrate to country X, the longer they have spent in country X, and the more acculturated they have become to country X. They would then design their study to test these multiple hypotheses.

Choosing a Method

Once the research question is developed, researchers should consider whether or not the case-control study is the most appropriate design. Case-control studies are not the most suitable study design for every research question, including evaluation of disease treatment, prophylaxis, or screening (Moss 1991; Hosek et al. 1996). In addition, case-control studies may be less efficient than cohort studies when the exposure of interest has a lower prevalence than the prevalence or incidence of the outcome of interest for a specific time period (Schulz and Grimes 2002). Data quality, study costs, and planned use of potential study results should all be considered in choosing a study design. Retrospective case-control studies can often be conducted quickly because the collection of historical exposure data can be a relatively straightforward process. This is an asset when the rapid identification of a potential disease-exposure association is needed to prevent the further spread of disease (e.g., in outbreak investigations) or when limited time and resources are available for conducting the study. However, differential misclassification bias can arise if cases recall potential exposures differently than controls, so the source of exposure data should be considered carefully in the design of the study. Also, retrospective data collection in a mobile population poses unique data collection challenges. Jones and Swerdlow (1996) found that migration had an impact on bias in a study of prenatal risk factors for childhood and adult diseases. Their results indicated that if more than 25% of controls migrated out of the study area between birth and the study time, statistically significant bias was introduced, although their conclusions had limited generalizability. Ideally, the potential exposures assessed in the case-control study should be relatively recent, or reliable medical or occupational records should be available for all study subjects for exposure assessment. In highly mobile, hard-to-reach migrant populations, follow-up visits and contact may not be possible, rendering prospective studies impractical or more time-consuming to conduct than retrospective case-control studies.

Case-control studies are usually more efficient and cost-effective than other forms of studies. Study efficiency depends on the proportion of the source population who have the disease, the population's distribution of exposure, the ratio of controls to cases in the study design, the magnitude of the disease-exposure association, and whether matching of cases to controls on one or more confounders is employed (matching will be discussed later in this chapter). When the disease is rare and exposure is common, a case-control study will usually be more efficient than a longitudinal study because a smaller sample size is sufficient for a given study power. However, if the exposure being studied is rare, a case-control study will require a larger sample size to ensure that an adequate proportion of subjects with the exposure(s) are represented in the study. In this circumstance, it may be preferable to use another study method (e.g., longitudinal study).

The only useful measure of association estimated directly from a case-control study is the odds ratio. However, under specific circumstances, the odds ratios calculated in case-control studies can estimate either a rate ratio or a risk ratio (Greenland and Thomas 1982). If incidence risk or rate measures are required for a particular study, case-control methods are not appropriate without information about case and control sampling proportions from the source population. The calculation and interpretation of the odds ratio is discussed in more detail later in this chapter.

Some basic questions to consider at the beginning of a case-control study can help clarify if the case-control design is an appropriate approach in a migrant health study. These issues should be thoroughly considered at the beginning of study design process to ensure that the appropriate study population is used and that the necessary data is collected. Some questions to consider early in the study design are as follows:

- Is there a particular population that is of interest? If so, how is that population defined? Can I identify migrants in this population? Defining a target population for a study is key in helping to decide the appropriate source population, study design, eligibility criteria, and variables that should be collected during the study. Studies can focus on migrants defined by country or region of birth, immigration status, length of time in the host country, occupation, and so forth. Immigration and emigration of study subjects to and from the study geographic area can have a strong influence on the source population. In the study of women from country Y with breast cancer, the population of interest is women who emigrated from country Y to country X, and the country of birth variable can identify members of this population.

- Is migration an exposure of interest? How should I define this exposure? Is the timing or duration of migration-related exposures important? What variables will I need to collect in order to assess these exposures? These questions will help define what questions need to be included in a data collection device or the data that should be extracted from existing records. The researchers from the hypothetical breast cancer study discussed above would want to collect data on the age at which participants migrated and how long they have lived in country X. In addition, they would want to identify and ask questions about variables that could be used to assess acculturation, such as language spoken at home, and consider potential confounders like age and socioeconomic status to test their hypotheses.

Source Population

The identification of the source population for a case-control study is a key component of the design (Miettinen 1985). Wacholder defines the study base, or source population, as the persons- or person-time from which diseased subjects enter a study as cases (Wacholder et al. 1992a). Stated another way, this population is the underlying population from which cases arise during the study period in which they would be eligible to be included as cases. The source population is affected by migration in and out of the study area, and control sampling in a dynamic population should be limited to those members who were present in the source population at the same time the case became a case (Wacholder et al. 1992a). This requirement limits selected controls to be members of the population at risk of becoming cases so that had they become cases, they would have been enrolled in the study. For example, in our hypothetical study on breast cancer and migration, the source population might consist of women from country Y residing in city Z, country X, between 2000 and 2010.

Case-control studies can be conceptualized as having either a primary base or a secondary base (Miettinen 1985). Primary base studies, also called population-based studies, have source populations that are explicitly defined a priori according to a time period and geographic region or occupational setting; cases and controls are sampled directly from this base. The primary base approach is usually the preferred method for identifying cases and controls to represent the disease and exposure experience of a well-defined population. However, identification of cases can be more difficult in this type of base. In our breast cancer study, if researchers want to conduct a population-based study, it is straightforward to identify the source population according to location (residents of Z city), country of origin (country Y), and time period of interest (2000–2010), but may be more difficult to identify all cases of breast cancer within this defined population since patients may be diagnosed by different sources—private physicians, hospitals, or even mobile screening clinics. For some diseases, registries are available at regional or national levels to facilitate the identification of cases in a population-based study.

Ideally, a complete population roster would exist for the source population defined in a primary base study, permitting random sampling of controls from the roster. Random sampling is the preferred method of control selection in a primary study base because this method reduces selection bias and increases the likelihood of representativeness of the sample, although in some cases matching (discussed later in this chapter) can improve study efficiency when controlling confounding.

A secondary base can be used when a primary base cannot be explicitly defined. A secondary base study identifies the sources for case selection a priori and then identifies controls from the same sources under the caveat that controls who may someday experience the outcome would be candidates for inclusion as cases in the study. For example, hospital-based case-control studies are secondary base studies, where cases as well as controls with conditions other than the outcome of interest are selected from the same hospital. In the breast cancer study, researchers could select breast cancer cases diagnosed in a particular hospital in Z city and choose patients without breast cancer from the same hospital as controls, making the assumption that these patients would also be treated at that hospital if they developed breast cancer. While case identification is usually easier in secondary base studies, this method of subject identification can result in inadequate representation of the underlying source population and potentially problematic selection of controls. Attendance at a particular clinic or hospital can be influenced by a number of factors (including migration-related factors) that result in a patient population that is not representative of the underlying population.

Case Selection

Selecting cases is a key step in the case-control study. Case selection can ideally consist of a count census of all cases from the source population. However, for efficiency, cases can also be sampled as long as the sampling is random (i.e., done independently of the exposure[s] of interest). In the scenario of women from country Y with breast cancer, researchers may choose to sample cases to keep the study smaller and less costly. In that instance, researchers should make sure that they randomly select cases from country Y independently of their arrival to country X and their ability to speak the language used in country X (both factors are associated with the exposures being assessed). They should choose a random sample that will be representative of the entire source population.

Cases can be identified from a number of sources, including hospitals, physician practices, health departments, clinics, disease registries, surveillance systems, screening programs, and vital records. There are some considerations to take into account in the selection of cases. First, if cases are selected from a single facility, the risk factors that are identified from these patients may be unique to the population served by that facility, so results of the study would not be broadly generalizable to all patients with the disease in the study area. If possible, it is preferable to select cases from all or most hospitals, clinics, or physician practices serving the broader study base, to improve generalizability. Second, patients selected from insurance provider or medical system records may have different risk factors than patients who do not have insurance or who are not present in the medical system, again limiting generalizability. This is an important issue for migrants (especially new arrivals and unauthorized immigrants) because they are less likely to have insurance coverage and may have limited access to care. Third, in most studies, it is far preferable to include incident (i.e., newly occurring) cases rather than prevalent cases because cases diagnosed farther in the past may have been identified by different and/or outdated diagnostic standards, and may have different exposures; further, prevalence is a function not only of incidence but also of duration of disease. Recently detected cases are more likely to have been diagnosed by way of consistent diagnostic methods. Using prevalent cases can introduce survivor bias because individuals who survive longer with the disease have a higher probability of selection into the study, leading to an unrepresentative sample if survival is influenced by the exposure factor(s). Finally, exposure recall may be more accurate among recently diagnosed cases.

It is important to establish very clear a priori criteria to define what a case is and to determine which cases should be included in the study. First, a standard case definition that explicitly states the clinical, diagnostic, and/or laboratory evidence defining a case should be used to identify and select all cases. In addition to the diagnostic criteria, eligibility criteria should be specified to further guide case selection, and the same eligibility criteria should be applied equally to the selection of controls (Poole 1986; Wacholder 1995). For example, in our hypothetical study of breast cancer in women from country Y, cases might be defined as women diagnosed with primary invasive breast cancer. Eligibility criteria might include the following: women born in country Y, between the ages of 25 and 79, residing in Z city at the time of diagnosis, and receiving a new diagnosis of a first occurrence of breast cancer between 2000 and 2010.

A significant challenge to conducting case-control studies in migrant populations is that many potential data sources for cases and controls do not include necessary information on country of birth or other migration-related factors. For example, in the breast cancer study scenario, hospital records used to identify cases and controls may lack information on country of birth. In some circumstances, researchers may be able to collect that information directly from patients by using contact information from records to follow up with patients. Ideally, cases and controls should be sampled from records that include all the required migration data.

In many circumstances, case definitions have varying degrees of confirmation. For example, some disease registries will capture suspected, probable, and confirmed cases of a disease based on the availability of clinical and laboratory evidence. Investigators must decide what degree of certainty they need when including cases in their study. In areas or populations that lack laboratory diagnostic capacity or that have differential access to confirmatory testing, excluding cases on the basis of laboratory results or missing information may result in incomplete case ascertainment, selection bias, and lowered study precision. For example, in a case-control study conducted in a Kenyan refugee camp, a case of cholera was defined as "any person suffering from watery diarrhea (at least three stools in a 24-hour period) who was admitted to the IRC cholera ward from April 1 through June 30." This definition is less specific but more sensitive than the WHO definition for a case of cholera, which is limited to individuals greater than five years of age. While there may have been some misclassification of disease status, the increased sensitivity was considered appropriate in the resource-limited setting (Shultz et al. 2009). If investigators feel uncertain about including cases that are not confirmed, they can categorize the disease outcomes by status in the analysis (e.g., suspect, probable, and confirmed) and analyze the strata separately.

Clear case definitions and eligibility criteria reduce misclassification and ensure that all cases are selected according to the same objective standards. Eligibility criteria can be applied either during case ascertainment or during the analysis phase. Applying eligibility requirements before the data collection phase may improve efficiency by reducing the collection of data that may be discarded during analysis, but eligibility requirements could also be applied later in the study, before analysis. Researchers should disclose at what point in the study eligibility requirements were used to select study subjects.

Matching

Matching during the design stage can be used to improve efficiency for the control of confounding (Rose and Laan 2009; Rothman et al. 2008). When controls are matched to cases on a potential confounder, the ratio of controls to cases will be the same over all the strata of that variable; for example, if age matching is used, each case should have at least one control present in the same age strata. Without matching, the distribution of the confounding variables in controls may be very different from the distribution in cases. The goal in matching is to make the case and control groups similar across the strata of matched variables. If matching is not used and a stratified analysis results in strata containing cases without controls or controls without cases, data in these strata would not be included in the analysis, reducing the available sample size for analysis and resulting in decreased study efficiency. Case-control matching is most useful when applied to known categorical confounders with several strata (Rothman et al. 2008).

Matching can be done individually or at a group level (also known as frequency matching). In individual matching, each case is matched to one or more controls on a specific value of one or more variables such as age, gender, and time of case occurrence. With frequency matching, the proportions of controls and cases included in the study sample with the potential confounding variables should be the same. For example, in a study using group matching on sex, if 20% of identified cases were female, investigators would match this by ensuring that approximately 20% of controls were also female, though perfect frequency matching does not have to be achieved to ensure study efficiency. Analysis of individually matched case-control studies will be different from analysis of unmatched or group-matched studies (discussed later in the chapter).

Control Selection

The controls selected for a case-control study will typically come from the same source population from which the cases were selected and should represent the exposure distribution found in that population. Controls should be selected independently of their exposure status and should be free of the disease or outcome of interest at the start of the follow-up period of the study (Wacholder 1995), although there are notable exceptions to this rule (e.g., matching). More than one control can be selected for each case, and in circumstances where there are few cases, selection of more than one control per case can increase the study's power and improve the precision of the effect estimates. While any number of controls can be selected for each case, there is little improvement in power if the control-to-case ratio is increased beyond 4:1 (Grimes and Schulz 2005), although counterexamples exist (Breslow and Day 1985). As much as possible, controls and cases should have comparable accuracy of information available to reduce nondifferential measurement errors (Wacholder et al. 1992a; Wacholder 1995).

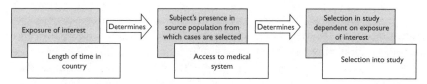

FIGURE 11.2. Study subject selection dependent on exposure of interest.

The eligibility criteria used to select cases should be applied equally to the selection of controls. An important consideration in the selection of controls is whether or not the identification of cases is dependent on a particular variable such as access to health care (Wacholder et al. 1992b). If cases identified in a source population have a higher probability than source population controls of being diagnosed with the disease because of a factor associated with the exposure of interest, this will introduce selection bias into the study. Returning to the example of the breast cancer risk study, if length of time in host country X is associated with access to health care systems, immigrants who have been in the country X longer are more likely to be captured by a study design that draws subjects from the health care system. Because length of time in country X is an exposure of interest, this will introduce bias because selection into the study is dependent on the exposure of interest (Figure 11.2)

This consideration is key in studies of migrants because their likelihood of being enrolled or accessing the health care systems that could be used for sampling these populations can vary widely depending on length of time in current country, immigration status, country of birth, and a number of other migration-related factors. Limiting a study to cases and controls from specific hospitals or clinics, or stratifying by key variables such as time in the host country can address this selection bias, though the controls may still not be representative of the broader migrant population of interest.

When a complete roster of the source population exists for a primary or population-based study, control selection can be accomplished with simple random sampling directly from the roster. In the absence of a complete roster, control selection is more difficult and prone to selection bias. In past studies, random-digit dialing (RDD) has been used to randomly select population controls in the absence of a roster, but this method is subject to increasing selection bias as more individuals have abandoned landlines and rely on cellular (mobile) phones. Also, RDD can be inefficient for targeting subpopulations within a study base. In an analysis of control selection techniques for a study base consisting of Latinos and African Americans in the United States, researchers spent an average of 18.6 hours per control recruited through RDD, compared with an average of less than an hour recruiting controls through other community-based recruitment methods, including recruitment presentations at churches, health fairs, senior centers, and outreach by university employees and physicians serving the target communities (Cabral et al. 2003). Relying on traditional RDD control selection techniques is likely to lead to selection bias, particularly with migrant populations that may have differing access to phone services and different participation rates and response bias.

Hospital, clinic, or registry records can be used to select controls from among those seen in the same treatment facilities or captured in the same registries as cases but that have conditions unrelated to the disease or exposures of interest. Investigators must make two assumptions in order to use hospital controls: (1) that selected controls would have been seen at the same hospital if the control also developed the outcome of interest, and (2) that the exposure of interest is unrelated to hospital admission in controls. Controls should ideally be selected from individuals who have diseases with symptoms and referral patterns similar to the disease of interest. This will help ensure that the study base is accurately represented. For example, if investigators intend to examine risk factors for breast cancer cases from a particular treatment hospital, controls taken from patients seen at the hospital for other, unrelated forms of cancer could be a good option since they will likely have referral patterns that are similar to cases, and patients with similar symptoms are likely to have comparable recall bias. However, use of other cancer cases for controls is based on the assumption that the risk factors for breast cancer are not risk factors for control cancer diagnoses, which may be unverifiable. An additional advantage to using hospital or registry controls is that hospital records and registry entries for both cases and controls should have similar data quality. In addition, obtaining specimens for testing or conducting physical exams will generally be easier in hospital controls. A significant potential problem with using controls from hospitals or registries is that control diseases could have different population catchments from the case diseases, particularly if the cases are from teaching hospitals that serve the local poor while also serving as tertiary referral centers for specific medical conditions. This problem could be dealt with by stratification based on the distance between the hospital and patient residence (Wacholder et al. 1992b).

The use of neighborhood controls can provide another option for control selection in case-control studies. In this method, controls are selected from residences in the same housing block or geographic area containing the case. Neighborhood controls can reduce variation in factors such as access to care and socioeconomic status if the neighborhood's population is relatively homogeneous, so confounding factors associated with location may be controlled for between cases and controls. This method is still subject to selection bias, particularly if it is used in a secondary base study where case selection occurred in a hospital that not all neighborhood residents are able to access (e.g., a military hospital).

With neighborhood controls, households can be randomly selected from a recent roster of homes that may be available from census data or neighborhood contact lists. In the case of refugee camps, maps and population lists are likely maintained by the agency managing the camp because resource distribution is dependent on knowledge of the population's location. These resources could be used as sampling frames for simple random or systematic selection of controls. If a roster for a neighborhood is not available or the population is very dynamic and the available roster is outdated, enumeration of households for the purpose of generating a sampling frame could be undertaken if resources and time allow. Alternatively, control households could be determined by using a systematic selection algorithm. This algorithm should be identified prior to the start of sampling to avoid bias that could arise when interviewers consciously or unconsciously select homes for ease of access, for example, if they skip a house to avoid an irritable dog. In a case-control study of typhoid fever in squatter settlements in Karachi, researchers enrolled neighborhood controls by selecting the third door to the left of the case's house. Interviewers started at this residence and moved to the next house until they identified a control meeting the eligibility requirements for the study (Siddiqui et al. 2008). In the case-control study in a Kenyan refugee camp, investigation team members selected controls by standing in front of the case's house, randomly selecting a starting direction, and then randomly selecting a number to determine the number of houses to pass in the chosen direction before selecting a home from which to interview the first control (Shultz et al. 2009).

Migration can play a significant role in the selection of controls from neighborhoods, and time and location eligibility requirements should be used for selecting neighborhood controls. Neighborhood controls should have been residents of their household at the time when the corresponding case was diagnosed. If neighborhood controls are chosen in a source population that is highly mobile, the study base may be significantly impacted by in- and out-migration, which reduces the number of eligible cases and controls. For this reason, carefully defining a source population in terms of time as well as location is necessary. Some migrant populations such as farmworkers or urban refugees may exist outside of easily accessible and well-defined neighborhoods, so methods of enumerating and selecting controls from these populations will have to be adapted to the setting in which the study is being conducted. Matching controls to cases by neighborhood of residence can result in selection bias with respect to the study exposures associated with residence, which would need to be addressed through conventional confounder control strategies for matched data (e.g., stratified or multivariable analysis). Other challenges to control selection include difficulty in determining the rate of nonresponse because the number of eligible subjects in homes without response is not known, and the potential for failing to obtain a random sample of controls from the people without disease from the study base.

Additional sources of controls for case-control studies include friends and family members of the cases. These types of controls can help address confounding from environmental and genetic variables. Use of friend and family controls to reduce confounding in a case-control study design is an example of individual matching in the study design and requires the use of a matched case-control analysis. In addition, these methods of control selection are nonrandom. Selection bias is a factor when friend controls are chosen by the case because friendship is related to exposure factor(s). For example, in a case-control study conducted in a migrant farmworker population with an occupational exposure of interest, there is a strong likelihood that friend controls nominated by the cases would be fellow migrant farmworkers who have similar occupational exposures, meaning that control selection would not be independent of the exposure (Flanders and Austin 1986). In some studies where the cases of interest are dead or too ill to be interviewed, proxy respondents such as spouses or family members can be used to collect information on exposures. Since in this case proxies will most likely be used more for cases than for controls, this approach can reduce the comparable accuracy between the two groups and should be approached with caution.

For a detailed discussion of control selection that explores in greater depth the strengths and weaknesses of each control type, see Wacholder's three-part series on control selection (Wacholder et al. 1992a, 1992b, 1992c).

Case-Control Design Variations

Another benefit of the case-control study is that it may be conducted within an existing cohort study. Once cases are identified in a well-defined cohort, a case-control study can be carried out by using people in the cohort who developed the disease as cases and by using a sample of the remaining at-risk cohort as controls. The resulting study can be either a nested case-control study or a case-cohort study depending on when and how the controls were sampled. In a nested case-control study, controls are sampled from the portion of the cohort at risk of the disease at the time when the case developed the disease; this is known as "risk-set sampling." In a case-cohort study, a subcohort is randomly selected from anyone included in the cohort at the study's start when all individuals are disease/outcome-free. Censored members of the subcohort (members without the outcome of interest at the end of the study period) serve as controls for the cases. All cases that develop in the cohort are included in the analysis regardless of whether they were members of the sampled subcohort or the remaining cohort. For more information on these types of studies, see Ernster's (1994) "Nested Case-Control Studies" and Barlow et al.'s (1999) "Analysis of Case-Cohort Designs."

ANALYSIS OF CASE-CONTROL STUDIES

Measure of Association

The odds ratio is the only effect measure that can be directly calculated from a case-control study. "Odds" is defined as the number of times an event occurs

TABLE 11.1 2 × 2 Table for Unmatched Case-Control Study

	Cases	Controls
Exposed	a	b
Not exposed	c	d

TABLE 11.2 2 × 2 Table for a Matched Pairs Case-Control Study

		Controls	
		Exposed	Not exposed
Cases	Exposed	W	X
	Not exposed	Y	Z

divided by the number of times that event does not occur. Because case-control studies are sampled based on outcome status and quantified exposure(s), the odds of a case or control having the exposure of interest is called the "exposure odds." The odds ratio in a case-control study is therefore the exposure odds among cases divided by the exposure odds among controls. The simple 2 × 2 table in Table 11.1 illustrates.

The odds of developing the disease can be compared between cases and controls in a simple ratio:

$$\text{Exposure odds ratio (OR)} = \frac{\text{exposure odds for cases}}{\text{exposure odds for controls}} = \frac{\frac{a}{c}}{\frac{b}{d}} = \frac{ad}{bc}$$

This calculation is also called the cross-product ratio because the value is calculated by multiplying diagonally across cells in a 2 × 2 table and dividing the products.

It is important to note that the exposure odds ratio is algebraically equivalent to the incidence (disease) odds ratio:

$$\text{Incidence odds ratio (OR)} = \frac{\text{disease odds among exposed}}{\text{disease odds among unexposed}} = \frac{\frac{a}{b}}{\frac{c}{d}} = \frac{ad}{bc}$$

The odds ratio is calculated differently for analyzing matched cases and controls. The orientation of a 2 × 2 table for a matched analysis is provided in Table 11.2.

Only the discordant matched pairs are compared (where the paired case and control have different exposure status), and the matched odds ratio is calculated with the following formula:

$$\text{Matched odds ratio (OR}_M) = \frac{X}{Y}$$

When more than one control is matched to a case, it is generally necessary to use multivariable statistical methods (e.g., conditional logistic regression) to perform matched analyses.

Interpretation of the Odds Ratio

If the odds are the same between the cases and controls, the odds ratio will equal 1, the null value. This would indicate that there is no association between the exposure and the outcome. If the odds ratio is greater than one, the odds of exposure are greater among cases than controls, and this would indicate a positive association between the exposure and the outcome. If the odds ratio is less than one, the odds of exposure are greater among controls than cases, and this would indicate a negative association between the exposure and outcome. Investigators may also say that such an exposure has a *protective effect* on disease outcome. Odds ratios can be adjusted for potential confounders during the analysis by means of either a stratified or multivariable analysis (e.g., logistic regression).

The odds ratio is less interpretively intuitive than other measures of association based on probability (e.g., risk ratio or rate ratio). Odds can range between zero and positive infinity, whereas probability measures range from zero to one. When the likelihood of an event occurring is low, the odds ratio approximates the risk ratio fairly closely. However, as the risk ratio rises above one, the odds ratio will increasingly overstate the likelihood of the event compared to the risk ratio. Conversely, when the risk ratio is less than one the odds ratio will be an underestimate of the risk ratio.

While case-control studies cannot directly calculate measures of risk, the odds ratio can estimate the relative risk depending on whether or not cases are incident or prevalent, if the source population is fixed or dynamic, how controls are selected, and what underlying assumptions are made during the study (e.g., if the disease is rare, i.e., less than 5% incidence in the time period under study in all strata of controlled variables). Use of prevalent cases always results in the calculation of a prevalence odds ratio. For incident cases, the odds ratio can estimate both the risk ratio and the rate ratio under specific conditions and depending on how controls are sampled. For further exploration, Knol et al. (2008) offer a detailed review of what measures can be estimated from odds ratios obtained from case-control studies according to study design.

Sample Size and Power Calculation

Sample size is an important consideration in study design. In some case-control studies with a limited number of cases, the investigator will not be able to influence the sample size beyond including multiple controls for each case, but in other studies that are based on sampled cases, sample size should be considered during the study planning. Larger samples produce more precise measures of effect but will usually require more resources and time. Power analysis can help decide an optimal sample size for a case-control study under specified constraints. Power is the probability that a statistical test will correctly reject the null hypothesis of a study when the null hypothesis is false (Rothman et al. 2008). The higher a study's power, the lower the chances of incorrectly failing to reject a null hypothesis (making a false negative decision). There are a number of free programs available online and for download that can be used to calculate sample size—or power, if a study has already been conducted and the sample size is known (see resources, below). Calculations of sample size and power for case-control studies are different from those used for cohort studies, so researchers must be sure to select the specific case-control calculator or formula when performing calculations. Such programs, however, may fail to account for the impact of confounder control on sample size calculations and power, underestimating the former and overestimating the latter. Because performing these calculations requires detailed information on associations between all confounders, exposures, and outcomes that will rarely be known with precision, sample size calculators should be regarded as rough estimates of study size that should be adapted based on investigator knowledge of study objectives, study design, and available resources.

SUMMARY/CONCLUSIONS

The case-control method is well suited for use in migrant populations because it does not require lengthy follow-up of subjects, can be used with newly or previously collected data, and generally requires a smaller sample size than other study designs, resulting in lower costs and greater efficiency. In cases where the target migrant populations or outcomes of interest are rare, case-control studies are useful because they can produce results with a much smaller sample size than other study types. The case-control study design can also be used to simultaneously assess multiple exposures related to migration for association with a particular outcome. Surprisingly, this accessible method has only rarely been reported in studies of migrant populations, but we believe it has a broad and valuable role for this area of research.

RESOURCES

- Epi Info™ (http://wwwn.cdc.gov/epiinfo/): A free suite of software tools developed and distributed by CDC, Epi Info™ can assist with the design and statistical analysis of multiple study designs. It can be easily used in areas with limited network connectivity, resources, and professional IT support. Epi info can be used to develop questionnaires for data collection and to perform data entry and analysis. To use the sample size and power calculator, select the StatCalc dropdown menu from the header bar on the menu page, choose the Sample Size and Power option, and select the Unmatched Case-Control option from the list that appears. The calculator that opens will list the data needed for the calculation.

- OpenEpi (http://www.openepi.com/OE2.3/Menu/OpenEpiMenu.htm): OpenEpi is free and open source software for epidemiologic statistics. It can be run from a web server or downloaded and run without a web connection. The OpenEpi . website lists available calculators on the left-hand side of the webpage. Sample Size and Power folders can be expanded to show links specifically for different study types, including an unmatched case-control study.

REFERENCES

Barlow, W. E., L. Ichikawa, D. Rosner, and S. Izumi (1999). Analysis of case-cohort designs [Comparative study research support, US government, PHS]. *Journal of Clinical Epidemiology* 52(12): 1165–72.

Bruno, G., G. Pagano, F. Faggiano, A. De Salvia, and F. Merletti (2000). Effect of Sardinian heritage on risk and age at onset of type 1 diabetes: A demographic case-control study of Sardinian migrants [Research support, non–US government]. *International Journal of Epidemiology* 29(3): 532–35.

Cabral, D. N., A. M. Napoles-Springer, R. Miike, A. McMillan, J. D. Sison, M. R. Wrensch, and J. K. Wiencke (2003). Population- and community-based recruitment of African Americans and Latinos: The San Francisco Bay Area Lung Cancer Study [Research support, US government, PHS]. *American Journal of Epidemiology* 15(3): 272–79.

Dos Santos Silva, I., P. Mangtani, V. McCormack, D. Bhakta, L. Sevak, and A. J. McMichael (2002). Lifelong vegetarianism and risk of breast cancer: A population-based case-control study among South Asian migrant women living in England [Research support, non–US government]. *International Journal of Cancer* 99(2): 238–44. doi: 10.1002/ijc.10300.

Ernster, V. L. (1994). Nested case-control studies. *Preventive Medicine* 23(5): 587–90. doi: 10.1006/pmed.1994.1093.

Flanders, W. D., and H. Austin (1986). Possibility of selection bias in matched case-control studies using friend controls [Research support, US government, PHS]. *American Journal of Epidemiology* 124(1): 150–53.

Greenland S., and D. C. Thomas. 1982. On the need for the rare disease assumption in case-control studies. *American Journal of Epidemiology* 116: 547–53.

Grimes, D. A., and K. F. Schulz (2005). Compared to what? Finding controls for case-control studies. *Lancet* 365(9468): 1429–33. doi: 10.1016/S0140-6736 (05)66379-9.

Hosek, R. S., W. D. Flanders, and A. J. Sasco (1996). Bias in case-control studies of screening effectiveness. *American Journal of Epidemiology* 143(2): 193–201.

John, E. M., A. I. Phipps, A. Davis, and J. Koo (2005). Migration history, acculturation, and breast cancer risk in Hispanic women [Research support, NIH; extramural research support, non–US government]. *Cancer epidemiology, biomarkers and prevention: A publication of the American Association for Cancer Research, cosponsored by the American Society of Preventive Oncology* 14(12): 2905–13. doi: 10.1158/1055-9965.EPI-05-0483.

Jones, M. E., and A. J. Swerdlow (1996). Bias caused by migration in case-control studies of prenatal risk factors for childhood and adult diseases. *American Journal of Epidemiology* 143(8): 823–31.

Knol, M. J., J. P. Vandenbroucke, P. Scott, and M. Egger (2008). What do case-control studies estimate? Survey of methods and assumptions in published case-control research [Research support, non–US government]. *American Journal of Epidemiology* 168(9): 1073–81. doi: 10.1093/aje/kwn217.

MacDonald, P. D., R. E. Whitwam, J. D. Boggs, J. N. MacCormack, K. L. Anderson, J. W. Reardon, et al. (2005). Outbreak of listeriosis among Mexican immigrants as a result of consumption of illicitly produced Mexican-style cheese. *Clinical infectious diseases: An official publication of the Infectious Diseases Society of America* 40(5): 677–82. doi: 10.1086/427803.

Miettinen, O. (1985). The "case-control" study: Valid selection of subjects. *Journal of Chronic Disease* 38(7): 543–48.

Mills, P. K., and R. Yang (2003). Prostate cancer risk in California farm workers [Research support, non–US government]. *Journal of Occupational and Environmental Medicine /American College of Occupational and Environmental Medicine* 45(3): 249–58.

Mills, P. K., and R. Yang (2005). Breast cancer risk in Hispanic agricultural workers in California [Research support, non–US government]. *International Journal of Occupational and Environmental Health* 11(2): 123–31.

Mills, P. K., and R. Yang (2007). Agricultural exposures and gastric cancer risk in Hispanic farm workers in California [Research support, NIH, extramural]. *Environmental Research* 104(2): 282–89. doi: 10.1016/j.envres.2006.11.008.

Mills, P. K., R. Yang, and D. Riordan (2005). Lymphohematopoietic cancers in the United Farm Workers of America (UFW), 1988–2001 [Comparative study evaluation studies research support, NIH, extramural]. *Cancer Causes and Control: CCC* 16(7): 823–30. doi: 10.1007/s10552-005-2703-2.

Moss, S. M. 1991. Case-control studies of screening. *International Journal of Epidemiology* 20: 1–6.

Poole, C. (1986). Exposure opportunity in case-control studies. *American Journal of Epidemiology* 123(2): 352–58.

Rose, S., and M. J. Laan (2009). Why match? Investigating matched case-control study designs with causal effect estimation [Research support, NIH, extramural]. *International Journal of Biostatistics* 5(1), Article 1. doi: 10.2202/1557-4679.1127.

Rothman, K. J., G. S. Poole, and T. L. Lash (Eds.). (2008). *Modern epidemiology* (3rd ed.). Philadelphia: Lippincott-Williams-Wilkins.

Schulz, K. F., and D. A. Grimes (2002). Case-control studies: Research in reverse. *Lancet* 359(9304): 431–34. doi: 10.1016/S0140-6736(02)07605-5.

Shultz, A., J. O. Omollo, H. Burke, M. Qassim, J. B. Ochieng, M. Weinberg, and R. F. Breiman (2009). Cholera outbreak in Kenyan refugee camp: Risk factors for illness and importance of sanitation. *American Journal of Tropical Medicine and Hygiene* 80(4): 640–45.

Siddiqui, F. J., S. R. Haider, and Z. A. Bhutta (2008). Risk factors for typhoid fever in children in squatter settlements of Karachi: A nested case-control study [Research support, non–US government]. *Journal of Infection and Public Health* 1(2): 113–20. doi: 10.1016/j.jiph.2008.10.003.

Wacholder, S. (1995). Design issues in case-control studies [Review]. *Statistical Methods in Medical Research* 4(4): 293–309.

Wacholder, S., J. K. McLaughlin, D. T. Silverman, and J. S. Mandel (1992a). Selection of controls in case-control studies. I. Principles. *American Journal of Epidemiology* 135(9): 1019–28.

Wacholder, S., D. T. Silverman, J. K. McLaughlin, and J. S. Mandel (1992b). Selection of controls in case-control studies. II. Types of controls. *American Journal of Epidemiology* 135(9): 1029–41.

Wacholder, S., D. T. Silverman, J. K. McLaughlin, and J. S. Mandel (1992c). Selection of controls in case-control studies. III. Design options. *American Journal of Epidemiology* 135(9): 1042–50.

12

Longitudinal Studies

Guillermina Jasso

INTRODUCTION

Migration occurs over time. And health unfolds over time. It is thus not surprising that longitudinal studies are the ideal approach for studying migration, health, and the two together. Longitudinal studies confer general advantages—making it possible to distinguish between cohort and duration effects, for example, and to obtain unbiased estimates in situations where cross-sectional data would yield consistent estimates at best. Longitudinal studies also confer specific advantages in the study of migration and health—making it possible to assess mechanisms of selection and integration with unprecedented sharpness.

This chapter begins with a brief overview of migration and health questions and of longitudinal studies and, after briefly summarizing the US immigration context, describes the US New Immigrant Survey (NIS), a multiple-cohort longitudinal study of persons newly admitted to legal permanent residence in the United States and their children, and provides a few illustrative examples of studying immigrant health. Additional description of immigrant longitudinal studies conducted in other countries can be found in the literature (Black et al. 2003; Morgan and Nicholson 2005). For an example of comparative research based on immigrant longitudinal data from two countries, see Jasso and Rosenzweig (2009).

MIGRATION AND HEALTH:
CENTRAL QUESTIONS AND GENERAL CHALLENGES

Four central questions arise in the study of migration:

1. What are the migrant's characteristics and behavior at entry?
2. How do the migrant's characteristics and behavior change with time in the destination country?
3. What are the characteristics and behavior of the children of immigrants?
4. What are the impacts of migration on the origin and destination countries?

The first question—the *selection question*—encompasses questions about the forces of selectivity (i.e., who migrates and why), including self-selection as well as economic, legal, and other inducements and restrictions at both exit and entry, and family dynamics. The second question—the *assimilation question*—pertains to the migrant's trajectory after immigration, including the extent and pace of adaptation as well as the decision to leave the destination country, either to return to the origin country or to go on to another destination. The third question—the *children-of-migration question,* covers everything that pertains to migrant children and the children of migrants, including the subset born in the destination country (the classic second generation). Finally, the fourth question—the *impacts question*—seeks to assess the myriad effects of migration on both origin and destination countries and their residents.

All four questions arise in the study of migration and health. The health selection question seeks to learn the direction of selection on health across different migration streams, specifically, whether the healthiest or the least healthy among an origin-country population seek to migrate. The health assimilation question explores health improvement or deterioration in the destination country, as well as the effect of health selection in the decisions to naturalize and/or to emigrate. The children-of-migration health question assesses parental transmission of health effects as well as health determinants and outcomes. The health impacts question seeks to understand the effects of migration on public health and health care costs in both origin country and destination country.

The selection question embeds several mechanisms, including the prospective migrant's *desire to move* and choice of a destination country, as well the actions of individuals and governments in both countries to encourage or discourage the move—in extremis, forcing or preventing it. A key element in the selection question is the connection between the prospective migrant's characteristics—such as socioeconomic location and health—and the desire to move, also called *migrant energy*. This apt phrase appears in several literatures. For example, the social scientist Aderanti Adepoju observes, "There is hardly any prosperous country that is not based on migrant energy" (Sawyerr 2010), and the historian Richard Gott (2005:45) discusses "the injection of migrant energy" in Cuba in the late eighteenth and early nineteenth centuries. Another key element in the selection question pertains to conditions in both the origin and destination countries, which may be linked to the prospective migrant's characteristics as well as to migrant energy, potentially giving rise to strong cohort effects. Finally, networks play an important part in self-selection, as shown by Massey (1987:1373–74) and Massey et al. (1993).

Meanwhile, the assimilation question also embeds several mechanisms, including the effects of sponsors (both family members and employers) and networks. There is keen interest in assessing the migrant's characteristics at specific periods of duration in the destination country—for example, at five, ten, fifteen, twenty years after migration—relative to the native population in the destination country and also to the migrant's counterparts who remain in the origin country.

Studying these questions is not easy. There is growing recognition that many factors intervene, including legal restrictions on migration, the family dynamics brought to widespread attention by Mincer (1978), and the migration process itself.

The classical research prescription was to compare movers and stayers. If there were no government restrictions on exit or entry and no interference from family dynamics, the contrast between movers and stayers in the population of an origin country would be fully informative about self-selection. But given government policies and family dynamics, the actual movers may (1) include tied movers and forced movers, and (2) miss tied stayers and forced stayers. Accordingly, a challenge in the study of selection is to correctly identify those who self-select into a move.

MIGRATION AND HEALTH: SPECIAL CHALLENGES

A key challenge is that the migration process itself affects health. The literature suggests that there are three sources of health change among migrants. First, the legal aspects of migration—the visa process—may be highly stressful, generating *visa stress* (Kasl and Berkman 1983; Vega and Amaro 1994; Jasso et al. 2004, 2005), one of the "emotional costs" of migration (Levine et al. 1985:3). Second, living in a foreign country may be highly stressful, generating *migration stress*. Third, each sociogeographic locale has its own *exposure effects* on health, such as effects associated with the food, altitude, environmental pollutants, climate, and so on. The visa stress and migration stress effects are negative; the exposure effects are a mix of positive and negative effects. Part of adaptation involves learning to mitigate harms and extract benefits from the new environment.

If there are no restrictions on migration, there is no visa stress. For example, persons from Puerto Rico who move to the United States experience migration stress but not visa stress; similarly, persons born in the United States but residing abroad since infancy experience migration stress but no visa stress. Visa stress may cause health to deteriorate, even if only temporarily. Thus, assessing immigrant health soon after arrival may be too late to obtain a pure and undistorted view of health selection; visa stress may have begun much earlier. For that reason, understanding health selection requires assessing immigrant health at an earlier time, such as at the time of the migration decision.

Conversely, a person may experience visa stress but not migration stress. Examples include a variety of persons raised from childhood in the United States—children of legal temporary residents, children of diplomats, children of unauthorized immigrants. The migration history is crucial for understanding the individual's health trajectory.

Note that while migration stress and exposure effects are tied to the destination country, visa stress can be experienced in the origin country—if the visa process occurs while the prospective immigrant is still in the origin country. Further, there are special sequences of effects. For example, if the prospective immigrant is living in the origin country throughout the visa process, visa stress ends before migration stress and exposure effects begin. In contrast, if the visa process starts after the prospective immigrant is already living in the destination country, all three effects may be experienced at the same time, exacerbating their negative effects—reminiscent of the classical conjecture about the stresses associated with reaching puberty and transitioning to middle school at the same time (Simmons and Blyth 1987).

Theoretical and empirical analysis of migration and health produces stylized stories. For example, in one such story—known as the healthy immigrant effect—new immigrants are healthier than stayers in the origin country and healthier than natives in the destination country but over time their health declines so that they lose the initial health advantage over natives in the destination country (Antecol and Bedard 2006; Biddle et al. 2007; Stephen et al. 1994). The decline may be associated with several mechanisms, including exposure to negative effects and inability to extract positive effects from the destination country environment.

However, given visa stress, the pervasive effects of legal status, and the dramatic diversity among the foreign-born—including, for example, naturalized citizens and illegals, world-class scientists and persons with no formal schooling—a more accurate story may follow two lines. First, among legal immigrants, health declines temporarily due to visa stress, migration stress, and exposure to the new health environment; but with the passage of time, visa stress and migration stress end, and the immigrant learns to navigate the new environment, mitigating its health harms and extracting its health benefits. Second, among the unauthorized, visa stress never ends, and the circumstances of daily life, coupled with deficits in the destination country language, may make it difficult to deal effectively with the new country's health environment.

That story, however, is premised on particular features of the legal environment and immigration climate. It may be that visa stress never ends, although it may become attenuated. For example, consider that a person may lose legal status and become deportable. Even a naturalized citizen can be stripped of citizenship and deported.

LONGITUDINAL STUDIES

A longitudinal study follows the same individuals over time, measuring characteristics, exposures, behaviors, and outcomes at several points in time. Once the sample is selected, and respondents agree to participate in the study, additional information is obtained that will make it possible to locate the respondents at a future time and reinterview them. Longitudinal studies have several strengths (Ashenfelter 2003:5, 262–74; Tourangeau 2004; Wooldridge 2006:448–509). First, they enable direct study of processes that occur over time, such as human development, attachments of all kinds (to the labor force, to a spouse, etc.), and immigrant assimilation. Second, they make it possible to study the uniqueness of individuals. Third, they make it possible to control the biasing effects of unobserved heterogeneity.

Statistically, longitudinal studies make it possible to estimate fixed-effects models (also known as differential-intercept models). These models hold constant the effects of time-invariant factors, enabling unbiased estimation of the effects of time-varying explanatory variables, even when they are correlated with the time-invariant variables. The textbook case pertains to estimates of the effects of schooling on earnings, which in cross-sectional data may be biased due to operation of the unobservable ability variable; fixed-effects models estimated on longitudinal data control for ability and thus yield unbiased estimates of the effect of schooling on earnings.

There are a number of equivalent approaches for estimating fixed-effects models. One approach is to include a dummy variable for each unit (as implied by the name "differential-intercept model"). Another is to transform the data into deviations from unit means. When the number of observations per unit is two, an equivalent procedure is to take first differences.

If there is a large number of observations per unit, it becomes possible to estimate a model that not only has differential intercepts but also has differential slopes, yielding a complete equation—a complete and distinctive pattern of effects—per unit, that is, permitting study of the uniqueness of individuals. As large panel datasets grow, it will become possible to estimate such fully heterogeneous models and test them against less heterogeneous models (e.g., using the Chow test to see whether the differential-intercept/differential-slopes model describes the data more faithfully than the common-intercept/common-slopes model). At the present time, distinctive equations for each respondent are largely confined to vignette studies (such as Jasso's 1988 study of judgments of the desirability of immigrants, which showed that each respondent had distinctive views of the criteria for the selection of immigrants, views expressed in a distinctive personal equation).

LONGITUDINAL DESIGNS FOR STUDYING
MIGRATION AND HEALTH

Beyond the generic strengths of longitudinal designs, there are special strengths that longitudinal designs impart to the study of migration. First, longitudinal studies make it possible to distinguish between the effects of cohort factors—such as conditions in the origin and destination countries at the time of migration—and the effects of experiences in the destination country. Second, longitudinal studies enable assessment of emigration selectivity and hence estimation of the true progress of immigrants, unconfounded by shifts over time, due to emigration decisions, in the composition of a cohort. Third, longitudinal studies make it possible to observe assimilation, which unfolds over time.

To illustrate how longitudinal studies make it possible to distinguish between cohort and duration effects, consider, for example, a cross-section study conducted in 2000. If persons who came to the United States in 1980 have higher earnings than persons who came in 1990, it is impossible to know whether (1) earnings increase with time in the United States (a duration effect), or (2) the immigrants who came in 1980 had higher earnings potential than those who came in 1990 (a cohort effect). Longitudinal study of multiple cohorts solves the problem by measuring each cohort's characteristics at entry and observing changes in characteristics (e.g., earnings growth) over time.

The ideal longitudinal design for studying migration and health starts with a probability sample of a birth cohort in an origin country. Health measures would be taken at regular intervals, as well as measures of schooling, employment, earnings, marriage, fertility, language skills, and so on. Migration histories would also be recorded, including spells in other countries, visa applications, and the desire to migrate. If and when migration occurs, the individual would continue to be interviewed regularly in the destination country. Such a design relies heavily on prospective data. It would yield data that could be used for addressing all the questions in the study of migration and health.

Less ideal but more feasible designs involve a mix of retrospective and prospective data. One possible design, based in the destination country, would begin with probability samples drawn from two populations: (1) persons newly admitted to legal permanent residence and (2) persons admitted for the first time with a temporary visa. The original design for the US New Immigrant Survey (NIS) proposed looking at both populations, but the second had to be eliminated as the requisite sampling frame for temporary migrants did not exist. Note that longitudinal study of first-time temporary entrants would make it possible to observe the process by which some among them decide to seek legal permanent residence, as well as the process by which some among them become illegal (by overstaying a

TABLE 12.1   Special Variables for Studying Migration and Health in a
Longitudinal Design

Year first wanted to visit destination country
Health at the time first wanted to visit destination country
Year first wanted to live permanently in destination country
Health at the time first wanted to live permanently in destination country
Date of first filing for each spell in destination country
Date of entry and exit for each spell in destination country
Entry documents for each spell in destination country
Schooling during each spell in destination country
Employment during each spell in destination country
Health at first filing, entry, and exit for each spell in destination country
Date of admission to another legal status during spell in destination country
Health at admission to another legal status during spell in destination country

NOTE: Further variables can be constructed from this basic set. For example, in the case of legal permanent residence, duration of the visa process can be calculated from the date when the first document was filed (e.g., application for labor certification in an employment-based case that requires labor certification or Form I-130, "Petition for an Alien Relative" in a family-based case) and the date of admission to LPR.

temporary visa or by violating the terms of their visa, say, by accepting unauthorized employment).

Table 12.1 lists some of the main variables that may be included in a longitudinal design for studying migration and health. These include a large number of dates—for example, in the case of legal permanent residence (LPR), dates of first wanting LPR, dates of all applications for LPR, date of admission to LPR—as well as schooling and employment during intervals in the destination country, together with comprehensive health measures at entry, exit, admission to LPR, naturalization, and any other key migration milestones. Many more variables can be constructed from this basic set, including duration variables such as duration of the visa process in the LPR case.

Of course, information would be collected on numerous other variables. These include variables that cover applying for and preparing for naturalization, sponsoring relatives and employees for immigration, sending and receiving remittances, and so on.

US IMMIGRATION CONTEXT

The United States admits about a million persons a year to legal permanent residence. This section briefly summarizes aspects of the visa allocation system that are relevant for understanding immigrant health.

Immigrant Class of Admission

The system of visa allocation provides numerically unlimited visas to the spouses, minor children, and parents of adult US citizens. Numerically limited visas are granted to three main categories of immigrants: (1) family immigrants, comprised of the adult children and siblings of US citizens and the spouses and children of legal permanent residents; (2) employment immigrants, comprised of five subcategories; and (3) diversity immigrants (winners of the lottery visas designated for persons from countries underrepresented in recent immigration). Two additional categories of LPR visas have subsets of both numerically limited and numerically unlimited type. These are (4) humanitarian immigrants (including refugees, asylees, and parolees) and (5) legalization immigrants, that is, illegal immigrants who are becoming legal, including registry-provision immigrants (who qualify by virtue of length of illegal residence) and cancellation-of-removal immigrants, plus immigrants who legalize under special legislation (such as the Nicaraguan Adjustment and Central American Relief Act of 1997, or NACARA). Unauthorized migrants may also become legal if they qualify for a visa under one of the other categories above.

Principals and Accompanying Relatives

The *principal* is the person who qualifies for the visa. The three categories of immediate relatives of US citizens—spouse, parent, minor child—are, with few exceptions, for principals only. Most other categories provide LPR visas not only for the principal but also for the spouse and minor children "accompanying, or following to join" the principal. Examples include spouses and minor children of employment principals and of sibling principals, and the nonrefugee spouses and minor children of refugees. Exceptions include the category for spouses of legal permanent residents and a few categories designated for unmarried principals, in which case accompanying-relative visas are available only for minor children.

New Arrivals and Adjustees

New legal permanent residents include both *new arrivals* and persons who are already in the United States with a temporary visa or in unauthorized status and adjust to LPR, known as *adjustees*. Over half of all new legal permanent residents are adjustees—55.8% in the 1996–2005 decade, 59.2% in the 2006–2010 period, and 54.6%, 53.1%, and 53.6% in 2011, 2012, and 2013.

Visa Availability

The number of visas available each year for the principal and accompanying spouse and minor children are approximately 226,000 in the numerically limited family categories, 140,000 in the numerically limited employment categories, and 50,000 in the diversity category.

Visa Volume

As noted above, about a million persons are admitted to legal permanent residence each year. The largest subsets of adult legal immigrants are spouses and parents of US citizens, about a third, and 12% of all new adult legal permanent residents, respectively.

Conditional Visas

Two sets of immigrants receive *conditional visas* as LPR. These are (1) spouses and children of US citizens and legal permanent residents whose eligibility for the visa is based on marriages of less than two years' duration, and (2) employment-based investor immigrants. The visas are conditional for two years and a special application is made for removal of the conditionality restrictions.

Duration of Immigrant Visa Process

The process of applying for an immigrant visa is arduous and time-consuming. Persons waiting for numerically limited visas may have to wait many years; the wait time depends jointly on the visa category and the origin country. The current upper extreme is around twenty-three years for persons from the Philippines approved for visas as the siblings of US citizens; at the other extreme, visas in some of the employment-based categories (such as that for priority workers, including world-renowned scientists, artists, and executives) are available immediately (US Department of State, *Visa Bulletin*). Besides the wait for numerically limited visas, all visa applications take processing time. In general, the visa process lasts from the date when the first application is filed to the date legal permanent residence is granted. For most immigrants the date of the first application is a convenient date to represent the date of the migration decision. Exceptions include refugees, whose migration decision, as well as admission to the United States with a nonimmigrant refugee document, predates the filing for LPR.

Health Requirements for an Immigrant Visa

The prospective immigrant must pass a medical examination to ensure that he or she is not inadmissible on medical grounds. The medical grounds for inadmissibility are grouped into four categories: (1) communicable disease of public health significance (e.g., tuberculosis or syphilis), (2) lack of required vaccinations (e.g., for polio and hepatitis B), (3) physical or mental disorders with harmful behavior, and (4) drug abuse or addiction. Thus, US immigration law plays a part in shaping the immigrant's health status at admission to legal permanent residence.

Temporary Visas

The United States also provides temporary visas for a large variety of persons and purposes, such as tourists for business or pleasure, students, temporary workers, musicians, athletes, representatives of foreign newspapers and broadcast media, and diplomats.

Unauthorized Migration

Several factors have led to substantial unauthorized migration. Many people around the world have no hope of legally visiting or living in the United States—for example, if they are poor (and thus inadmissible on public charge grounds) or do not qualify for one of the visa categories. Further, persons who do qualify for immigrant visas may have to wait many years for them—currently, there are 4,322,575 applicants waiting for the approximately 366,000 numerically limited LPR visas available annually (US Department of State 2013).

Foreign-Born Population in the United States

Currently, the population of foreign-born people living in the United States is estimated to be about 40 million. The average number in 2012 was estimated by the Census Bureau at 40,824,658. The US Department of Homeland Security (DHS; US Department of Homeland Security 2002–2013) provides estimates of the noncitizen resident foreign-born. Table 12.2 combines information from DHS and the Census Bureau on the resident foreign-born on January 1, 2012. As shown, the total foreign-born is estimated at 40,601,259. The Census Bureau provides estimates of the entire foreign-born population and for the subsets who are and are not citizens. DHS provides estimates of legal permanent residents, temporary residents, and the unauthorized. The two sets of estimates reveal a discrepancy. The number of citizens implied by the DHS estimates is about 4 million lower than the estimate of citizens estimated by the Census Bureau. This means that one or more of the following holds: the Census Bureau overestimates the number of citizens; DHS overestimates the number of noncitizens—legal permanent residents, temporary residents, and/or unauthorized migrants.

ILLUSTRATION OF A LONGITUDINAL STUDY: THE US NEW IMMIGRANT SURVEY

The New Immigrant Survey (NIS) is a multiple-cohort longitudinal study of new legal immigrants to the United States and their children. The objective of the NIS is to provide a public-use database that will be useful for addressing scientific and policy questions about migration behavior and the impacts of migration. The basic design calls for taking representative samples of cohorts of new legal immigrants and following them over time, with new cohorts selected every four or five years, or whenever developments in US immigration policy or in conditions worldwide warrant. The sampling frame for each cohort, to be described below, is based on the electronic administrative records compiled for new legal permanent residents

TABLE 12.2 Foreign-Born Population in the United States, by Legal Status: 1 January 2012

	DHS Office of Immigration Statistics 1 January 2012		DOC Bureau of the Census Average 2011–2012
Legal status	Published	Implied	Published
All foreign-born	—	—	40,601,259
US citizen	—	—	18,413,215
Not a US citizen	—	GT 26,600,000	22,188,045
Legal permanent residents who have not become citizens	13,300,000	—	—
Legal temporary residents (omits refugees, asylees, and parolees)	1,870,000	—	—
Unauthorized	11,430,000	—	—

NOTE: Both the legal temporary residents and the unauthorized include persons who are on the track to legal perma-nent residence (LPR) and persons aspiring to LPR as well as persons who are not interested in LPR. The implied DHS estimate of noncitizen foreign-born is a lower bound because the component with legal temporary residents omits refugees, asylees, and parolees. The Department of Commerce (DOC) estimate of foreign-born who have become citizens is based on a question about naturalization; foreign-born who acquire citizenship in other ways (chiefly by "deriving" it from their parents) may or may not be included.
SOURCE: Baker 2014; Baker and Rytina, 2013, Rytina, 2013; US Census Bureau 2012, 2013.

by the US government (via, formerly, the US Immigration and Naturalization Service [INS; US Immigration and Naturalization Service 1979–2001] and now its successor agencies, the US Citizenship and Immigration Services [USCIS] and the Office of Immigration Statistics [OIS]). The sampling frame consists of all adult immigrants admitted to legal permanent residence during a specified period and two types of child immigrants who would not be found in the households of adult immigrants. Accordingly, the sampling frame includes both new-arrival immigrants—immigrants arriving in the United States with immigrant docu-ments acquired abroad—and adjustee immigrants—immigrants who are already in the United States with a temporary nonimmigrant visa (or, in some cases, ille-gally) and adjust to lawful permanent residence.

Thus, for the first time, the NIS obtains longitudinal information on nationally representative cohorts of new legal immigrants in the US.

Interviews are conducted with sampled adult immigrants and their spouses and with the sponsor-parents of sampled child immigrants and the spouses of the sponsor-parents; sampled children and other children (both foreign-born and US-born children) in the households of both sampled adult and child immigrants are interviewed and/or given assessments based on an age-eligibility schedule.

Two key elements of the design are that interviews for the baseline round are conducted as soon as possible after admission to lawful permanent residence, and that immigrants are interviewed in the language of their choice (e.g., 95 languages were used in the baseline round of the first full cohort, NIS-2003). The survey is made possible by the fact that the administrative records in the sampling frame include the address to which the immigrant has requested that the "green card"—the paper evidence of legal permanent residence—be mailed; this is the best possible address for locating sampled immigrants.

New rounds of data collection are to be conducted regularly for each cohort. The NIS design calls for reinterview every three to five years (e.g., round 2 of NIS-2003 was in the field in 2007–2009).

Because the NIS design, based on sampling named individuals from administrative records, with its attendant challenges of locating specific, named individuals and providing instruments and interviewers in many languages, had never been tried before, a pilot—the NIS-Pilot (NIS-P)—was carried out in 1996. The NIS-P confirmed the soundness of the design, highlighted the importance of contacting sampled immigrants as soon as possible after admission to permanent residence (while they are still at the address on the immigrant record), and provided new information on immigrants never before available (Jasso et al. 2000).

All aspects of the design of NIS-2003 were developed with information from two sources: (1) the NIS-Pilot of 1996 and (2) the public-use immigrant records for fiscal years 1996–2000. Data from the NIS-Pilot and from the first and second rounds of NIS-2003 are available for public use. Data and documentation are posted on the NIS website at http://nis.princeton.edu.

NIS-2003 SAMPLE DESIGN

NIS-2003 Sample Design at Round 1

The first full cohort to be surveyed as part of the NIS project consists of new legal immigrants whose administrative electronic immigration records were compiled in the seven-month period May to November 2003.

Adult and Child Samples. Two samples of new legal immigrants were drawn—the Adult Sample and the Child Sample. The two samples are defined in terms of immigration category and age.

The Adult Sample covers all immigrants who are eighteen years of age or older at admission to LPR and who have visas as principals or as accompanying spouses. The Child Sample covers immigrants with child-of-US-citizen visas (except self-petition immigrants) who are under eighteen years of age and adopted orphans under five years of age.

The NIS thus excludes from the sampling frame accompanying children, accompanying adult offspring, and other accompanying nonspouse/nonchild relatives; these are covered as household members of sampled immigrants in the Adult

Sample. The NIS also excludes adopted orphans five years of age and over, self-petition child-of-US-citizen immigrants, and children under eighteen who hold principal visas other than child-of-US-citizen or adopted-orphan visas. Self-petition child-of-US-citizen immigrants may be covered as household members of self-petition immigrants in the Adult Sample; the other excluded children are relatively few, so it would not be possible to obtain large enough sample sizes to permit reliable inference (additionally, rules for the protection of human subjects preclude contacting unaccompanied minors such as some self-petition children).

The target sample sizes were set at 12,500 immigrants in the Adult Sample and 1,250 in the Child Sample. Nonresponse would still leave healthy sample sizes. Table 12.3 provides an overview of the NIS Adult and Child Samples.

Sample Stratification.   There is substantial scientific and policy interest in comparing immigrant characteristics and behavior across immigration visa categories. Immigration visa categories provide information about the way in which LPR was acquired—whether, for example, by dint of employment or through marriage to a US citizen, and so forth. Immigrant visa categories signal particular types and amounts of human and social capital. Importantly, they are policy levers. The most recent restructuring of immigrant visa categories occurred in 1990 with passage of the Immigration Act of 1990, whose provisions took effect in 1992. Of course, the numbers admitted vary substantially across visa categories. Immigrants admitted as spouses of US citizens constituted between 27 and 33% of adult immigrants in the 1996–2000 period; in contrast, diversity principals, in whom there is great interest as the visa is acquired by lottery, constituted 4–5%. Similarly, adopted orphans are one-fourth to one-fifth of the child sampling frame. Accordingly, the Adult and Child Samples were stratified in order to obtain reliable information on the visa categories of major interest.

In the Adult Sample, four strata were defined: spouses of US citizens, employment principals, diversity principals, and other immigrants. Spouses of US citizens were undersampled and employment principals oversampled, with spouses of US citizens sampled at approximately half their natural occurrence and employment principals at approximately twice their frequency. Diversity principals were sampled at about three times the natural rate. In the Child Sample, equal numbers were sampled of the under-five adopted orphans and the minor children of US citizens.

Sample Geography.   The United States covers a vast area, and it would be prohibitively expensive to attempt to locate and interview all sampled immigrants regardless of where they reside. However, a representative sample of new immigrants cannot be constrained by location choices. Fortunately, immigrants display substantial geographic clustering, and thus it was possible to design the geographic aspect of the NIS without sacrificing representativeness or spending astronomical sums.

TABLE 12.3 Overview of NIS-2003 Samples, by Visa Type and Age

Visa type	Sample	
	Adult	Child
A. *Principals*		
Spouse of US citizen	18+	—
Spouse of permanent resident	18+	—
Employment	18+	—
Diversity	18+	—
Other principal	18+	—
Child of US citizen	18+	<18
Adopted orphan	—	<5
B. *Accompanying, or following to join*		
Spouse of new immigrant	18+	—
Child of new immigrant	Excluded	Excluded
Other relative of new immigrant	Excluded	Excluded

NOTE: 1. Principal and accompanying immigrants. The United States grants immigrant visas to individuals who meet the eligibility criteria set forth for the various classes of admission; such immigrants are called principals. Examples include the spouses of US citizens, refugees, workers of several kinds, and winners of the diversity visa lottery. The United States also grants immigrant visas to the spouses and minor children "accompanying, or following to join" principals in certain classes of admission. Examples include spouses and minor children of employment principals and of sibling principals, and the nonrefugee spouses and minor children of refugees; principals for whose spouses and minor children visas are not available include, not surprisingly, spouses and parents of US citizens.

2. NIS-2003 Samples

a. The NIS Adult Sample covers all immigrants who are 18 years of age or older and who have visas as principals or as accompanying spouses.

b. The NIS Child Sample covers immigrants with child-of-US-citizen visas (except self-petition immigrants) who are under 18 years of age and adopted orphans under 5 years of age.

c. The NIS excludes accompanying children, accompanying adult offspring, and other accompanying nonspouse/nonchild relatives; these are covered as household members of sampled immigrants in the Adult Sample. The NIS also excludes adopted orphans 5 years of age and over, self-petition child-of-US-citizen immigrants, and children under 18 who hold principal visas other than child-of-US-citizen or adopted-orphan visas; self-petition child-of-US-citizen immigrants may be covered as household members of self-petition immigrants in the Adult Sample.

d. Age refers to age at admission to legal permanent residence.

Analysis of the initial residence (the address to which the green card would be mailed) for the full immigrant cohorts in the five-year period FY 1996 to FY 2000 showed that approximately 89% of the immigrants in the defined sampling frames reside in the top 85 Metropolitan Statistical Areas (MSAs) and another 4–5% in the top 38 counties, with about 1% overseas. Accordingly, the geographic sample design called for including all top 85 MSAs and all top 38 counties and to select a random sample of 10 MSAs from among the rest of the MSAs and a random sample of 15 county pairs from among the rest of the counties. The segment with an initial overseas address was excluded because of the high locating cost. Of course, respondents with a non-overseas address in the administrative record who were overseas during the field period would still be interviewed.

Monthly Replicates. The NIS-Pilot had confirmed that immigrants are a highly mobile population and that locating them requires contacting them as soon as possible after admission to LPR—while the addresses to which they have requested that the green cards be mailed are still fresh. Accordingly, the NIS-2003 round 1 design called for sampling once a month from the government administrative records on new immigrants. As events unfolded, the survey organization, which needed one month's lead time for location and mailing activities prior to the first actual interview, was ready to start interviewing on 14 June 2003. Accordingly, the first replicate drawn covered the half-month 1-15 May. This was followed by six monthly replicates and a final half-month replicate.

Procedures for Selecting the Sample. The procedures consisted of three steps. First, the Office of Immigration Statistics prepared an electronic file with the immigrant records for all new legal immigrants whose records were compiled in the specified period (e.g., May 1–15, 2003) and sent it to the NIS principal investigator (PI) team. Second, the PIs selected the Adult and Child Samples according to the specifications described above; sample selection was carried out using a random-number statistical routine. Third, the PIs sent the Samples to the survey organization, the National Opinion Research Center.

Duplicates, Retentions/Deletions, Replacements. The original sampling design, as described above, did not recognize relationships between individuals selected into the sample (the administrative record does not provide information on relationships, but does, of course, provide addresses, which could be the same for several new immigrants, as well as visa codes, which in some cases signal family relationships). Thus, if a husband and wife both fell in the sample, the original idea was to keep both of them as sampled immigrants. However, the field procedures developed by the survey organization made this impossible to implement efficiently. Accordingly, to maximize the smoothness of the field operation, the PI team decided to define as duplicates three kinds of multiple immigrants selected in the samples: two adults married to each other; two minor children; and a parent and a minor child.

Duplicates were identified at two points, first, at the sampling stage, and second, in the field. Duplicates identified in the field could come from the same replicate or from different replicates (principals and accompanying spouses and children need not arrive on the same date, for example). The rules followed for retentions and deletions were as follows: (1) if the two (or more) duplicates are in the same replicate, retain the one with the earlier sampling number; and (2) if the duplicates are in different replicates, retain the one in the earlier replicate.

Replacements for duplicates found in the field for replicates 1–7 were made at the time of the subsequent replicate. Duplicates found in the field after delivery of replicate 8 were not replaced. It would have been extremely costly to launch the field operations for these cases, which numbered twelve adults and one child.

Size of Selected Samples. The final number of cases selected was 12,488 in the Adult Sample and 1,249 in the Child Sample. Note that in all duplicate cases, the "deleted" case remains in the NIS as a spouse, child, or sibling of the sampled immigrant.

Sampling Weights. The public-use documentation includes, for each replicate and for each stratum within each replicate, the number in the sampling frame, the number sampled, the number located, and the number interviewed. Design weights are included with the data. Additionally, researchers can construct weighting schemes appropriate to the particular topic and approach.

NIS-2003 Sample at Round 2

The design called for locating and reinterviewing all sample members from round 1 except divorced or separated spouses of the sampled immigrant and sponsor-parents of sampled child immigrants who had reached the age of eighteen. Sampled immigrants who were now eighteen were treated as adults (and administered the adult immigrant schedule from round 1). Spouses and sponsor-parents who did not participate in round 1 were invited to participate in round 2 if they were eighteen or older. Also invited to participate were new spouses and new age-eligible children. As in round 1, round 2 participants were interviewed even if they were living overseas.

NIS-2003 LANGUAGE DESIGN

As noted, the key principle is that every respondent—sampled immigrant, spouse, child—is interviewed in his or her preferred language. Interviewing respondents in the language of their choice maximizes response rate and data quality. However, it presents new challenges in questionnaire preparation and field operations.

NIS-2003 Language Design in Round 1

The design for round 1 classified languages into several tiers and designed a treatment for each tier. The language classification was based on (1) the expected origin-country distribution, (2) the expected native-language distribution, and (3) the expected preferred languages by country. Information on these elements was developed using the NIS-Pilot of 1996 and the public-use immigrant records for fiscal years 1996–2000.

Language Tiers.   Tier 0 was English. In the NIS-P, although only about 20% of the respondents came from a country one of whose official or dominant languages is English, over 40% preferred English (almost 46% in the unweighted sample). Tier 1 was Spanish; in the NIS-P, 26% in the unweighted sample preferred Spanish. Tier 2 comprised the next six languages expected to be most often requested—Chinese, Korean, Polish, Russian, Tagalog, and Vietnamese. In the NIS-P, each of the tier 2 languages was requested by more than 1% of the sample; the language most requested was Chinese, by 9%, followed by Russian, by 7%. Tier 3 included the next nine languages expected to be most requested—Arabic, Croatian, Farsi, French, Gujarati, Hindi, Serbian, Ukrainian, and Urdu. Finally, tier 4 included all other languages.

Language Treatments by Tier.   Spanish (tier 1) received the same treatment as English—not only translation but also full computer-assisted personal interviewing (CAPI) implementation. For tier 1 and tier 2 languages, the instruments were translated. For tier 3 languages, a set of key concepts was translated.

Interviews in tier 1 and tier 2 languages, plus Amharic, French, and Haitian Creole, were conducted by bilingual interviewers. Interviews in all other languages were conducted by a team of interviewer and interpreter. Additionally, in languages for which bilingual interviewer treatment had been specified, if bilingual interviewers were not available, interviewer-interpreter teams conducted the interviews.

Key Concepts (Tier 3).   Two sets of key concepts were identified, one related to immigration, the other not. These were presented to the respondents in both translation and English original.

Translation of Instruments and Key Concepts.   A professional translation firm translated the instrument into the tier 1 and tier 2 languages and the key concepts into the tier 3 languages. In addition, translations were assessed by NORC teams of bilingual translation and survey experts.

NIS-2003 Language Design in Round 2

Round 1 provided precise information on language requirements for the NIS-2003 cohort. Accordingly, survey instruments were translated into ten languages—the seven tier 1 and tier 2 languages from round 1 plus Amharic, Arabic, and Creole. For other languages, interpreters participated in a three-way interview process with a trained interviewer and the respondent.

NIS-2003 QUESTIONNAIRE CONTENT

NIS-2003 survey instruments for the baseline round obtained information on a wide range of topics, including a complete migration history and comprehensive information on health, schooling, marriage and family, skills, languages and English-language skills, labor force participation, earnings, remittances and help received, use of government services, networks, travel, and religion. A large component of the NIS survey instruments is comparable to instruments used in the major US longitudinal surveys, such as the National Longitudinal Studies of Labor Market Experience (NLS) and the Panel Study of Income Dynamics (PSID), thus facilitating comparison of immigrants and the native-born. Other information is specific to immigrants, such as information on sponsorship of new immigrants and on naturalization. Special attention is paid to immigrant children and the children of immigrants, including assessment of their academic abilities, skills, and achievements. In addition, the instruments seek immigrants' ideas about the migration process, including assessment of the helpfulness of various sources of information.

The round 2 instruments tracked changes over time in the information collected at round 1. Sampled child immigrants who were now eighteen were administered the adult immigrant schedule from round 1.

The child assessments at both rounds consisted of the Digit Span for Memory test and the Woodcock Johnson III Tests of Achievement (tests 1, 5, 9, and 10). The Digit Span for Memory test and the WJIII Tests 1 (Letter-Word Identification) and 10 (Applied Problems) were given to children aged 3 to 12, inclusive. Children aged 6 to 12, inclusive, also received the WJIII Tests 5 (Calculation) and 9 (Passage Comprehension) (Mather et al. 2001).

NIS-2003 RESPONSE RATES AND DATA AVAILABILITY

Round 1 was in the field from June 2003 to June 2004. In the Adult Sample, interviews were completed with 8,573 main sampled immigrants—for a response rate of 68.6%—plus 4,334 spouses and 1,072 children age 8–12. A total of 2,551 children age 3–12 in the Adult Sample received cognitive assessments. In the Child Sample, interviews were completed with 810 sponsor-parents of the main sampled immigrant children—for a response rate of 64.8%—plus 579 spouses and 194 children 8–12 years of age. Cognitive assessments were carried out with 483 children in the Child Sample.

Round 2 was in the field from June 2004 to December 2009. The number of completed interviews with main sampled immigrants in the Adult Sample was 3,902, for a response rate of 45.5%, plus 1,557 spouses. Adjusting for 69 deceased and 48 incapacitated main respondents, the response rate is 46.1%. Among sponsor-parents in the Child Sample and now-adult main children, the response rates are 53.3% and 28.1%, respectively.

As noted above, data from rounds 1 and 2 of NIS-2003 are available for public use. Documentation and further information are available at the NIS website: http://nis.princeton.edu.

A CLOSE LOOK AT VISA STRESS IN THE
NIS-2003 COHORT

Above we introduced the three sources of health change among immigrants—visa stress, migration stress, and US exposure effects. In the case of legal permanent residence, a convenient way to define the duration of visa stress is by the duration of the visa process, which begins when the first document is filed and ends with admission to LPR. For new legal immigrants with conditional visas, however, visa stress does not end until removal of conditionality restrictions two years later. Moreover, visa stress resurfaces during the immigrant's application for naturalization. And, as noted above, some form of visa stress, possibly a low-grade form, may remain, given that a naturalized citizen can be stripped of citizenship and deported.

New-arrival immigrants—immigrants who apply abroad for LPR and arrive in the United States with an LPR visa—experience visa stress by itself, before arrival. In contrast, adjustee immigrants experience all three sources of health change at the same time. Building on the classic insight of Simmons and Blyth (1987) about the stress adolescents face if they must go through puberty and a school transition simultaneously, we would expect the overall negative effects to be greater for adjustee immigrants than for new-arrival immigrants. Further, visa stress may be easier to endure in the origin country.

Of course, there are many special cases that may operate differently—for example, refugees and asylees may endure very little LPR visa stress because for them the daunting part of the migration process was obtaining the initial refugee or asylee status, with the subsequent adjustment to LPR being somewhat pro forma. Similarly, an LPR visa applicant who is a longtime "temporary" resident (say, someone who spent ten years on a student visa and is now in the sixth year of a temporary work visa) may have completed the process of adjustment to the United States before beginning the LPR visa application process.

The questions thus arise: How long does visa stress last? Where is visa stress experienced? Is visa stress experienced jointly with migration stress and exposure to the US environment? Further, the longitudinal nature of the NIS will make it possible to estimate the proportion of conditional visa cases in which the conditionality restrictions are removed.

How Long Does LPR Visa Stress Last?

Setting aside the longer duration of visa stress among conditional immigrants and the possible permanency of a low-grade form of visa stress, the major form of visa stress—LPR visa stress—lasts for the duration of the visa process. As noted above, the visa process lasts from the filing of the first document to the granting of legal permanent residence. A priori there are several mechanisms affecting duration of the visa process, some of which work at cross purposes. First, the visa process should be longer for numerically limited visas, which are backlogged—in 2003 these were family preference visas (US Department of State, *Visa Bulletin*). Other visas are not subject to waiting for a visa number; moreover, diversity visas must be processed within the fiscal year. Second, the visa process should be longer for adjustment-of-status cases than for new-arrival cases, because the volume is larger stateside (Jasso 2011) and the per-case resources appear to be lower than in US consulates abroad. Third, however, the visa process should be longer for new-arrival cases because, while among adjustees approval leads immediately to LPR (indicated by a stamp in the passport), among new arrivals that same approval is only the first of two approvals, yielding a visa that is valid for six months as the prospective immigrant prepares to travel to the United States, where a US agent conducts an inspection and provides the second approval, authorizing admission to LPR (again indicated by a stamp in the passport). Fourth, within visa categories that provide visas for both principals and accompanying spouses, new arrivals granted LPR as spouses of principals should have a shorter visa process than principals because the marriage might have occurred after the initial petition was filed. Fifth, however, new arrivals granted LPR as spouses of principals should have a longer visa process because they are allowed an additional six months for "following to join" the principal. Sixth, employment cases requiring labor certification (second and third preference categories) should have a longer visa process than cases not requiring it. Finally, country of birth also affects the duration of the visa process in the numerically limited preference categories.

Note that the second and third mechanisms have opposite effects, as do the fourth and fifth. Which mechanism is stronger is an empirical question.

Table 12.4 (reprinted from Jasso 2011) reports the duration of the visa process in the NIS-2003 cohort, separately for new arrivals and adjustees, for principals and spouses, and by gender. The first result that hits the eye is a result not anticipated from the mechanisms listed above: in each of the four subsets, visa processing takes longer for spouses of foreign-born US citizens than for spouses of native-born US citizens. The reason is not immediately obvious. Inspection of the requisite Form I-130 ("Petition for an Alien Relative"), which must be filed by the sponsor, indicates that the only difference between the two types of sponsors pertains to the evidence of their citizenship that must be presented, namely, while both native-born and foreign-born citizens can present a passport, other evidence includes a birth certificate for a native-born citizen and a certificate of naturalization (or of citizenship) for a foreign-born citizen. Thus, there are two further avenues to explore: (1) whether marriage cases involving foreign-born US citizens are more complicated in an immigration sense (e.g., they are higher-order marriages for one or both spouses; the sponsored spouse has difficulty accessing the requisite documents, such as military and police records; or the documents have to be

TABLE 12.4 Average Years of Immigrant Visa Processing Time, by Visa Characteristics and Sex: NIS-2003 Cohort

Immigrant class of admission	New arrival				Adjustee			
	Principal		Spouse		Principal		Spouse	
	M	F	M	F	M	F	M	F
Spouse of native-born US citizen	1.23	1.11	NA	NA	2.39	2.15	NA	NA
Spouse of foreign-born US citizen	1.88	1.88	NA	NA	3.60	2.78	NA	NA
Parent of US citizen	2.65	2.38	NA	NA	2.54	2.58	NA	NA
Minor child of US citizen	2.80	3.74	NA	NA	4.78	4.59	NA	NA
Adult single child of US citizen	6.96	6.41	NA	NA	8.17	9.06	NA	NA
Adult married child of US citizen	7.71	8.19	6.45	6.69	8.93	8.84	—	—
Sibling of US citizen	13.2	13.7	12.4	12.7	10.39	13.8	—	—
Spouse of legal permanent resident	6.34	7.70	NA	NA	7.73	8.54	NA	NA
Child of legal permanent resident	9.09	8.85	NA	NA	11.5	11.3	NA	NA
Employment	2.67	2.25	2.50	3.76	4.04	4.73	4.48	3.36
Diversity	2.01	2.27	2.32	2.29	2.15	2.04	—	—
Refugee/asylee/parolee	NA	NA	NA	NA	5.82	5.45	6.57	6.43
Legalization	NA	NA	NA	NA	7.08	5.95	NA	NA
Other	—	—	—	—	—	—	—	—
All immigrants	4.58	4.18	6.48	6.59	4.89	3.90	5.80	4.59

SOURCE: Jasso 2011.

NOTE: Sample size is 8,573. Estimates based on weighted data. Combinations that either do not arise in immigration law or do not appear in the sample are denoted "NA." Dashes indicate cells with observations fewer than 20.

translated from a non-Roman alphabet), and (2) whether marriage cases involving foreign-born US citizens receive greater scrutiny from US officials.

Other results illuminate the mechanisms described above. As expected, numerically unlimited cases (spouses, parents, and minor children of US citizens), diversity cases, and employment cases have the shortest visa process. Sibling cases have the longest visa process.

Contrasting adjustee and new-arrival visa process times within subsets of principals indicates that in almost every visa type, the adjustee process is longer than the new-arrival process, suggesting that the agency mechanism trumps the behavioral mechanism (new arrivals taking up to six months to settle affairs before traveling to the United States). For example, the visa process for spouses of native-born US citizens lasts 1.23 and 1.1 years, on average, for men and women, respectively, who are new arrivals, but almost twice as long for adjustees—2.39 and 2.15 years for men and women, respectively. These figures also provide an empirical grounding for the policy of permitting employment-based visa applicants residing in the United States to choose consular processing (as shown in Form I-140, "Petition for Alien Worker"), as well as the associated perennial discussion among visa applicants and immigration lawyers on the relative merits of adjustment of status and consular processing.

Within new arrivals, spouses of principals have a shorter visa process than principals among numerically limited married children and siblings of US citizens—indicating that they may have married after the principal entered the visa queue. Differences in duration of the visa process between principals and spouses are trivial among employment and diversity immigrants, except among employment new-arrival women, who exhibit the opposite pattern—longer visa process for spouses of principals—presumably because the visa wait is shorter and the spouses follow later.

Thus, there is considerable variation in duration of visa stress across visa situations. In general, then, the effect of duration of the visa process on health change and other health outcomes may be approached in two ways: (1) by including each respondent's actual visa process duration as a regressor in the health equation and (2) by including in the health equation the determinants of visa process duration—namely, visa category, whether the immigrant is a principal or an accompanying person, whether the immigrant is a new arrival or an adjustee, and whether the country of origin is one of the four countries with distinctive (and longer) waits for numerically limited visas (China, India, Mexico, and the Philippines).

Where Is LPR Visa Stress Experienced?

As an initial exploration of the question of where LPR visa stress is experienced, and focusing on the major form of visa stress associated with the process of obtaining legal permanent residence, consider the subset of new legal permanent residents in the NIS-2003 whose very first time in the United States was the day they arrived with their new immigrant visa. NIS-2003 data include a history of trips lasting more than sixty days, as well as a question on shorter visits to the United States. Preliminary calculations indicate that approximately 24.5% of the adult immigrants had never set foot in the United States and thus experienced the totality of their visa stress outside the US—possibly with the comforts of home and certainly without the further effects of migration stress and US exposure.

Other immigrants experience visa stress in the United States or in both the United States and one or more other countries. For example, adjustees who did not leave the United States during the entire visa process would experience all of their visa stress in the United States.

Is LPR Visa Stress Experienced Jointly with Migration Stress and US Exposure?

Adjustee immigrants—57.4% of the adult immigrants in the NIS-2003—experience all three sources of health change simultaneously, for at least a part of the time. Among the subset of new-arrival immigrants who had never set foot inside the United States before obtaining LPR, visa stress would end before the start of migration stress and US exposure. However, the remaining new-arrival immigrants, who may have spent part of the visa process time in the United States—18%—may also have had spells of all three sources of stress simultaneously.

LPR Visa Stress and Removal of Conditionality Restrictions

Of the 326 respondents who were identified at round 1 as having conditional visas and who were interviewed at round 2, 60.7% had had the conditionality restrictions removed. The remainder are as follows: (1) did not admit they had conditional visas (18.9%); (2) had not filed (8.05%); (3) had filed but application was pending (3.34%); (4) had filed and been denied (2.61%); and (5) did not answer the question (6.04%). These figures suggest that up to 39% of the immigrants with conditional visas may have lapsed into illegality.

Among spouses of US citizens, those married to native-born US citizens had a substantially higher rate of removal of the conditionality restrictions than those married to foreign-born US citizens—67.9% versus 51.8%. Further research is warranted to explore this difference. Note that this result may be linked to the result reported above that the visa process lasts longer for spouses of foreign-born citizens than for spouses of native-born citizens. It is too early to speculate, but these results raise the possibility that marriage fraud may differ by nativity of the US citizen sponsor.

Using data from both round 1 and round 2 of NIS-2003 will make it possible to assess the health trajectory of new legal immigrants in the first several years after admission to legal permanent residence and to discern more sharply the operation of visa stress, migration stress, and US exposure, gauging the effects of the duration of visa stress and of whether it was experienced in the origin country or in the United States (and alone or jointly with migration stress and US exposure), assessing the determinants of the duration of migration stress, and exploring the conditions under which US exposure effects are negative, positive, or shift from one to the other.

CONCLUDING NOTE

It is by now well established and accepted that longitudinal surveys provide the best approach for studying migration and other dynamic processes (Morgan and Nicholson 2005; Tourangeau 2004). The years ahead will bring both new longitudinal data on migration and new analyses of longitudinal data. Together, these will provide advances in substantive and methodological knowledge, stimulating creativity in data collection and analysis and further waves of new knowledge on migration.

REFERENCES

Antecol, Heather, and Kelly Bedard. 2006. "Unhealthy Assimilation: Why Do Immigrants Converge to American Health Status Levels?" *Demography* 43:337–60.

Ashenfelter, Orley, Phillip B. Levine, and David J. Zimmerman. 2003. *Statistics and Econometrics: Methods and Applications.* New York: Wiley.

Baker, Bryan. 2014. "Estimates of the Size and Characteristics of the Resident Nonimmigrant Population in the United States: January 2012." DHS-OIS Population Estimates.

Baker, Bryan C., and Nancy Rytina. 2013. "Estimates of the Unauthorized Immigrant Population Residing in the United States: January 2012." DHS-OIS Population Estimates.

Biddle, Nicholas, Steven Kennedy, and James Ted McDonald. 2007. "Health Assimilation Patterns amongst Australian Immigrants." *Economic Record* 83:16–30.

Black, Richard, Tony Fielding, Russell King, Ronald Skeldon, and Richmond Tiemoko. 2003. "Longitudinal Studies: An Insight into Current Studies and the Social and Economic Outcomes for Migrants." Sussex Migration Working Paper no. 14. Sussex Centre for Migration Research, University of Sussex.

Gott, Richard. 2005. *Cuba: A New History.* New Haven, CT: Yale University Press.

Jasso, Guillermina. 1988. "Whom Shall We Welcome? Elite Judgments of the Criteria for the Selection of Immigrants." *American Sociological Review* 53:919–32.

Jasso, Guillermina. 2011. "Migration and Stratification." *Social Science Research* 40:1292–1336.

Jasso, Guillermina, Douglas S. Massey, Mark R. Rosenzweig, and James P. Smith. 2000. "The New Immigrant Survey Pilot (NIS-P): Overview and New Findings about US Legal Immigrants at Admission." *Demography* 37:127–38.

Jasso, Guillermina, Douglas S. Massey, Mark R. Rosenzweig, and James P. Smith. 2004. "Immigrant Health—Selectivity and Acculturation." Pp. 227–266 in Norman B. Anderson, Randy A. Bulatao, and Barney Cohen (eds.), *Critical Perspectives on Racial and Ethnic Differences in Health in Late Life.* Washington, DC: National Academies Press.

Jasso, Guillermina, Douglas S. Massey, Mark R. Rosenzweig, and James P. Smith. 2005. "Immigration, Health, and New York City: Early Results Based on the US New-Immigrant Cohort of 2003." *Economic Policy Review* 11:127–51.

Jasso, Guillermina, and Mark R. Rosenzweig. 2009. "Selection Criteria and the Skill Composition of Immigrants: A Comparative Analysis of Australian and US Employment Immigration." Pp. 153–183 in Jagdish Bhagwati and Gordon H. Hanson (eds.), *Skilled Immigration Today: Prospects, Problems, and Policies.* New York: Oxford.

Kasl, Stanislav V., and Lisa Berkman. 1983. "Health Consequences of the Experience of Migration." *Annual Review of Public Health* 4:69–90.

Levine, Daniel B., Kenneth Hill, and Robert Warren (eds.). 1985. *Immigration Statistics: A Story of Neglect.* Washington, DC: National Academies Press.

Massey, Douglas S. 1987. "Understanding Mexican Migration to the United States." *American Journal of Sociology* 92:1372–1403.

Massey, Douglas S., Joaquin Arango, Graeme Hugo, Ali Kouaouci, Adela Pellegrino, and J. Edward Taylor. 1993. "Theories of International Migration: A Review and Appraisal." *Population and Development Review* 19:431–66.

Mather, Nancy, Barbara J. Wendling, and Richard W. Woodcock. 2001. *Essentials of WJ III Tests of Achievement Assessment.* Hoboken, NJ: Wiley.

Mincer, Jacob. 1978. "Family Migration Decisions." *Journal of Political Economy* 86:749–73.

Morgan, Beverley, and Ben Nicholson (eds.). 2005. *Immigration Research and Statistics Service Workshop on Longitudinal Surveys and Cross-Cultural Survey Design: Workshop Proceedings*. London, UK: Crown. Accessed 3 January 2014: http://s3.amazonnaws.com /zanran storage/www.nyu.edu/ContentPages/6619011.pdf.

Rytina, Nancy. 2013. "Estimates of the Legal Permanent Resident Population in 2012." DHS-OIS Population Estimates. Accessed 3 January 2014: http://www.dhs.gov/xlibrary/assets /statistics/publications/ois lpr pe 2012.pdf.

Sawyerr, Stella. 2010. "Workshop: Reducing Tears of Migration." Tell Magazine. www. telling.com

Simmons, Roberta G., and Dale A. Blyth. 1987. *Moving into Adolescence: The Impact of Pubertal Change and School Context*. New York: Aldine.

Stephen, E. H., K. Foote, G. E. Hendershot, and C. A. Schoenborn. 1994. "Health of the Foreign-Born Population: United States, 1989–90." *Advance Data: Vital and Health Statistics*. No. 241. National Center for Health Statistics.

Tourangeau, Roger. 2004. *Recurring Surveys: Issues and Opportunities*. Arlington, VA: National Science Foundation.

US Census Bureau. 2012. The New American FactFinder, Table S0501, Selected Characteristics of the Native and Foreign-Born Populations, 2011 American Community Survey 1-Year Estimates. Accessed 3 January 2014: http//factfinder2.census.gov/faces/tableservices/jsf/pages/productview.xhtml?pid=ACS 09 1YR S0501&prodType=table.

US Department of Homeland Security, Office of Immigration Statistics. 2002–2013. *Yearbook of Immigration Statistics*. Washington, DC: Government Printing Office.

US Department of State. Various issues. *Visa Bulletin*. Posted online. Accessed 3 January 2014: http://travel.state.gov/visa/bulletin 1360.html.

US Department of State. 2013. *Annual Report of Immigrant Visa Applicants in the Family-sponsored and Employment-based Preferences Registered at the National Visa Center as of November 1, 2013*. Updated report accessed 3 January 2014: http://www.travel.state.gov /pdf/WaitingListItem.pdf.

US Immigration and Naturalization Service. 1979–2001. *Statistical Yearbook of the Immigration and Naturalization Service*. Washington, DC: Government Printing Office.

Vega, William, and Hortensia Amaro. 1994. "Latino Outlook: Good Health, Uncertain Prognosis." *Annual Review of Public Health* 15: 39–67.

Wooldridge, Jeffrey M. 2006. *Introductory Econometrics: A Modern Approach*. 3rd ed. Mason, OH: Thomson South-western.

Qualitative Methodological Approaches

Section Editor: Xóchitl Castañeda

13

Ethnographic Research in Migration and Health

Seth M. Holmes
Heide Castañeda

INTRODUCTION AND LAYOUT

This chapter explores the methodological approach of ethnographic research and its importance in migration and health studies. It serves as an introduction to the methodology of ethnography for those new to this approach, helping such readers become familiar with the ways in which their understanding of migration and health could be expanded by reading ethnographic studies, collaborating with ethnographic researchers, or embarking on the path of conducting ethnographic research themselves.

Ethnography is the long-term study of a group of people, their interactions and experiences, and the meanings through which they understand their lives. However, ethnographers should not assume unchanging, static cultures or groups of people. Rather, contemporary ethnography focuses on the effects of history, politics, economics, social inequalities, and interaction (Clifford 1998; Pratt 1992). It is an overarching, multifaceted, and holistic qualitative research method based on participant observation (see chapter 14, by Aguilera and Amuchástegui, in this volume) and often supplemented by complementary methods such as interviews, life histories, and the review of media, archival, and clinical records. Ethnography requires the long-term, in-depth immersion of the researcher in a particular social, economic, political, and historical context. This methodology is especially helpful in understanding complex and power-imbued social and cultural interactions in context, without simplifying reality into easily analyzable questions, dichotomies, or scales.

Due to its contextual nature, ethnography is a useful strategy in answering questions associated with health issues in the setting of migration. Because of its strong emphasis on exploring the complex nature of social phenomena, ethnography is especially useful for analyzing the systems of concepts, beliefs, and perceptions of risk and vulnerability related to practices or behaviors (Holmes 2011; Quesada, Hart, Bourgois 2011). At the same time, ethnographers must keep in mind that patterns and issues associated with migration and health exist within specific social, economic, political, and historical conditions. Ethnography is especially helpful in answering research questions focused on the interrelationships between the micro illness experiences and health-related practices or behaviors of individuals and the macro social, political, economic, and cultural conditions influencing those experiences and behaviors. For instance, ethnographic research can illuminate the effects of specific health and social policies, which is important because even efforts that are intended to be beneficial may contribute to marginalization and exacerbate inequalities. Embedded within a particular context, ethnography helps to link local specificities with transnational perspectives.

This chapter will consider the ways in which ethnography differs from other research methodologies, the specifics of ethnographic data collection and analysis, the advantages and limitations of this method, as well as brief case study examples to illustrate the value of this approach. The main points include the following:

- Ethnography provides in-depth investigation of multiple levels related to health and inequality, from individual experiences and practices to sociocultural structures influencing those individuals, their experiences, and their practices.
- Ethnography is especially useful in research with "hidden" and stigmatized populations, such as many immigrant groups.
- Ethnographic research does not provide for the calculation of incidence and prevalence of specific health problems, but rather seeks to understand their production and expression in the larger context of daily life.

THE UNIQUE CONTEXTUAL NATURE OF ETHNOGRAPHY

Ethnography helps us understand social and cultural phenomena from the perspective of participants in the social setting under study. Ethnography explicitly acknowledges the context in which research is performed. In order to avoid ethnocentrism—that is, perceiving and judging the social world one observes according to the meanings from one's own cultural milieu—ethnographers actively seek to understand and set aside their own assumptions as much as possible. This allows ethnographic researchers to be open to understanding new meanings and realities that they might not have conceptualized before entering the field. In this way, ethnographic research is more inductive—coming from the context being investigated—than most forms of research. As a result, ethnographers should not formulate the answers to their questions before entering the field, as this would involve bringing too many assumptions from a potentially different social and cultural context. In addition, as with all research, ethnographic projects are undertaken only after the researchers and the research subjects engage together in the process of informed consent, which entails outlining the goals of the study.

One related key difference between ethnographic research and quantitative research, in particular, is its flexibility. Ethnography is an iterative process, occurring through successive and overlapping research segments. Thus, ethnographers can change or further refine their questions during the long-term immersion of participant observation or as the data they collect compel them to do so. Most other research methods require that research questions be enumerated and codified before the beginning of formal data collection. This relates to the relative dearth of information about some migrant populations in the health disparities literature, a field that often relies heavily on quantitative information. Because there may be no reliable epidemiological data for some populations, they may be excluded entirely. Ethnographic studies are helpful partially because they aid in the understanding of particular experiences of disparities from the perspectives of particular groups about whom it may be difficult to collect reliable quantitative data.

Whereas many other research methods seek to "generalize from" one group to all similar groups of people (to be able to say, for example, "Latino immigrants have higher rates of [a specific health problem] than does the general U.S. population"), ethnography seeks to "generalize within." This phrase, used by Clifford Geertz (1973), one of the founders of the field of cultural anthropology, implies not a generalization to all people of a given category, but rather a generalization of theories, analyses, concepts, or phenomena. As a result, an ethnographer might be more focused on understanding the manner in which power, hierarchy, stigma, or the dismantling of the social safety net functions in the world rather than on making generalizations about specific populations. For example, rather than focusing on alleged cultural characteristics such as "machismo" or "familism" among Mexican migrants and their effects on health prevention efforts, the ethnographer might instead focus on how these concepts emerged within historical power relations in Mexican society and became reinforced or changed through migration processes, as well as how and why their expressions have been so readily taken up by medical and public health practitioners in the US. In this way, ethnography is often understood to be "interpretive" in that it tends to focus on interpreting the meaning of symbols and the functions of power. Rather than positing that reality is stable and can be observed in one objective way, an interpretive approach recognizes that there are many subjective understandings of reality, processes, or events, and that these are vital components of the phenomena under study. Ethnographic methods can be critical to investigating disparities in migrant health without simplifying the complex reality in which those disparities are embedded (sidebar 13.1).

SIDEBAR 13.1 ETHNOGRAPHIC FIELD RESEARCH: EXAMPLE
OF US-MEXICO MIGRATION AND OCCUPATIONAL HEALTH

The following field example from our own work yields fruitful and relevant insights to research questions that would not have been as deeply understood through less in-depth and experiential methods.

The first example relates to ethnic hierarchies and health among indigenous Mexican farmworkers in the United States (Holmes 2007; Holmes 2013). This ethnographic research took place over the course of one cycle of migration from a mountain village in Oaxaca, Mexico, through central California, to northwestern Washington State. This multisited project provided a full analysis of the multiple occupational conditions and living conditions in Mexico and the US that play into the health problems of this group of people. The long-term immersion in the sociocultural context of one particular farm in Washington State allowed for an understanding of multiple perspectives simultaneously, including subtle meanings of race and power that differ depending on one's social position. For example, the hidden yet robust hierarchy of workers on this farm relates not only to the quality of work and housing one has access to but also directly to one's ethnicity, citizenship status, and gender. This subtle yet deeply important reality that partially determines health and disease was uncovered only by living in labor camps, picking fruit, observing interactions, celebrating birthdays and baptisms, and interviewing various people on the farm for several months. The particularly subtle hierarchical meanings attached to different ethnic groups, including different indigenous groups, would have been extremely difficult to apprehend through a less immersive and in-depth method.

ETHNOGRAPHIC DATA COLLECTION

Ethnographic research involves building conceptual models through participant observation supplemented by other specific methods and then validating them qualitatively and sometimes quantitatively. The ways in which ethnographic data are collected are distinct from other research techniques. Not only is ethnography most often a longer-term observation of the social world of the study subjects, but it is also a more holistic immersion into that world via participant observation. Whereas most research methodologies involve an inanimate research tool (for example, a survey instrument or a pipette), the instruments utilized in ethnographic research are the ethnographers themselves. This means that the researchers collect not only cognitive but also bodily and sensory observations about the social world they are studying. Ethnographers analyze what they see and hear, along with what they experience, in a more bodily fashion, such as spatial relationships, daily rhythms, seasonal shifts, even odors and tastes. This allows for a more complex, nuanced, and "thick" description of the data (Geertz 1973).

Participant observation takes place in community settings that have direct relevance to the research questions. While this methodology may include data collection from interviews and surveys, it differs significantly from other methods of research in that it is performed and analyzed within the situational knowledge provided by long-term participation, observation, and relationship-building. The researcher approaches and builds rapport with participants in their own environment; in the case of migration and health, these environments might include migrant camps, clinics, day laborer centers, churches, or community organizations. For example, one of the authors (SMH) spent approximately eighteen months full-time migrating with a group of indigenous Mexican farmworkers, living in a migrant camp in Washington State and picking berries alongside participants, migrating to California and visiting migrant clinics, migrating to the hometown of participants in rural Mexico, and then crossing the border desert into Arizona with participants (Holmes 2007; Holmes 2013).

Researchers write detailed accounts of what they see and hear, recording all observations as field notes. Field notes are written either discreetly during or following the activity, depending on how much the researcher is participating, and expanded upon as soon as possible before memory of the details fades. Ethnographers quickly learn that they must take field notes on everything they notice in the early part of their fieldwork, especially the first few weeks or months, because, soon, many details will no longer stand out or even be noticed at all. For example, in one study, gaining the trust of migrant backstretch workers (i.e., people who labor in the stable areas behind racetracks, feeding and grooming horses and mucking stalls) required becoming accustomed to the rhythm of the horseracing world through regular visits. This included unique experiences of time (workers are "on the clock" 24/7, and all activities are dictated by racing schedules), space (living, cooking, and socializing only feet from the animals), and social hierarchies based on specific occupational roles (Castañeda et al. 2010). Once the ethnographer becomes accustomed to the new social world, aspects of this reality that seemed interesting initially may be perceived as normal to the point that they are no longer consciously perceived. Thus, writing field notes is not only a vital source of material for later analysis, but also a means for ethnographers to reflect upon their experiences as part of the iterative process that allows for the refinement of research questions (Rosaldo 1993).

Along with the explicit acknowledgment of context, ethnography requires researchers to be reflexively aware of their own social position. Researchers must be cognizant of and document power hierarchies not only in the field they study, but also in their interactions with research subjects. This includes recording the ways in which people respond to them given their particular social position, including gender, race, nationality, and social class. In this way, the particularity of the context of research and of the researchers themselves becomes an opportunity for further data collection.

Within ethnographic work, formal and informal interviews are often used to supplement participant observation field notes. Interviews tend to be utilized once rapport with a research subject has been built in order to further address sensitive topics. Interviews are appropriate for eliciting individual experiences, opinions, and feelings, and they provide the opportunity to collect in-depth responses, with all of the nuances and contradictions, connections and relationships, that a person sees among particular events, phenomena, and beliefs. Face-to-face interviews (often called "direct administration") are preferred, since they create more rapport between the interviewer and the respondent and avoid problems stemming from illiteracy, poor comprehension, and mixed language ability. The context of the interview, including any potential distraction or involvement of others, should be noted. As in any interview, the ethnographer should avoid preconceptions or leading questions that are worded in such a way as to influence participants' responses. Asking open-ended questions can also encourage more in-depth responses. Interviews—as well as natural conversations within participant observation more generally—are often audio-recorded and transcribed later for analysis.

In the context of migration and health, ethnographic research can be especially helpful in exploring social interactions and categories, symbolic meanings of health and health-related activities, power hierarchies, and the social and cultural workings of prejudice and exclusion. For example, the research of one of the authors (SMH) reveals social hierarchies and health disparities organized around immigration status, ethnicity, and labor position as well as the ways in which these hierarchies and disparities come to be understood as normal and natural in society. These unofficial social dynamics and subtle meanings would have been complicated and difficult to explore using less in-depth, long-term, and contextual research methods.

In the last decade, more ethnographers have been calling for the practice of "multisited ethnography" (Stoller 1997; Tsing 2008; Falzon 2009). This practice involves research in multiple, usually geographically dispersed, sites and is understood to allow for deeper understandings as well as comparative analyses of a particular problem. In the study of migration and transnationalism, multisited ethnography can be especially helpful because events and experiences often span multiple locations. For example, this could mean engaging in research on the US farms where Mexican migrants live as well as in their hometowns in Mexico, which could allow for further conceptualization of the reality of transnational immigration (Holmes 2007; Holmes 2013) (sidebar 13.2).

SIDEBAR 13.2 ETHNOGRAPHIC FIELD STUDY: EXAMPLE OF AFRICAN IMMIGRATION TO GERMANY AND REPRODUCTIVE HEALTH

Ethnography encourages long-term involvement with individuals over time in order to understand the particular trajectories of their experience. For instance, in one study (Castañeda 2008), it was useful to follow firsthand the case of "Sarah," a thirty-three-year-old undocumented woman from Ghana living in Berlin, Germany. The original research questions focused on access to medical care for undocumented migrants; however, during the course of participant observation of experiences with patients of a migrant clinic, the unique analytical potential of studying reproduction became evident and thus influenced the course of the rest of the project. Because the ethnographer gained rapport with Sarah, she was invited to accompany her during visits to clinics for prenatal care, to the hospital when she gave birth, and to various government offices in failed attempts to secure a birth certificate for her (undocumented) child. She was also introduced to a large West African expatriate community, which supported Sarah and related similar experiences of social marginalization and exclusion from health care services. The various elements of Sarah's experience, like those of many other pregnant undocumented women encountered in the larger study, came together only over the course of over a year and a half of formal and informal conversations, visits to clinics, shared meals, and so forth. This underscores the value of longitudinal ethnographic fieldwork in following individuals over time to draw out their complex and often contradictory experiences.

ETHNOGRAPHIC RESEARCH STAGES OF ANALYSIS

As described above, ethnographic methods involve long-term immersion in a particular social and cultural context. Through participant observation, the researcher participates in everyday life during an extended period of time, while observing interactions and listening to conversations in order to identify significant practices, ideological and political economic forces, and cultural concepts. Ethnography involves data from observations, conversations, and interviews, as well as from the social interactions and bodily experiences of the ethnographer. Data collection involves the taking of field notes, often supplemented by audio-recorded conversations and interviews and sometimes by other methods, such as clinical chart reviews. In general, these different methodologies and their analysis within the ethnographic research project take place in two overlapping stages.

The first stage focuses on the in-depth, thick description of background, context, and important social actors and institutions related to the research question. This stage involves a broad review of detailed field notes with descriptions of everything possibly related to the topic. In this stage, the researcher may ask many "naïve" questions of all the participants in order not only to understand the general layout of the social world, but also to gain perspective about his or her particular vantage point.

The second stage of ethnographic field research, which often begins as the first stage is still under way, involves what might be described as a process of iterative hypothesis testing, which should lead to more and more precise and inductive, reality-based questions and observations. This stage focuses more directly on the research question; hypotheses are developed based on the background contextual research of the first stage and extant findings and social theory already understood from previous literature. The researcher develops a hypothesis, asks questions, and continues to conduct participant observation related to the research question. Next, the researcher analyzes the data, refines or completely transforms the hypothesis, and undergoes another round of data collection aimed at further exploration and refinement. This continues until the researcher (or research team) is confident in the ongoing reproduction of findings. For example, mainstream media portrayals of Mexican migration imply a voluntary, economic decision-making process. However, ethnographic research led one of the authors (SMH) to question this assumption based on repeated conversations and interviews with Mexican migrants indicating that Mexican migrants experience the migration process as involuntary and brought about by political as well as economic forces (Holmes 2011).

The analysis of ethnographic data is multifaceted and depends on the individual methods utilized. Because the goal is to examine complex social processes and meanings, data interpretation often involves reading and rereading notes and transcripts, reflecting, asking additional questions of participants to clarify issues that may be confusing, and comparing issues both within the study's data and between the current project and other related literature. As an example of one common method of analysis, qualitative data from interviews, focus groups, and field notes can be coded into domains or variables. As a next step in analysis, the researcher (or research team) may conduct a componential analysis of themes, along with the selection of illustrative quotes related to those themes. The researcher can analyze the qualitative data with a data management program such as ATLAS.ti or MAXQDA or simply by hand, marking different sections according to the related code. Data within a single code are then compiled and analyzed for their characteristics and meanings, and may also be coded axially, which means focusing on connections among different categories. The technique known as "triangulation" allows for the verification of results and the integration of qualitative and quantitative data. This involves reviewing the results of several kinds of data from the same sources over time as well as from independent sources in order to increase the validity (sometimes called "internal validity") of the findings.

The model of grounded theory can be particularly useful in ethnographic studies (Strauss and Corbin 1990). Despite the term, grounded theory is a technique for analysis rather than a theoretical orientation. It focuses on inductively allowing the codes and related analysis to emerge from the data, instead of imposing preformulated possibilities. In ethnography, analysis often begins during fieldwork, as investigators systematically analyze and code field notes and interviews in order to test the primary hypotheses of the study and develop more precise questions for the next rounds of interviews and participant observation. In some cases, the researcher will leave the field site and then reenter after some period of reflection and refinement of the research questions. This method allows for ongoing contextual development of more and more precise understandings.

Many ethnographic researchers invite study participants themselves to look over and comment on the analysis and conclusions of a project. This can work to increase the validity of findings by minimizing the a priori bias of the outsider and can sometimes bring complicated negotiations. This process of consultation with study participants may sometimes lead to further awareness of power hierarchies and different social positions and perspectives in the midst of potential complications and negotiations.

ADVANTAGES AND LIMITATIONS

Ethnography has many advantages as a research technique. First, it provides for in-depth, long-term understanding of specific case studies. The specific length of an ethnographic study will depend on the researcher's familiarity with the community and specific research questions. Another strength of this type of research is extremely strong internal validity, or the degree and depth of understanding and verification of the data and analysis being presented. Triangulation with different social actors as well as with the same person over time allows for further understanding from multiple vantage points and through processes of change. In addition, ethnography allows for understanding of complex, subtle, and power-imbued social, cultural, and symbolic interactions in vivo, in context, and without the requisite simplification that is necessary in the formulation of easily analyzable questions, dichotomies, or scales.

Ethnography is especially helpful for research among stigmatized and hidden populations, with whom rapport takes significant time and comprehension improves with rapport. For example, undocumented migrants are often hidden populations, limiting the feasibility of many other methods. Among this particular population, no sampling frame exists since the size of the population is often unknown, and membership involves stigmatized behavior that may lead to mistrust and low response rates with other methods of inquiry. For this reason, ethnographic methods built around participant observation are ideal; they offer more depth than the surface examination provided by more short-term methods (Walter et al. 2002).

Another primary benefit of ethnographic field research in the study of hidden populations is "the potential of limiting the artificiality of group definitions by grounding research parameters within the context of actually observed behaviors; insider understandings . . . [and] self-reported identities of the target group" (Singer 1999: 172). Other research methods may lend themselves, unfortunately, to the reproduction of preconceived understandings and questions regarding the hidden or stigmatized group. This can occur through the use of juridical constructions such as "legal" and "illegal," "voluntary economic migrant" or "involuntary political refugee" or even through definitions of the community under study according to preconceived identities and boundaries (such as "Latino" instead of utilizing categories employed by the study participants, for example, indigenous Mexican groups).

In addition, ethnography allows the researcher to gain access to locations and activities that might otherwise be closed to surveys or one-time interviews, along with a long-term commitment to a field site to capture change over time. This allows the researcher to investigate subtle forms of prejudice, assumption, and meaning that are often difficult to assess with quantitative methods or interviews alone. In addition, ethnography emphasizes in-depth investigation of the various levels influencing health and inequality, what Nader (1969) has called a "vertical slice." For example, a health issue such as HIV/AIDS in a particular migrant population requires the investigation of power interactions at multiple levels, including interpersonal relationships, structural factors, stereotypes and prejudice, access to testing, access to care, economic and political factors influencing migration, and national and international policy.

At the same time that ethnography allows for these many possibilities, it does not allow for the incidence and prevalence calculation of specific health issues. In addition, due to the nature of in-depth, long-term participant observation, ethnography generally involves a relatively small number of research participants. While this allows for strong internal validity, it does not provide for as strong external validity, or the degree to which the data are representative of other populations in other places and times. This can be partially overcome through triangulation, or the cross-verification of multiple sources of data in order to facilitate comparative analysis and validation. However, given the focus of most ethnography on "generalizing within" as opposed to "generalizing from," this limitation is not of primary concern to most ethnographic research questions. In addition, ethnography, like any research method, requires perseverance and humility as it may take time and patience to build rapport.

PRESENTATION AND PUBLICATION

Ethnographic research is published both in traditional health sciences venues (such as public health, medical, and nursing journals) and in social science journals or books. Ethnographic articles are often longer than what is typical for the presentation of quantitative or survey-based data. An article based on ethnographic research will look very different depending on whether it is published in a journal focused on the health sciences or the social sciences. Health science journals require the author to separate the iterative and inductive process of ethnographic research into different predetermined sections (such as Methods, Analysis, Results, and Discussion). Ethnographic articles published in social science journals often take a different, more narrative format. This format allows the author to remain closer to the iterative process of data collection and analysis most common to ethnographic research, and allows the reader more narrative flow, providing reflexive description of the research methods alongside the description and analysis of the observations. Those in the health sciences may be unfamiliar with this format, but many ethnographers find it a helpful means for presentation. Ethnographers often briefly describe themselves, where they were, and what was going on as they relay their observations and analysis. This allows for a more full recognition of the interpretive nature of ethnography and, indeed, of all research.

Many ethnographers write books with multiple chapters about the same long-term research project in order to allow the reader the most in-depth understanding. The writing of such a book also allows for more detailed narrative development of the characters of the research subjects, their relationships with one another, and the power dynamics involved, as well as an in-depth analysis of different topics in each chapter. Such books, published with peer-reviewed academic presses, are highly respected (often more so than articles) by many ethnographers, anthropologists, and sociologists. These books may also reach different and sometimes broader audiences than academic articles alone.

Regardless of the format, the presentation or publication of ethnographic research allows for an impressive degree of human everyday life to be revealed. The presentation of in-depth descriptions of a small group of people along with related direct quotes and/or descriptions of events allows the reader to imagine the reality being described and analyzed. One might argue that this form of presentation invites the reader to feel more interest and compassion than with the presentation of statistics. For these reasons, ethnographic research should be considered seriously when one is interested in effecting policy, public opinion, and/or behavioral change. Finally, because of the long-term, in-depth involvement with a specific community that ethnography fosters, this approach allows for a better understanding of how research findings might be translated into efforts at improving health. For this reason, many health ethnographers argue that this research method is truly and deeply "community based." As described above, the practice of discussing findings and interpretations with research participants can be helpful in increasing awareness of the ideas and goals of the research participants themselves.

SUMMARY/CONCLUSION

This chapter has provided a basic understanding of ethnographic research, its advantages and limitations for research on migration and health, and its data collection, analysis, and presentation. We anticipate that after reading this chapter, you will have strengthened interest, desire, and confidence to begin planning and conducting your own important research into the critical area of migration and health. If you plan to use primarily quantitative or other nonethnographic research methods, we hope you now have a stronger understanding of the ways in which reading ethnography or collaborating with ethnographers in mixed-methods team research will expand the possibilities of your investigations. Alternatively, if this chapter has sparked further interest in beginning on the path to becoming comfortable engaging in ethnographic research, we hope you will explore some of the resources below. Through ethnographic research, you can contribute meaningfully to the further understanding of the reality and experience of health and sickness among the many migrants around the world.

RESOURCES

Qualitative Data Analysis Software/Computer Assisted Qualitative Data Analysis (CAQDAS):

- ATLAS.ti (www.atlasti.com)
- NVivo (www.qsrinternational.com)
- MAXQDA (www.maxqda.com)
- Dedoose (www.dedoose.com)

Websites:

- Migrant Clinicians Network (http://www.migrantclinician.org)
- Indigenous Mexicans in California Agriculture (http://www.indigenousfarmworkers.org)
- National Center for Farmworker Health, Inc. (http://www.ncfh.org/)
- Platform for International Cooperation on Undocumented Migrants (PICUM) (www.picum.org)
- Migration Policy Institute (MPI) (www.migrationpolicy.org)
- Center of Expertise on Migration and Health (http://ccis.ucsd.edu/programs/coemh)

- AccessDenicd: A Conversation on Unauthorized Im/migration and Health (http://accessdeniedblog.wordpress.com)

REFERENCES

Castañeda, Heide. 2008. "Paternity for Sale: Anxieties over 'Demographic Theft' and Undocumented Migrant Reproduction in Germany." *Medical Anthropology Quarterly* 22(4):340–59.

Castañeda, Heide, Nolan Kline, and Nathaniel Dickey. 2010. "Health Concerns of Migrant Backstretch Workers at Horse Racetracks." *Journal of Health Care for the Poor and Underserved* 21(2):489–503.

Clifford, James. 1998. *Routes: Travel and Translation in the Late Twentieth Century.* Cambridge: Harvard University Press.

Falzon, Mark-Anthony. 2009. "Introduction: Multi-Sited Ethnography: Theory, Praxis and Locality in Contemporary Research." In *Multi-Sited Ethnography.* M.-A. Falzon, ed. Pp. 1–24. Surrey, England: Ashgate.

Geertz, Clifford. 1973. "Thick Description: Toward an Interpretive Theory of Culture." In *The Interpretation of Cultures: Selected Essays.* Pp. 3–30. New York: Basic Books.

Holmes, S. M. 2007. "Oaxacans Like to Work Bent Over: The Naturalization of Social Suffering among Berry Farm Workers." *International Migration* 45(3):39–68.

Holmes, S. M. 2011. "Structural Vulnerability and Hierarchies of Ethnicity and Citizenship on the Farm." *Medical Anthropology* 30(4):425–49.

Holmes, S. M. 2013. *Fresh Fruit, Broken Bodies: Migrant Farmworkers in the United States.* Berkeley: University of California Press.

Nader, Laura. 1969. "Up the Anthropologist—Perspectives Gained from 'Studying Up.'" In *Reinventing Anthropology.* Del Hymes, ed. Pp. 284–311. New York: Pantheon.

Pratt, Mary Louise. 1992. *Imperial Eyes: Travel Writing and Transculturation.* London: Routledge.

Quesada, James, Laurie K. Hart, Philippe Bourgois. "Structural Vulnerability and Health: Latino Migrant Laborers in the United States." Medical Anthropology 30(4):339-62.

Rosaldo, Renato. 1993. *Culture and Truth: The Remaking of Social Analysis.* Boston: Beacon Press.

Singer, Merrill. 1999. "Studying Hidden Populations." In *Mapping Networks, Spatial Data and Hidden Populations, Book 4, The Ethnographer's Toolkit.* J. Schensul, M. LeCompte, R. Trotter, E. Cromley, and M. Singer, eds. Pp. 125–91. Walnut Creek, CA: Altamira Press.

Stoller, Paul. 1997. "Globalizing Method: The Problems of Doing Ethnography in Transnational Spaces." *Anthropology and Humanism* 22(1):81–94.

Strauss, Anselm C., and Juliet M. Corbin. 1990. *Basics of Qualitative Research: Grounded Theory Procedures and Techniques.* Sage.

Tsing, Anna. 2008. "The Global Situation." In *The Anthropology of Globalization.* J. X. Inda and R. Rosaldo, eds. Pp. 66–98. Malden, MA: Blackwell.

Walter, N., P. Bourgois, H. M. Loinaz, and D. Schillinger. 2002. "Social Context of Work Injury among Undocumented Day Laborers in San Francisco." *Journal of General Internal Medicine* 17(3):221–29.

14

Participant Observation and Key Informant Interviews

Rosa María Aguilera
Ana Amuchástegui

INTRODUCTION

Our times are characterized by increasing complexities associated with globalization. Human migration is as complex as its study, both because of its quantitative dimensions—the present century has been called the "century of migration"—and because it is occurring within the context of growing economic, political, and sociocultural globalization, which has introduced tension into classical categories like those of "nation-state," "identity," "citizenship" and "multiculturalism." These complexities also produce tension for research methods and pose specific epistemological challenges.

In this context, the present chapter reflects on the use of two qualitative research techniques: participant observation and key informant interviews, and evaluates their usefulness for the study of mobile populations. It also emphasizes the importance of researchers making their theoretical and political positions explicit, given that those positions can limit the point of view from which researchers set out to do their fieldwork and, moreover, can undermine the whole research process.

Given that this volume explores different research techniques for the study of migrant populations, we consider it essential to reflect critically on how information about these groups is currently produced, especially from a *transnational perspective*.

TRANSNATIONAL PERSPECTIVES ON INTERNATIONAL MIGRATION

Migrant populations are conceived as populations in movement within transnational social spaces that escape the universal logic of the nation-state. It does not matter which expelling or receiving states are involved; the *transnational character of international migration* refers to "the economic, political and sociocultural practices linked to and confined to a logic of more than one nation state characterized by the constant crossing of borders . . . which simultaneously affect the migration process in the country of origin and in the country of destination" (Suárez 2008:911).

This approach has generated some debate because it questions the "economic" point of view, which considers international migration as an individual strategy that takes advantage of the supply-demand imbalance in the labor market. It alerts against the danger of what Suárez calls *"methodological nationalism"* (Suárez 2008: 914, 927), which considers only one of the poles of the migration circuit, assuming that the territory of nations does shape and limit social phenomena. The units of analysis are thus defined within the borders of the nation-state, preventing the recognition of transnational processes.

These assumptions lead to *methodological individualism,* which relies on concepts like "integration," "assimilation," and "acculturation" as the only adaptation strategies used by migrants. In contrast, the transnational perspective looks at the emergence of new identities based upon dual nationalities, in which the dominant political model of national citizenship becomes inadequate (Cordero Díaz 2007:63).

This critique has emerged through the study of the *social networks* migrants create as bridges between the social fields of origin and destination, which allow them to access information, support, and resources. Analyses of these networks show there are multiple differences within migrant systems, regions, groups, and individuals. The transnational perspective actually disclaims the notions that ethnicity is the "essence" of subjects and that concepts of "nation" can be used without concrete historical and geographical referents.

The transnational approach recognizes social networks as a form of social capital. Even though social networks are effective because they mobilize resources on both sides of a border and are based on trust and previous family, friendship, and neighborhood relationships, to simply naturalize them as "blood" ties between equals and relatives leads to biologist notions of the social sphere that tend to romanticize networks and prioritize them over other relationships. Migration scholars agree that there is a risk of reifying concepts that are in fact analytical instruments: networks based on kinship cannot be considered "primary" networks, or the "first phase or level" in the evolutionary chain of transnational migration (Besserer 2004:21; Suárez 2008:925).

The transnational perspective not only conceives of social networks as relations between "equals" and forms of "reciprocity" but also introduces the analysis of the *power* that is present in gender, generational, clientelistic, sex, and race relationships produced in the transnational space.[1]

The analysis of power allows for the visualization of what is being played out in the transnational social field, that is, the *governability of mobile populations,* as Suárez makes clear:

> The *transnational social field* is not limited to a space containing social networks, but to a set of dynamics that emerge from the impact of the process of globalization in the labor market and in the governability of populations, which are decreasingly rooted in a single territory. In the creation and maintenance of a transnational field of migration, what is at play is the creation of mobile subjects and of logics of incomplete belonging. Mobility not only refers to physical movement in space, since within such a field there are also sedentary and not-mobile subjects, for whom the capital generated by the transfers between the poles of the transnational field is instrumental, not only on the economic, but also on the cultural and political level. (2008:930)

Lastly, the transnational perspective views concepts such as "the construction of differences" and "nation" as sociocultural constructs and considers "culture" to be a process that is not necessarily linked to a particular territory.

WHAT IS PARTICIPANT OBSERVATION?

All scientific knowledge is the result of some kind of observation. Participant observation is a qualitative technique placed in the micro-social level; it is interested in looking at social relations and interactions, the meanings that subjects give to their actions and practices within the existing social context and structures that condition their actions (Amezcua 2000; Sánchez 2004). It intends to grasp cultural influences, power in group relations, beliefs, symbols and rituals, customs, values, community lifestyles, the identity of social movements, social hierarchies, and forms of organization. It shows in great detail the social practices of daily life: conversations and participation; but also silence and caution, that which remains unsaid and implicit, and that which is a given—informal, interstitial, not documented and contradictory.

This is a disciplined qualitative technique used for producing detailed information in order to generate knowledge, in our case, *about* and *with* mobile populations. It is closely linked to anthropological research practices and certain sociological traditions such as the Chicago school.[2] Participant observation (PO) embraces ethnographic work as a way of approaching reality, and it is most often complemented with other techniques such as interviews, where the researcher plays a part in the situation being studied.

PO calls for an interdisciplinary approach and allows looking at the object of research from different theoretical traditions such as phenomenology, ethnomethodology, symbolic interaction, and, more recently, critical theory, feminist thinking, and constructivism. It is possible to promote community development through the use of the knowledge produced in the hope that it will help in the solution of complex human social problems (Denzin and Lincoln 2011; Rosaldo 1989).

According to Gutierrez and Delgado (1995), participant observation is the most representative method of external observation (or *etic*) procedures, since it is developed by an external-to-the-community subject who introduces him- or herself, albeit unobtrusively, into a sociocultural context different from his or her own, with the objective of understanding the internal point of view of a group (the *emic* perspective). This double perspective is perhaps the reason why, paradoxically, these authors also define it as "internal or participant active observation" (Gutierrez and Delgado 1995:144). PO requires the researcher to reside for a time in the chosen setting so that the information produced can reflect both the *emic* and *etic* perspectives.

The researcher thus plays a triple role: to develop a social interaction with the informants, to record the information, and to interpret the information obtained in a controlled and systematic way. Inevitably a dialogue is initiated between the two cultures, that of the researcher and that of the informants (Sánchez 2004).

As mentioned earlier, participant observation is carried out within social processes that require direct contact with social actors. It is possible for the researcher, though it seldom occurs, to specify to readers the theoretical assumptions that he or she is working with, that is to say, the way in which he or she conceives of society and people. The assumption of the existence of a "real, objective, and external" world is different from the assumption that the researcher is actually a part of the social processes under study. For example, researchers will produce a certain kind of knowledge if they believe that migrants "deprive" natives of certain jobs that they feel entitled to, or that those who have entered a country without proper permission deserve sanctions, or that a "vulnerable" population always needs the help of supportive people. They will produce very different findings if they consider migrants to be social actors whose human rights have been violated, but who are still capable of changing their limiting social conditions. These notions constitute the *ontological* aspect of a study, that is to say, the researcher's ideas on the *nature of reality, society, and people.*

There are three general perspectives regarding ontology in social science: the first assumes that social, economic, and political structures influence the social life of people (macro-structural theory); the second holds that it is people in their agency who produce structures through their interactions (micro-social theory); and the third tries to connect the two by considering that, when people act according to their own motivations and react to existing structures, they both reproduce *and* modify them.

Researchers will also have to specify their conception of themselves and their concepts of reality, society, and people, as well as the kind of relationship they will establish with them. These are the *epistemological* aspects of research: for example, if reality is considered to be "objective," then it will be necessary to keep a "distance" and produce equally "objective" and "unbiased" findings. However, if society is considered to be a historical-cultural construction, in which both researcher and social actors participate—with their beliefs, values, and wishes, that is, with their subjectivity—the findings will be the product of that analysis of subjective interpretations of *all* participants. If the researchers think of themselves as "experts" dedicated to finding out *about* mobile populations, their appraisal of the subjectivity of migrants will be different than if they set out to produce findings *in collaboration with* mobile populations.

The previous considerations affect the *methodological* aspect of research: if one is seeking "objective" findings, the bias supposedly brought about by the subjectivity of the researcher is expected to be "controlled" and protected from "confusing variables" that may limit the generalization of findings. However, if researchers consider that reality can only be known through interaction with others and by way of the self-reflective capacity of all participants, that is, of the subjective dimension, they will have to find mechanisms that will foster the interpretation of interactions (Castro 1996; Sánchez 2004).

STRENGTHS AND WEAKNESSES OF PARTICIPANT OBSERVATION

The strengths and limitations of participant observation depend on their epistemological bases. Guber (2004) discusses whether PO components—observation and participation—are practiced equally in fieldwork or whether the field seems to favor one over the other.

Approaches that favor observation point out that it should be "neutral" and that the researcher should not become emotionally involved with participants. When participation is rendered inevitable, it should be looked upon as a "necessary evil." The concrete experience of interaction and research should be limited to a series of "procedures" allegedly free of judgment.

Other approaches believe that participation is key to understanding because then the researcher experiences social meanings firsthand.[3] This way, participation turns from a necessary evil to the *condition for knowledge* (Guber 2004). Understanding is as much a methodology for research as a particular form of experience in which common sense is used to understand the sociocultural world.

One of the strengths of PO is what Guber calls "the actor's perspective": "that universe of shared reference—not always verbalized—which underlies and orchestrates the set of practices, notions and sense organized by the interpretation and the activity of social subjects" (Guber 2004:41). Such a notion is close to what

Giddens calls "mutual knowledge" and Schutz calls "common sense" (in Guber 2004:41). PO thus becomes a symbolic space in which an "encounter between pre-interpreted worlds" takes place: that is, the social actor's world within the reference framework of the social group to which he or she belongs and the researcher's world within the framework of his or her perspective. Just like migrants, researchers will make the journey of "coming and going" between their assumptions and the social actors' reference framework, until they discover a viewpoint that will allow them to understand the phenomena from the perspective of those who experience it. This procedure entails a reflexive process since "the knowledge constructed by the researcher is not disconnected, but rather intrinsically tied to the knowledge he produces about himself and which the informants also produce about him" (Guber 2004:113).

VALIDITY AND RELIABILITY OF PARTICIPANT OBSERVATION

Often the main objection to PO is the alleged difficulty of observing in the field what is called "collective subjectivity" (Gutierrez and Delgado 1995), illustrated in international migration by the notion of the "culture of migration."[4] For example, is said "culture" experienced in the same way by a Mexican migrant as by a Moroccan migrant? In the globalized societies where these movements take place, cultures lose their "essence" and no longer function as "cognitive models and unique operations." It is necessary to ask, then: What is the "cultural distance" that researchers should try to diminish? Are there commonalities between the worlds of the observer and the participants?

While these are valid concerns, criteria for validation and representation in qualitative methodology must be addressed through the recognition of the nature of social phenomena: "Depth rather than frequency of the phenomena is privileged, understanding (sense and meaning) rather than description, the depiction of a context rather than statistic representativity" (Szasz and Amuchástegui 1996:22).

In PO, the researcher is the main tool, and thus the validity of his or her production is related to skill, competence, commitment, and knowledge of the context of multicultural processes, which are themselves influenced by class, race, gender, and ethnicity. PO's main challenge is not to produce generalizations, but to generate theoretically significant knowledge (Sánchez 2004). Researchers need to use triangulation together with other methods—as well as teamwork—so that their work can be placed within the academic domain, rather than within literature or journalism. Participant observation demands that the observer perform constant reflection and flexibility, and replace notions of validity and trustworthiness with those of credibility and coherence.

HOW TO CARRY OUT PARTICIPANT OBSERVATION

Participant observation is an *art* that demands qualities such as patience, empathy, rapport, and prudence. But it is also a *technique* that requires knowing how and when to use it (Amezcua 2000:32). It is necessary to create an atmosphere that allows for the most spontaneous communication possible and to produce a presence and participation in the diverse aspects of daily life, including exceptional situations, that will allow for the *construction* of relevant information. Sánchez (2004) believes it is necessary for the researcher to stay at a distance in order to avoid the illusions of the group and maintain a critical attitude: presence implies social interaction and the production of reciprocity, making it necessary to also observe reactions such as curiosity, solidarity, support, distrust, aversion, and hostility.

The following sections describe the steps to follow in PO.

Preparing the Scene

The "field" is the place where the researcher places him- or herself as an observer: it may be a community, a neighborhood, a health center, a street corner, a bar, an asylum, a business, a school. This is the time when the researcher chooses and sets up the borders of the scene of observation, defines the object of study, and builds up preliminary ideas about the phenomena to be observed. He or she also constructs categories of analysis and the instruments needed to gather information. The researcher must in and out of the field and double-check preconceived ideas, because the field usually produces surprises, and new theoretical and practical questions may come up, allowing for fine-tuning of overall research questions. Sensitivity to the process can be increased by not setting up the objectives beforehand and by not having a preconceived notion of what a "theoretical sample"[5] should look like. Actually, the final design will emerge as the research develops and in reaction to the vicissitudes of fieldwork.

Rosaldo (1989) recommends that in order to define the social situations to be observed, researchers should assume that they are "situated subjects" who hold a structural place in which their age, gender, condition as a foreigner, and relationship to the neocolonial regime molds their everyday experiences, a molding that allows or inhibits the possibility of observing certain aspects in the field. Guber (2004) maintains that the only way for observers to access the field is with their own interpretive concepts and framework, which should be submitted to an ongoing reflective process.

Access

Accessing transnational social fields and being accepted in them can prove difficult. At first, the researcher may not be familiar with the people, alliances, or conflicts happening in the place of observation. The informants do not know why the researcher is there, what he or she wants, or what his or her intentions are. Thus, fieldwork is usually carried out in situations where there are many unknowns that need clarification. It is necessary to be diligent and patient, and prepared to negotiate.

In many settings access is complicated by the potential presence of organized crime, which may operate along the same clandestine routes and borders used by undocumented migrants. For example, the "war" on drugs in Mexico has created an atmosphere of growing distrust of "strangers" in rural communities in the country, which complicates the observer's ability to access the scene.

In such situations it is necessary to try to get the cooperation of *key informants* (KIs), who can guide the researcher and act as a source of basic information on meaningful topics of a given culture and social context. KIs are people who also often serve as "gatekeepers" because of their hierarchical position (community or religious authorities, members of councils of elders). It often takes time to find a "social godfather" who may alert the researcher to possible mistakes that might obstruct the process. Guber (2004) insists that face-to-face contact is the only way to guarantee real communication between the researcher and the informant, through what she calls "intersubjectivity."[6]

Relationships in the Field

The very presence of the researcher within a different sociocultural context is itself a kind of participation. However, the character of the social interactions established with participants will allow, or in some cases prevent, the possibility of understanding them as complex producers of meanings, as well as their potential for transformation. Mere presence in the field does not entail full access to the object of study. According to Guber (2004), it is through *mediation* performed by *informants* that reciprocal understanding between cultural worlds may be achieved. It is necessary to find volunteers who will work at finding other *informants* through what is usually called "the snowball effect" (Johnston and Sabin 2010).[7] Once accepted in the field, the researcher should explore the points of view of new participants/collaborators and establish relationships with different and even opposing groups in order to contrast diverse perspectives that often depend on an informant's position in the social context or on individual and situational variations.

There are several recommendations about the kinds of interactions that should take place in the field: the literature points to problematic[8] and sometimes even contradictory accounts. Researchers will have to make their own decisions, depending on the object of study, their common sense, their personal criteria, and ethical issues. However, the observer is not a passive subject and, without losing sight of his or her sources' *critical sense,* he or she may find it necessary to reconcile definitions and narratives of complex situations observed in fieldwork with his or her informants.

Since researchers' subjective and emotional experiences[9] are real and legitimate tools that can be used for producing knowledge, helping out and doing favors when needed is not ruled out. It must be remembered, however, that PO creates ties between the observer and the actor, and that the difference between them is one of *positions;* it is not a *personal* one.[10] The researcher is just another actor in the social context, who may at times observe and at others be observed because, indeed, at times key informants can become "observers of the observer."

Production of Information

Researchers need to associate with key informants, who also function as companions, in order to introduce themselves to the scene. Informants can also help researchers hone their reflective capacities and heighten awareness of their own ideological and cultural baggage. When informants contribute in this way, they can become coauthors of the research findings. This can happen even if such a contribution brings theoretical or political tension into the academic, cultural, and social world of the researcher. At this stage, the researcher can define his or her own categories by constantly coming and going between theory and data, in order to reach new meanings, new contextual relations, and new interpretations (Guber 2004).

Ruiz and Ispizúa (1989) distinguish between different kinds of informants depending on the relationships established in the field. The *stranger* does not meddle in the social group's issues; the *reflexive subject* enjoys social legitimacy as a carrier of innovative ideas; the *intellectual* is socially acknowledged and well educated; the *displaced individual* has lost his position; the *old wolf* manages a lot of information and does not mind making it public; and the *needy one,* in exchange for certain forms of support, is willing to reveal information and keep the researcher company. There are also "non-informants," who may be hostile to the process and make fieldwork more difficult.

In PO the number of scenes to be observed and people to be interviewed must be set depending on the amount of information needed, or until a *saturation point* is reached, that is, when new interviews or PO records repeat the information and data already produced and no longer contribute new information.

The Art of Questioning

"Before asking questions, it is necessary to learn to listen; the best observer is not the person who talks the most, but rather the one who lets and makes others talk . . .; it is as important to know how to ask, as it is to detect what not to ask" (Amezcua 2000:33). The main thing is to approach with an understanding of the actors' perspectives. It is recommended not to begin with loaded questions or value judgments. Developing sensitivity in order to be aware of and avoid forbidden issues is important. It is better to wait until something significant comes up and then probe it cautiously, avoiding aggressive methods such as doing audio/video recording, presenting questionnaires, or expressing conflicting opinions. Discrepancies can be assessed and addressed subtly as the investigation continues.

Recording Information and the Field Notebook

For fieldwork a diary is fundamental because it is the instrument the researcher uses to make detailed notes about his or her observations. Writing down detailed notes after each observation session calls for enormous discipline and is not an easy task. Observations make practical sense when an ethnographic monograph is finally written,[11] because the reflexive and critical information is organized in such a way that it will support the interpretations of the findings. However, findings only reach theoretical significance if they are able to capture key aspects of the observed phenomena and reveal its development possibilities. It is suggested that neither informants nor geographical characteristics of the field be identified in the final document unless they are explicitly requested.

WHY SHOULD PO BE USED WITH MOBILE POPULATIONS?

PO is relevant for the study of mobile populations because it renders stigmatized and *hidden populations* visible ("illegal aliens," "sudacas," "refugees"). It is especially effective with mobile populations whose rights have been violated and who live on the margins of society, forced to remain hidden and surviving as *disposable labor*. The main purpose of PO is to unveil the symbolic spaces in which these populations move, since it is there that stigma and violation are fostered; thus the intention is to "look from the inside out and integrate the "native/stranger point of view" (Atkinson and Hammersley 1994).

WHAT ARE WE GOING TO FOCUS ON AS RESEARCHERS USING PO?

Researchers who adopt the participant observation methodology should focus on the following:

- on *key actors* who exert control over these transnational fields, such as nation-state representatives who have the power to open up borders for those who have proper documents and to close them down for those who do not (e.g., governors, congresspersons, and representatives)
- on the employers of migrants who exploit new forms of labor based on the precariousness, insecurity, and instability brought about by the processes of economic globalization and flexibilization

- on the people who live off the "business" of migration, such as smugglers, some government employees on both sides of borders, and employees of human rights nongovernmental organizations (NGOs) and associations
- on civic groups who may turn migrants into targets for aggression, and on the government institutions in charge of controlling such situations
- on the organized crime sectors that make up "de facto juridical instances,"[12] which may see migrants as an opportunity to make easy money through kidnappings, extortion, or forced participation in illegal activities (selling drugs, human trafficking, etc.)
- on new kinds of migrants who experience displacement in different ways: women, young people, children, the elderly, ecological migrants, and refugees
- on new social actors who have been forced to migrate, not so much for economic reasons but because of internal wars and conflicts with drug-trafficking organizations
- on the ways in which analytical categories are transformed due to the life experiences of social actors who create and reproduce transnational spaces. These categories include power, gender, generational relations, bodies and corporealities, families, the market, nation-states, notions of sovereignty, the reconfiguration of ethnic identities, the arising of new postnational identities, dual citizenship, voting in foreign countries, integration, and assimilation
- on the organizations that migrants create as a form of resistance and struggle for their rights, as well as on those social practices that entail accepting the values of the receiving society (levels of consumerism, lifestyles, cultural values, etc.)
- on the transformations of subjectivity of those displaced, due to the gains and losses experienced along with displacement; on the cultural dilemmas they may face, and on the emotional effects related to their mental health
- on researchers as key actors and producers of discourse and knowledge about mobile populations, who are positioned in particular geopolitical sites and specific statements, and whose situated knowledges may show how relations of domination and exploitation are present in transnational social fields (Cerda et al. 2009)

ETHICAL CONSIDERATIONS: WHO IS THE RESEARCH BEING DONE FOR?

Participant observation is not free of ethical dilemmas. For instance, the issue of deception is one of the main debates regarding research in which participants do not go through an "informed consent" process. Some authors justify deception when investigating powerful groups who would not consent to being "observed" (Sánchez 2004:109).

There is no consensus in the literature about whether "the end justifies the means": does the making of a "good study" justify actions that would be immoral or amoral in other contexts? Being an accomplice to illegal or reproachable activities with key informants is one example. There are those who decide to advocate for other people in the face of any abuse. Others approve of certain moral ambiguity in order to carry out their fieldwork. Legally, researchers are not required to report illegal acts, although it is a civic duty to testify and provide information in legal proceedings. For example, in the US new anti-immigration laws invite the general public to provide information about anyone suspected of being in the country illegally. Authorities in charge of immigration control may thus see researchers as potential "key informants," placing them in positions of personal risk and ethical dilemmas.

Since there is no consensus about existing normative ethical frames, researchers face many dilemmas. In the US, for example, a dominant ethics of principles is in place, one that renders researchers as bearers of principles of non-maleficence and beneficence, where informants are seen as enjoying their autonomy, and where the state is responsible for maintaining justice. In most countries in the European Economic Community, ethics emphasizes values of responsibility, justice, and equality as ways to ameliorate the unfair distribution of wealth (Schramm and Kottow 2001).

Researchers are expected to consider if their social responsibility ends when they publish their findings (Aguilera-Guzmán et al. 2008) or if they should participate in organized social movements, in this case those that advocate for migrants' views. Some may even consider becoming leaders of such organizations in their eagerness to change abusive migration conditions (Amezcua 2000). This is the time to answer not only the question of who this research is being done for but also the question of the "place" of participants as actors committed to changing social conditions. In the end, we need to ask: what are the benefits for each of the parties involved?

It is important to remember that social relations established among research participants always carry a *dimension of mutual power,* and that the human relations created in PO tend to stir emotional processes that require proper attention. Szasz and Amuchástegui believe that "researchers should be prepared, ethically and technically, to respond to the unavoidable effects that their interventions generate in both themselves and in the subjects of the research. An awareness of the emotions which may be set off in the researcher him/herself, the emotional attention to the subjects interviewed and the way in which inter-subjectivity affects the process of generating information, should all be a part of the research agenda" (1996:20).

It only remains to be said that the interest in mobile populations entails looking at the "main character of the twentieth century: the foreigner," and also paying close attention to the injustice generated by the fear of difference, so present in many societies today. "The other" is the one who makes us question the value of "our own." Reflecting on what is foreign to our point of view involves an ethical stance and constitutes "a call for assuming one's responsibility in relation to others" (Cohen and Martínez de la Escalera 2002:7–8).

ACKNOWLEDGMENTS

The authors wish to thank Reyna Gutierrez Reynaga for the critical revision of the first draft of this chapter and the librarian Rosario Infante Rodriguez for her support in the search for pertinent information.

NOTES

1. The Ecuadorian social networks analyzed in Spain, for example, showed structures historically rooted in clientelism and patronage (Suárez 2008).

2. The Chicago School—named because it was initially based in the universities around the Chicago area—was the first major body of work to specialize in urban sociology, introducing innovative methods by combining theory and ethnographic fieldwork. It emerged during the 1920s and 1930s.

3. A good example of this process is the case of the Mexican American anthropologist Renato Rosaldo (1989), who reflects on how his experience of the death of his wife gave him the means to better understand the ire that may arise from devastating losses, thus helping him to better understand the experiences of his informants in the Philippines.

4. The theory of the accumulative causation of migration (Arango 2003; Herrera 2006) affirms that if displacement is repeated and perpetuated due to the influence of the multiple factors that initiated it, a "culture of migration" is created, explaining its reproduction. At a subjective level, this culture of migration is usually lived as an option that is preferential to development in the communities of origin, that is to say, it is the construction of migration as a destination.

5. According to Glaser and Strauss (1967), a theoretical sample is a sample that seeks to represent a theoretical problem by selecting social situations that offer observations that generate as many categories and characteristics as possible that relate it with the theory by way of minimizing differences between cases in order to make basic characteristics of a certain category visible and then maximizing the differences between cases in order to increase the categories and narrow the incidence of the theory (Martin-Crespo and Salamanca 2007). Guber (2004) talks about the "significant" sample in contrast to the "representative" sample in quantitative investigation.

6. We use this term to describe the space in which the interaction between researcher and research participants allows for the interpretation of meanings co-constructed in the field.

7. This consists of each informant recommending one or more people in his or her circle of confidence to the investigator.

8. For example, the degree of affective involvement of the investigator with the informants, the use of deceit, the aspect of prioritizing, the success of the investigation, or the benefits for the participants.

9. Impressions, feelings, intuition, and all that may be called subjective are not obstacles for objective findings, since subjectivity is social; thus what is real is integrated/produced by what is subjective (Guber 2004).

10. All human beings have the same stature as people. What differentiates us is the position we have within social structures.

11. See chapter 13 of this volume, on ethnographic studies, by Holmes and Castañeda, for a detailed description of the subject.

12. Body guards, mercenaries, hitmen, paramilitaries who vie with the state for the monopoly on military operations, use of violence, coercion, and the right to kill (Mbembe 2003:31).

REFERENCES

Aguilera-Guzmán, Rosa María, Liliana Mondragón Barrios, and María Elena Medina-Mora. 2008. "Consideraciones éticas en intervenciones comunitarias: La pertinencia del consentimiento informado." *Salud Mental* 31: 129–38.

Amezcua, Manuel. 2000. "El trabajo de campo etnográfico en salud: Una aproximación a la observación participante." *Index de Enfermería* 9(30): 30–35.

Arango, Joaquín. 2003. "La explicación teórica de las migraciones: Luz y sombra." *Migración y Desarrollo* 1: 4–22.

Atkinson, Paul, and Martyn Hammersley. 1994. "Ethnography and Participant Observation." In *Handbook of Qualitative Research,* edited by Norman Denzin and Yvonna Lincoln, 248–61. Thousand Oaks, CA: Sage.

Besserer, Federico. 2004. *Topografías transnacionales: Hacia una geografía de la vida transnacional.* Mexico City: UAM-I and Plaza y Valdés.

Castro, Roberto. 1996. "En busca del significado: Supuestos alcances y limitaciones del análisis cualitativo." In *Para comprender la subjetividad,* edited by Ivonne Szasz and Susana Lerner, 57–85. Mexico City: El Colegio de México, 1996.

Cerda, Alejandro, María del Consuelo Chapela, and Edgar Jarillo. 2009. "Acontecimiento, sentido y referencia: Claves para comprender la experiencia de los sujetos en procesos globales." *Argumentos, Nueva Época* 22(61):29–47.

Cohen, Esther, and Ana María Martínez de la Escalera. 2002. *Lecciones de extranjería: Una mirada a la diferencia.* Mexico City: UNAM and Siglo XXI.

Cordero Díaz, Blanca Laura. 2007. "Ser trabajador transnacional: Clase, hegemonía y cultura en un circuito migratorio internacional." PhD diss. Benemérita Universidad Autónoma de Puebla.

Denzin, Norman K., and Yvonna S. Lincoln. 2011. *El campo de la investigación cualitativa.* Barcelona: GEDISA.

Glaser, B., and A. Strauss. 1967. *The Discovery of Grounded Theory.* Chicago: Aldine.

Guber, Rosana. 2004. *El salvaje metropolitano: Reconstrucción del conocimiento social en el trabajo de campo.* Buenos Aires: Paidós.

Gutiérrez, Juan, and Juan Manuel Delgado. 1995. "Teoría de la observación." In *Métodos y técnicas cualitativas de investigación en ciencias sociales,* edited by Juan Manuel Delgado and Juan Gutiérrez, 141–73. Madrid: Editorial Síntesis.

Herrera, Roberto. 2006. *La perspectiva teórica en el estudio de las migraciones.* Mexico City: Siglo XXI Editores.

Johnston, Lisa G., and Keith Sabin. 2010. "Sampling Hard-to-Reach Populations with Respondent Driven Sampling." *Methodological Innovations Online* 5: 38–48.

Martín-Crespo, Cristina, and Ana Belén Salamanca. 2007. "El muestreo en la investigación cualitativa." *Nure Investigación* 27.

Mbembe, Achille. 2003. "Necropolitics." *Public Culture* 15(1):11–40.

Rosaldo, Renato. 1989. *Cultura y verdad: Nueva propuesta de análisis social.* Mexico City: Grijalbo.

Ruiz, José, and María Ispizúa. 1989. *La descodificación de la vida cotidiana: Métodos de investigación cualitativa.* Bilbao: Universidad de Deusto.

Sánchez, Rolando. 2004. "La observación participante como escenario y configuración de la diversidad de significados." In *Observar, escuchar y comprender: Sobre la tradición cualitativa en la investigación social,* edited by María Luisa Tarrés, 97–131. Mexico City: Miguel Ángel Porrúa, Colegio de México, and FLACSO México.

Schramm, Fermin Roland, and Miguel Kottow. 2001. "Principios bioéticos en salud pública: Limitaciones y propuestas." *Cadernos de Saúde Pública* 17(4): 949–56.

Suárez, Navaz Liliana. 2008. "La perspectiva transnacional en los estudios migratorios: Génesis, derroteros y surcos metodológicos." *Inmigración Española* 7(1): 911–40.

Szasz, Ivonne, and Ana Amuchástegui. 1996. "Un encuentro con la investigación cualitativa en México." In *Para comprender la subjetividad,* edited by Szasz Ivonne and Susana Lerner, 17–30. Mexico City: El Colegio de México.

15

Focus Groups/Group Qualitative Interviews

Patricia Zavella

INTRODUCTION

This chapter discusses the origins of focus groups (occasionally called group qualitative interviews), illustrating how they are helpful in different research projects and describing the process of recruiting, organizing, and conducting them for health research that involves migrant populations. Complex issues often arise when focus groups are used with migrant populations and these issues are explored in depth. An extended case study of best practices describes a project that negotiates many of the complications involved in conducting focus groups with migrants.

Focus groups allow researchers to convene multiple subjects and ask them to respond to a set of questions and discuss issues related to the topic being investigated. The subjects may be recruited because of relevant personal experiences or because of membership in a particular population or group. These methods are increasingly used to incorporate more women, racial/ethnic groups, or migrants into health research. The development of focus groups can be traced to Merton and Kendall (1946:541), who suggest that interviews be focused by introducing a common experience and then conducting "content analysis of what has been said as well as . . . omissions," which can provide "a major cue for the detection and later exploration of private logics, personal symbolisms, and spheres of tension."[1] Group qualitative interviews allow investigators to understand how subjects conceptualize and reflect on specific topics and can aid in the development of an appropriate language to describe participants' experiences or perceptions. These methods can provide researchers with a deeper understanding of the social context of health problems and help identify important questions for further research.

The new knowledge and information developed through these methods can also have significant health policy implications.

Focus groups have been used extensively in market research to obtain feedback from consumers on product launches or advertising campaigns, and firms often target specific consumers, including migrants (Dávila 2001).[2] Perhaps because of the use of focus groups for marketing purposes, critics of the method often express concerns about the reliability of the data collected and suggest that focus groups need to be "triangulated" with other forms of data collection. While it is usually a good idea to collect data in multiple ways, the notion that focus group data are somehow incomplete follows positivist logic. As with other qualitative methods, focus groups are not designed to secure the objective truth but to provide a rich source of information that should be evaluated and analyzed systematically. As Reed and Payton (1997:766) caution, "This methodology needs careful considera- tion when making decisions about what sort of data are appropriate to a study, what analysis is needed, and how issues of validity can be addressed." Focus groups are often perceived as a more time-conserving and inexpensive way of collecting qualitative data than more traditional ethnographic methods such as participant observation, which ideally entails full-time research over a much longer duration.

As far back as the 1980s, there has been increasing use of focus group methods in public health research in general and, more specifically, in health research involving migrant populations. These methods are particularly useful for investi- gating migrant populations because they employ inductive techniques that aim to elicit knowledge where little or no previous research has been conducted and there are no validated measures available. They are also appropriate when research sub- jects feel intimidated by participating in a research project or when members of a disempowered group feel the need for research that addresses social disparities; both these conditions can be true of migrant groups.

Focus groups are especially useful for addressing values, norms, and percep- tions related to culturally sensitive health problems such as unpacking the stigma related to sexually transmitted infections or contagious diseases (Dodds 2006; Yamada et al. 1999). They can be helpful for understanding the sociocultural fac- tors associated with medical examinations deemed embarrassing by migrants, such as mammograms or pap smears, or when used with migrant populations who believe in alternative notions of illness and healing (Garcés et al. 2006; Liang et al. 2004; Lantz et al. 1994; Kahn and Manderson 1992). They are also helpful in under- standing self-care practices, as Hjelm and her colleagues (2001) found when com- paring Yugoslavian migrants and native diabetic females in Sweden.

Focus groups are also good for uncovering background information that can be useful for constructing questionnaires and protocols in studies with large samples or random sampling that allow for generalizability (Ruppenthal et al. 2005). Focus groups have been used effectively with migrant children as young as eight years old whose perspectives are often crucial in pilot research (Cooper et al. 2001). For example, Young and Ansell (2003) found that the consequences of losing parents to AIDS in southern Africa often makes migrants of children, whose views on optimal ways to stage their relocation are crucial in multimethod research. Attention should be given to addressing perceptions based on home country experiences as well as how a new context creates different perceptions about health (Polonsky and Renzaho 2011). This knowledge in turn may help establish credibility in the community, which can help further other research goals.

Focus groups are also useful with migrants who have low literacy levels, particularly in dominant languages, and cannot participate in research that requires written responses. Often migrants have experienced insensitive treatment and outright discrimination for their "backward" beliefs and practices in their countries of origin and destination, and are acutely aware that they are outsiders in terms of language and culture. In this context, focus groups can be "safer" spaces where participants feel free to articulate what is meaningful to them in terms of causes of health problems, appropriate interventions (including spiritual ones), and particular ways in which they want to communicate with their families, support networks, and health care practitioners. Among migrants, farmworkers are highly mobile, moving from crop to crop following various harvest seasons, and they include transnational as well as internal migrants who return home after each work season (Perilla et al. 1998). Migrant farmworkers may also be socially vulnerable, with high numbers of the unauthorized and those who are poor, which requires that researchers be "especially vigilant in protecting them from the potential harms of research and in ensuring that the special ethical issues that arise in research with this population are identified and addressed for every project" (Cooper et al. 2004:1).

Focus groups may be used in conjunction with other methods, such as telephone surveys or individual interviews, and are helpful in multiphase research projects where the initial methods indicate the need to understand cultural processes in more detail in relation to nuances of meaning (Scarinci et al. 2003). They are particularly useful for identifying culturally appropriate intervention practices and processes of providing information to migrants, whose information needs often differ from those of the dominant culture, or in instances where they are dissatisfied with their care. For example, in a study with Chinese migrant cancer patients in Australia in which patients wished to incorporate culturally specific treatments into their care, the focus group participants stressed the need for interpreters and psychological and spiritual support in addition to medical interventions (Huang et al. 1999). In countries where migration is relatively recent and migrants' needs are little understood, focus groups have identified the importance of support from organizational structures and national policies to develop better models of caring for migrants. For example, within Swedish health settings, simple routines and facilities to communicate with foreign-language-speaking asylum-seeking refugees were developed along with a training program for staff to provide a deeper understanding of individual needs in the light of varied migrational histories and cultural backgrounds (Hultsjö and Hjelm 2005). Focus groups may also work well in cities in which there are many language groups. In a Canadian study with thirteen migrant groups, preliminary work applying focus group methods to mixed ethnocultural groups of women yielded valuable information on the appropriateness of planned research. The women recommended consent and interpretation procedures, counseling to develop trust in the research process, home visits after births, specific approaches to sensitive topics, the inclusion of discrimination variables in the research, and reimbursement of participants (Ruppenthal et al. 2005).

CONDUCTING SUCCESSFUL FOCUS GROUPS WITH MIGRANTS

Focus groups should be fairly small, ideally about six to eight participants. However, often because of contingencies, they may end up being larger, which makes them more challenging to run. The groups should be formed with the help of local staff or participants in a community setting, such as a center, clinic, church, university, or other venue where participants feel comfortable. An advisory committee made up of members of the community is often advisable. The advisory committee can help the researchers avoid pitfalls in conceptualization or language use, recruit participants who initially may be reluctant or fearful to get involved with outsiders, and ensure that the community's needs are included in the research project. It is a good idea to offer refreshments to set an informal atmosphere in which the subjects feel comfortable and a modest incentive to encourage subject participation. It is advisable to have an introductory period during which the facilitator clarifies the purpose of the research and the ground rules, which usually include the importance of confidentiality and courtesy (e.g., everyone gets the opportunity to speak and only one person speaks at once). Focus groups may be more formally organized, where the subjects sit around a table and respond to the facilitator, or they may sit more informally and respond directly to one another. There is debate about whether focus groups should be relatively homogenous (e.g., include those who know one another) or include strangers of diverse origins. Researchers should make a decision about the composition of focus groups based on their research purpose. Focus groups composed of young children often work better when they are allowed to play on the floor or move around rather than sit still. The formality of the setting affects the relationship between the facilitator and participants and whether the "rules" of the discussion are followed, which can ultimately affect the styles of storytelling within the group and the degree to which debate and discussion are encouraged (Green and Hart 1999).

It is important to have a strong facilitator who establishes rapport with the participants. He or she should be fully bilingual if the discussion is conducted in another language and have good knowledge of the participants' ethnic background and dialects. The facilitator should establish his or her trustworthiness so the participants do not worry that they are being judged and therefore can be more forthright and relaxed. Dialogic materials such as a film, poster, health promotion materials, artifacts, cartoons, or drawings can help elicit responses that lead to deeper reflection about the issues at hand. Previously established formal and informal power relationships are difficult to control, and some members may try to dominate the discussion. In these instances, the facilitator should feel comfortable intervening, mindful that some are well known for their storytelling abilities and verbal skills, which may provide important survival mechanisms for migrants (Guerra 1998). The facilitator may find that introducing debate to stimulate discussion is helpful or that repeatedly reframing questions is useful if the discussion gets off track (Kahn and Manderson 1992; Cooper et al. 2001).

Researchers may need to make culturally appropriate adaptations to focus group techniques such as organizing single-gender groups with gender-matched facilitators. Other considerations, such as age, sexual identities, disabilities, or other markers of difference among the participants or between participants and the facilitator(s), also need to be taken into account. Ideally, there should be more than one facilitator so the second one can take notes on group dynamics and formulate questions to pursue in the discussions that the lead facilitator may overlook. Those who organize focus groups with migrants should be well versed in local gender norms related to attending public events or speaking in public. In a research project on health promotion with indigenous Oaxacan migrants, Rebecca Hester (2014) found that focus groups intended for women were frequently attended by their male spouses and partners. The men spoke on behalf of the women since that was considered more culturally appropriate, especially since migration can erode men's sense of respect and authority.

Audiotaping or videotaping the focus group is advisable so the facilitator can avoid taking notes and pay closer attention to the discussion and explore ideas as they come up. Organizers should design a focus group guide that includes the main questions and any issues to be explored based on the project's purpose as well as literature reviews and preliminary field research. The facilitator should also pursue issues/questions that emerge during the discussion, as this is a significant advantage to the focus group method. It is also helpful to prompt the participants by asking provocative questions or by raising issues that have not been mentioned. Another useful technique is to raise indirect questions about the larger social and cultural context so as to elicit additional information that might prove useful (Cooper et al. 2001). While each discussion has its own dynamic and it may be more appropriate to follow up on issues that get raised rather than go through the questions as listed, it is a good idea to ask for a quick time-out so you can check and make sure that all your questions are addressed.

Once participants get into it, the discussion itself is often fast-paced, loud, and fun. Participants with great verbal facility may take the lead in sharing stories or humorous incidents, so the facilitator should take care to make sure that everyone gets to speak and to draw out the shy participants without making them feel targeted. One way to do this is to ask a question that everyone is asked to respond to. This technique breaks the ice for the quiet participants, and repeating this strategy often provides a space for those who do not feel comfortable interjecting their views. Another strategy is to have the participants write or draw something that they can later report to the group.

I co-organized focus groups in north-central California about Mexican migrant women's perceptions of changing gender norms and HIV risk, some in school or university settings and some in community clinics (Castañeda and Zavella 2003; Zavella and Castañeda 2005). All these focus groups began with the screening of a film about HIV risk in Mexico that provided a springboard for discussion about HIV risk for migrant women in the United States. Mindful that talking about sexual behavior in public could be fraught, we clarified that we were not asking them to disclose their risky behavior but to share their observations of changes they had witnessed in their communities. One of the focus groups included women who had been meeting regularly on issues related to literacy, self-esteem, and self-care, and they requested that our discussions on sexuality and risk continue because they had been enjoyable and enlightening. For example, the women decided that condom use could be culturally rationalized as a means of spacing children, which would make the women less vulnerable to criticism from their partners for being sexually loose.

After focus groups are concluded, researchers should take notes of their observations to help contextualize data analysis, and audiotapes or videotapes should be transcribed. There is some debate about transcription, with some researchers suggesting transcription is sometimes unnecessary. However, Bloor and his colleagues (2001) advocate strongly that analysis without transcription leads to selective and superficial analysis, and they discuss strategies related to capturing every word, using grammatically correct speech, and so on.[3] (Selective transcription may be helpful if there is some irrelevant material.) The transcripts, along with the notes, can be organized by using qualitative software programs to identify patterns, hypotheses, or outlying issues that could be pursued further in other focus groups or through other methods.[4] The data then can be analyzed like other qualitative data; care must be taken to contextualize the study and participants, and illustrate the patterns and diversity in findings that support the argument (Krueger and Casey 2000). Bloor and colleagues (2001) suggest analytical induction, in which explanatory hypotheses are revised in relation to unusual cases; they also suggest that longer quotations be used to contextualize the speaker's meanings. Whether the participants know one another is an important theoretical consideration and should be reported in data analysis since it may affect group dynamics (Reed and Payton 1997). It is also important to examine the discussion in sequence and to identify the people speaking; this illustrates how views are modified and developed in relation to subjects' experiences rather than coding only for content (Reed and Payton 1997).

CHALLENGES AND LIMITATIONS

Despite the enthusiasm by those who have successfully used focus groups, the approach entails some challenges, especially with migrants, and there can be limitations to their effectiveness. Focus groups can be difficult to organize precisely because they explore sensitive issues, but they are especially challenging to organize with migrants, who are often adapting to entirely new surroundings and may feel constrained about expressing their views openly. Focus groups are also time-consuming for subjects, who have many demands on their time. Furthermore, recordings are more time-consuming to transcribe than interviews since the "don't all speak at once" rule is often violated, which makes it hard to hear what is being said by whom. Recording the discussions may frighten some migrants from participating, especially if they have migrated without authorization, or from sharing information fully, so the researcher must weigh carefully whether to record focus groups or not. Despite confidentiality agreements, subjects may repeat private information they hear in focus groups to outsiders. In the project I participated in, some women did describe their own behavior, creating potential tensions outside the focus group if someone breached confidentiality. Another possible problem is the sharing of misinformation about particular health problems within focus groups. Researchers should anticipate this possibility and be prepared to intervene, which requires that they have the best health knowledge themselves and bring educational materials to distribute if needed (Culley et al. 2007).

Increasingly scholars are emphasizing the ways in which focus groups are less of a "window" onto people's attitudes and opinions. Instead, scholars are acknowledging the ways in which perceptions are actively negotiated and constructed during the course of the focus group itself, and the dialogic, processual, rather than fixed, nature of the data. Michele Crossley (2002) suggests that the process of interaction within focus groups is inextricably linked to social considerations and moral notions such as blame and the allocation of responsibility. In her research on health promotion in a northern British city, different focus groups came with completely opposing stances about health promotion, and certain members of the groups based these stances on personal considerations. She reminds us that focus groups are sites of "constant negotiation of meanings, identities and stances over a limited period of time" (1472).

Focus groups also provide particular challenges related to data analysis. Focus group data may be more difficult to analyze than data from individual interviews, as it is often hard to attribute ownership to any one speaker. Reed and Payton (1996) suggest that researchers pay attention to the sequence of focus group discussions, the individuals involved, and the social context of the focus groups. In their study, they conducted the patients' focus groups prior to separate staff focus groups. This allowed them to discuss the patients' concerns with staff in relation to suggestions for policy changes regarding moving older people into nursing and residential homes. Several scholars (Reed and Payton 1996; Culley et al. 2007) have concluded that focus groups are not a "quick and easy" method of collecting qualitative data. As with other qualitative research methods, researchers should report fully the logic of organizing, recruiting, and administering focus groups, as well as the group dynamics, including whether the subjects know one another, so that others can evaluate the findings for themselves.

Other methodological complications may arise when the focus group method is applied in a cross-cultural setting. When researchers are investigating migrant populations comprised of multiple ethnic groups, it is crucial to have facilitators who are fluent in particular dialects and who understand nuances of translation. For example, in working with South Asian migrants in England and South Asia who spoke five languages, Culley, Hudson, and Rapport (2007) had focus group guides translated by community members, who could ensure they were linguistically accurate and culturally sensitive. Culley et al. concluded: "For this kind of work to be successful, researchers need to take into consideration not just the costs of interpreting or translating but additional resources for participation in designing data collection tools, involvement in data analysis, and training" (107). Another project, in Victoria, Australia, used focus groups to explore an ethnically diverse sample of mothers about their beliefs concerning sudden infant death syndrome. Yelland and Gifford (1995) found that some methodological difficulties were related to culturally specific notions about blame and cautioned researchers to consider whether focus group discussions are appropriate research methods in cross-cultural public health research.

Another concern about using focus groups relates to validity of the data garnered in settings where power dynamics are situational. Instead of viewing focus group data as representing facts about the real world, another positivist leaning, it is more appropriate to see them as sites where processes of constructing a perspective among a particular set of people are taking place (Reed and Payton 1996). This perspective may include debate, negotiation, and remaining differences of opinion, where the validity lies in illuminating the collective process of constructing meaning.

BEST PRACTICES

An exemplary use of focus groups is the study conducted by Sharon Cooper and her colleagues (2001) with Mexican migrant farmworkers that investigated children's exposure to pesticides. The study compared migrants from northeastern Colorado and southern Texas, two locations with very different crops and histories of migration. Those from Texas often travel great distances, such as to Illinois or California, and return to their homes in Texas so the children can attend school, while Colorado migrants often migrate to work on more local crops or with cattle within Colorado. Cooper and her colleagues were interested in sources of early and chronic exposures, and the little preliminary research available suggested there were multiple sources and pathways of exposure for children. Additionally, because children may have enhanced susceptibility to exposures because of their size, metabolism, and rapid growth, studies on adults were of limited value. Cooper et al. hoped eventually to construct questionnaires that uncovered a range of activities that may expose migrant and seasonal farmworker children to pesticides directly rather than through prenatal or take-home routes of exposure via their parents.

During the first phase of the project, the researchers designed and conducted five focus groups with migrant farmworker mothers and their children, ages eight to sixteen years of age, who participated in same-sex groups. The mothers in this study reported migrant histories of two to forty-two years, confirming the view that farmworkers are extremely mobile. They carefully planned that the mothers' focus groups would be staged first since they were designed to elicit any concerns about inappropriate issues, and they wanted the women's advice about the best ways to obtain information about pesticide exposure from their children. Mothers' consent for their children's participation was confirmed before the researchers approached the children. The children gave oral consent to participate when not in the presence of their mothers, and some children were allowed to be present but not actually participate once the discussions began (Cooper et al. 2004:36). The researchers recruited and worked with bilingual community facilitators as well as a researcher with fifteen years of experience working in the community. The mothers' groups were mainly conducted in Spanish while the children's groups were in English. The Texas focus groups were held at a middle school and the Colorado focus groups were held at a community clinic, and all the families were provided a stipend of $25. The audiotapes were transcribed and enhanced by notes taken during the focus groups; the data was analyzed using Krueger and Casey's (2000) descriptive methods.[5]

In their study, Cooper and her colleagues present a table with the guided (rather than general) questions they used and suggestions for follow-up questions in slightly different form, which is helpful to those who are considering working with children. They had a number of interesting and unexpected findings, including the following: children sometimes were working in the fields when pesticides were being administered; children reported working in the fields at much younger ages than their mothers reported; it took follow-up questions with mothers and children to elicit a list of chemicals to which children had been exposed; both groups did not always wash produce that had been sprayed or wash their hands before consuming produce in the fields. The researchers reported on questions that made the participants feel uncomfortable. For example, mothers did not consider questions about breastfeeding, smoking habits of children or lice to be off limits, but mothers and children felt uncomfortable when asked about hand-washing practices and the young age at which children began working. Cooper et al. provide a table summarizing activities that might increase children's exposure to pesticides as well as a table on their recommendations to researchers using focus groups on migrant farmworker children's pesticide exposure so as to acquire better information in future studies. In sum, this project is a model of transparency and allows other researchers to judge the quality of the data and assess the analysis and recommendations.

CONCLUSION

Like any qualitative research method, with thoughtful planning "focus groups and group qualitative interviews can be a powerful, versatile, and effective research tool in accessing community attitudes" (Culley et al. 2007:110). Conducting this type of research with migrants adds another layer of complexity, and researchers will need to be attentive to a variety of practical, analytical, social, and ethical issues to ensure effectiveness.

NOTES

1. Drawing on studies of the psychological effects of mass communications, Merton and Kendall (1946) emphasize the situation or experiment that stimulates the discussion in which the questions initially are relatively unstructured and the interviewer should take care not to impose his or her own views.

2. There are important differences between focus groups organized for marketing research, which often rely on homogenous subjects who do not know one another, and social science research that is attuned to diverse perspectives among subjects as well as the social context and interactional dynamics of the focus group itself (Reed and Payton 1997).

3. Bloor and his colleagues (2001) suggest some conventions for indicating in the transcript when there is overlapping speech, unintelligible speech, loud utterances, or indications of bodily movements.

4. Computer-assisted qualitative data analysis software (CAQDAS) may be helpful to those conducting focus groups since it provides support for tasks such as transcription

analysis, coding and text interpretation, content analysis, discourse analysis, grounded theory methodology, and so forth. However, CAQDAS has been criticized for establishing rigid processes, privileging of coding and retrieval methods, and being time-consuming to learn. For excellent discussions of the possibilities and shortcomings of qualitative software programs, see St. John and Johnson (2000) and Banner and Albarran (2009). Bear in mind that those using Macintosh computers (as I do) will find that not all software programs for qualitative data analysis are Mac-friendly. I find that HyperRESEARCH works well on a Mac; there are many other programs for use on PCs, including The Ethnograph, NUD*IST, Atlas Ti, NVIVO, and QUALRUS.

5. Because focus groups generate an extraordinary amount of qualitative data, researchers have focused on the process of data analysis. Kruger and Casey's (2000) descriptive methods are cited as a good model (Rabiee 2004). They suggest a systematic process of examining the data, including listening to the tapes and reading the transcripts and observational notes. Then researchers should reduce extraneous material, identify themes, and return to the original intentions and purpose of the study before formulating conclusions. Thus there is an analysis continuum from raw data to descriptive statements to interpretation that is influenced by the context of the focus groups. Krueger and Casey (2000) suggest that scholars clarify the process used for data analysis with enough detail that others can verify the findings, which safeguards against selective perception.

REFERENCES

Banner, D. J., and J. W. Albarran. 2009. "Computer-Assisted Data Analysis Software: A Review." *Canadian Journal of Cardiovascular Nursing* 19(3): 24–31.

Bloor, Michael, Jane Frankland, Michelle Thomas, and Kate Robson. 2001. *Focus Groups in Social Research*. London: Sage.

Castañeda, Xóchitl, and Patricia Zavella. 2003. "Changing Constructions of Sexuality and Risk: Migrant Mexican Women Farmworkers in California." *Journal of Latin American Anthropology* 8(2): 126–51.

Cooper, Sharon, Amy R. Darragh, Sally W. Vernon, Lorann Stallones, Nancy MacNaughton, Tracy Robinson, Craig Hanis, and Sheila Hoar Zahm. 2001. "Ascertainment of Pesticide Exposures of Migrant and Seasonal Farmworker Children: Findings from Focus Groups." *American Journal of Industrial Medicine* 40(5): 531–37.

Cooper, Sharon, Elizabeth Heitman, Erin E. Fox, Beth Quill, Paula Knudson, Sheila H. Zahm, Nancy MacNaughton, and Roberta Ryder. 2004. "Ethical Issues in Conducting Migrant Farmworker Studies." *Journal of Immigrant Health* 6(1): 29–39.

Crossley, Michele. 2002. "'Could You Please Pass One of Those Health Leaflets Along?' Exploring Health, Morality and Resistance through Focus Groups." *Social Science and Medicine* 55: 1471–83.

Culley, Lorraine, Nicky Hudson, and Frances Rapport. 2007. "Using Focus Groups with Minority Ethnic Communities: Researching Infertility in British South Asian Communities." *Qualitative Health Research* 17(1): 102–12.

Dávila, Arlene. 2001. *Latinos Inc.: The Marketing and Making of a People*. Berkeley: University of California Press.

Dodds, Catherine. 2006. "HIV-Related Stigma in England: Experiences of Gay Men and Heterosexual African Migrants Living with HIV." *Journal of Community and Applied Social Psychology* 16: 472–80.

Garcés, Isabel C., Isabel C. Scarinci, and Lynda Harrison. 2006. "An Examination of Sociocultural Factors Associated with Health and Health Care Seeking among Latina Immigrants." *Journal of Immigrant Health* 8: 377–85.

Green, Judith, and Laura Hart. 1999. "The Impact of Context on Data." In *Developing Focus Group Research: Politics, Theory and Practice,* edited by Rosaline S. Barbour and Jenny Kitzinger, 21–35. London: Sage.

Guerra, Juan C. 1998. *Close to Home: Oral and Literate Practices in a Transnational Mexicano Community.* New York: Teachers College Press.

Hester, Rebecca J. 2014. "Bodies in Translation: Health Promotion in Indigenous Mexican Migrant Communities in California." In *Translocalities/Translocalidades: Feminist Politics of Translation in the Latin/a Américas,* edited by Sonia E. Alvarez, Claudia de Lima Costa, Verónica Feliú, Rebecca J. Hester, Norma Klahn, Millie Thayer, and Cruz C. Bueno. Durham: Duke University Press.

Hjelm, Katarina, Per Nyberg, Ake Isacsson, and Jan Spelqvist. 2001. "Beliefs about Health and Illness Essential for Self-Care Practice: A Comparison of Migrant Yugoslavian and Swedish Diabetic Females." *Journal of Advanced Nursing* 30(5): 1147–59.

Hultsjö, S., and K. Hjelm. 2005. "Immigrants in Emergency Care: Swedish Health Care Staff's Experiences." *International Nursing Review* 52(4): 276–85.

Huang, X., P. Butow, B. Meiser, and D. Goldstein. 1999. "Attitudes and Information Needs of Chinese Migrant Cancer Patients and Their Relatives." *Australian and New Zealand Journal of Public Health* 29(2): 207–13.

Khan, Me, and Lenore Manderson. 1992. "Focus Groups in Tropical Diseases Research." *Health Policy and Planning* 7(1): 56–66.

Kruger, Richard A., and Mary Anne Casey. 2000. *Focus Groups—A Practical Guide for Applied Research.* 3rd ed. Thousand Oaks, CA: Sage.

Lantz, Paula, Laurence Dupuis, Douglas Reding, Michelle Krauska, and Karen Lappe. 1994. "Peer Discussions of Cancer among Hispanic Migrant Farm Workers." *Public Health Reports* 109(4): 512–20.

Liang, Wenchi, Elaine Yuan, Jeanne S. Mandelblatt, and Rena J. Pasick. 2004. "How Do Older Chinese Women View Health and Cancer Screening? Results from Focus Groups and Implications for Interventions." *Ethnicity and Health* 9(3): 283–304.

Merton, Robert K., and Patricia K. Kendall. 1946. "The Focused Interview." *American Journal of Sociology* 51(6): 541–57.

Perilla, Julia L., Astrid H. Wilson, Judith L. Wold, and Lorine Spencer. 1998. "Listening to Migrant Voices: Focus Groups on Health Issues in South Georgia." *Journal of Community Health Nursing* 15(4): 251–63.

Polonsky, Michael Jay, and Bianca Brijnath Renzaho. 2011. "Barriers to Blood Donation in African Communities in Australia: The Role of Home and Host Country Culture and Experience." *Transfusion* 51(8): 1809–19.

Rabiee, Fatemeh. 2004. "Focus-Group Interview and Data Analysis." *Proceedings of the Nutrition Society* 63: 655–60.

Reed, Jan, and Valerie Roskell Payton. 1996. "Focus Groups: Issues of Analysis and Interpretation." *Journal of Advanced Nursing* 26(4): 765–71.

Ruppenthal, Luciana, Jodi Tuck, and Anita J. Gagnon. 2005. "Enhancing Research with Migrant Women through Focus Groups." *Western Journal of Nursing Research* 27(6): 735–54.

Scarinci, Isabel C., Bettina M. Beech, Kristen W. Kovach, and Terry L. Bailey. 2003. "An Examination of Sociocultural Factors Associated with Cervical Cancer Screening among Low-Income Latina Immigrants of Reproductive Age." *Journal of Immigrant Health* 5(3): 119–28.

St. John, Winsome, and Patricia Johnson. 2000. "The Pros and Cons of Data Analysis Software for Qualitative Research." *Journal of Nursing Scholarship* 32(4): 393–97.

Yamada, Seiji, Jeff Caballero, Doris Segal Matsunaga, Graciela Agustin, and Marichu Magana. 1999. "Attitudes regarding Tuberculosis in Immigrants from the Philippines to the United States." *Family Medicine* 31(7): 477–82.

Yelland, Jane, and Sandra M. Gifford. 1995. "Problems of Focus Group Methods in Cross-Cultural Research: A Case Study of Beliefs about Sudden Infant Death Syndrome." *Australian Journal of Public Health* 19(3): 257–63.

Young, L., and N. Ansell. 2003. "Young Aids Migrants in Southern Africa: Policy Implications for Empowering Children." *AIDS Care* 15(3): 337–45.

Zavella, Patricia, and Castañeda Xóchitl. 2005. "Sexuality and Risks: Young Mexican Women Negotiate Gendered Discourse about Virginity and Disease." *Latino Studies* 3(2): 226–45.

16

Full Circle

The Method of Collaborative Anthropology for Regional and Transnational Research

Bonnie Bade
Konane Martinez

INTRODUCTION

Collaborative anthropology is a new paradigm in ethnographic research that involves long-term community-based research projects with community partners living regionally. Fundamental to the collaborative anthropology method is that research—the topics to be examined, the purpose of the research, the data resulting from the research, and the organization and presentation of the results of the research—are determined collaboratively, with the needs and priorities of the community directing the goals of the researchers. Depending on the site of the researchers, appropriate community partners for collaborative anthropological research projects might include farmworker and other occupationally based communities, grassroots organizations, indigenous migrant associations, health care agencies, tribal communities, nonprofit philanthropy organizations, and health/social service agencies.

In this chapter we present a model of collaborative anthropology that is relevant, mindful, horizontal, integrative, reciprocal, sustainable, and ethical, and describe how this model has great potential to inform and drive research initiatives related to migrant and transnational communities. We also demonstrate the collaborative anthropology research model using examples from the anthropology program at California State University, San Marcos, and research collaborations with nonprofit and service agencies.

COLLABORATIVE ANTHROPOLOGY IS RELEVANT

A mainstay of the Department of Anthropology at California State University, San Marcos, has been its collaborative relationships with local migrant communities.

The department has developed and implemented a collaborative anthropology research program with the goal of shifting the traditional vertical paradigm of scientific research with migrant and indigenous communities both locally and regionally. The university's proximity to the US-Mexico border and San Diego's productive agricultural industry have contributed to the development of the department's robust, relevant, and collaborative research program. At CSUSM the training of undergraduate student anthropologists is purposefully united with anthropological research goals and community needs. The program has a local focus and long-term collaborative research projects that address regional needs and incorporate multiple perspectives by working collaboratively with community and interdisciplinary academic partners. Community partners have diverse histories of connection to the region, with some having their origins locally, others having binational and transnational identities, and yet others having institutional service delivery origin, such as health and social service agencies. Interdisciplinary partners include researchers from the sciences, social sciences, arts, and humanities.

Collaborative anthropology is a response to some of the inherent problems that have challenged anthropology and other research disciplines involving people, such as "verticality" (Kearney 2004:43–48) in which the researcher "studies down" by studying characteristics of a specific population—migrants, farmworkers, urban poor—but "writes up" in order to professionally validate findings in peer-reviewed, theoretically focused journals not accessible to the communities upon which they focus, but rather geared to a specialized audience of academic researchers. Verticality manifests as research projects determined relevant by the researcher and the researcher's disciplinary orientation, without consultation with the community under investigation. In contrast, collaborative anthropology transforms the "ethnographic other," otherwise known as informants or subjects, into participating collaborators by including them in the research design, execution, analysis, production, and presentation, thereby ensuring the relevance of the research to the community under investigation. The objective of collaborative anthropology is to promote the complementary exchange of resources to examine global phenomena happening locally and generate on-the-ground cultural, social, political, and economic tools to address issues of health and community well-being.

COLLABORATIVE ANTHROPOLOGY IS MINDFUL

A key component of collaborative anthropological research is the tool of self-reflection. Self-reflection furthers the discipline of anthropology and research in general through change toward mindful practice. Self-reflective research involves changing the ways we conceptualize research design and train new researchers. The concept of collaborative anthropology has emerged as a twenty-first century expression of this disciplinary self-reflection and awareness of a need for change.

Several scholars have commented on the ways in which collaborative anthropology addresses this need for change. For example, Lassiter (2005) discusses the ethical and moral responsibility inherent in collaborative anthropology, while Fluehr-Lobban (2008) argues that collaboration is key to the sustainability of fieldwork and the discipline of anthropology itself. Lamphere (2004) suggests training graduate students in collaborative anthropology methods, while Choy et al. (2009), Austin (2003), Hann and Paradise (2009), and Homchampa and Moreno-Black (2008) examine various contributions of collaborative anthropology that enhance the quality of the research and the discipline. Menzies (2012) discusses collaborative anthropology from the perspective of indigenous anthropology and the benefits of researchers studying phenomena in their own communities. Arguably, however, the degree to which these discussions have translated to reality has been limited, and the practice of collaborative anthropology has principally taken place among individual graduate students bucking the system within a traditional vertical research environment. The appropriate model for collaborative anthropology unites the education of all new researchers with the purpose of qualitative and quantitative research and the needs of the local community.

Collaborative anthropology is similar to community-based participatory research (CBPR) in that it seeks to design a structure for participation by communities in all aspects of the research process (Viswanathan et al. 2004; also see chapter 19, by Minkler and Chang, in this volume). Collaborative anthropology, however, differs from CBPR in several ways. Collaborative anthropology employs a "holistic" perspective as a way to understand human health and behavior. This approach emphasizes the "whole" of the human condition, taking into account the ways in which history, economics, politics, religion, kinship, gender, ethnicity, and class impact all aspects of human life. Anthropological research, therefore, is grounded analytically within the context of these conditions. Another key difference is that a collaborative anthropology project, by its location in a university or social service agency, is uniquely positioned to establish and sustain longitudinal research in local communities. CBPR projects tend to wax and wane within a community depending on funding availability, research priorities of both funders and researchers, and the inherent structure and timeline of any intervention. A collaborative anthropology research program makes a long-term commitment to work with the community with or without funding, making sustainability of partnerships possible. Finally, the anthropological method of fieldwork allows collaborative research to be locally grounded, driven, and relevant. Data collected through in-depth fieldwork provides timely and relevant data that can be used to quickly identify pressing health issues, rapidly assess cross-cultural communication through direct observation, and identify culturally competent solutions to improving health outcomes. These differences between CBPR and collaborative anthropology have implications for the ways in which research is conducted in the areas

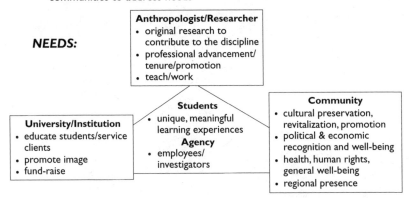

Program of Collaborative Anthropology
- Graduate and undergraduate levels at universities
- Long-term collaborative research projects involve partnerships with local communities to address needs

NEEDS:

Anthropologist/Researcher
- original research to contribute to the discipline
- professional advancement/ tenure/promotion
- teach/work

University/Institution
- educate students/service clients
- promote image
- fund-raise

Students
- unique, meaningful learning experiences

Agency
- employees/ investigators

Community
- cultural preservation, revitalization, promotion
- political & economic recognition and well-being
- health, human rights, general well-being
- regional presence

FIGURE 16.1. Addressing needs of collaborative research partners in a collaborative research program.

of immigrant and migrant health. Health research projects specific to migrant and transnational communities that emerge from a collaborative anthropology perspective have the potential to be historically grounded, complex, long term, and deeply invested in working collaboratively with local communities.

COLLABORATIVE ANTHROPOLOGY IS HORIZONTAL

Collaborative anthropology involves researchers, including undergraduate and graduate students at universities, agency employees, and/or nonprofit affiliates, united through long-term collaborative research projects involving partnerships with local communities to address regional needs. A pragmatic approach recognizes the needs and priorities of the parties engaged in collaborative research projects, namely the researcher, the community, and the university or public/private agency whom the researcher represents. Figure 16.1 illustrates the various needs of the entities engaged in a collaborative research project and the horizontal nature of the interaction between the entities.

The researcher working at a university, health agency, or other institution has specific needs that must be met during research. These needs revolve around the researcher's academic and professional career and include performance expectations from the academic discipline and the university/institution.

The community collaborators have needs that can be met through engagement with the researchers, such as cultural preservation, revitalization and promotion,

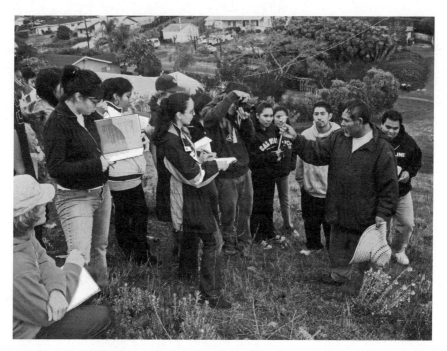

FIGURE 16.2. Erasto Camacena with students.

political and economic recognition, health and health care, general well-being and human rights, and the establishment or fortification of a regional and therefore global presence. At the same time, the needs of the university (the education of students, promotion of image through community engagement and faculty achievements, and development of community support) and the needs of the agency (name recognition, positive press, marketability to funding sources) are met through collaborative anthropological research projects that focus on regional communities. The needs of the researcher, university/agency, and community are united by the students or agency workers conducting the research, who gain a unique and meaningful learning experience in the field with the community (figure 16.2).

An example of the horizontal nature of collaborative anthropological research can be found in ANTH 430 (Medical Ethnography), taught once a year by the CSUSM Department of Anthropology. This upper-division field research course partners with the Binational Indigenous Organizations Front, the Coalition of Indigenous Oaxacan Communities, and the Center for Binational Oaxacan Indigenous Development. These regional community partners are parts of transnational migrant communities with strong links and constant communication with their communities of origin in Mexico, as well as Oaxacan indigenous communities throughout California and the United States. CSUSM has increasing numbers of students from the Oaxacan and Mexican indigenous communities who have enrolled in CSUSM anthropology courses because of the curricular focus on their own communities. A significant number of these students have family relations with members of the collaborative research partners and thus are engaged in another new paradigm in anthropology, indigenous anthropology, in which the researcher comes from the community being researched. Indigenous anthropology is a logical extension of—and directly manifests the goals of—collaborative anthropology.

Through the ANTH 430 course the anthropology department has created the Community Ethnobotany Garden Laboratory, a campus garden where edible and medicinal plants are cultivated and harvested. All plants found in the garden laboratory have been identified over a period of several years by Mexican indigenous herbalists and traditional medicine practitioners representing the course's community research partner, the Center for Binational Oaxacan Indigenous Development (CBDIO). Local community residents interested in a tea of *pericón* flower, a traditional medicinal treatment for stomachache used by transnational Mixtec migrant communities, can go to the garden and take cuttings from the many pericón (Mexican tarragon, *Tagetes lucida*) plants there. Additionally, the garden has prickly pear cactus, *gordo lobo, yerba buena,* and other medicinally and nutritionally useful plants available for community needs. The garden also serves as a laboratory for the university, providing research opportunities for biology, chemistry, geography, native studies, and visual arts projects involving plants, habitat, medicine and nutrition, sustainable agriculture, and endangered ecosystems (figure 16.3).

Original research produced by the ANTH 430 class collaboration generates tangible and relevant research products and resources available and accessible to the students, to the university, and, most importantly, to the community. Perhaps one of the most beneficial products of the collaborative anthropological research that is taking place in ANTH 430 is the Mexican Indigenous Medicinal Plants Database. Over the last five years the course has documented the medicinal and nutritional uses of plants identified by local traditional medical practitioners and herbalists. These community research collaborators attend courses and research training sessions as instructors and are compensated for their time via support from the laboratory budget of the course. Currently the database has a record of more than 160 plants, with detailed notes about the plant names (scientific, common, indigenous), uses, parts used, cultivation methods, harvest times and techniques, and the cultural background of each plant. In addition to the database, the course has produced ethnographic and scientific analyses of the medicinal uses of Mexican indigenous plants that have been made available to collaborative community research partners. These analyses manifest in the forms of videos, posters,

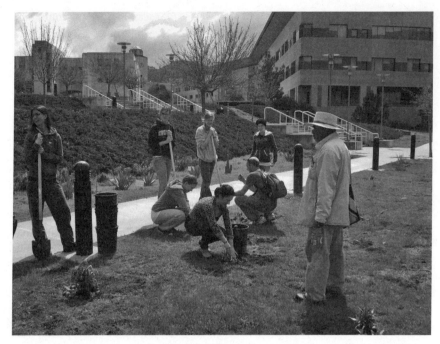

FIGURE 16.3. CSUSM Community Ethnobotany Garden.

and books and are made available and accessible to the community; they have been used by the community in public presentations to health care agencies, government offices, and granting foundations.[1] The research products from the community partner–university collaboration described above constitute cultural, social, and political capital for community partners.

COLLABORATIVE ANTHROPOLOGY IS INTEGRATIVE

Collaborative anthropology as a method identifies and integrates available resources to accomplish research goals. For collaborative research projects, each participating entity, from the university or agency/institution to the community to the students, brings to the table valuable and useful resources applicable to the research design, execution, analysis, write-up and distribution. Figure 16.4 illustrates the integration of diverse resources that emerge in a collaborative research project, including those of the anthropologist/researcher, who brings qualitative and quantitative research training, acts as teacher/trainer to students and other participants, and serves as a liaison between the community and local health/social service agencies. In addition, the collaborative research project

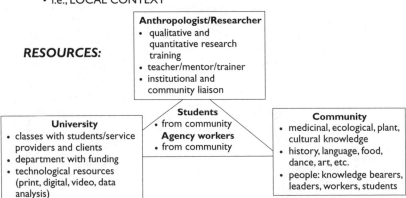

Collaborative Anthropology is **Integrative**
- Mobilize research to link with institutional resources and community resources
- i.e., LOCAL CONTEXT

RESOURCES:

Anthropologist/Researcher
- qualitative and quantitative research training
- teacher/mentor/trainer
- institutional and community liaison

University
- classes with students/service providers and clients
- department with funding
- technological resources (print, digital, video, data analysis)

Students
- from community
Agency workers
- from community

Community
- medicinal, ecological, plant, cultural knowledge
- history, language, food, dance, art, etc.
- people: knowledge bearers, leaders, workers, students

FIGURE 16.4. Integrating respective resources of collaborative researchers.

integrates the resources of the community, including knowledge bearers, cultural and political leaders, and cultural knowledge involving everything from health to history to organization, with the resources of the institution, such as a university or a health care agency with technological and monetary resources and access to a workforce, such as students and agency workers, to contribute to the accomplishment of the research.

An example that serves as a model for the collaborative anthropology research method and demonstrates the integration of resources to achieve meaningful and tangible research products is ANTH 440, Farmworker Health Ethnography, taught at CSUSM in the anthropology department. This course partners with local and transnational organizations, including Vista Community Clinic, North County Health Services, Palomar Pomerado Health, the Coalition of Indigenous Oaxacan Communities, the National Latino Research Center, and Community Housing Works, to conduct research concerning migrant and farmworker health and health care, living conditions, working conditions, and community well-being. Each time the course is taught the instructor meets with local health care agencies, health advocacy groups, and farmworker associations to determine an appropriate and focused topic of research for a four-month period. Projects suggested by both health care agencies and farmworker and migrant organizations have centered on the documentation of health, living, and working conditions for farmworkers, health care access and utilization, and the development of culturally and linguistically appropriate services for migrant communities.

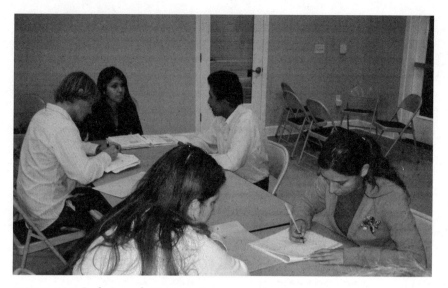

FIGURE 16.5. Students conducting interviews.

Health status data is one critical area of need related to migrant and farmworker health in the region and has been the focus of research through this collaborative anthropology course for over six years. In tandem with farmworker community–based organizations and health service providers, health status data has been collected through the California Agricultural Workers Health Survey (CAWHS), a statistically valid and tested survey instrument developed in 2000 by an interdisciplinary team of researchers from the California Institute for Rural Studies, the University of California Davis, and California State University, San Marcos (Villarejo et al. 2000). While the CAWHS instrument has served as the backbone of survey data gathered to assess the health status in the farmworker/migrant community, the course has also gathered substantial qualitative data through ethnographic work in local communities. The lead researcher works in collaboration with community associations and local agencies to tailor the questions to best meet the needs and priorities of the local communities as well as to ensure that the survey and/or ethnographic research can be completed over a sixteen-week semester. Student researchers in the course, trained in qualitative and quantitative research methods, work in teams of two to five, with at least one member being fluent in Spanish, and partner with community members, health educators, and outreach workers to conduct survey and ethnographic interviews with farmworkers in the North San Diego County region (see figure 16.5).

The course to date has revealed pertinent and timely data related to the health status of migrants and farmworkers in North San Diego County. Over the course of six years students have interviewed and surveyed over 150 farmworkers. Student researchers also are responsible for data entry, analysis, and write-up, which are used to develop a health status report that is reviewed and edited by the collaborating research partners. Results from this research reveal the extent and frequency of dental, respiratory, musculoskeletal, digestive, and urinary problems suffered by North County farmworkers, as well as accidents at work and clinically identified chronic illness. The collaborative research has been used by local health care agencies to provide supporting data in grant applications focused on illness and special populations as well as by the CBDIO to seek support from The California Endowment to conduct health and medicine workshops for the transnational Mexican indigenous community. The ANTH 440 collaborative research resonates with previously voiced attributes of the collaborative anthropology method, including the argument by Choy et al. (2009), Austin (2003), Hann and Paradise (2009), and Homchampa and Moreno-Black (2008) that collaborative anthropology enhances both the research quality and the discipline.

COLLABORATIVE ANTHROPOLOGY IS RECIPROCAL

The method of collaborative anthropology invokes relevance to research and the discipline. Collaboration with community partners in research design, objective, execution, analysis, write-up, and distribution ensures that the interests of both the community and the researchers are addressed. Collaborations with migrant and immigrant communities, occupational and health communities, and tribal and indigenous communities tend to focus on leveraging resources and raising awareness to address such issues as human rights, health, and community well-being. By working closely with locally based communities, collaborative anthropological research addresses regional needs, thus enhancing the position of the university or research institution in terms of its significance to the larger community in a given region as well as to the international and transnational communities in which migrant populations operate.

The first statewide study of California farmworker health and health care, the Suffering in Silence study,[2] supported by The California Endowment, utilized the collaborative anthropology method to study the health and health care of farmworkers living and working in California. The study found that farmworkers suffer from comparatively higher levels of high glucose, hypertension, body mass index, dental problems, respiratory problems, and other chronic and acute illness. The results of this landmark study constitute the only existing statewide data on farmworker health and health care and are still being used by farmworker organizations, migrant associations, health clinics, and county health departments to validate the need for health interventions and programs throughout California. The interdisciplinary team of coprincipal investigators of the study first met with organized farmworker groups, individual farmworker families, and farmworker advocacy groups to determine the principal interests that these groups have regarding farmworker health. Focus groups and key interviews with community members revealed that concerns about the impact of housing on health, environmental and pesticide exposure, access to clinical health care, and job security were among the issues that the farmworker community finds relevant. The team also met with health care providers of local clinics and hospitals, who indicated a need for data regarding the occurrence of specific health conditions such as diabetes, asthma, obesity, hypertension, and cancer. The core research team then developed a survey instrument and physical exam incorporating the expressed needs of the community partners. The instrument was reviewed by the community partners and edited accordingly.

After research sites in agricultural regions throughout California were determined by means of statistically rigorous methods, research teams enumerated households within postal district units, purposefully including nonconventional housing such as tents, trailers, sheds, and other dwellings found in yards, fields, and along rivers in order to increase the opportunity for all local farmworker households to participate in the study. Site coordinators identified local clinic options to determine the health provider research collaborator and organized transportation, the research base of operation, and the partnering with health providers to conduct the physical exam portion of the research.

In accordance with the collaborative nature of the study, at each of the seven sites core research staff worked with local farmworker organizations, high schools, colleges, and neighborhood organizations to identify bi- and trilingual researchers from the farmworker community to conduct the two-hour interview. These community researchers attended training workshops to more closely examine the goals of the study and to learn skills in quantitative methods, field interviewing, documentation of responses, appropriate and ethical behaviors in field research, random selection of household participants, procedures for requesting consent, and organization and submission of research documents. Farmworker participants in the California Agricultural Workers Health Survey were compensated monetarily for their time and were provided with the formal results of their physical exam as well as a follow-up appointment at the collaborating site clinic.

According to the collaborative anthropology goal of reciprocal exchange between research partners, at the end of the one-year study and analysis of data, draft reports were submitted to community partners throughout the state for review. After the final report, the study was published by The California Endowment, and coprincipal investigators launched a statewide tour with the report. Led by the collaborating partners at each site, the co-PIs held community and town hall meetings to present the findings not only to the communities in which the study took place but also to counties and regions where agricultural labor is a significant portion of the population.

The collaborative anthropology method works to sustain communities, nonprofit health and social service agencies, and university and research institutions in numerous ways. By integrating the needs and resources of all the parties involved and sharing the goal of community well-being, the method ensures continuation of research and collaboration. The data published in 2000 from the Suffering in Silence collaborative research project on the health and health care of California's farmworkers provoked significant change in the state through the allocation of funding by nonprofit foundations toward farmworker health, sparking the development of farmworker health advocacy programs involving diverse entities, including California Rural Legal Assistance, migrant clinics, hospitals, Community Housing Works, the Oregon Law Center, and many other agencies and community health promotion entities. The study has been used by transnational migrant associations such as the Coalition of Indigenous Oaxacan Communities, the Center for Binational Oaxacan Indigenous Development, the United Mixtecs, and other grassroots indigenous migrant associations to support applications for community development grants, cultural revitalization projects concerning indigenous health care practices, and community well-being projects.

Reciprocity in collaborative anthropology projects occurs in many ways. Migrant community-based organizations have practical needs such as needing space for meetings and events, recruiting volunteers for special events, and collaborating with outside agencies and individuals on boards or committees. Working collaboratively with migrant communities means working to coordinate research as well as resources for the betterment of the migrant community. Another example of the reciprocity that occurs in the collaborative anthropology program at CSUSM is the hosting of the Oaxacan "Guelaguetza," a festival that has emerged among migrant groups in the US as a key form of cultural expression. The Oaxacan community, the anthropology department, and the university have spent huge amounts of time and resources in the planning of this event, which brings 3000–5000 local Oaxacan indigenous community residents to campus. The collaboration that has emerged from this event is just one example of the type of reciprocal relationship that has been established from the department's long-term vested partnership with the Oaxacan migrant community.

COLLABORATIVE ANTHROPOLOGY IS SUSTAINABLE

By envisioning research projects as integral to the community in which they take place and by addressing the needs of all collaborating partners, the collaborative anthropology method makes research sustainable, with immense potential to generate long-term longitudinal research with migrant communities. Two collaborative anthropology projects at CSUSM best illustrate the sustainable nature of this approach to research with migrant and transnational communities.

Poder Popular (People's Power) in North San Diego County, a rural leadership program led by the National Latino Research Center (NLRC) at CSUSM, is a long-time partner with the anthropology department. The Poder Popular program exemplifies the potential of sustainable collaborative research to positively impact community health in immigrant communities. The project was initiated in 2005 when The California Endowment launched a statewide strategy to build the leadership capacity of the farmworker community at the grassroots level. The NLRC, in collaboration with Community Housing Works, a provider of affordable housing, and Vista Community Clinic, a community clinic, partnered to implement the project in North San Diego County.

The majority of approximately 25,000 farmworkers live in the northern region of San Diego County. Farmworkers and their families face more than their fair share of economic, structural, and geographical barriers to health care, low-income housing, stable jobs, and healthful food (Martinez et al. 2005; Bade 2005). As is the case with farmworkers nationwide, farmworkers in San Diego County are working poor families whose annual family income averages between $5,000 and $7,000 (Bade 2005). Farmwork is an intensive, precarious, and unstable industry in San Diego. Many community members state that they live in a constant state of uncertainty about their jobs, which are impacted by the economy, the weather, and the industry's access to water (Campbell 2011). Exposure to pesticides, harsh weather, and dangerous agricultural equipment puts farmworkers at risk for debilitating occupational health problems. Due to the lack of low-income housing, farmworkers and their families in the region are pushed to live in overcrowded and substandard housing. A large percentage of farmworkers in San Diego live in apartments within suburban communities and share housing as a way to afford the costly rent. Given the high cost of living, working poor farmworker families have to make tough decisions when it comes to funding costs related to health care, education, and safety. Health care in the region is available on a sliding-fee scale for adults and often at no or low cost for children and pregnant women. During the current economic downturn families have often had to go without needed health care and preventative health care, and screenings often take a backseat to more pressing individual and family needs such as rent, food, and transportation. For an undocumented immigrant, trying to access medical services in San Diego County is difficult. Both Bade (1994) and Martinez et al. (2005) have documented the institutional barriers that keep undocumented indigenous Mixtec immigrants from Mexico away from services. Cost, limited clinic hours, bureaucratic complexity, and the lack of culturally and linguistically appropriate services all play a role in limiting access to and utilization of health care services (Bade 1994; Martinez et al. 2005). The structural barriers outlined above have led to a lack of trust on the part of the community, and many do not utilize the services offered by the clinics; many immigrants delay treatment and avoid preventative screenings to which they may have access.

The core philosophy of the Poder Popular project is that all activity—such as research, health education, community events and health interventions—emerges from and involves the farmworker community at every level. Since 2005 Poder Popular has trained and integrated 120 *líderes comunitarios*—community leaders—into the program. The community leaders participate in a core training where they acquire a wide range of skills, including community organizing, effective communication, and conflict resolution. This core training positions the leaders to be critical intermediaries between their farmworker neighbors, friends, and family and local community and governmental agencies. Community leaders have been key members of several research projects and have been trained on data collection and ethics related to research. As a result, the community leaders have participated in needs assessments, asset mapping, and survey research in their communities. Working with the community leaders has allowed the research sample to be diverse and inclusive of historically invisible community members. The project has seen a remarkable transformation of community members through the collaborative process of organizing and action. Community leaders are the key catalysts of action and are regarded as the experts in their own community. Community residents have used this opportunity to take ownership of the project and are key consultants for any new research or intervention targeting the local farmworker community. Leaders from the key project sites have established working groups with specific tasks and goals, for example, working groups on immigration issues, disaster preparedness, special events, and food access.

Several initiatives have emerged from the collaborative partnership. One initiative includes an HIV/AIDS education project that trained community leaders on how to educate community residents on HIV and AIDS prevention and the importance of screening. A second initiative and perhaps the largest to date involves disaster preparedness in the farmworker community. The 2007 wildfires that raged through San Diego County exposed the especially vulnerable position of farmworker communities in the region. During the fires farmworkers and their families were often the last to be evacuated, were excluded from immediate and long-term relief, and experienced widespread discrimination (Martinez 2009). After the fires, Poder Popular community leaders, together with agency representatives, worked to set in place a plan of action to ensure that the lack of preparedness and inequities experienced in 2007 would not be repeated. This effort involved partners at every level. The organizing and partnering agencies and institutions collaborated with the American Red Cross and the County Office of Emergency Services to design and test an incident command structure that could be used to coordinate an effective response during a disaster. At the community level, farmworker leaders received training on how to set up a shelter and how to help fellow residents prepare for emergencies. Community residents were also trained in first aid, and in one region of Poder Popular developed the first Spanish-based community emergency response team in the county. Together the community and the agencies tested the strength of the system by participating in a disaster simulation in spring of 2011. The simulation best exemplifies the success of the collaborative project; during this one-day event individuals representing the American Red Cross, the National Latino Research Center, the Department of Anthropology at CSUSM, Vista Community Clinic, Community Housing Works, and Poder Popular came together for a common purpose, cause, and vision.

A final initiative that has emerged from Poder Popular further illustrates how a collaborative research model ensures sustainability. Research conducted by the NLRC in collaboration with Poder Popular leaders identified that one of the most profound and pressing impacts of the current economic downturn is food security among farmworker families in San Diego. This research finding has allowed the collaborative partners to seek out immediate solutions to the problem. The first mobile pantry in San Diego is currently being piloted among the farmworker community in three Poder Popular sites as a result of the collaborative research and intervention. Community leaders have been integral to the design and implementation of the pantry and are directly responsible for working with all partners involved and in the distribution of food twice a month.

The Poder Popular program is sustainable because it directly involves community residents—from a community with tremendous needs—who are committed to making immediate and lasting improvements in the daily lives and the health of themselves, their families, and their neighbors. The synergy from the partnership among the community, local agencies, and researchers is the direct result of the collaborative research method. In the case of Poder Popular, the collaborative research model has yielded critical and pertinent health data about farmworker families and has led to the development and implementation of timely, relevant, and culturally appropriate interventions that positively impact the health and well-being of farmworkers and their families in San Diego County.

The second project is a more recent course based upon our ongoing relationship with a local community clinic in San Diego County. Anthropology 460—Cultural Competency in Health Care—aims to educate new researchers (students) about the important role that language and culture (of both the patient and the health care institution) play in the delivery of health care services. Students worked directly in partnership with a local community clinic to investigate the cultural and linguistic barriers in accessing colon, breast, and cervical cancer screenings among the clinic's largely Latino im/migrant patient population. The clinic asked the student researchers to facilitate a set of focus groups and provide community-based data related to the cultural and linguistic barriers encountered. The students and clinic worked collaboratively to design and plan the focus group logistics as well as the structure and content of the focus groups themselves. Six focus groups in two different languages brought together forty community residents who gathered for a "Cena y Plática" (Dinner and Discussion) to share opinions and experiences related to cancer screening. Students were responsible for greeting patients, inviting them to participate, gaining informed consent, and moderating the focus group. Following the data collection, the students transcribed and analyzed the focus group results. A hundred-page report authored by the students was presented to the clinic. The report contained an extensive literature review of key health areas, relevant local statistics gathered from the AskCHIS dataset, focus group results, and recommendations related to cultural and linguistic competency in the key health areas. The clinic expressed its intention to apply the results of the research to improving their outreach strategies and delivery of services in the health areas of focus. The course will be offered every two years and we are confident that it will prove to be yet another sustainable research effort that involves anthropology student researchers, local institutions, and community residents. The course will provide timely data related to the cultural and linguistic patterns of the Latino im/migrant community in North San Diego County. The im/migrant community in the region is large, complex, and ever changing. It is of utmost importance for health care agencies to stay abreast of the cultural and linguistic issues impacting patient-provider communication, as well as service design and delivery. Sustaining these types of research efforts depends on the partnership of the collaborative anthropology department, local health care agencies, and the community.

Important to the development of collaborative anthropology research projects is the consideration of place. The unique position of the CSUSM anthropology program in the region is vital to the implementation and sustainability of collaborative research projects such as these. No matter where the place, local communities, agencies, organizations, and nonprofits exist that serve or seek to improve the lives of migrant and immigrant communities and that share common goals with researchers and communities. The health and vitality of migrant communities is contingent on the collaborative philosophies of local research institutions and agencies. Sustainability occurs when partnerships that make the most of the respective resources and needs are forged and reciprocal benefits are accomplished.

COLLABORATIVE ANTHROPOLOGY IS ETHICAL

The collaborative anthropology method consciously seeks to cultivate an approach to research that places the researcher's goals in line with the interests and needs of community collaborators. Field research in migrant and local communities takes time and, even when participants are compensated, becomes tiresome to the community if not linked to tangible benefits that are accessible to the community. Researchers must carefully cultivate and maintain collaborative links to the community they investigate; otherwise, they will expend valuable social and cultural capital and can negatively impact future research about crucial issues ranging from vaccinations to frequency of diabetes. Regional and transnational migrant communities are technologically and culturally sophisticated in promoting their interests and needs via acquisition of nonprofit status, celebration of culture and history, and advocacy for social, economic, and cultural justice. Contemporary researchers must recognize the value of the indigenous and community perspective, incorporate relevant and tangible components into their research projects, and generate studies that invite collaboration and community contribution.

Collaborative anthropology is mindful of the historic role of researchers, and in particular research anthropologists, in the lives of indigenous and other communities, and of the fact that much research knowledge generation has occurred in the context of a continued colonial mentality in which the researcher extracts resources—cultural knowledge, demographic data, and so forth—from the community in the form of qualitative and quantitative data. Without the cultivation of collaborative links with the community, researchers can damage the prospects of future research with a community when their research projects involve a helicopter approach that dips into the community for resources (information), extracts those resources, and then disappears from community view as the results are published in journals and periodicals that do not advocate change or produce tangible effects from the perspective of the studied community. Purposeful collaboration deconstructs the hierarchical structure in which research and the production of research knowledge take place. Collaborative anthropology transforms the ethnographic "self" and the ethnographic "other" into the ethnographic we.

A logical extension of collaborative anthropology is indigenous anthropology.[3] Students and researchers from collaborating communities engage in the study of their own communities through collaborative anthropology methods and, through representation of their communities, can influence research design, implementation, and outcomes in new and exciting ways.

USING THE COLLABORATIVE ANTHROPOLOGY METHOD

Collaborative anthropology methods provide multiple perspectives to the goals, design, implementation, execution, and production of research and research outcomes. It incorporates the needs of collaborators into a mutually beneficial partnership from which all gain—the researcher, the students and agencies, and the community partners. This in turn ensures more accurate and meaningful data. We outline below key steps for designing and implementing a collaborative anthropology or collaborative research program.

1. ENGAGE IN SELF-REFLECTION

- Principal investigators (PIs) create list of potential research topics and goals. This list should be part of an overall process of self-reflection by the researcher. Why does the researcher want to research this community or issue? How will the PI work with the community? What sort of relationship does the PI want to have with the community? How will the PI negotiate challenges that arise related to power, control, or division of labor?
- PIs identify the intended population to be studied and document everything they know about the community—where its members live, what they do, with whom they engage, migration history and trends, principal activities they undertake, special characteristics or attributes they have, political or economic barriers they may face, any organizations or associations they may have, and so forth.
- PIs identify agencies, organizations, and institutions that engage with the community—social service agencies, health care facilities, school districts, nonprofit organizations, and so forth.

2. RECRUIT RESEARCH PARTNERS

- PIs should recruit collaborative research partners from both the community and the community that services them, from the list of potential collaborative partners identified in step 1.
- PIs meet with representatives from the community to open a dialogue about the nature of potential collaboration and research products.
- PIs meet with representatives of agencies that service the community to discuss potential collaboration and research products.
- PIs and students invest time and interest in getting to know the community through participant observation in local community events and forums.
- A collaborative team composed of community representatives, service agency representatives, and PIs generates draft research goals, planning the design, scope, analysis, research product, and dissemination. We suggest that the results be made accessible to multiple audiences, including academia, funding agencies, government agencies, policy makers and, most importantly, the community. Collaborative research tends to be immediately applicable to solving problems in a community and can be made quickly available to funders and service organizations for that purpose.

3. IDENTIFY RESOURCES

- The collaborative team identifies resources that each partner brings to the research project: PIs may bring funding, institutional and technological support, space for meetings, field researchers, field research training programs, and so forth. Community collaborators may bring field researchers, cultural and language interpreters, and political and social organizational structures that link to the community, organizations and associations, cultural knowledge, knowledge bearers, and key informants, and so forth. Service community collaborators may bring funding, field researchers, diverse links to community members, technological and personnel support, space for meetings, office and paperwork support, and so forth.

4. REFINE NEEDS, GOALS, AND RESEARCH PRODUCTS

- The collaborative team conducts focus groups and key informant interviews. We consider this step critical to ensuring that all voices in the community are included in the research design. This step is especially needed to determine and align all community partner needs; determine details of research topics, goals, scope, design, analysis, product, and dissemination; and determine roles of each collaborative entity in the initiation and execution of each phase of the research.
- The collaborative team produces the final draft of the research instrument and design, which is reviewed by all entities of the collaboration and revised accordingly.

5. IMPLEMENT RESEARCH AND DISSEMINATE RESEARCH RESULTS

- According to the roles of each collaborator, as determined in step 4, the collaborative team implements the field research, manages data collection, initiates data analysis, and generates the draft research product. Research products can be more than reports or academic articles; digital projects, film, recordings, and photo books are highly effective ways to present the results of the collaborative research endeavor.
- All entities of the collaborative team review the draft research product and changes are made accordingly.
- The final research product is reviewed and edited by the collaborative research team.
- The final research product is presented to the communities of each entity of the collaborative research team.
- The final research product is disseminated according to draft plans made in step 2.

6. SUSTAIN COLLABORATION OVER TIME

- The collaborative research team makes plans for continued and ongoing research that meets respective needs and continues collaborative work indefinitely.
- The collaborative research team regularly reflects upon the partnership's goals and trajectory.

CONCLUSION

Collaborative anthropology links the community with institutions and agencies that service them and provides voice to underrepresented groups in academic, health provider, social service, education, governmental, and legal agencies. The collaborative anthropology method is relevant, mindful, horizontal, integrative, reciprocal, sustainable, and ethical, and has great potential to inform and drive research initiatives related to migrant and transnational communities. It is guided by the needs of the community and incorporates the resources and voices of all participating collaborators. The method of collaborative anthropology addresses regional needs and cultivates long-term collaborative relationships with community and institutional partners. The products of collaborative anthropological research have tremendous potential to reach beyond academic publications to impact policy, advocacy, and services related to im/migrant communities.

NOTES

1. See, for example, http://www.youtube.com/watch?v=QmHa-QColXc; http://www.blurb.com/bookstore/detail/1307860, and http://www.blurb.com/books/1303692-restoring-equilibrium for some of the products of this research.

2. The Suffering in Silence Study took place in seven agricultural regions of California. The towns in which farmworkers were interviewed were randomly selected, as were the dwellings and participants. The study reports the findings of from 652 interviews and 971 physical exams of farmworkers.

3. For further discussion of native anthropologists working with First Nations see Menzies (2012).

REFERENCES

Austin, Diane E. 2003. "Community-based Collaborative Team Ethnography: A Community-university-agency Partnership." *Human Organization* 62: 143–52.

Bade, Bonnie L. 1994. *Sweatbaths, Sacrifice and Surgery: The Practice of Transnational Health Care by Mixtec Families in California*. Riverside: University of California at Riverside.

Bade, Bonnie L. 2005. "Farmworker Health in Vista." In *The Ties That Bind Us: Mexican Migrants in San Diego County*, edited by Richard Kiy and Christopher Woodruff. La Jolla: Lynne Rienner. 45–62.

Campbell, Kate. 2001. "Water Costs Squeeze San Diego County Farms." *AgAlert*. Sacramento: California Farm Bureau Federation.

Choy, Timothy, Lieba Fair, Michael Hathaway, Miyako Inoue, and Anna Tsing. 2009. "A New Form of Collaboration in Cultural Anthropology: Matsutake Worlds." *American Ethnologist* 36: 380–403.

Fluehr-Lobban, Carolyn. 2008. "Collaborative Anthropology as Twenty-first-century Ethical Anthropology." *Collaborative Anthropologies* 1: 175–82.

Hann, Mariette, and Ruth Paradise. 2009. "Responsibility and Reciprocity: Social Organization of Mazahua Learning Practices." *Anthropology and Education Quarterly* 2: 187–204.

Homchampa, Pissamai, and Geraldine Moreno-Black. 2008. "Collaboration, Cooperation, and Working Together: Anthropologists Creating a Space for Research and Academic Partnerships." *National Association for the Practice of Anthropology Bulletin* 29: 87–98.

Kearney, Michael. 2004. *Changing Fields of Anthropology: From Local to Global.* Lanham: Rowman and Littlefield.

Lamphere, Louise. 2004. "The Convergence of Applied, Practicing, and Public Anthropology in the Twenty-first Century." *Human Organization* 63: 431–43.

Lassiter, Luke Eric. 2005. "Collaborative Ethnography and Public Anthropology." *Current Anthropology* 46: 83–106.

Martinez, Konane. 2009. "Thirty Cans of Beef Stew and a Thong: Anthropologist as Academic, Administrator and Activist in the U.S.-Mexico Border Region." *National Association for the Practice of Anthropology Bulletin* 31: 100–113.

Martinez, Konane, David Runsten, and Alejandrina Ricárdez. 2005. "Salir Adelante—Getting Ahead: Recent Mexican Immigrants in San Diego County." In *The Ties That Bind Us: Mexican Migrants in San Diego County,* edited by Richard Kiy and Christopher Woodruff. La Jolla: Lynne Rienner. 63–98.

Menzies, Charles. 2012. "Putting Words into Action: Negotiating Collaborative Research in Gitxaala." *Canadian Journal of Native Education* 28: 15–32.

Villarejo, D., B. Bade, D. Lighthall, D. Williams, A Souter, R. Mines, S. Samuels, and S. McCurdy. 2000. "Suffering in Silence: A Report on the Health of California's Agricultural Workers." Los Angeles: The California Endowment.

Viswanathan, Meera, et al. 2004. "Community-based Participatory Research: Assessing the Evidence." Prepared for the Agency for Healthcare Research and Quality. Evidence Report/Technology Assessment no. 99. Agency for Healthcare Research and Quality Publication no. 04–E022-2.

17

Photovoice as a Methodology

Regina Day Langhout

INTRODUCTION

Photovoice is a methodology in which participants take pictures based on a prompt and discuss their photographs following a specific structured format. The goal is to take a grassroots approach to study a community-based issue and to move toward social action. Photovoice has been used as a stand-alone methodology, but also in conjunction with other methods, such as community mapping, individual interviews, and focus groups. It has also been used as a form of community-based participatory research or participatory action research.

In this chapter, I position photovoice as a methodology that can facilitate critical consciousness, empowerment, and social action. Then, I describe the steps of photovoice and detail how my research team and I have modified the procedure for use with young immigrants and children of immigrants. Next, I provide examples of how photovoice has been used to address immigrant and migrant health issues in the US, Uganda, and Finland. I then move into challenges with photovoice. I end with providing resources for more information.

HEALTH-RELATED INTERVENTIONS, EMPOWERMENT, AND SOCIAL ACTION

Interventions that are intended to lead to better health outcomes are varied in focus and scope. For example, health-related issues can be defined as specifically as a particular medical condition—such as diabetes—or as broadly as community wellness, which is personal, relational, organizational, and community thriving

(Prilleltensky 2012: 2). Due to the far-reaching nature of health-related interventions, and because of the links between wellness and equity (Prilleltensky 2012), many researchers and practitioners prefer approaches that attend to social justice.

When considering health-related interventions oriented to social justice, one might examine how the intervention relates to empowerment (Prilleltensky 2012: 4; Rappaport 1990: 52). Empowerment is "an intentional, ongoing process centered in the local community, involving mutual respect, critical reflection, caring and group participation through which people lacking an equal share of valued resources gain greater access to and control over those resources" (Cornell Empowerment Group 1989: 2). Empowerment includes group-based critical reflection and action that leads to increased control over psychological and/or material resources. It is an especially important goal when researchers and practitioners are working with subordinated communities, such as many migrant and immigrant populations.

Empowerment-centered interventions should use methodologies, and therefore paradigms, that are aligned with social justice. One such paradigm is critical theory (Denzin and Lincoln 2011: 1; Lincoln et al. 2011: 98), where knowledge is considered a co-constructed resource within social, historic, political, and economic structures. Social positioning also is highlighted because people are situated differently in society based on their race, ethnicity, social class, gender, sexuality, citizenship status, and so forth; people working together who are differently positioned facilitates better science, interventions, and social action (Fals Borda 2008: 3). The goal of this intervention-focused research is to transform the status quo by altering social structures.

Methodologies within critical theory tend to be collaborative, with researchers or practitioners working side by side with everyday people (i.e., not just those labeled as community leaders), especially those who are affected by the issue of concern (Clandinin and Connelly 1994: 414; Fals Borda 2008: 28; Martín-Baró 1994: 29; Rappaport 1990: 55). Collaboratively, the group decides on the issue to be addressed, the conclusions from the inquiry, and possible interventions. Interventions based on such methods create socially just change by combining community- and university-based knowledge (Fals Borda 2008: 33).

PHOTOVOICE AS A TOOL FOR EMPOWERMENT AND SOCIAL ACTION

Photovoice was developed by Caroline Wang and Mary Ann Burris (1994, 1997) for use with rural Chinese women to document their health- and work-related experiences. Since its development, photovoice has enjoyed wide use in public health and social sciences research. Participants are given a camera and a prompt, with the goal of recording and examining their experience. They take pictures and then have group conversations, using the photos as the starting point for the conversations.

Photovoice has been used with many populations for various purposes. Preschoolers (e.g., Clark 2010), young people of color (e.g., Wilson et al. 2008), and immigrants (Rhodes et al. 2009; Stevens 2010) have used the methodology. Common uses include needs assessments, asset mapping, and program evaluation (Wang 1999: 189).

Photovoice was designed as a feminist methodology (Wang 1999: 185), but is used much more broadly now. Nevertheless, at least some defining characteristics of feminist methodologies remain embedded in most photovoice projects. These include highlighting women's experiences from their perspectives, considering participants as collaborators, and moving toward social action by developing critical consciousness. Specifically, those taking pictures have control over the images they photograph, show, and discuss, thus enabling community members to highlight experiences of their choosing. Also, the methodology is collaborative because participants are collecting the data. Moreover, critical consciousness is facilitated when participants critically reflect on their lives, including how structural issues shape their subjectivities and everyday experiences (Freire 1988).

Photovoice facilitates critical consciousness, empowerment, and social action through a deep examination of experience. First it enables a critical understanding of how problems are defined. Images and the stories linked to them provide a starting point for defining problems. Communities that do not control the narratives about them, however, usually have little say over how problems are conceptualized. Indeed, when powerful dominant groups set problem definitions, those problems tend to be individualized, and subordinated communities are blamed for the problems in their communities (Ryan 1972: 4). Photovoice addresses this problem by putting cameras in the hands of people so that they can tell, or author, their stories. Through this process, people confront what Ignacio Martín-Baró calls "the Social Lie," or stories told by dominant groups that are not based in the realities of subordinated groups (1994: 188; see also Stewart 2011). Instead, through photovoice, these groups are asked to use art to tell stories that are grounded in their realities, thereby taking control of an important psychological resource and helping to shape civic life (Finley 2011: 446; Thomas and Rappaport 1996: 320). Because images help shape how we think about our realities (Wang 1999: 186), this is especially important in communities where people have little control over dominant stories.

Photovoice has two other elements that help facilitate critical consciousness, empowerment, and social action. First, structured conversations are designed to move the group discussion from individual experience to broader structural issues (Wang and Burris 1994: 188); these discussions will be described in more detail in delineating the steps of photovoice. Second, information is shared with policy makers to produce knowledge and influence public policy (Wang and Burris 1994:

186). Overall, photovoice is well aligned with the development of critical con-sciousness, empowerment, and social action.

PHOTOVOICE STEPS

The steps involved in photovoice can vary depending on the level of community collaboration in setting the problem definition (Catalani and Minkler 2010). Sometimes, a problem definition has already been set. Although this might not be ideal for a fully collaborative model, it can be advantageous, as decision makers (e.g., elected officials, physicians) are more likely to serve on a photovoice board if there is consensus around an established problem definition. This step can create the target audience for the results, as these stakeholders will be in the position to implement recommendations (Wang 1999: 187). When a problem definition is not set, participants can be recruited first. Wang (1999: 187) recommends seven to ten participants. Yet, in reviewing thirty-seven public health photovoice projects, Cat-alini and Minkler (2010: 439) concluded that the size of the group did not alter participation, although the length of the project did (longer projects had more participation). The size of the group may be dependent on the researcher's goals.

Once the group is assembled, the first session should introduce the project. Topics covered should include the nature of the project, the methodology, poten-tial risks and benefits to participants, how to use the camera, the ethics of taking pictures, how to take pictures safely, and how to frame an image to get the desired effect. It is imperative to discuss approaching people to take their pictures, the eth-ics of taking pictures of people without their knowledge, what might happen with the pictures (in terms of public displays and research reports), and when people should not be photographed (e.g., when involved in illicit behavior or when in a private place, without consent; Wang 1999: 188). Depending on the research design and the level of collaboration, the group might be given a prompt for taking pic-tures (e.g., "What do you like about your neighborhood? What would you like to change about your neighborhood?"), or the group might collaboratively brain-storm a prompt.

Participants then take pictures, turn the film (or digital images) in for process-ing, and then reassemble to view their photos and select one to two for group discussion. The group discussion—facilitated through the chosen pictures—uses the SHOWED method (Wang 1999: 188). Questions are as follows: "What do you see here? What is really *h*appening here? How does this relate to *o*ur lives? Why does this situation, concern, or strength *e*xist? How could this photo be used to *e*ducate policy makers? What can we *d*o about it?"

Next steps include theme discernment and planning, and holding an exhibi-tion. After several sessions, participants codify their knowledge by determining themes based on their pictures and conversations. They then decide which photos they would like to use to illustrate their themes in an exhibit, and what medium might be best. Some possibilities include slide shows, simple frames on walls, storytelling, and/or written narratives to accompany the photos. All stakeholders should then be invited to the exhibition with time allotted for advancing a dialogue with community decision makers. Other social actions may also be appropriate.

MODIFICATIONS FOR YOUNG IMMIGRANTS

In this section, I describe in depth the curriculum we use in our photovoice research; our participants are largely nine- to eleven-year-old fourth- and fifth-grade students who are immigrants and/or children of immigrants. Their families are mostly from Mexico and Central America. I have chosen to provide a detailed methodological account because it can help others avoid rushing into picture taking and discussions. Without a solid background, young people—including young migrants and immigrants—may have difficulty developing a structural and critical analysis because their school settings have not prepared them to do so (Green and Kloos 2009: 478). Additionally, few researchers report in detail on their photovoice process, making replication difficult. Finally, participatory projects—which are more likely to facilitate individual empowerment—require building community capacity around photography and research (Catalani and Minkler 2010: 440). Although conceptualized as changes necessary for young people, some of these alterations may be appropriate for other groups who have also, for structural reasons, had little exposure to cameras or dialogic discussions.

Phase 1: Building Capacity for Photovoice

In our first lesson, we give an example of young people who changed something in their community using photovoice. We discuss a news story describing how young people who were mainly homeless used photovoice to advocate for their city's park district to clean up a park (Baker 2006). Two weeks after their presentation, the park district installed new playground equipment and added additional trashcans. The park district then partnered with the young people to create artwork. Next, we have a conversation about who the young people were, what they identified as the problem, what they did, and the outcome. We then explain how photovoice works and provide a timeline for our use of the methodology.

Next, we focus on how to "read" a picture. We use Helen Levitt's photo from Ewald and Lightfoot's book on teaching photography to children (2001: 19). We ask the young people to list everything that they see. We then have a guided discussion about the photograph. Questions include the following: "What is happening outside of the frame of the photograph? Who are the people in the picture? What do you learn about the community when you study this picture? How are the people in the photograph different from one another? Where was the picture taken? When was the picture taken? Have things changed since this picture was taken? Who is the photographer? Is she or he an insider or outsider? Where is the camera? What happened just before the picture was taken? What do you think happened just after the picture was taken? Why was this picture taken?" (Ewald and Lightfoot 2001: 18). We then explain symbolism and ask the young people to draw symbols that represent the following: happiness, home, and birthday.

In our second lesson, we review the main ideas from the previous lesson (e.g., What is photovoice? What is symbolism?) and then we focus on framing. First, we describe the prompt question for their pictures (e.g., What are your hopes and dreams for your school? What does community wellness look like to you?). Then, young people write a paragraph to answer the question, and they discuss their paragraphs. Next, they develop a shot list by writing their idea in one column and then the picture they would take to represent that idea in the next column. Adult researchers can answer the same question from their perspectives and then share their shot list with the young people. This can model openness and taking chances.

After the shot list has been developed, the young people are given a square piece of cardboard with a smaller square cut out of it (so that it resembles a frame). They take their shot list and frame on a field trip where they practice looking for images that might convey their shot list ideas. They examine what different pictures could look like by moving their frame. Adult researchers ask the following types of questions: "What is inside your frame? What is outside your frame? What did you intentionally leave out? What did you intentionally leave in? If someone did not know what idea you were trying to show, how do you think they would interpret this if it were a real picture? Is there anything you could change about this picture to make your idea clearer?" Young people discuss their potential images and modify their shot lists.

After the short field trip, young people learn about the ethics of taking pictures. They learn first about the word "ethical" and then apply it to their picture taking. Adult researchers act out skits where the photographer is behaving ethically and unethically, and young people discuss what was (un)ethical about the behavior. If it was unethical, they discuss what to alter. Adult researchers act out the unethical skit again, using the young people's ideas for how to behave more ethically. Students are given cameras at the end of the session. They are told when and where to return the cameras. Adult researchers get the film developed before the next session.

Phase 2: Taking Pictures and Discussing Images

In lesson 3, young people are given their pictures and asked to choose one to three pictures for small-group discussion. In small groups, they answer the following questions, which we have modified from Ewald and Lightfoot (2001: 18), and

Wilson et al. (2007: 246), who found that young people had difficulty answering the original SHOWED questions. Our questions are as follows: "Who's/What's in the picture? What are they doing? What's happening? Why was the picture taken? What happened before this picture was taken? What happened after this picture was taken? What does this tell you about your school/neighborhood/community? Why did you want to share this photo? What is important for people to understand about this photo?" Additional clarifying questions might include these: "What did it mean to you to experience that? What is important for others to understand about your experience? What do you think could be done to change the problem you identified? How could this picture be changed to more clearly represent the idea the photographer was trying to present?" These discussions can elicit deep sharing and new perspectives.

Small groups then choose one picture to discuss with the entire group. After each photo is described and the small-group conversation is summarized, all young people engage in the following discussion: "Have you experienced what the photographer described? Do you agree with the photographer's and/or group's interpretation of the topic/event? What do you think could be done to address this issue?"

In our experience, the first round of pictures is often not usable because young people have taken photos of their friends posing. In other words, the cameras are treated as they are normally within a US context. After the photovoice discussion, however, young people begin to see how the pictures can serve a different purpose. Photos taken after the first round are generally more usable. Young people modify their shot lists and are given a second camera, with instructions on how and when to return it for processing.

Lesson 4—and all lessons where new pictures are taken—follows the format of lesson 3. Some photovoice projects vary the prompt question from session to session. It is our experience that the same prompt question should be used for at least two sessions, as this enables deeper exploration.

Phase 3: Codification

After all pictures have been taken, the project moves into the codification phase, which includes discerning themes from the pictures and conversations. We begin with a candy-sorting activity, developed by Foster Fishman et al. (2010: 76). Young people get into small groups and are given a pile of candy. They are told they own a candy store and they have candy to sell. They have three minutes to organize the candy into piles that make sense to them. They need to organize and label the piles. After they have sorted the candy, they are asked why they put the candy into these specific piles, if this task was hard, if they had disagreements and how they solved them, and how they named each pile. Adult researchers connect young people's language with the language of qualitative data analysis by using words like "themes" and "categories."

Next, the adult researchers inform the young people that they have lost shelf space and they need to sort their candy into three piles. After the new sorting, the adult researchers ask the young people to say how the candy was reorganized, if there are other ways to organize the candy, to think of benefits of creating fewer piles, and to look for similarities and differences between how the different groups organized their candy. They then discuss how this process might be similar to sorting messages in their photovoice data.

Next, the young people sort their pictures individually. They then discuss their piles and as a group decide on an area of focus based on the pictures they have and what they find interesting. They separate these pictures from the others.

In the following lesson, the young people submit photos that fit the focus area. In smaller groups, they sort pictures based on the themes they discern from their photos. Pictures of similar themes are combined at this point, so each group has the pictures for one theme. Subthemes are constructed. They then develop the story they wish to tell for that subtheme. We have had success with young people gluing pictures to poster board and writing accompanying narratives. Sometimes, there is one poster board per theme, and other times each poster board has the same three to five themes.

Young people should then consider possible solutions to the problems they define. We encourage solutions that engage power in one of three ways. They can think of possible solutions that they (1) can engage in on their own, (2) can enact but that they need help in implementing, often because of the way that society is hierarchically structured, and (3) cannot enact because it is not within their power, but they can advocate and/or organize for these solutions. The conceptualization of power on these three levels is useful because it draws attention to individual agency and structural forces. This phase generally takes two to six sessions.

Phase 4: Action

The final phase deals with moving into action, which begins with presentation preparation. The young people put together their presentation, practice it, and practice answering questions that exhibition attendees might pose. The young people and the adult researchers collaboratively identify and invite stakeholders, decide how the presentation should take place, and determine if they think media should be present. This final phase can take four to eight lessons.

The students in our program have created a variety of presentations. Fourth- and fifth-grade students in our program created posters, for example. Students were first given cameras with the prompt, "What are your hopes and dreams for your school?" They took pictures and sorted them into themes. They then developed their problem definition, which was that they did not have a strong sense of belonging in the school because the stories told about them and their communities were inconsistent with their experiences (Kohfeldt and Langhout 2012). One

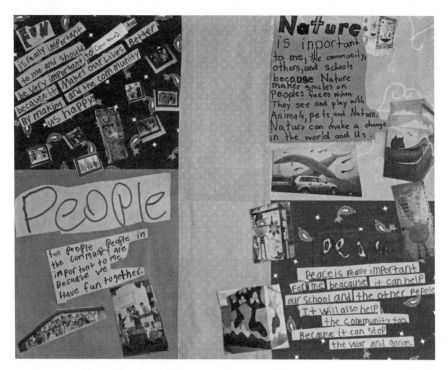

FIGURE 17.1. Photovoice theme poster 1.

of the actions they decided to take was to create a mural at the school to tell a story about them that was rooted in their community. The mural would be a permanent marker of an alternative narrative. Empowerment includes people having control over the psychological resources that affect them; the stories we tell ourselves and that are told about our communities are important psychological resources.

In the second photovoice round young people took pictures of ideas they wanted to include in the mural. Based on their data analysis, their themes included family, fun, nature/environmental justice, valuing diversity, and peace. Figures 17.1 and 17.2 are pictures and narratives that helped the young people create images and symbols for their mural. Figure 17.3 shows the final mural, which they codesigned and painted together.

OTHER EXAMPLES

Photovoice has been used in several immigrant and migrant communities, inside and outside of the United States, to address health-related issues. Topics covered range from the psychological distance between elder Liberian refugees in the US

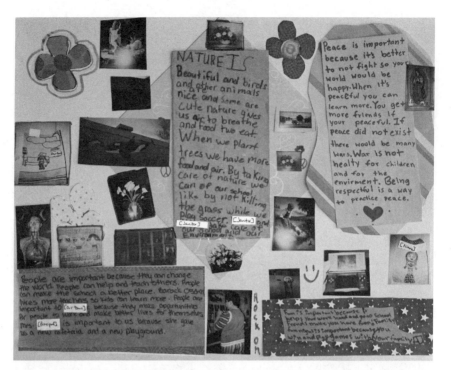

FIGURE 17.2. Photovoice theme poster 2.

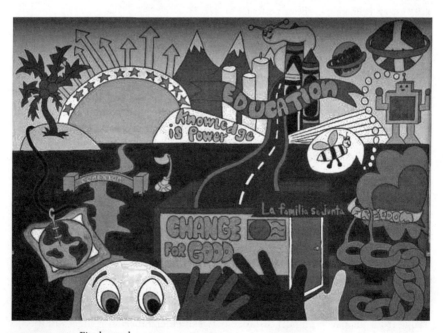

FIGURE 17.3. Final mural.

and their communities in Liberia (Chaudhry 2008), to sexual health behaviors of recent immigrant Latino men (Rhodes et al. 2009), to neighborhood influences on immigrants' health (Haque and Rosas 2010), to how immigrants experience smaller cities in Canada (Sutherland and Cheng 2009), to youth experiences with forced migration in northern Uganda (Green and Kloos 2009), to immigrant women's lives in Finland (Janhonen-Abruquah 2010). Four short examples are provided below, two based in US contexts and two outside of North America.

Isolation is a common experience for elderly Liberian refugees in the United States, and a photovoice study was conducted to connect these immigrants with people in their current communities, as well as in their Liberian home communities (Chaudhry 2008). Goals included highlighting strengths around survival and safekeeping, enhancing social networks within and across countries, and providing information to health service providers around the Liberian refugee context. The study took a strengths-based approach to address psychosocial health issues while also providing important information to resource providers. Eight elder Liberians participated in this study, all living in Staten Island, New York. Common settings for building community were Liberian-owned businesses and African churches. Support was also found in informal networks that provide resources for those in most need. Additionally, social support and networks were expanded on the basis of the research, buttressing connections for those in Staten Island and across the diaspora. Finally, service providers gained insight into the cultural adaptations that Liberian refugees had to undergo to live in the United States (Chaudhry 2008: 67). Overall, this project benefitted displaced Liberian refugees by helping to strengthen their connections to each other, family, friends, and service providers, thus likely facilitating better health outcomes and culturally appropriate services. Photovoice was key because it facilitated communication and expression that probably would not have occurred otherwise.

Another example of photovoice in the US examined constructions of masculinity as they relate to the sexual health behaviors of newly arrived Latino men to the southeastern US (Rhodes et al. 2009). Eight immigrant Latino men (from El Salvador, Guatemala, and Mexico) living in North Carolina, most of whom were undocumented, were participants. Results were coanalyzed by the university research team and community members. Preliminary analysis was shared with all participants. Overall, increased sexually risky behavior was associated with (1) the loss of power that came with immigration, including increased experiences of racism, reduced connection with family, substandard housing, harsh working conditions, and minimal access to health care, and (2) changing roles that challenged their sense of masculinity, including feeling that they needed to prove their masculinity because they were engaging in traditionally female gender roles like cooking and cleaning. Participants also reported community strengths that mediated risky sexual behavior and promoted wellness. Strengths included (1) strong networks in their new communities where people helped with job and housing placement, (2) soccer leagues, which helped maintain, broaden, and deepen connections, (3) the growing Latino economic community, which offered a sense of community through selling familiar foods and merchandise, (4) strong job opportunities, and (5) a network of Latino organizations with culturally appropriate services and bilingual staff (Rhodes et al 2009). Results provide a structural analysis by showing how social conditions influence behavior and by indicating which community strengths are most helpful in mediating risky sexual behavior.

Photovoice has also been used with migrants and immigrants outside of the United States. In one example, twelve young people (12–16 years old) who were forced migrants living in a displacement camp in northern Uganda were the participants (Green and Kloos 2009). Students took pictures of their school life and the images were used for advocacy. Through publicizing the photos, participants and researchers amassed resources by encouraging people in the US to donate money for laptops and secondary school fees for students (see www.displaced-communities.org).

In a second example, photovoice was used to study the experiences of women who immigrated to Finland from places as varied as India, Iran, Russia, Somalia, and Afghanistan (Janhonen-Abruquah 2010). Through photos, women told stories about (1) starting independent lives, including the accompanying challenges and joys, (2) the demands of being a single mother in a new country with a different culture, (3) difficulties with the labor market, partially due to the complexities of the Finnish language and perceived disposability of their labor, and (4) their (newfound) reliance on religion as a place for accessing social support and creating connections with other immigrants. Here, the pictures were one form of data collection, but a form that elicited different information compared to more traditional data-gathering techniques.

In sum, photovoice has been used to better understand the lives of immigrants and migrants, and to promote better health outcomes. What makes this technique unique is the participant's ability to control the data and the depth and breadth of conversation. Even with these benefits, however, there are important limitations that must be considered.

PHOTOVOICE CHALLENGES

Like all data-gathering methods, photovoice brings with it a set of challenges. For example, being part of a photovoice project takes skill and time. Participants must learn how to take and be comfortable with taking ethical pictures, turn in their cameras, and have hours-long discussions about their photos. For community members who are already juggling many commitments, the additional time required to participate in photovoice can be prohibitive. Yet, attempts to lessen the commitment may move away from some of the goals of photovoice, including critical consciousness raising and empowerment, as these processes require time (Catalani and Minkler 2010: 445).

A second issue is money. Researchers might address time requirements by paying participants and providing meals and child care during meetings. These expenditures can add up. Also, given the nature of photovoice, fewer people generally participate than in some other study types, which may make photovoice projects less attractive to funders, who may be judging the research by an inappropriate set of standards (e.g., needing a large sample for generalizability) that are not rooted in the paradigmatic perspective best aligned with photovoice (i.e., critical theory).

Third, there may be issues around group dynamics, which can take the form of language barriers and difficulties with collaboration. Specifically, some projects include immigrants from many different language-speaking communities (Janhonen-Abruquah 2010; Stevens 2010). Even when translators are employed, there can be language barriers that make it difficult to have in-depth conversations (Green and Kloos 2009: 466). Additionally, participants discuss their experiences, and these experiences are embedded within their relationships to one another and to the research team (Clandinin and Connelly 1994: 419). Sometimes, however, experiences are challenged as insignificant, irrelevant, unimportant, or just plain wrong; other times, researchers think they know more about participants with whom they have engaged collaboratively than they actually do (Clandinin and Connelly 1994: 419). Indeed, interpreting experience for participants and researchers can be challenging. Yet, for photovoice to facilitate critical consciousness and empowerment, participants need to have in-depth group conversations that link experience to structural aspects (Freire 1988).

For specific immigrant communities, there is another set of limitations involved with photovoice. First, the technique might not be culturally appropriate. In certain communities, cameras might be reserved for men or tourists. Asking groups to use cameras who do not normally have access to them can create family and/or community tensions (Lykes 2006: 274; Stevens 2010: 280). In other cases, participants may not take pictures for fear of reprisal (Stevens 2010: 279). The lesson here is that it is a good idea to build relationships with the community before beginning photovoice so that stakeholder groups can assess the cultural fit of the project and make appropriate modifications (Catalani and Minkler 2010: 440).

For those working with displaced or forced migrants, there can be other limitations. Displaced people are often used to dealing with outsiders within a nongovernmental organization model based on needs to be met. If photovoice researchers wish to take a strengths-based perspective and explore community assets, conversations will need to be structured so that new expectations can be set in such a way that strengths can arise, rather than only needs (Green and Kloos 2009: 477).

SUMMARY

Photovoice can be a powerful tool for data collection, deep discussions, critical consciousness raising, empowerment, and social action. Its flexibility allows it to be used across settings (e.g., schools, clinics, displaced persons camps), with various populations (e.g., young people, immigrants, the elderly), and for many different reasons (e.g., asset mapping, program evaluation). Furthermore, it has the potential to bring communities together in ways that few other methodologies can. Yet, one must keep in mind that challenges should be expected. For example, time must be allotted for skill building, and group dynamics (among both participants and researchers) must be navigated. Taken together, it is often worthwhile to problem-solve likely challenges and collaborate with community members on a photovoice project.

RESOURCES

Articles

Catalani, Caricia, and Meredith Minkler. "Photovoice: A Review of the Literature in Health and Public Health." *Health Education and Behavior* 37 (2010): 424–51.

Wang, Caroline, and Mary Ann Burris. "Empowerment through Photo Novella: Portraits of Participation." *Health Education and Behavior* 21 (1994): 171–86.

Wang, Caroline, and Mary Ann Burris. "Photovoice: Concept, Methodology, and Use for Participatory Needs Assessment." *Health Education and Behavior* 24 (1997): 369–87.

Books

Ewald, Wendy, Katherine Hyde, and Lisa Lord. *Literacy and Justice through Photography: A Classroom Guide.* New York: Teachers College Press, 2011.

Ewald, Wendy, and Alexandra Lightfoot. *I Wanna Take Me a Picture: Teaching Photography and Writing to Children.* Boston: Beacon Press, 2001.

Women of PhotoVoice/ADMI, and M. Brinton Lykes. *Voces e imágenes: Mujeres Mayas Ixiles de Chajul / Voices and images: Mayan Ixil women of Chajul.* Guatemala: Magna Terra, 2000.

Palibroda, Beverly, Brigette Krieg, Lisa Murdock, and Joanne Havelock. *A Practical Guide to Photovoice: Sharing Pictures, Telling Stories and Changing Communities.* Winnipeg: The Prairie Women's Health Centre of Excellence, 2009. Can be downloaded at http://www.pwhce.ca/photovoice/pdf/Photovoice_Manual.pdf

Webpages

http://www.photovoice.org/
http://www.photovoice.ca/
http://ctb.ku.edu/en/tablecontents/chapter3_section20_main.aspx
http://www.theinnovationcenter.org/files/doc/D5/CLW%20pp%20164%20Photovoices
 .pdf

REFERENCES

Baker, Jenna. 2006. "Colfax Kids Ask, Aurora Parks Listens." *Denver Post,* August 17, 2006. Accessed December 7, 2011. http://yourhub.denverpost.com/aurora/colfax-kids-ask-aurora-parks-listens/tLK7zLeJbT1Ak2is2gdWaI-ugc.

Catalani, Caricia, and Meredith Minkler. 2010. "Photovoice: A review of the Literature in Health and Public Health." *Health Education and Behavior* 37: 424–51.

Chaudhry, Serena. 2008. "Coming Home: Connecting Older Liberians in the Diaspora with the Family and Friends at Home." *Refugee* 25: 60–68.

Clandinin, D. Jean, and F. Michael Connelly. 1994. "Personal Experience Methods." In *Handbook of Qualitative Research,* edited by Norman K. Denzin and Yvonna S. Lincoln, 413–27. Thousand Oaks, CA: Sage.

Clark, Allison. 2010. "Young Children as Protagonists and the Role of Participatory, Visual Methods in Engaging Multiple Perspectives." *American Journal of Community Psychology* 46: 115–23.

Cornell Empowerment Group. 1989. "Empowerment and Family Support." *Networking Bulletin,* October, 2.

Denzin, Norman K., and Yvonna S. Lincoln. 2011. "Introduction: The Discipline and Practice of Qualitative Research." In *Handbook of Qualitative Research,* 4th ed., edited by Norman K. Denzin and Yvonna S. Lincoln, 1–20. Thousand Oaks, CA: Sage.

Ewald, Wendy, and Alexandra Lightfoot. 2001. *I Wanna Take Me a Picture: Teaching Photography and Writing to Children.* Boston: Beacon Press.

Fals Borda, Orlando. 2008. "Participatory (Action) Research in Social Theory: Origins and Challenges." In *Handbook of Action Research: Concise Paperback Edition,* edited by Peter Reason and Hilary Bradbury, 27–37. Thousand Oaks, CA: Sage.

Finley, Susan. 2011. "Critical Arts-Based Inquiry: The Pedagogy and Performance of a Radical Ethical Aesthetic." In *Handbook of Qualitative Research,* 4th ed., edited by Norman K. Denzin and Yvonna S. Lincoln, 435–450. Thousand Oaks, CA: Sage.

Foster Fishman, Pennie G., Kristen M. Law, Lauren F. Lichty, and Christina Aoun. 2010. "Youth ReACT for Social Change: A Method for Youth Participatory Action Research." *American Journal of Community Psychology* 46: 67–83.

Freire, Paulo. 1988 (1970). *Pedagogy of the Oppressed.* Translated by Myra Bergman Ramos. New York: Herder and Herder.

Green, Eric, and Bret Kloos. 2009. "Facilitating Youth Participation in a Context of Forced Migration: A Photovoice Project in Northern Uganda." *Journal of Refugee Studies* 22: 460–82.

Haque, Nasim, and Scott Rosas. 2010. "Concept Mapping of Photovoices: Sequencing and Integrating Methods to Understand Immigrants' Perceptions of Neighborhood Influences on Health." *Family and Community Health* 33: 193–206.

Janhonen-Abruquah, Hille. 2010. "Gone with the Wind? Immigrant Women and Transnational Everyday Life in Finland." PhD Diss., University of Helsinki.

Kohfeldt, Danielle, and Regina Langhout. 2012. "The 5 Whys: A Tool for Defining Problems in yPAR." *Journal of Community and Applied Social Psychology* 22: 316–29.

Lincoln, Yvonna S., Susan A. Lynham, and Egon G. Guba. 2011. "Paradigmatic Controversies, Contradictions, and Emerging Confluences, Revisited." In *Handbook of Qualitative*

Research, 4th ed., edited by Norman K. Denzin and Yvonna S. Lincoln, 97–128. Thousand Oaks, CA: Sage.

Lykes, M. Brinton, in collaboration with the Association of Maya Ixil Women–New Dawn. 2006. "Creative Arts and Photography in Participatory Action Research in Guatemala." In *Handbook of Action Research,* edited by Peter Reason and Hilary Bradbury, 269–78. Thousand Oaks, CA: Sage.

Martín-Baró, Ignacio. 1994. *Writings for a Liberation Psychology.* Translated by Adrianne Aron and Shawn Corne. Cambridge: Harvard University Press.

Prilleltensky, Isaac. 2012. "Wellness as Fairness." *American Journal of Community Psychology* 49: 1–21.

Rappaport, Julian. 1990. "Research Methods and the Empowerment Social Agenda." In *Researching Community Psychology: Issues of Theory and Methods,* edited by Patrick Tolan, Christopher Keys, Fern Chertok, and Leonard A. Jason, 51–63. Washington, DC: American Psychological Association.

Rhodes, Scott D., Kenneth C. Hergenrather, Derek M. Griffith, Leland J. Yee, Carlos S. Zometa, Jamie Montaño, and Aaron T. Vissman. 2009. "Sexual and Alcohol Risk Behaviors of Immigrant Latino Men in the South-eastern USA." *Culture, Health, and Sexuality* 11: 17–34.

Ryan, William. 1972. "The Art of Savage Discovery: How to Blame the Victim." In *Blaming the Victim,* by William Ryan, 3–30. New York: Vintage Books.

Stevens, Christine A. 2010. "Lessons from the Field: Using Photovoice with an Ethnically Diverse Population in a HOPE VI Evaluation." *Family and Community Health* 33: 275–84.

Stewart, J. Eric. "On Voice: Difference, Power, and Change." 2011. In *Empowering Settings and Voices for Social Change,* edited by Mark S. Aber, Kenneth I. Maton, Edward Seidman, and James G. Kelly, 193–206. New York: Oxford University Press.

Sutherland, Cheryl, and Yang Cheng. 2009. "Participatory-Action Research with (Im)migrant Women in Two Small Canadian Cities: Using Photovoice in Kingston and Petersborough, Ontario." *Journal of Immigrant and Refugee Studies* 7: 290–307.

Thomas, R. Elizabeth, and Julian Rappaport. 1996. "Art as Community Narrative: A Resource for Social Change." In *Myths about the Powerless: Contesting Social Inequalities,* edited by M. Brinton Lykes, Ali Banuazizi, Ramsay Liem, and Michael Morris, 317–36. Philadelphia: Temple University Press.

Wang, Caroline. 1999. "Photovoice: A Participatory Action Research Strategy Applied to Women's Health." *Journal of Women's Health* 8: 185–92.

Wang, Caroline, and Mary Ann Burris. 1994. "Empowerment through Photo Novella: Portraits of Participation." *Health Education and Behavior* 21: 171–86.

Wang, Caroline, and Mary Ann Burris. 1997. "Photovoice: Concept, Methodology, and Use for Participatory Needs Assessment." *Health Education and Behavior* 24: 369–87.

Wilson, Nance, Stefan Dasho, Anna C. Martin, Nina Wallerstein, Caroline C. Wang, and Meredith Minkler. 2007. "Engaging Youth Adolescents in Social Action through Photovoice: The Youth Empowerment Strategies (YES!) Project." *Journal of Early Adolescence* 27: 241–61.

Wilson, Nance, Meredith Minkler, Stefan Dasho, Nina Wallerstein, and Anna C. Martin. 2008. "Getting to Social Action: The Youth Empowerment Strategies (YES!) Project." *Health Promotion Practice* 9: 395–403.

Crosscutting Issues

Section Editors: Marc B. Schenker, Alfonso Rodriguez-Lainz,
and Xóchitl Castañeda

18

Ethical Issues across the Spectrum of Migration and Health Research

Kevin Pottie
Patricia Gabriel

INTRODUCTION

We all use stories, beliefs, and rituals to create a sense of community, to enrich our experiences, and to sustain us during difficult times. Stories also reflect how people of different cultures explain the cause of illness, the types of treatment they believe in, and to whom they will turn if they become ill (Helman 1997). Secular Western societies often have identities and stories linked to science and technology while traditional societies have stories based more on religion and community belonging (Giddens 1991). The search for ethics or answering the question "Is it right?" is complex when societies lack a shared story, or a collection of shared values, principles, and beliefs (Somerville 2000).

Inequality of power can prevent the sharing of stories, opportunities, and knowledge, and can leave vulnerable members of a society dependent on the decisions of others (Farmer 2005). As migrant health researchers, we need to be aware of these inequalities of power and to be aware that in our engagement with migrant populations we will be entering into or creating forums for shared values. In this engagement process, we must be willing to allow variation and pluralism, and appreciate constraints of social position (Kleinman 1995). Across different worlds of experience, we must be aware of the process of ethics, the process of building trust and accommodating and respecting people's conscience, religion, and beliefs. Indeed, a foundation of trust is an essential component for valid research results regardless of the methods being employed.

When researchers are faced with complex realities it is tempting to oversimplify "research ethics" and consider them to be a mere set of rules to follow when

TABLE 18.1   Continuum of Research Creation and Translation

Knowledge creation	Knowledge translation
Research team setup	Publication and authorship
Partnerships with communities	Sustained knowledge use (conflicts of interest)
Research design	Evaluation of application and barriers
Funding (public/private)	Equity in implementation
Ethics review board application	Adaptation of knowledge for local context
Informed consent process	Prioritization of topics for evidence reviews
Recruitment, data collection, and analysis	and summaries

applying to research ethics boards. However, if we limit our attention to the process of acquiring ethics board approval we miss the opportunity to acquire an understanding and appreciation of the philosophical underpinnings of ethical approaches to research. Further, we are apt to take shortcuts, miss opportunities for novel approaches, and risk inadvertently causing harm to research participants. Ethical issues in research also emerge in setting up teams and developing partnerships, selecting research priorities, seeking funding, determining research design and approaches to analysis, selecting venues for presentation and publication, and supporting implementation equity and adaptation for local context (see table 18.1). As an alternative, we favor an approach to research ethics that rigorously and honestly integrates ethical thinking into research across the continuum of knowledge creation and knowledge translation (implementation science).

When researchers are seeking ethically sound approaches to vulnerable populations, there are both theoretical and practical considerations. Theoretical considerations help us to understand the underlying values, principles, and frameworks that drive research ethics. Practical considerations in the research process help us to translate and utilize theories in the challenging realities of research on migration and health. This chapter will start by stepping back and reflecting on the values and norms that inform ethically sound research and will then engage with these theoretical concepts to consider how traditional theories apply to migrant populations. Second, using two case studies, it will take a practical look at the interface of ethics and research processes to provide practical guidance on the implementation of ethically sound practices for research in migration and health.

THEORETICAL ISSUES

Research with Vulnerable Populations

The theoretical approach to research ethics with migrant populations is embedded within a larger framework of research ethics with vulnerable populations. Research conducted in Western countries has a dark history in regard to vulnerable populations and is fraught with examples of exploitation and injustice. There are inherent ethical and humanitarian concerns for research with disadvantaged groups due to often gross power imbalances between researchers and participants. This impacts the ability to acquire true informed consent, ensure participant autonomy, and prevent mistreatment of participants (Lott 2005). Thus, research involving vulnerable populations such as migrant populations requires special consideration and quality assurance.

Why Are Migrants Considered Vulnerable?

Among migrants, vulnerability is variable between internally displaced persons, individuals in refugee detainment camps, irregular migrants (illegal aliens, non-status persons), refugee claimants (asylum seekers), government-assisted refugees, and other immigrant categories. These vulnerabilities, as discussed elsewhere, are a result of premigration, migration, settlement, and personal and social factors. Irregular migrants are persons without official authorization or status to stay in the country; this group is often forced to live in a clandestine fashion and may be significantly marginalized from local health and social services.

In regard to the interface of vulnerability and engaging in research, concerns can emerge from language and cultural barriers, lack of education, financial burdens, perceived lack of rights, dependency on host country governments, endemic hostility, and a history of physical or emotional distress (Lott 2005). As a result, some migrants may be at risk of engaging in research without understanding the nature of the research, engaging in research despite known risks due to a lack of perceived alternatives, or at worst, being coerced against their will to participate in research.

Western Bioethics

Researchers have tended to look toward medical ethics as a scholarly framework to guide engagement with participants. For clinical research with human subjects, thirty-five specific principles are described in the World Medical Association's Declaration of Helsinki, last updated in 2008. The basic principles of ethical medical research are simplified in the Belmont Report and include beneficence, nonmalfeasance, justice, and autonomy (DHEW 1979). We will discuss each of these principles in relation to the conduct of research with migrant populations.

Beneficence. The hope that research will be beneficial to the population being studied is, or should be, the driving force motivating research. More often it is reasonable to expect long-term benefits to a population as a result of a subset of that population participating in research; for example, a subset of a population may participate in a qualitative study to determine access-to-care barriers. The knowledge gained from this study can potentially be translated into long-term benefits to the migrant population en masse. The potential benefits include the emergence of a health care system that has improved understanding of the population's health care needs and improved delivery of health care services to the population. Whether or not research benefits the study participants themselves over the short and long term is more difficult to ascertain. For individual migrant participants, while system-level changes may primarily benefit new migrants on arrival, system changes may also benefit participants or their families in the future. There is a possibility that participants will gain new learning and relationships during the research process or will benefit from system changes that occur as a result of the actual research. In some studies, participants may benefit from tangible rewards in a study in the form of free medical assessment, treatment, or material and financial compensation in the form of honorariums. Given the uncertainty that participation in research will benefit the participant in the short term, and the potential for loss of time and resources to participants, tangible rewards often play an important role in ensuring benefits to migrant populations who face economic constraints.

Migrant participants may also benefit from the opportunity to share their stories, as described in studies of residents with limited access to health care in the United States and refugee detainees enthusiastically sharing their stories with researchers in the UK (Grady et al. 2006; Bloom 2010). In the focus group study of a vulnerable urban population by Grady et al., participants stated that they found participation valuable and appreciated the opportunity to be heard. Bloom draws examples from a study of detainees in the UK who, despite their precarious status, elected to use their names and even photographs in a research study. In fact, "the majority of the interviewees responded with enthusiasm and commitment to the opportunity to publicly articulate their perspectives and experiences." Participating in research, even for the vulnerable, can be empowering. Depending on the type of research study, participants may also benefit from engagement in social activities such as focus groups, or skill development and employment opportunities through participatory action research.

Nonmalfeasance. The principle of nonmalfeasance means to do no harm. There are many instances of research causing harm to participants. One has only to remember the research crimes committed in Nazi concentration camps brought to light during the Nuremberg trials or the notorious Tuskegee syphilis studies in the US, which followed the natural course of syphilis in black males without offering treatment. The types of potential harm vary greatly with the type of research being done, varying from potential harms due to medical examinations, screening, investigations, or treatment, to the more subtle potential psychological harms from research questioning in the form of interviews, focus groups, or surveys. The potential for harm increases with the power imbalance between researchers and participants, as the possibility for exploitation, loss of autonomy, and inadequate informed consent become more likely (Lott 2005).

Research with migrants has the same potential to cause harm as other forms of research, but in addition there are often population-specific perils to consider. For example, we must consider the human rights and political context of migrants (Beyrer 2002). If research is done in countries where governments and institutions do not guarantee participant confidentiality or in recipient nations where a refugee's legal status is perilous, researchers must consider the safety and privacy rights of participants to prevent research data and results from being used against participants (Lott 2005). For example, misuse of information collected during research can result in exploitation, persecution, or deportation of migrants.

This challenge is highlighted by Bernhard et al.'s research with refugees with precarious status in Canada. They were unable to promise participants complete confidentiality as the Canadian legal framework only permitted the maintenance of confidentiality to the "fullest extent possible by law," which may have actually permitted research records to be used in court. The possibility for "policing of knowledge production" requires further exploration but should be considered in all migrant research.

Many migrants, especially refugees, have a history of physical and sexual abuse (Kirmayer et al. 2011). Inappropriate questioning on these topics, especially when there may be background issues such as posttraumatic stress, can lead to psychological harm (Rousseau et al. 2011). Lack of measures to ensure that participants are well informed as to the nature of the study may lead to confusion, fear, and uncertainty. Risk factors for research studies that may cause harm include the provision of material or financial incentives and the provision of a lower standard of care for participants. These are often mediated by participant poverty, which leads to a lack of other options (Lott 2005).

Justice.   Considering justice when designing and conducting research helps to ensure equality in who benefits from research and who bears the burden. Justice requires that we as researchers assess, on the one hand, which individuals will potentially bear the burdens or accrue the benefits of being research participants and, on the other hand, which populations will potentially suffer or benefit due to the outcomes associated with research findings.

If equality is used as a lens and we assume that, overall, research benefits society, justice supports including migrant populations in research so that they have the opportunity to benefit from its fruits. In fact, given the relative paucity of research on migrant populations, one might argue that there is an even greater need for research in this population. However, considerations of justice make us aware of the need to assess the burden on research participants as well. Some researchers question whether or not research should be done with vulnerable populations such as migrants at all. Such concerns are raised due to the often unequal power relations between participants and researchers, which can be further accentuated with migrant populations. In studying refugees, for example, research may inadvertently contribute to human rights abuses and the worsening of conditions for refugees (Zion et al. 2010). Advocates for research with vulnerable populations argue that scientific investigation is needed to help end inhuman and cruel conditions, and they further argue that denying these populations the right to participate in research is paternalistic (Bloom 2010; Justo 2010; Rousseau and Kirmayer 2010; Strous 2010). Within this debate, a balance is proposed wherein it is recognized that research is necessary, but that we must be aware of the ethical pitfalls and devise new research tools and approaches to ameliorate potential harms (Rousseau and Kirmayer 2010; Justo 2010; Strous and Jotkowitz 2010).

In regard to migrant research, justice reminds us to determine if our approach to the research maintains the same rights for participants as research with other populations. This is not to be confused with doing things the exact same way, for treating people justly is not always the same as treating them equally. For example, research ethics boards often require written consent from participants. The purpose of this is to help ensure that participants have been appropriately informed about the study and are participating voluntarily. However, some migrant populations have high illiteracy rates, and requiring participants to read and sign a consent form to participate may be inherently unjust. Stepping back and considering the underlying values guiding research ethics may result in different approaches to migrant populations in order to maintain equality. We must always consider the inequalities between populations in our approach to research and try to make adjustments to account for these differences.

Autonomy (Respect for Person).   Ensuring autonomy in research means that individuals must be capable of deliberation and able to act under their own direction without obstruction (DHEW 1979). The Declaration of Helsinki discusses elements of autonomy in at least nine of its thirty-six principles (11, 22, 24–29, 34) (WMA 2010), articulating the need for participants to be adequately informed of the aims, methods, risks, and benefits of the research and their right to refuse participation. Additionally, it requires that participants act voluntarily and provide informed consent, preferably in writing.

Maintaining autonomy in medical research is facilitated through the process of informed consent. For research involving migrant populations, there are numerous reasons to suspect that the standard Western informed consent processes are inadequate for maintaining autonomy for nonwestern populations. For these populations there is a higher risk of individuals consenting without understanding their rights or refusing to participate due to a lack of understanding of the value of the proposed research (Wong and Song 2007).

The major principles of informed consent are disclosure, comprehension, capacity, voluntariness, and consent (Nakkash et al. 2009). At each step, there is potential for inefficacy when these principles are applied in the context of research with migrants. Disclosure, that is, insuring that participants are adequately informed, is often complicated by language barriers (Johnson et al. 2009) and by insufficiently trained research assistants (Nakkash et al. 2009). Inappropriate translation of research material and lack of professional interpretation of verbal interactions can result in the inaccurate exchange of information. Research personnel who lack appropriate cultural competency or familiarity with endemic concepts of health and research may be unable to convey information appropriately or accurately to participants, thus preventing them from being truly informed.

Comprehension refers to a participant's ability to understand the purpose of the research and the implications of participating in the research. Comprehension can be compromised in migrant populations. On the one hand, participants may struggle with understanding due to illiteracy, lack of education, and lack of familiarity with research. On the other hand, as with any population, comprehension becomes increasingly challenging with the complexity of the research (Nakkash et al. 2009). Assessing comprehension in vulnerable populations, where there is often a power differential, may also be difficult if participants are unwilling or unable to disclose a lack of understanding due to fear, embarrassment, or a desire to please.

Capacity broadly implies an individual's ability to reason and make his or her own decisions. Capacity in migrants, as with any population, can be affected by age and mental status. With certain vulnerable migrants, capacity can also be impacted by real or perceived extraneous cultural or political circumstances that may limit an individual's liberty (Nakkash et al. 2009).

Voluntariness means that an individual agrees to participate in research under conditions that are free of undue influence and coercion. In migrant research, voluntariness can be impacted by a power imbalance between researchers and participants (Mkandawire-Valhmu et al. 2009) and contextual issues (Nakkash et al. 2009) such as a desire to please, threats of harm, or promises of reward that might lead to coercion.

The final step in ensuring the principle of autonomy involves the act of actually giving consent. This is a culmination of all of the aforementioned issues and refers to the step where an individual indicates that he or she is willing to participate. This can take the form of written, oral, or implied consent. This step can be impacted by all of the issues outlined above. Additionally, it can be negatively impacted by a participants' literacy level in the case of written consent or by their suspiciousness of signing official documents (Karwalajtys et al. 2010).

In summary, the theoretical considerations in research ethics include assessing the potential benefits and harms to participants, considering justice by reflecting on equity in the distribution of research efforts, and ensuring the protection of participant autonomy throughout the informed consent process. General principles must be considered for migrant research in addition to population-specific measures reflective of potential vulnerabilities due to political, linguistic, and cultural variations.

PRACTICAL AND ETHICALLY SOUND APPROACHES IN RESEARCH

Research and scholarship entail knowledge creation and knowledge translation. Knowledge creation refers to new knowledge derived through research, and knowledge translation refers to the methods used to ensure that new knowledge is shared, implemented into systems, and considered in further knowledge creation research (Straus et al. 2009a, 2009b). To engage in ethically sound knowledge creation and translation with migrant communities, it is important to consider the following guiding principles (Waters 2006):

1. Engage individuals and communities throughout the process.
2. Ensure reciprocal relationships when possible and share responsibility for creating effective partnerships.
3. Use leadership and accountability to create sustained change.
4. Build on the strengths of the community—know the community well and build on what works with that community

Setting up Teams and Developing Partnerships

Research usually begins with an idea, and the next step is often the formation of a team to refine that idea into a viable research question. In this early stage there will be an opportunity to invite team members from other disciplines for collaboration, and it will also be important to form partnerships with relevant knowledge users and members of the migrant communities that will be asked to participate. Knowledge translation principles highlight the importance of engaging knowledge users and community members early in the research process, and many argue that this should begin during the initial development of the research team (Straus et al. 2009a, 2009b).

Community participatory methods can be used to inform one's approach to setting up a research team (Ellis et al. 2007; Guruge and Khanlou 2004; Johnson et al. 2009). Engaging community members aids not only in improving the ethical rigor of research studies but also in enhancing the quality of the methods. Trust is a central theme for research teams in migrant health. Trust can be enhanced through full disclosure of information and involvement of advocates, physicians, and trusted religious or community leaders (Grady et al. 2006).

Selecting Research Priorities

Early in the research process there should be discussions aimed at determining and refining research priorities. All members of the team, including research partners from the community, should consult in order to develop a clear consensus about those priorities (Swinkels et al. 2011). Another ethical consideration at this stage is to undertake high-quality background synthesis and comprehensive literature reviews to ensure that the project is building on prior research. This will prevent redundancy and maximize the potential scholarly advances from the research. For the most vulnerable migrant populations such as irregular migrants, asylum seekers, and internally displaced persons, we suggest that studies be restricted to those questions that cannot be addressed in any other way, that only studies that are urgent and vital to the health and well-being of the researched population be undertaken, and that studies provide important direct benefits to either study participants or their communities (Leaning 2001).

Seeking Funding

For many research projects, consideration of private or public funding opportunities may be part of the process. Researchers should be aware of the risks and benefits of various funding sources and be alert to any potential conflicts of interest. Research priorities should consider the needs of migrant populations first and should not be unduly influenced by individual researchers' career goals, publication interests, grant opportunities, or other self-motivated priorities that may risk undermining the study population's priorities.

Determining Research Design, Recruitment, and Approaches to Analysis

A research team that has determined its research priorities and drafted its research questions will then begin to determine the best research design to answer its questions. Traditionally the research question is the main determinant of the research design. However, the potential risks and benefits to participants inherent in different methodologies should also be considered. Researchers must ensure that the study design imposes the absolute minimum of additional risk (Leaning 2001). Recall that harm may be caused by asking about rape, reproductive health, and mental health, or through undue attention, humiliation, and emotional upset during questioning (Leaning 2001). The potential risks and benefits inherent in different research designs can be influenced by contextual factors related to language, culture, power structures, political environments, and the practical circumstances specific to each migrant community engaged in research. Acknowledging any oppressive realities of participants within the context of the research design helps to avoid further marginalization of participants and may offer opportunities to improve participants' life situations (Mkandawire-Valhmu et al. 2009). Procedures to assess, minimize, and monitor the risks to individual subjects, their community, and their future security must be embedded within the research design (Leaning 2001).

Elements of the research design subsequently influence recruitment approaches. Careful attention to language barriers and consideration of the insider-outsider status of the researchers is vital (Olgivie et al. 2008). Recruitment must be negotiated with awareness of potential power imbalances, institutional discrimination, and trauma associated with premigration, migration, and settlement experiences (Olgivie et al. 2008). Study participants should be selected based on sound methodology, not ease of accessibility and potential malleability of participants (Leaning 2001).

Research design and recruitment methods together will influence inclusion and exclusion criteria. The principle of justice should be considered. For example, quantitative research often requires participants who can read and write. Due to harsh circumstances, refugees and internally displaced persons are often illiterate and may be unjustly excluded from the benefits of research participation. Adjustments to research design should thus be explored.

For research analysis the importance of engagement with knowledge users and community members can play an important role in ensuring that outcomes and results are both relevant and of high quality. Many research tools are not culturally valid, and endemic knowledge may be necessary to aid in the interpretation of research findings to aid in internal and external validity of results.

Prior to data collection, the research protocol, recruitment information, questionnaires, and informed consent forms should be reviewed by members of the proposed study population to identify potential ethical concerns as outlined above. Pilot testing, if possible, is also recommended.

Ensuring Informed Consent for Participants

Research projects that involve direct contact with participants will require an informed consent process. Ensuring informed consent across linguistic and cultural barriers can be challenging.

Strategies for facilitating ethically sound informed consent can be used at each stage of the process, including disclosure, comprehension, capacity, voluntariness, and consent (Nakkash et al. 2009). Disclosure can be improved through careful selection of research assistants, clear explanations of the importance of informed consent, and training in conducting informed consent.

Participant comprehension can be addressed by using diagrams and pictures to help explain the steps in the study, simplifying the vocabulary used in the consent form, and adapting the language and concepts with consideration of the local context.

In addition to traditional considerations, capacity in some migrant populations may be affected by limitations to autonomous choice based on the cultural setting. Some cultures may have power structures in families with unexpected or multiple guardians and decision makers, and may have beliefs that children or women are not able to give informed consent independently. This can be addressed by understanding who is involved in giving consent, seeking consent from all concerned, and explaining the value of informed consent and assent to guardians and family decision makers.

Voluntariness can be ensured by assessing power structures in the community, between academia and the community, or between academics and participants that may unduly impact autonomous decision making. These can then be addressed by choosing comfortable locations for informed consent taking and recruiting research assistants from the community with whom participants would be comfortable asking questions and declining participation if desired.

The final act of recording consent, traditionally by signing an informed consent form, can be hindered by participants' inability to write or fear of official documents. Adaptations can be made by requesting oral consent or implied consent by other ethical means, following a rigorous informed consent process.

Selecting Venues for Presentation and Publication

In the presentation of research in progress or completed research results, it is important to consider again the participants and the populations that are implicated in the research, and to ensure that the results are put in a form that is accessible and meaningful for stakeholders. While peer-reviewed publication remains an important product of research, it is now recognized that other knowledge translation products will be important to ensure that research both reaches the right audience and plays a role in creating action.

Supporting Implementation Equity and Adaptation for Local Context

Finally, the results of research may require adaptation to local contexts for appropriate implementation. This knowledge translation often will benefit from a consideration of how implementation may affect various populations and how the knowledge can be applied to local contexts. There are many methods that can be used at this stage, and again the central idea is to ensure that the research plays a role in contributing to further research, community action, or policy and practice. Individual research efforts are not necessarily expected to change policy and practice, as such change often requires a larger body of evidence (Lavis et al. 2005). However, we feel that all migrant research should at least inform future research and play a potential role in raising awareness in academic and migrant communities.

CASE STUDY 1: RESEARCH ON REFUGEES ARRIVING IN A HIGH-INCOME COUNTRY

You are working at an inner-city community health care center that provides primary health care for underserved populations in a large urban center. Over the last year you have noticed a large number of Somali patients and discover that there has been an influx of Somali refugees settling in the surrounding neighbourhood. From speaking with the local settlement agency, you learn that there will be an additional hundred Somali refugees arriving over the next year.

Your clinic is staffed by two doctors, two nurses, and a social worker. At a staff meeting you are reflecting on some of the observations you have made about this population at the clinic. There have been some challenges to providing quality ' care. Some factors are related to the patient population, the care providers, and the health care system. With an aim to better prepare for the arrival of refugees, you propose a research study to retrospectively evaluate patients' files and to host a series of focus groups with your Somali patients to better understand the health needs and health care challenges for this population.

Before clarifying your research questions, you decide to engage the community from the beginning and invite past and current Somali patients to an evening meeting at the clinic. You advertise through the clinic that there will be an opportunity to be involved in a research project on the health of Somali refugees. You wonder how much the community knows about research, what their attitudes toward the research process will be, and what factors may hinder or enable their participation.

Only two bilingual Somali women come to the evening session, but they are very keen and well informed. They are both invited to join the research team. Your group decides to host focus group sessions to assess Somali patients' challenges with their health and access to appropriate health care services in their first year in Canada. You apply for ethical approval through your health authority Research Ethics Board. The application process is helpful for clarifying your recruitment plans, but you are frustrated by the necessity to stick to a cumbersome and lengthy consent form.

For recruitment you decide not to offer any financial incentive, but your posters advertise that dinner will be provided. Your posters are colorful and translated into Somali. Nevertheless, you struggle with recruitment of participants through the clinic, even when the nurses and doctors give personal invitations to patients. You end up relying heavily on Somali team members, who know most members of the community and call to invite individuals personally to the focus group sessions.

At the focus groups sessions, you wonder what group composition is appropriate and consider having groups based on age and gender. You reflect as a team about what questions might be inappropriate. You decide on a semistructured interview guide and ask one of your Somali research assistants to interpret for you as you facilitate the group session.

At the start of the focus group sessions you have one of your Somali research team members explain independently the English consent form in Somali. The time taken seems very brief and you are left wondering what exactly was disclosed. None of the participants ask any clarifying questions. You discover that only half of the participants are literate, and when asked to sign the consent forms, some participants ask a neighbor to sign their form on their behalf.

Your first group is composed of seven Somali women. The atmosphere quickly lightens after the consent form is done and there is a lot of laughter and smiling over dinner. Once the first few questions have been asked, the participants speak candidly about their experiences and the session runs an hour longer than expected, but nobody wants to leave. As the participants leave, two women stop and give you a big hug and thank you for the opportunity to participate.

CASE STUDY 2: CONDUCTING A NEEDS ASSESSMENT OF INTERNALLY DISPLACED PERSONS

It is 1995 and Médecins Sans Frontières (MSF) is working in the postwar Republic of Georgia. As a result of the war in the breakaway Republic of Abkhazia, ethnic Georgians have fled south into Georgia and set up residences in hotels and communities along the coast of the Black Sea. MSF has set up a drug distribution program to support the internally displaced population. In its distribution of essential medical supplies, it has become apparent that the supplies may not be reaching the displaced populations, and also it becomes unclear whether the need for medical services between the local population and the internally displaced population is significantly different. To ensure it is reaching the most vulnerable population with its medical supplies and services, MSF decides to conduct a needs assessment survey.

The research team includes two international MSF physicians (Canadian and French), a Georgian physician, two Georgian nurses, and internally displaced person (IDP) camp leaders, with some technical support from the Centers for Disease Control, USA. As the team begins to design the research project they discover that several students, some with epidemiology research backgrounds, are available. They also discover Soviet-era detailed maps of neighborhoods in the area.

There are no functioning ethics review boards in the Republic of Georgia. Nor has MSF established its own internal ethics review board. But it does have coordinators in Amsterdam who are able to review the research protocol and provide funding for the research. The research team adapts and translates into Georgian a health needs assessment questionnaire that was recently used for an MSF project in Bosnia. University students who speak the language of the population to be surveyed are recruited and trained to conduct door-to-door surveys employing a sampling method used by UNICEF to determine rates of vaccination in a population. The Soviet-era neighborhood maps are used to enable stratified random sampling to reduce the risk of bias.

With the funding support and leadership of MSF and national staff, the research survey is conducted over a three-week period, and then field epidemiology software from CDC—EpiInfo—is used to analyze the results. It is discovered that health needs and access to health services are an issue, but that access to services and essential medications does not differ significantly between the IDPs and the local population. MSF publishes the results of the research in the only operating Georgian publication, the Save the Children Newsletter, and presents the results to the Ministry of Health and other nongovernmental organizations who are also interested in the research methods. The research is used to help ensure ongoing humanitarian assistance, but rather than focusing only on IDPs, the assistance targets the communities themselves for essential services and essential medication distribution. The national Georgian staff is able to repeat the survey in three years to monitor the situation. As a result of the research experience, one of the Georgian staff is recruited for additional epidemiology training in Atlanta at the CDC (Pottie et al. 1995).

CONCLUSION

In this chapter we highlight the tension between medical bioethics and medical anthropology, showing how, in approaching research across cultures, it is important to consider the process of building trust and partnerships with communities, sharing stories and opportunities that arise from research results, and recognizing cultural variations and power inequities. We also wish to broaden the meaning of ethics in research on migration and health to be more than just a focus on getting ethical approval for projects or achieving informed consent for participation; rather, ethics involves seeing ethically sound approaches as processes within the various steps of the knowledge creation and knowledge translation continuum.

REFERENCES

Beyrer, C, and NE Kass. 2002. "Human rights, politics, and reviews of research ethics." *Lancet* 360(9328):246–51.

Bloom, T. 2010. "Asylum seekers: Subjects or objects of research?" *American Journal of Bioethics* 10:59–60.

Department of Health, Education, and Welfare (DHEW). 1979. *The Belmont Report: Ethical Principles and Guidelines for the Protection of Human Subjects of Research.* Washington, DC: OPRR Reports. http://www.hhs.gov/ohrp/humansubjects/guidance/belmont.html.

Ellis, BH, M Kia-Keating, SA Yusuf, A Lincoln, and A Nur. 2007. "Ethical research in refugee communities and the use of community participatory methods." *Transcultural Psychiatry* 44:459–81.

Farmer, P. 2005. *Pathologies of Power: Health, Human Rights and the New War on the Poor.* Berkeley: University of California Press.

Giddens, A. 1991. *Modernity and Self-Identity: Self and Society in the Late Modern Age.* Stanford: Stanford University Press.

Grady, C, LA Hampson, GR Wallen, MV Rivera-Goba, KL Carrington, and BB Mittleman. 2006. "Exploring the ethics of clinical research in an urban community." *American Journal of Public Health* 96:1996–2001.

Guruge, S, and N Khanlou. 2004. "Intersectionalities of influence: Researching the health of immigrant and refugee women." *Canadian Journal of Nursing Research* 36:32–47.

Helman, C. 1997. *Culture, Health and Illness.* 3rd ed. Oxford: Butterworth-Heinemann, Oxford.

Johnson, CE, SA Ali, and MP Shipp. 2009. "Building community-based participatory research partnerships with a Somali refugee community." *American Journal of Preventive Medicine* 37:S230–36.

Justo, L 2010. "Consent while hanging from a cliff?" *American Journal of Bioethics* 10(2):61–62.

Karwalajtys, TL, LJ Redwood-Campbell, NC Fowler, LH Lohfeld, M Howard, JA Kaczorowski, and A Lytwyn. 2010. "Conducting qualitative research on cervical cancer screening among diverse groups of immigrant women: Research reflections: Challenges and solutions." *Canadian Family Physician* 56(4):e130–35.

Kirmayer, LJ, L Narasiah, M Munoz, et al. 2011. "Common mental health problems in immigrants and refugees: General approach in primary care." *Canadian Medical Association Journal* 183(12):E959–E967.

Kleinman, A. 1995. *Writing at the Margins: Discourse between Anthropology and Medicine.* Berkeley: University of California Press.

Lavis, J, H Davies, R Gruen, K Walshe, and C Farquhar. 2005. "Working within and beyond the Cochrane collaboration to make systematic reviews more useful to healthcare managers and policy makers." *Healthcare Policy* 1(2):21–33.

Leaning, J. 2001. "Ethics of research in refugee populations." *Lancet* 357:1432–33.

Lott, JP. 2005. "Module three: Vulnerable/special participant populations." *Developing World Bioethics* 5:30–54.

Mkandawire-Valhmu, L, E Rice, and ME Bathum. 2009. "Promoting an egalitarian approach to research with vulnerable populations of women." *Journal of Advanced Nursing* 65:1725–34.

Nakkash, R, J Makhoul, and R Afifi. 2009. "Obtaining informed consent: Observations from community research with refugee and impoverished youth." *Journal of Medical Ethics* 35:638–43.

Ogilvie, LD, E Burgess-Pinto, and C Caufield. 2008. "Challenges and approaches to newcomer health research." *Journal of Transcultural Nursing* 19:64–73.

Pottie, K, C Greenaway, J Feightner, et al., and co-authors of the Canadian Collaboration for Immigrant and Refugee Health. 2011. "Evidence-based clinical guidelines for immigrants and refugees." *Canadian Medical Association Journal* 183(12):E824–E925.

Pottie, K, N Malakmadze, and B Piquemal. 1995. "Access to health care, Kobuleti Region, Republic of Georgia." Technical Report for MSF and Publication in "Save the Children Georgian Newsletter."

Rousseau, C, and L. Kirmayer. 2010. "From complicity to advocacy: The necessity of refugee research." *American Journal of Bioethics* 10(2):65–67.

Rousseau, C, K Pottie, BD Thombs, et al. 2011. "Post-traumatic stress disorder: Evidence-based clinical guidelines for immigrants and refugees." *Canadian Medical Association Journal* 183(12):E876–E878.

Somerville, M. 2000. *The Ethical Canary: Science, Society and the Human Spirit.* Toronto: Viking.

Straus, S, T Tetroe, and I Graham (Eds.). 2009a. *Knowledge Translation in Health Care: Moving from Evidence to Practice.* Oxford: Wiley-Blackwell.

Straus, S, J Tetroe, and I Graham. 2009b. "Defining knowledge translation." *Canadian Medical Association Journal* 181(3–4):165–68.

Strous, RD, and A Jotkowitz. 2010. "Ethics and research in the service of asylum seekers." *American Journal of Bioethics* 10:63–65.

Swinkels, H, K Pottie, P Tugwell, M Rashid, and L Narasiah. 2011. "Development of guidelines for recently arrived immigrants and refugees to Canada: Delphi consensus on selecting preventable and treatable conditions." *Canadian Medical Association Journal* 183(12): E928–E932.

Waters, E (Ed.). 2006. *Cultural competency in health: A guide for policy, partnerships and participation.* Canberra, ACT: Commonwealth of Australia.

Wong-Kim, E, and Y Song. 2007. "Obtaining informed consent for research on immigrant populations." *Journal of Empirical Research on Human Research Ethics* 2:83–84.

World Medical Association (WMA). 2010. "Declaration of Helsinki: Ethical principles for medical research involving human subjects." 59th WMA General Assembly, Seoul 2008.

Zion, D, L Briskman, and B Loffa. 2010. "Returning to history: The ethics of researching asylum seeker health in Australia." *American Journal of Bioethics* 10(2):48–59.

19

Community-Based Participatory Research

A Promising Approach for Studying and Addressing Immigrant Health

Meredith Minkler
Charlotte Chang

INTRODUCTION

An alternative approach to inquiry known as community-based participatory research (CBPR) holds substantial value for work with immigrant populations (Arcury et al. 2001; Farquhar and Michael 2004; Tandon and Kwon 2009). An *orientation to research,* rather than a particular research method, CBPR is concisely defined as "systematic inquiry, with the participation of those affected by the problem, for the purposes of education and action or affecting social change" (Green et al. 1995). Unlike most investigator-driven approaches, CBPR emphasizes equitable engagement of all partners throughout the research process, from problem definition through data collection and analysis, to dissemination and use of findings, to help effect change (Israel et al. 1998, 2005).

In this chapter, we begin by summarizing the key principles of CBPR and the value that may be added to immigrant health research processes and outcomes when this orientation is utilized. We then briefly describe the Restaurant Worker Health and Safety Study, an ecologic CBPR project undertaken in San Francisco's Chinatown District, which then is used to illustrate each of CBPR's potential benefits. We review the challenges and limitations that frequently arise when a CBPR approach is utilized, as well as some ways in which these problems may be mitigated. We offer web-based and other resources for academic, community, and other partners interested in employing a CBPR approach, and conclude by suggesting that while CBPR may not be well suited to all immigrant health research, when it is appropriate, it can make a real difference in both the processes and outcomes of this work.

CBPR: CORE PRINCIPLES AND RELEVANCE FOR WORK
WITH IMMIGRANT POPULATIONS

The core principles of CBPR developed by Israel and her community and academic colleagues in Michigan (1998, 2005) are arguably the most widely utilized in health and related CBPR research. Briefly, these principles emphasize (1) recognizing the community as a unit of identity; (2) all partners participating equitably in the research process, emphasizing empowerment and power sharing; (3) identifying and building on community strengths; (4) focusing on an issue of strong relevance to the community; (5) facilitating capacity building and systems change; (6) balancing research and action; and (7) committing to the long haul for sustainability. Finally, and of particular relevance in work with immigrant populations, CBPR should embody the concept of cultural humility (Minkler and Wallerstein 2008). As described by Tervalon and Murray-Garcia (1998), cultural humility acknowledges that while we can never be truly competent in another's culture, we can engage in critical self-reflection, maintain openness to others' cultures, and commit to redressing power imbalances and developing genuine and respectful partnerships.

The emphasis of CBPR on empowerment, individual and community capacity building, and translating research findings into action makes this approach particularly advantageous in work with immigrant populations. As noted in earlier chapters, these groups tend to have disproportionate health needs, to be understudied and underserved (Abe-Kim et al. 2007; Takeuchi et al. 2007), to have limited education and second-language proficiency, and to be economically and politically disadvantaged—often comprising much of the low-wage job sector (Bernhardt et al. 2009). They also tend to have low rates of political participation (Junn 1999; Ramakrishnan and Espenshade 2001; Wong et al. 2011), often exacerbated by undocumented status in the host country (Tandon and Kwon 2009).

At the same time, characterizing health status, concerns, socioeconomic status, and other risk and protective factors for immigrant populations and subpopulations is itself a challenging task given that much of the available health data in the US is collected and organized under broad racial and ethnic demographic categories such as "Asian," "Hispanic or Latino," "African American," "white," and "other," which obscures large differences between subpopulations. These diverse immigrant populations are becoming increasingly dispersed geographically as well, and smaller communities outside of areas of traditionally large immigrant settlement, such as California, New York, and Texas, often are not captured in national health data. The local contexts for health for linguistically isolated immigrant communities in different parts of Ohio, Alabama, and California are likely to differ quite substantially from each other, particularly as more states pass anti-immigrant legislation.

Further, traditional "outside expert–driven" research approaches often have proven ill-suited to work with immigrant populations, whose members may be distrustful of research and fearful of disclosing information or participating in interventions due to immigration status, fear of retaliation, or earlier life experiences (Tandon and Kwon 2009; Minkler et al. 2010; Arcury et al. 2001; Farquhar and Michael 2004). As noted above, a growing number of research studies have demonstrated the promise of CBPR for collaboratively studying and addressing problems of local relevance in immigrant communities. These range from epidemiological and survey research (Minkler et al. 2010; Schulz et al. 2001) to ethnography, focus groups, and other qualitative approaches (McQuiston et al. 2005; Rhodes et al. 2009), to intervention studies using randomized controlled designs to assess the effects of environmental and behavioral health interventions on health outcomes. The latter have included community-engaged intervention studies in areas such as pesticide exposure (Salvatore et al. 2009), HIV/AIDS prevention (Rhodes et al. 2009), and asthma (Krieger et al. 2005). We now turn to a more detailed look at the ways in which CBPR can add value to research with immigrant populations, drawing on an ecological study with immigrant restaurant workers in San Francisco's Chinatown District.

CBPR AND IMMIGRANT WORKER HEALTH: WHAT'S THE VALUE ADDED?

Numerous authors have elucidated the ways in which CBPR can add value to health research in underserved communities, including, importantly, immigrant communities (Cargo and Mercer 2008; O'Fallon and Dearry 2002; Israel et al. 2005; Minkler 2005). Briefly, these include (1) helping insure that the research question comes from, or is of genuine importance to, the local community; (2) increasing community buy-in and trust, which can in turn increase response rates; (3) enhancing the cultural acceptability of study instruments, often improving their validity; (4) improving the design and implementation of interventions, increasing the likelihood of success; (5) improving data interpretation; (6) identifying and using new channels for dissemination; (7) helping translate the findings into action that will benefit the community; and (8) building individual and community capacity and leaving behind a community better able to study and address other health and social issues of local concern. Each of these is illustrated below.

OVERVIEW OF THE CHINATOWN RESTAURANT WORKER HEALTH AND SAFETY STUDY

The Chinatown Restaurant Worker Health and Safety Study (CRWHSS) began in 2007 with the overarching goal of conducting and evaluating an ecologic CBPR study to examine and address the occupational health conditions of immigrant workers in a densely populated San Francisco neighborhood. As in the nation as a whole, restaurants are the single largest employer of immigrants in Chinatown, with fully a third of its workers employed in this sector (US Census Bureau 2000). Restaurants have historically had among the highest numbers of reportable injuries and illnesses as well as the highest percentage of reportable injuries and illnesses among private industry in the nation (Webster 2001). Injuries from burns, cuts, and falls, as well as elevated rates of psychosocial problems related to on-the-job stress (Woo et al. 2003) are common in the industry. Of even greater concern to many immigrant restaurant workers, however, are such economic vulnerabilities as failure to receive minimum wage, delayed or nonpayment of wages, and lack of job security (Chinese Progressive Association 2010; Bernhardt et al. 2009; Restaurant Opportunities Center of New York 2005).

The partnership that conducted the Chinatown study consisted of a prominent community-based organization, the Chinese Progressive Association (CPA); two universities (the Labor Occupational Health Program [LOHP] at the University of California, Berkeley, School of Public Health, and the University of California, San Francisco, School of Medicine); and the Occupational and Environmental Health Section of the San Francisco Department of Public Health. A steering committee comprised of all project partners and several subcommittees with representatives of each partner organization met regularly to provide project oversight and decision making. Nine worker partners were hired and extensively trained during the course of the project, and received much follow-up training while meeting regularly on a weekly to biweekly basis to facilitate members' in-depth participation throughout the project. In addition to this core group, seventeen members of the Chinese immigrant community were hired and trained as surveyors, with many also receiving training for subsequent work as organizers with CPA. A grant from the National Institute for Occupational Safety and Health (NIOSH) and a subsequent grant to the community partner from The California Endowment supported partnership development, the multifaceted study, and a participatory evaluation of the partnership, as well as dissemination and action activities. The research component included initial focus groups with workers; a detailed survey of 433 current and former Chinatown restaurant workers; the development and use, by the health department partner, of an observational checklist to study working conditions in 106 of Chinatown's 108 restaurants; and interviews and surveys conducted with participating study partners. All partners, including immigrant worker members, actively participated in working groups to develop data collection protocols and study instruments. Through subsequent biweekly meetings, the immigrant worker partners provided additional feedback on study instruments, developed a recruitment plan for surveys, and helped pilot-test the study instruments.

University partners took the lead in preparing and analyzing survey data, and health department partners did so for the observational restaurant-level data.

During the analysis period, preliminary results were routinely shared with all partners, who were asked for their insights, and monthly data interpretation workshops were held with the worker partners. Conducted in Chinese by CPA staff and the project coordinator with participation of different university and health department partners, these sessions enabled additional co-learning, with immigrant worker partners acquiring skills in data interpretation and providing other partners with many insights into the data that were not originally apparent. For example, in interactive data interpretation sessions, worker partners were sometimes surprised that the data on health and social problems were not starker; for instance, 8% of workers reported being owed back wages and 13% reported having their initial pay withheld for one or more pay periods. Academic, CPA, and other partners responded that such practices are unacceptable at any level. More in-depth discussions further revealed the worker partners' belief that many of those responding "don't know" to other wage theft issues, such as stolen tips, were simply afraid to respond because they feared possible retribution from employers.

The health department took the lead on dissemination of findings, including reporting on the utility of a new checklist tool for gauging restaurant safety from a worker perspective; this checklist was made available online to other health departments and stakeholders around the country (Gaydos et al. 2011; http://www .sfphes.org/publications/Restaurant_Health_Safety_Checklist.pdf). The health department also followed up with action, writing a number of letters to relevant government regulatory agencies citing the findings and pressing for greater enforcement of existing laws while offering the health department's assistance.

But it was the community partners—CPA and the worker partners—who took the lead in disseminating survey and other study findings through nonacademic means and using the findings as the basis of the key action component of the study. As discussed below, a widely attended press event at which key study findings and a data-driven action plan were unveiled, plus subsequent base building and organizing, played a key role in the development and passage of the second municipal anti-wage theft ordinance in the nation in September 2011. The sharing of study findings through both scientific and lay channels (e.g., monthly worker teas and community events) continues; adoption of the study's action plan and the creation of a new cross-ethnic and cross-industry organization involving many other immigrant workers—the Progressive Workers Alliance—are also high points of the work's outcomes to date.

VALUE ADDED: ILLUSTRATIONS FROM THE CHINATOWN IMMIGRANT WORKER HEALTH STUDY

The Chinatown study clearly illustrates each of the ways in which CBPR can add value to research processes and outcomes.

Relevant Research Question

CBPR can help insure that the research question comes from, or is of genuine importance to, the local community. For more than thirty-five years CPA, the community partner, had organized campaigns for worker rights in Chinatown restaurants and other venues, and was particularly concerned about the problem of wage theft, both in the community and beyond its borders. CPA staff increasingly realized, however, that scientific data were needed to help make the case for policy level action. By adopting a broader definition of health (WHO 1946) and expanding the traditional research topic (health and safety conditions in restaurants) to put a heavier accent on wage theft and related issues, the academic and health department partners validated the community partner's concern and helped facilitate its investigation.

Fostering Community Trust

CBPR can increase community buy-in and trust, which can in turn increase response rates. Previous collaborative work by some of the partners, and the bridging role played by the university-based project director, who was born in Chinatown and was a founding member of the CPA, helped provide important groundwork for the establishment of trust. Also of major importance was the long track record of the CPA in organizing campaigns for worker rights in Chinatown and beyond its borders. Yet even with these advantages, much front-end trust building among the community, university, and health department partners occurred. This included early and candid discussions about the various partner groups' excitement—and concerns—about working together, and the development and structure of an active steering committee, the involvement of the worker partners, and other subcommittees to facilitate equitable partnership. The hiring and intensive training of over two dozen actual community members, including the active involvement of the original core group of current and former restaurant workers throughout the research process, also greatly increased community buy-in and trust. The collection of detailed (103 items) survey data from 433 workers in little over a month can be attributed in large part to this active community engagement and the trust building at its core.

Improved Cultural Validity

CBPR can improve the cultural acceptability of study instruments, often enhancing their validity. Both the CPA and the worker partners made substantial improvements to the draft worker survey that was provided as a template by the university researchers. This review and revision process greatly increased the survey's cultural relevance and insured that we asked "the right questions." New items recommended by workers were added (e.g., about whether or not workers who did not smoke were called in earlier from breaks, and whether workers had experienced a variety of forms of wage theft, such as failure to get minimum wage, delayed or nonpayment of wages, including during a "probationary period," and bosses taking a portion of their tip money). Validated scale items that did not translate well into Chinese (such as the Center for Epidemiological Studies Depression Scale (CES-D), which includes idioms like "butterflies in my stomach") were also flagged by worker partners and brief explanations were subsequently included to make them more easily understandable to immigrant respondents taking the survey in Chinese (Minkler et al. 2010). Such culturally and socially appropriate additions resulted in a final product that was far more likely to achieve both accurate responses and to include issues that were of substantial interest in the community.

Laying the Groundwork for Policy Change

The use of CBPR can improve the design and implementation of interventions, increasing the likelihood of success. As Minkler and Salvatore (2012: 200) note, "In keeping with its CBPR orientation, the Chinatown project kept the 'final' phases of CBPR—dissemination and translation of findings into action—at the forefront of planning from the study's onset." Although this preliminary study was not designed to develop and test an intervention, we had hoped to lay the groundwork for subsequent community-level interventions, such as a possible city-backed program to incentivize "good employers" by giving them "seals of approval" and encouraging diners to patronize these establishments. Our community partners pointed out, however, that while some restaurants would like such recognition, and indeed were receiving it through an existing local community-based organization's guide to "guilt-free eating" in the city, many would not want to be singled out and risk the wrath of fellow restaurant owners. As indicated below, the policy intervention that the community partner eventually took the lead in developing, based in part on the study findings, proved far more important and feasible. A key step in this process involved the community partner's creating its own report focused on the research findings for the specific audience and purposes of organizing for future policy change, discussed below (www.cpasf.org). Similarly, the health department partner provided invaluable feedback on what sorts of health department interventions were within its purview and realistic, particularly in a time of severe budget and staffing cutbacks.

Improving Data Interpretation

Using CBPR can improve data collection. Community partners greatly enhanced the accuracy of data interpretation on multiple fronts. They pointed out, for example, that the proportion of workers reporting that they got "paid sick leave" (58%) was likely quite inflated, reflecting the fact that for many in this community, paid sick leave simply means that one can take a day off when ill or caring for a sick relative and make it up later with no pay (Minkler and Chang 2013). Similarly, when the observational checklist data revealed that almost 90% of cooks failed to wear long sleeves—a fact academic partners attributed solely to the heat of the kitchen—workers added that burn marks and scars received while cooking were for many considered "badges of honor."

Identifying and Using New Channels for Dissemination

Use of CBPR can facilitate the identification and use of new channels for dissemination. Although the importance of traditional academic and professional vehicles for dissemination of findings cannot be minimized, community partners can play an important role in determining how best to reach the community "end users" of findings, as well as policy makers. As noted above, the CPA held bimonthly "worker teas" in the community to help provide education and training based in part on study findings. They also worked with another community organization, the Data Center, to package study findings, highlight quotes from workers, and advance recommendations for action in an eye-catching booklet entitled, "Check, Please!" (Chinese Progressive Association 2010). The report was released at a press conference attended by a packed crowd of 170, including close to two dozen representatives of the mainstream and ethnic press, and four of the city's eleven supervisors. These and other events (e.g., two rallies on city hall steps and worker testimony at hearings) helped disseminate findings in ways that could make a profound impact long before journal articles appeared in print.

Translating Findings into Action

CBPR can help translate research findings into action that will benefit the community. The Chinatown study was focused, since its inception, on developing policy- and practice-relevant data that could help promote change. The health department partner played an important role in writing letters to several key agencies, citing study findings and urging far stronger compliance with existing labor laws as well as verifying workers compensation insurance in the issuance of new business licenses (Gaydos et al. 2011). Concurrently, the community partner co-created a new coalition, the Progressive Workers Alliance; together these partners crafted a "low-wage worker bill of rights" grounded in study findings and ultimately pushed for an ordinance that would codify key elements of the "bill of rights"—a wage theft ordinance—into law. Through effective partnership building, rallies, and testimony, as well as considerable work with policy allies in government, the legislation was unanimously passed by the board of supervisors and signed by the mayor in fall 2011.

Empowering the Community

CBPR can help build individual and community capacity and leave behind a community better able to study and address other health and social issues of local concern. A major outcome of the Chinatown study was the individual, organizational, and community capacity built through the training and active engagement of two dozen immigrant restaurant workers in the study and action components of the work. While the CPA gained new visibility and benefited from a major new grant, of greater importance was the cultivation and training of a new generation of worker leaders, many of whom have remained active with the organization and in other efforts to improve their community. In the words of one core leader, "When I first got involved in this survey project, I thought it was impossible to change anything in Chinatown. But now that we have done so much work in the community and helped other workers recover wages, I see that change is possible. We can improve things. We must!"

CHALLENGES AND LIMITATIONS IN CBPR WITH IMMIGRANT WORKERS

Many challenges and obstacles are encountered by partners engaging in CBPR, and these often are intensified when immigrant community partners are involved. We describe some of the key challenges below.

Time- and Labor-Intensive

Building and maintaining partnerships takes substantial time both early on and throughout the research and action process (Israel et al. 2006; Seifer 2006). This often is compounded with immigrant workers, who frequently work long hours and return home to serve as primary caregivers across generations. Translation costs and time delays, and the extra training time needed to work with partnerships that vary dramatically in education, social class, and racial/ethnic background, also add to the time and costs incurred (Minkler and Chang 2013). Finally, CBPR's call to include action as part of the research process itself often requires the engagement of outside researchers and their partners well beyond the funded project period.

Conflict and Power Dynamics

Partners who engage in a CBPR project must be comfortable dealing with conflict. Struggles over power, the just allocation of resources, and elements of the study design and implementation are part of the process itself. Developing initial ground rules and memorandums of understanding (MOUs), as well as being clear about such fixed parameters as institutional review board (IRB) requirements, may help address such concerns early on. Further, a strong process evaluation, with evaluators reporting back to the group periodically and "calling time" when project process needs to be attended to more directly, can be of significant value (Chang et al. 2012).

Some immigrant group partners may be reluctant to openly air their concerns when doing so means challenging partners with more education and better command of English, particularly in areas related to research. Contexts of reception or opportunity structures immigrant communities face in terms of labor market constraints and economic vulnerability, as well as experiences with racial or linguistic prejudice and exposure to a hostile immigration discourse, can shape a community's readiness and willingness to participate fully in civic and political activities, including CBPR (Chang 2010). Demonstrated openness and valuing of the immigrant partners' contributions on the part of the academic and other partners is a strategy that has proven effective in this regard. Similarly, small-group meetings incorporating critical reflection and action, which allow immigrant (and other) partners to talk among themselves, and then having a representative speak to the larger body on behalf of their group also has demonstrated utility.

Scientific versus Community Concerns

The enhanced cultural sensitivity and relevance of research instruments made possible by high-level community collaboration may also at times conflict with outside research partners' desires for the most rigorous possible research designs and study instruments. Community partners may question the relevance of certain validated scales or may oppose on the grounds of fairness intervention designs such as randomized controlled trials (RCTs) since not all gain equal benefit (Buchanan et al. 2007; Israel et al. 2005; Minkler and Chang 2013). Early and continuing discussions about the meaning of concepts like "validity" from a science and a community perspective, as well as discussions of the need for both scientifically strong data and findings that matter locally and reflect local knowledge, can help address, yet often not fully resolve, these conflicts.

Disagreements over the Dissemination and Use of Findings

Not infrequently in CBPR and related approaches, community partners may wish to move more quickly from preliminary findings to action, including advocating for changes in programs, practices, and policies, while academically trained research partners may wish to move more slowly, insuring the accuracy of any findings put forward and in some cases waiting for peer review. Conversely, findings may emerge that could cast the community in an unfavorable light, and community partners might not want to have to "go public" (Flicker et al. 2007). Continued dialogue and MOUs may be helpful in anticipating such "what-ifs" and deciding on ways to deal with them early on, but such methods are not likely to preclude unanticipated issues from arising that will require the utmost care as they are addressed.

Challenges to Evaluation

Although a strong process and outcomes evaluation is integral to effective CBPR, this component of the work will also take time and resources that may be in short supply. Discussing early and often the importance of evaluation to the project's continued progress and achievement of its goals, and where possible, having a designated evaluator and creating an evaluation subcommittee with members representing different partnership groups, may increase both the appreciation and the efficacy of the evaluation component of the work.

IMPLICATIONS AND LESSONS LEARNED

CBPR involves many challenges, from the substantial time and labor involved through the compromises that must sometimes be reached over research design and other key aspects of the work. As suggested above, these challenges may be intensified when immigrant community partners, often with limited command of English and severe time and income constraints, are involved as key partners. The added fiscal burdens that may be incurred simply in relation to adequate translation, for example, are worthy of note. Yet as illustrated through the Chinatown study described above, the potential of CBPR for improving the relevance of the research and the validity of data collected, and for enhancing the dissemination and implementation of findings, may well outweigh the limitations involved. Based on this and other CBPR case studies with immigrant populations, we present several key lessons learned and their implications for research and practice.

1. Involve multiple stakeholders, including, where possible, a strong autonomous and well-respected community partner with deep roots in the immigrant community. As illustrated in the Chinatown case study, having as a partner a local health department can also be important for gaining entrée into the community and environments (e.g., immigrant worksites) that otherwise would likely be "off limits."

2. Include "bridge people." Different partners on the project served as vital bridges between the community and academic and health department professionals, and between the community-based organization and the community. These bridging individuals facilitate collaboration while partners are still getting to know each other and building trust.

3. Through secondary grants or other means, insure from the outset substantial funds for translation so that non-English-speaking immigrant partners will be actively involved from the beginning. Conducting partnership meetings in languages other than English allows for more spontaneous participation by partners with limited English proficiency and can provide some counterbalance to language power dynamics within the partnership.

4. Collaboratively develop ground rules, MOUs, or other devices (e.g., subcommittee meetings) to help ensure equitable participation, even (and especially) when difficult or contentious issues are being discussed.

5. Emphasize co-learning throughout, including discussion of topics such as research rigor and validity, different ways of knowing, and how to balance and accommodate the need for strong science with the equally important need for action, and balancing "stories and statistics" for maximum policy impact.

6. In data collection and analysis, as well as dissemination and use of findings, pay primary attention to issues of greatest relevance to immigrant and other community partners (in the Chinatown study, although data were collected on problems such as slips and falls, "wage theft" was by far the topic of greatest local importance, and many questions therefore were added in this area). Provide adequate time and resources for in-depth, participatory project evaluation from the outset, with a well-trained lead evaluator who can effectively engage the full team (and ideally an evaluation subcommittee) throughout the process.

7. Plan for sustainability through continued training and leadership development of community partners, helping the community partner find new funding streams, seeking out policy mentors and cultivating those relationships, and having all partners commit to the long haul by being present and active as needed beyond the funded project period.

8. Expand your base throughout, hiring and training new immigrant community members to help build the community partner organization, identifying new policy and other stakeholders, and "building alliances across differences" (Chavez et al. 2008). Recognition and sharing of the relevance of your group's findings to those of other immigrant and worker groups (e.g., Latino day laborers and domestic workers from a variety of backgrounds) is critical to building coalitions for united action.

RESOURCES

The following resources may be useful to partnerships or coalitions interested in exploring or conducting community-based participatory research with immigrant and other underserved populations.

- Community Campus Partnerships for Health (www.ccph.info/): This national organization, with a strong online presence, frequent webinars, and an active listserve, as well as national meetings and trainings, is particularly helpful for learning about potential funding, training, and other resources for CBPR, including work with immigrant populations.

- The community tool box (http://ctb.ku.edu.): Developed by the Work Group for Community Health and Development at the University of Kansas (KU), the community toolbox is an extensive Internet-based support interface for participatory research and evaluation, community assessment, and related endeavors.

- PolicyLink (www.policylink.org): A national organization committed to health and social equity and using the lessons of community building "on the ground" to help effect policy-level change, PolicyLink is a strong supporter of CBPR. Its website includes numerous resources on this and related topics, and it hosts meetings and webinars, as well as an active listserve, for those interested in working with immigrants and other underserved populations.

- *Research for Organizing: A Toolkit for Participatory Action Research from the Community Development Project.* http://www.researchfororganizing.org.

- *Speaking Truth, Creating Power: A Guide to Policy Work for Community Based Participatory Research Practitioners.* Workbook by C. Ritas, 2003. http://futurehealth.ucsf.edu/pdf_files/Ritas.pdf (accessed January 15, 2011).

- *Community-Based Participatory Research: Assessing the Evidence.* By M. Viswanathan, A. Ammerman, E. Eng, G. Gartlehner, et al. Evidence Report/Technology Assessment No. 99. Rockville, MD: RTI–University of North Carolina, 2004.

- "Community-Based Participatory Research." By S. D. Tandon, and S. C. Kwon. In *Asian American Communities and Health: Context, Research, Policy and Action,* edited by C. Trinh-Shevrin, N. S. Islam, and M. S. Rey (pp. 464–503). San Francisco: Jossey Bass, 2009.

- *Community-Based Participatory Research for Health: From Process to Outcomes.* By M. Minkler and N. Wallerstein (2nd ed.). San Francisco: Jossey-Bass, 2008.

- *Methods in Community Based Participatory Research for Health.* By B. Israel, E. Eng, A. Schulz, and E. A. Parker. San Francisco: Jossey-Bass, 2005.

- "The Value and Challenges of Participatory Research: Strengthening Its Practice." By M. Cargo and S. Mercer. *Annual Review of Public Health* 29(1) (2008): 325–50.

- "Promoting Environmental Justice through Community-Based Participatory Research: The Role of Community and Partnership Capacity." By M. Minkler, V. A. Brechwich, M. Tajik, and D. Petersen. *Health Education and Behavior* 35 (2008): 119–37.

REFERENCES

Abe-Kim, J., David T. Takeuchi, Seunghye Hong, Nolan Zane, Stanley Sue, Michael S. Spencer, Hoa Appel, Ethel Nicdao, and Margarita Alegría. 2007. "Use of Mental Health–Related Services among Immigrant and US-Born Asian Americans: Results from the National Latino and Asian American Study." *American Journal of Public Health* 97 (1):91–98.

Arcury, Thomas A., Sara A. Quandt, and Allen Dearry. 2001. "Farmworker Pesticide Exposure and Community-Based Participatory Research: Rationale and Practical Applications." *Environmental Health Perspectives* 109 (Suppl. 3):429–34.

Bernhardt, Annette, Ruth Milkman, Nik Theodore, Douglas Heckathorn, Mirabai Auer, James DeFilippas, Ana Luz Gonzalez, Victor Narro, Jason Perelshteyn, Diana Polson, and Michael Spiller. 2009. *Broken Laws, Unprotected Workers: Violations of Employment and Labor Laws in America's Cities.* New York: National Employment Law Project.

Buchanan, David R., Franklin G. Miller, and Nina Wallerstein. 2007. "Ethical Issues in Community-Based Participatory Research: Balancing Rigorous Research with Community Participation in Community Intervention Studies." *Progress in Community Health Partnerships* 1 (2):153–60.

Cargo, Margaret, and Shawna L. Mercer. 2008. "The Value and Challenges of Participatory Research: Strengthening Its Practice." *Annual Review of PublicHealth* 29 (1): 325–50.

Chang, Charlotte. 2010. "Evaluation and Adaptations of a Community-Based Participatory Research Partnership in San Francisco's Chinatown." DrPH dissertation, School of Public Health, University of California, Berkeley. Berkeley: ProQuest/UMI. (Publication No. AAT 3413544).

Chang, Charlotte, Alicia Salvatore, Pam Tau Lee, Shaw San Liu, and Meredith Minkler. 2012. "Popular Education, Participatory Research, and Community Organizing with Immigrant Restaurant Workers in San Francisco's Chinatown: A Case Study." In *Community Organizing and Community Building for Health and Welfare,* edited by M. Minkler. Piscataway, NJ: Rutgers University Press. 246–68.

Chavez, Vivian, Bonnie Duran, Quinton E. Baker, Magdalena M. Avila, and N. Wallerstein. 2008. "The Dance of Race and Privilege in Community-Based Participatory Research." In *Community-Based Participatory Research for Health,* edited by M. Minkler and N. Wallerstein, 2nd ed., 91–103. San Francisco: Jossey-Bass.

Chinese Progressive Association. 2010. "Check, Please! Health and Working Conditions in San Francisco Chinatown." San Francisco: Chinese Progressive Association.

Farquhar, Stephanie A., and Yvonne L. Michael. 2004. "Poder es Salud/Power for Health: An Application of the Community Health Worker Model in Portland Oregon." *Journal of Interprofessional Care* 18 (4):445–57.

Flicker, Sarah, Robb Travers, Adrian Guta, Sean McDonald, and Aileen Meagher. 2007. "Ethical Dilemmas in Community-Based Participatory Research: Recommendations for Institutional Review Boards." *Journal of Urban Health* 84 (4):478–93.

Gaydos, Megan, Rajiv Bhatia, Alvaro Morales, Pam Tau Lee, Charlotte Chang, Alicia Salvatore, Shaw San Liu, Niklas Krause, and Meredith Minkler. 2011. "Promoting Health Equity and Safety in San Francisco's Chinatown Restaurants: Findings and Lessons Learned from a Pilot Observational Survey." *Public Health Reports* 126 (Suppl. 3):62–69.

Green, Lawrence W., M. Anne George, Mark Daniel, C. James Frankish, Carol P. Herbert, William R. Bowie, and Michel O'Neill. 1995. *Study of Participatory Research in Health Promotion: Review and Recommendations for the Development of Participatory Research in Health Promotion in Canada.* Vancouver, BC: Royal Society of Canada.

Israel, Barbara A., Eugenia Eng, Amy J. Schulz, and Edith A. Parker. 2005. "Introduction to Methods in Community-Based Participatory Research for Health." In *Methods in Community-Based Participatory Research for Health,* edited by B. A. Israel, E. Eng, A. J. Schulz, and E. A. Parker, 3–26. San Francisco: Jossey-Bass.

Israel, Barbara A., James Krieger, David Vlahov, Sandra Ciske, Mary Foley, Princess Fortin, J. R. Guzman, R. Lichtenstein, Ann-Gel Palermo, and Gary Tang. 2006. "Challenges and Facilitating Factors in Sustaining Community-Based Participatory Research Partnerships: Lessons Learned from the Detroit, New York City and Seattle Urban Research Centers." *Journal of Urban Health* 83 (6):1022–40.

Israel, Barbara A., Amy J. Schulz, Edith A. Parker, and Adam B. Becker. 1998. "Review of Community-Based Research: Assessing Partnership Approaches to Improve Public Health." *Annual Review of Public Health* 19:173–202.

Junn, Jane. 1999. "Participation in Liberal Democracy: The Political Assimilation of Immigrants and Ethnic Minorities in the United States." *American Behavioral Scientist* 42 (9):1417.

Krieger, James W., Tim K. Takaro, Lin Song, and Marcia Weaver. 2005. "The Seattle-King County Healthy Homes Project: A Randomized, Controlled Trial of a Community Health Worker Intervention to Decrease Exposure to Indoor Asthma Triggers." *American Journal of Public Health* 95 (4):652–59.

McQuiston, Chris, Emilio A. Parrado, Julio Cesar Olmos-Muniz, and Alejandro M. Bustillo Martinez. 2005. "Community-Based Participatory Research and Ethnography: The Perfect Union." In *Methods in Community Based Participatory Research for Health*, edited by B. A. Israel, E. Eng, A. J. Schulz, and E. A. Parker. San Francisco: Jossey-Bass. 210–29.

Minkler, Meredith. 2005. "Community-Based Research Partnerships: Challenges and Opportunities." *Journal of Urban Health* 82 (2 Supp 2):ii3–ii12.

Minkler, Meredith, and Charlotte Chang. 2013. "Engaging Communities in Participatory Research and Action." In *Oxford Handbook of Public Health Practice*, 3rd ed., edited by Charles Guest, Walter Ricciardi, Ichiro Kawachi, and Iain Lang. Oxford: Oxford University Press. 198–209.

Minkler, Meredith, Pam Tau Lee, Alex Tom, Charlotte Chang, Alvaro Morales, Shaw San Liu, Alicia Salvatore, Robin Baker, Feiyi Chen, Rajiv Bhatia, and Niklas Krause. 2010. "Using Community-Based Participatory Research to Design and Initiate a Study on Immigrant Worker Health and Safety in San Francisco's Chinatown Restaurants." *American Journal of Industrial Medicine* 53 (4):361–71.

Minkler, Meredith, and Alicia L. Salvatore. 2012. "Participatory Approaches for Study Design and Analysis in Dissemination and Implementation Research." In *Dissemination and Implementation Research in Health*, edited by R. C. Brownson, G. A. Colditz, and E. K. Proctor, 192–212. New York: Oxford University Press.

Minkler, Meredith, and Nina Wallerstein, eds. 2008. *Community-Based Participatory Research for Health: From Process to Outcomes*. 2nd ed. San Francisco: Jossey-Bass.

O'Fallon, Liam R., and Allen Dearry. 2002. "Community-Based Participatory Research as a Tool to Advance Environmental Health Sciences." *Environmental Health Perspectives* 110 (Suppl. 2):155–59.

Ramakrishnan, S. Karthick, and Thomas J. Espenshade. 2001. "Immigrant Incorporation and Political Participation in the United States." *International Migration Review* 35 (3):870–909.

Restaurant Opportunities Center of New York. 2005. *Behind the Kitchen Door: Pervasive Inequality in New York City's Thriving Restaurant Industry*. New York: Restaurant Opportunities Center of New York and the New York City Restaurant Industry Coalition.

Rhodes, Scott D., Kenneth C. Hergenrather, Fred R. Bloom, Jami S. Leichliter, and Jaime Montano. 2009. "Outcomes from a Community-Based, Participatory Lay Health Adviser HIV/STD Prevention Intervention for Recently Arrived Immigrant Latino Men in Rural North Carolina." *AIDS Education and Prevention* 21 (Suppl. 5): 103–8.

Salvatore, Alicia L., Jonathan Chevrier, Asa Bradman, José Camacho, Jesús López, Geri Kavanagh-Baird, Meredith Minkler, and Brenda Eskenazi. 2009. "A Community-Based Participatory Worksite Intervention to Reduce Pesticide Exposures to Farmworkers and Their Families." *American Journal of Public Health* 99 (S3):S578–S581.

Seifer, Sarena D. 2006. "Building and Sustaining Community-Institutional Partnershipsfor Prevention Research: Findings from a National Collaborative." *Journal of Urban Health* 83(6): 989–1003.

Schulz, Amy J., Barbara A. Israel, Edith A. Parker, Murlisa Lockett, Yolanda Hill, and Rochelle Wills. 2001. "The East Side Village Health Worker Partnership: Integrating Research with Action to Reduce Health Disparities." *Public Health Reports* 116 (6):548–57.

Takeuchi, David T., Margarita Alegría, James S. Jackson, and David R. Williams. 2007. "Immigration and Mental Health: Diverse Findings in Asian, Black, and Latino Populations." *American Journal of Public Health* 97 (1):11–12.

Tandon, S. Darius, and Simona C. Kwon. 2009. "Community-Based Participatory Research." In *Asian American Communities and Health: Context, Research, Policy, and Action*, edited by C. Trinh-Shevrin, N. Islam, and M. J. Rey. San Francisco: Jossey-Bass. 464–503.

Tervalon, Melanie, and Jane Murray-Garcia. 1998. "Cultural Humility versus Cultural Competence: A Critical Distinction in Defining Physician Training Outcomes in Multicultural Education." *Journal of Health Care for the Poor and Underserved* 9 (2):117–25.

US Census Bureau. 2000. Summary file 3: P49: Sex by Industry for the Employed Civilian Population 16 Years and Over. Accessed January 5, 2014. https://www.census.gov /population/www/cen2000/sfiles/SF3-pop.html#top.

Viswanathan, Meera, Alice Ammerman, Eugenia Eng, Gerald Gartlehner, Kathleen N. Lohr, Derek Griffith, Scott Rhodes, Carmen Samuel-Hodge, Siobhan Maty, Linda Lux, Lucille Webb, Sonya F. Sutton, Tammeka Swinson, Anne Jackman, and Lynn Whitener. 2004. "Community-Based Participatory Research: Assessing the Evidence." Evidence Report/Technology Assessment No. 99. Rockville, MD: Agency for Healthcare Research and Quality.

Webster, Timothy. 2001. "Occupational Hazards in Eating and Drinking Places." *Compensation and Working Conditions* (Summer):27–33.

Wong, Janelle., S. Karthick Ramakrishnan, Taeku Lee, and Jane Junn. 2011. *Asian American Political Participation: Emerging Constituents and Their Political Identities*. New York: Russell Sage Foundation.

Woo, Shinoff C., and N. Krause. 2003. *Working Conditions and Health of Hotel Kitchen Workers in San Francisco*. Unpublished Report, San Francisco. ·

World Health Organization (WHO). 1946. Preamble to the Constitution of the World Health Organization as Adopted by the International Health Conference, New York, 19–22 June 1946; signed on 22 July 1946 by the representatives of 61 States (Official Records of the World Health Organization, no. 2, p. 100) and entered into force on 7 April 1948.

The findings and conclusions in this chapter are those of the authors and do not necessarily represent the views of the National Institute for Occupational Safety and Health.

20

Occupational Health Research with Immigrant Workers

Michael A. Flynn
Donald E. Eggerth

INTRODUCTION

Work is the principal driver of current international immigration. Over half of the 214 million international immigrants are labor migrants actively participating in the workforce; their families account for an additional 40% of the global immigrant population (ILO 2009). The globalization of the world economy is characterized by increased flows of labor across international borders and has contributed to an increasingly complex pattern of international migration as well. While traditional immigration patterns persist (e.g., Mexicans migrating to the United States), new ones have also emerged in the past thirty years (e.g., immigrants now represent 92% of the workforce in Qatar) (IMI 2006; ILO 2009). Despite the increasing complexity of labor migrations or differences in destinations, one thing remains constant—the vast majority of immigrants are employed in what have come to be known as "3-D"—dirty, demanding, and dangerous—jobs (Connell 1993). Despite the centrality of work to the lives of immigrants and the often difficult and dangerous jobs they perform, little attention has been paid by researchers to the occupational health of immigrants. Ahonen et al. (2007) reported that a search of the literature on occupational health and migration yielded only forty-eight articles in English or Spanish from 1990 to 2005. This chapter discusses central themes and methodological considerations for doing occupational health research with immigrant populations. While the chapter is written from the perspective of current research with Latino immigrants in the United States, the themes are applicable worldwide.

Immigration from Latin America to the United States has experienced tremendous growth over the past twenty years, and there are about 19 million Latino immigrants living in the United States today (Pew 2011). This growth has been accompanied by geographic expansion into nontraditional settlement areas such as the Midwest and Southeast regions of the United States as immigration patterns have responded to job opportunities in the service, construction, and meat processing industries in these areas of the country (Pew 2005; Striffler 2007). This rapid and unanticipated growth in areas without bilingual infrastructure or a history of a Latino community presents unique challenges and opportunities for immigrants, employers, and the communities at large (Pew 2005). Although most immigrants from Latin America are authorized to be in the United States, increasing numbers of recent Latino immigrants are here without legal status. For example, the Pew Hispanic Center estimated that roughly 80% of Mexican immigrants coming to the United States in the last decade were undocumented (Passel and Cohn 2009).

The recent increase of Latino immigration has been accompanied by growing occupational health disparities for Latino immigrant workers. Latino immigrants to the US have a workplace fatality rate of 5.9 per 100,000 person-years, which is almost half again as much as the rate for all workers (4.0) and even greater when compared to Latinos born in the United States (3.5) (CDC 2008). Richardson, Ruser, and Suarez (2003) report that as a group, Latinos have higher rates of nonfatal occupational illness and injury than non-Latinos. Unfortunately, the data reported in this study did not distinguish between immigrant and native-born Latinos. However, the fatality rates mentioned above suggest that immigrants may be the driving force behind these elevated rates of injuries and illnesses. These rates are not only an affront to core values of our society such as equal opportunity and equal protection, but they are of significant concern on a practical level as well. As the US population ages, immigrants, particularly Latinos, will make up an increasing percentage of the workforce. The Pew Hispanic Center (2008) estimates that immigrants will make up roughly 23% of adults of working age in 2050, up from 15% in 2005. Occupational injury and illness currently represent one of the highest health-related economic burdens in the United States. The combined direct and indirect cost of occupational injury and illness in the United States in 2007 was $250 billion, up from an inflation-adjusted $217 billion in 1992 (Leigh 2011). If occupational safety and health (OSH) disparities are not reduced or eliminated for Latino immigrant workers, these costs to society will increase as Latino immigrant participation in the workforce grows over time.

Latino immigrants make up roughly 7% of the workforce in the United States and are concentrated in four industry sectors: services 43%, warehousing 16%, construction 16%, and manufacturing 13% (Pew 2009). Despite this, the majority of the limited research related to Latino immigrants has focused on the agricultural sector, which represents about 5% of the Latino immigrant workforce. Over the past ten years the construction sector has been increasingly represented in the literature and to a lesser degree meat and poultry processing plants (Smith-Nonini 2003; Stuesse 2009; Quandt et al. 2006; Dong and Platner 2004; Loh and Richardson 2004). While research in these industry sectors should continue, it is imperative that additional research be conducted to ensure that the industries employing the majority of Latino immigrants are represented.

RESEARCH AREAS

Eliminating occupational health disparities for immigrant populations requires improved knowledge in three key areas. First, further surveillance needs to be conducted to give a more accurate picture of what is going on with OSH among immigrants (i.e., who is getting hurt, how it is occurring, and what is being done in response to the injuries). Second, there is a need to better understand those aspects of the immigrant experience that lead to increased occupational morbidity and mortality compared to other workers. Finally, research is needed to find effective ways to prevent occupational injuries and illnesses among immigrants and to eliminate these disparities.

Surveillance

Data for identifying and tracking occupational health disparities can come from a variety of sources, such as primary surveillance programs, secondary sources, convenience sampling, and targeted smaller studies.

Primary Surveillance.   Primary surveillance entails efforts whose specific purpose is to collect data related to occupational safety and health. The US Department of Labor's Census of Fatal Occupational Injuries (CFOI) and the Survey of Occupational Injuries and Illness (SOII) are the principal occupational health surveillance systems in the US on a national level. The CFOI is an example of active surveillance because it searches out data from over twenty-five types of sources, whereas the SOII is considered a passive surveillance system because it relies primarily on reviewing employer records of injuries (Souza et al. 2011). While these systems are the most comprehensive data that exist, they are not perfect tools. The CFOI collects a significant amount of demographic data, including country of birth; however, it does not include variables such as immigration status of the victim or duration of time living in the US. It would be helpful to include that information in the future because immigration status has long been hypothesized as contributing to OSH disparities for immigrants (Schenker 2010). Conversely, employer records used by SOII are often missing basic demographic data such as race/ethnicity. Additionally, the SOII data is acknowledged to be incomplete because employees, especially vulnerable ones like immigrant workers, likely do not report every injury to their employers for fear of reprisals, and employers likely do not record every injury so they can avoid negative consequences such as Occupational Safety and Health Administration (OSHA) fines or increased workers' compensation premiums (Azaroff et al. 2002; Ruser 2008; Souza et al. 2010).

Another form of primary surveillance involves inclusion of occupational health items in larger population-based surveys. An example of this would be inclusion of occupational health items in the US Department of Labor's National Agricultural Workers Survey (NAWS), which is administered annually to between 1,500 and 4,000 crop workers (Steege et al. 2009). NAWS generates important information on the occupational health of farmworkers in part because of the considerable effort to ensure that the data collection instruments and methods address the unique characteristics of this workforce. However, even these extensive efforts cannot guarantee a truly representative sample, which ultimately threatens generalizability (Souza et al. 2010). Another limitation to including OSH items in population-based surveys such as NAWS is the restriction it puts on the number of items that can be included in the instrument, thereby reducing the amount of data that can be collected on any one topic. Despite these limitations, efforts such as NAWS generate substantial data and are essential tools for understanding the occupational health of immigrant workers.

Chronic occupational illnesses are perhaps the hardest to track given the current surveillance systems. In part, this is because of the lag time separating occupational exposure to toxins and the emergence of the attendant illness. In some cases, this period is so long that neither worker nor health care provider thinks to make a connection. Consequently, the OSH community is advocating for occupational data fields to be included in electronic medical records, which could potentially provide a wealth of data on occupational illness as well as injuries (Filios et al. 2008).

Secondary Surveillance.   Secondary surveillance efforts involve mining datasets that did not initially target occupational health. Souza et al. (2010) point to several studies (Fleming et al. 2003; Caban-Martinez et al. 2007) using data from the National Health Interview Survey (NHIS) that have been employed to document occupational health disparities. Secondary data can be particularly useful in studying immigrant populations because national health studies may target or oversample groups, such as immigrants and ethnic minorities, which are often underrepresented in current occupational health surveillance (Souza et al. 2010). However, Schenker (2010) cautions that national population-based surveys such as the Hispanic Health and Nutrition Examination Survey often run into sampling errors due to issues such as language, residential stability, and a tendency to focus on urban populations.

Convenience Sampling.   Due to barriers of language, culture, and immigration status, Latino immigrant workers are often very difficult to recruit as research participants. Consequently, many studies, both quantitative and qualitative, rely upon convenience samples. Although convenience samples have the advantage of making recruitment easier, there are almost always questions regarding the representativeness of the sample and consequently the extent to which the study results are generalizable to the population of interest. The most common recruitment strategies typically fall into one of two categories. One strategy is to recruit from naturally occurring gatherings of immigrants, such as workplaces, church services, or community festivals. The other strategy is to work with organizations that already have the trust of the immigrant community and that are willing to endorse study participation to their constituents.

When a group is poorly represented in the literature, it is clear that nearly any systematically collected information is better than no information at all. However, when interpreting study results, one must always bear in mind the limitations to generalization of findings. For example, the Health Foundation of Greater Cincinnati (2006) recruited a sample of over five hundred Latinos at a large community festival sponsored by a church-affiliated community service organization. The participants were surveyed on a wide variety of health-related topics via items from standardized questionnaires. Nearly all of the items were also used in the foundation's health survey of the Greater Cincinnati area, which used a sophisticated sampling technique to ensure that the participants were representative of the area's population. This approach provided a rare opportunity to contrast Latino immigrant responses to those of the host community. However, because convenience sampling was used for the Latino sample, it is difficult to draw clear conclusions as there is no way of knowing if the sample is representative of the population.

Recruiting from workplaces not only involves difficulties related to representativeness of the participants, but also poses issues related to the validity of the responses. Many Latino immigrants report that they feel very vulnerable to job loss and/or retaliation from employers (Walter et al. 2002; O'Connor et al. 2000; CPWR 2004). Consequently, many are reluctant to respond in a manner they fear might somehow anger their employers. O'Connor, Gildner, and Easter (2000) report that many Latino immigrants believe that the basis of their attractiveness to American employers is that Latinos "work hard" and "don't complain"—breaking this stereotype risks reducing their employability.

Partnering with organizations that are trusted by the immigrant community can sometimes help to broaden the subject pool for an investigation. However, representativeness remains an issue. For example, working with a labor union that is trusted by its immigrant members can help increase access, but Latino immigrants might be underrepresented as they are far less likely to be union members (Dong and Platner 2004). Working with community service agencies or advocacy groups has its own set of constraints. These organizations are often staffed by members of the community they serve. Consequently, fearing breaches of confidentiality, participants may be hesitant to respond truthfully when surveyed regarding sensitive topics. In addition, these organizations frequently initiate recruiting with the community members who are most involved with its activities. Expansion beyond this initial pool typically utilizes the "snowball" sampling method, wherein participants are asked to recommend others who might be interested in participating (Goodman 1961). These recommendations are frequently family members, friends, or neighbors. Again, representativeness of the sample becomes an issue. Response-driven sampling is a nuanced version of snowball sampling that attempts to reduce its inherent biases while maintaining its usefulness in reaching "hidden" populations such as undocumented immigrant workers (Heckathorn 1997).

Targeted Smaller Studies. The move to a more temporary and mobile workforce, underrepresentation of immigrants in traditional sampling techniques, and the lack of data fields specific to immigrant workers (i.e., primary language, time in the United States, immigration status, etc.) often reduce the effectiveness of traditional occupational epidemiology methods in documenting the health status of immigrant workers. This has led researchers to utilize more targeted and tailored efforts, often referred to as "shoe-leather" epidemiology, to further understand the occupational health of immigrants. In an attempt to better understand the occupational health of immigrant workers, Gany et al. (2011) developed a survey that specifically looked at history of workplace injuries, access to resources, and reporting behaviors. The survey was administered in person to Mexican nationals seeking services at the Mexican consulate in New York City. Gany and colleagues found that respondents were at high risk for occupational illness and injury, were not receiving adequate safety training, and were underreporting occupational injury. Targeted local efforts like this are an important complement to national surveillance efforts because they allow for a deeper and more nuanced examination of the occupational health of immigrant workers and are essential in gaining a better understanding of occupational injury, illness, and service utilization in the local immigrant community.

Methods used for occupational epidemiology need to reflect the changing nature of work and the demographics of the workforce (Schenker 2010). In an attempt to identify and address some of the deficiencies discussed above, the National Institute for Occupational Safety and Health organized the "Workshop on Improving Surveillance for Occupational Health Disparities" in April of 2008. One of the outcomes of the workshop was identifying four key methodological challenges: defining the disparity, obtaining adequate data on exposures, correctly estimating denominators, and avoiding bias in the use of an occupation variable (Souza et al. 2010). While a detailed discussion of the findings at this meeting is beyond the scope of this chapter, the topic is explored in greater detail in a special issue of the *American Journal of Industrial Medicine* (Baron et al. 2010). It is clear that much still remains unknown about the occupational health of immigrants in the United States.

Barriers to OSH

A second area needing increased research efforts involves identifying why immigrants are injured at higher rates. Potential explanations can be grouped into three general categories: knowledge, culture, and structural barriers. This section provides an overview of each of these categories.

Knowledge.   All workers have a right to know the potential health risks their job presents and the measures that can be taken to avoid these risks. Immigrant workers are no different, but for several reasons they are often at a disadvantage when compared with native-born workers. Immigrants coming to the United States often find themselves working in an industry they did not have experience with back home (Eggerth et al. 2012). For example, many recent Latino immigrants come from the countryside, where they worked as subsistence farmers. Yet, upon arrival to the United States the majority find themselves in urban areas working in the manufacturing, service, and construction industries. They are often required to use machines, chemicals, and tools that are foreign to them, and they are unaware of how to use the tools of their new trade safely. Even those who worked in similar industries in their home country often face unfamiliar materials and technologies on the job in the United States. Additionally, immigrant workers are often unfamiliar with safety procedures and regulations common to the US workplace. Standard safety procedures, across a wide range of industries, may be different or nonexistent in the immigrant's home country. Furthermore, safety regulations and the level of enforcement differ from one country to the next. What may be considered safe or allowable in Mexico, for example, may be against regulations in the United States.

Culture.   While there have been increased efforts to address culture in public health research and interventions with immigrant workers, often these efforts, implicitly or explicitly, adopt a limited definition of culture. Culture is often reduced to a short list of static characteristics used to describe a particular group. For example, Latino culture is often characterized as being family oriented, fatalistic, and deferential to authority (Antshel 2002). While it is beyond the scope of this chapter to discuss the merits of these characterizations, we suggest that investigations using a broader understanding of culture are essential in understanding its contribution to occupational health disparities.

Generally speaking, research on culture and occupational health of immigrant workers should explore their shared set of beliefs, behaviors, and understanding of symbols, and how these impact safety and health at work. This represents a wide range of topics, but some areas of importance include the lived experience of immigrants and how they understand themselves as workers and members of society, their common assumptions about the role of employees and employers and the proper way to relate to coworkers and supervisors, and perceptions regarding dangers at work and how they address these risks. A recent ethnographic study of Latino immigrant workers in Chicago suggests that being perceived as "a hard worker" is a cultural adaptation to help them compete for jobs (Gomberg-Muñoz 2010). Maintaining this image often requires immigrants to work faster and harder than their native-born counterparts. This often gives these workers a competitive edge in the labor market but can also place them at increased risk for injury. Individuals who attempt to slow down and work at a sustainable pace are often coerced by other immigrants to work harder. A second study looked at how the commonly accepted understanding of the etiology for arthritis put Latino immigrant farmworkers at risk for increased pesticide exposure (Quandt et al. 2001). Specifically, hand-washing stations were provided to workers in the field as a way of avoiding transmission of pesticides from the hands to the mouth when the workers ate lunch. However, workers were reluctant to wash their hands with the cold water because they believed that exposure to cold water, especially after physical activity, contributed to developing arthritis. These examples highlight how shared beliefs, either brought from home or developed after arrival, can impact the occupational health of immigrant workers.

Language is perhaps the most commonly identified cultural trait that could potentially impact the safety and health of immigrant workers on the job. The inability of supervisors, management, and coworkers to communicate effectively with their immigrant coworkers and vice versa is frequently identified as contributing to occupational health disparities (NRC 2003). This is particularly common in areas of the United States such as the Midwest and South, which have little to no bilingual infrastructure. The lack of bilingual infrastructure in a company often leads managers to identify the "best" English speaker among the immigrant workers and have that person translate for the other workers. This presents several problems. First, it is likely that this person does not speak English well and therefore the manager is not clearly understood. Second, it creates a dependence on this person and enables him or her to exploit that position for his or her own gain, if the person is so so inclined, by telling the employer one thing and the workers another. Employers often assume a natural affinity between all individuals of a minority ethnic/racial group. However, the Latino community is not homogeneous, and immigrants who are more proficient in English frequently come from or have obtained a better socioeconomic status than those who are not. These employees can exhibit a range of attitudes from unintended paternalism to intentional bigotry toward immigrants from a lesser station in life. Their familiarity with the culture and lived immigrant reality allows them to more easily control and exploit their coworkers. This might be referred to as the "dark side of cultural competence." This is not to suggest that all privileged Latinos treat immigrants poorly or that Caucasian employees treat immigrants any better, but rather that ethnicity or race cannot be seen as a proxy for solidarity and/or homogeneity.

Structural Barriers.   While knowledge and culture may contribute to occupational health disparities, some researchers have expressed concern that focusing on these two factors has inadvertently shifted the burden of workplace safety from the employer to the immigrant worker (Cole and Brown 1996). They argue that structural barriers such as workplace policies and practices, social norms of the dominant group, and laws have a significant impact on workers being exposed to riskier situations and their capacity to address unsafe situations at work. The changing nature of work and how it is organized, discrimination, and increased vulnerability resulting from undocumented immigration status (i.e., not having permission to live and work in the United States) are examples of the structural barriers to occupational safety and health (OSH) that many Latino immigrant workers face on a daily basis.

Workplace Policies and Practice.   Government and industry policies and practices that influence how work is done and who does what work have changed dramatically in the past thirty years. The globalization of the economy has led to increased job insecurity, an increased power differential between employer and worker based on declining union participation, increased concentration of wealth, and increased stratification of the labor market (Quinlan and Sokas 2009; Siqueira et al. 2011; Landsbergis et al. 2011). A common explanation for the occupational health disparities of Latino immigrants has been that they are employed in more dangerous jobs. A recent study analyzed data from the Contingent Work Supplements in the Current Population Survey, along with the Quality of Employment Survey, and found that nonstandard work arrangements and lack of US citizenship may be more important than race and sex in channeling workers into less desirable, more dangerous jobs (Hudson 2007). Similarly, analysis of data from the American Community Survey and the Bureau of Labor Statistics Injuries, Illnesses, and Fatalities Program found that immigrants have a very limited range of employment opportunities and work in more dangerous jobs compared to native-born workers (Orrenius and Zavodny 2009). While these findings suggest that labor market segmentation is likely a contributing factor to occupational health disparities, they may not account for all the differences. Dong and Platner (2004) found that Latino construction helpers and roofers had far higher rates of fatal injuries than did non-Latinos who held the same positions. These disparities between workers with the same job may be the result of what is commonly referred to in Europe as "precarious employment" (Porthe et al. 2010). Undocumented immigrants in Spain identified several characteristics of precarious employment. including high job instability, lower wages, and difficulty exercising their rights, all of which directly or indirectly contribute to the occupational safety and health of an individual or group (Garcia et al. 2009).

Social Norms of the Dominant Group.   Discrimination based on racist or sexist societal norms that perpetuate power differentials between groups can negatively impact the physical and emotional heath of workers (Okechukwu et al. 2011). Workers not of the dominant group may be given harder or more dangerous tasks than their coworkers. For example, immigrant respondents in focus groups reported that they were often asked to work faster than their US-born counterparts or were denied basic protective equipment such as stools or gloves that their coworkers received (Flynn 2010). In addition, workers may often face reduced opportunities for advancement, increased chance of harassment or bullying, and unfair treatment, all of which contribute to occupational stress (Krieger et al. 2006). Eggerth et al. (2012) used focus groups and individual interviews to explore the work experience of Latina immigrants. Respondents reported that they not only faced occupational hazards similar to their male counterparts but also often had to contend with gender-specific concerns such as sexual harassment or increased employment insecurity because of pregnancy or child care. Additionally, they reported complications in their relationship with their husbands related to cultural expectations concerning the division of labor in the household as well as the challenges their increasing economic independence presented to the traditional family roles.

Legal Restrictions.   Federal and state laws and regulations can directly (e.g., OSHA regulations) and indirectly (e.g., immigration laws) impact the occupational health of workers (Siquiera et al. 2011). Undocumented immigration status is one of the most often mentioned legal barriers to occupational health for many Latino immigrants. In 2008 it was estimated that undocumented immigrants comprised 5.4% (8.9 million) of the total labor force (165 million) in the United States, up from 4.3% just five years earlier (Pew 2009). Undocumented immigrants come from all corners of the globe; however, the majority (80%) is from Latin America. While this topic is often mentioned as contributing to the occupational health disparities of immigrant workers, surprisingly little research has been conducted on it (Schenker 2010). In qualitative interviews with day laborers in San Francisco, Walter et al. (2002) found that undocumented status was related to occupational health in two ways. First, upon arriving to the United States immigrants often reported feeling pressure to repay the money they had borrowed to pay human smugglers to guide them across the border. This often led them to accept dangerous working conditions rather than turn down a day's wages. The second impact was the stress resulting from the constant fear of deportation. Another qualitative study with immigrants found that fear of job loss or deportation often results in immigrant workers not addressing dangerous situations at work (Flynn 2010). In addition, this study found that the recent wave of anti-immigrant legislation at the state and local level has not only legally excluded immigrants from some services and benefits but has also led many immigrants to believe they are ineligible for any legal protections, which leads many immigrants to avoid all institutions that might otherwise provide benefits. While this strategy of disengagement protects workers against deportation, in some circumstances it also prevents them from accessing resources they are entitled to, such as workers' compensation and OSHA protections.

Ironically, while structural barriers to OSH are often the most frequently identified by immigrant workers, they are the least studied in the literature. This suggests that while there is a need to develop a better understanding of all the barriers mentioned above, special attention should be paid to identifying and overcoming structural barriers.

Health Promotion

By law, in the United States, all workers must be trained regarding the occupational hazards associated with their jobs and the safety procedures used to avoid those hazards. However, research has generally found that Latino immigrant workers do not have access to effective safety training on the job either because training is not provided or because the training that is provided is of poor quality (NRC 2003). Recent efforts to improve OSH training for immigrant workers and other vulnerable worker populations are discussed at length in O'Connor et al. (2011). Two challenges to effectively promoting occupational safety and health for immigrant workers include the changing nature of work and the need for training to address barriers to safety beyond workers' knowledge and motivation. Research is needed to find effective ways of promoting OSH with immigrants in light of these and other challenges.

Changing Nature of Work.   Safety training has traditionally been provided on the job by the employer, a labor union, or both. As mentioned above, structural changes to the economy have led to a decline in the unionized workforce and a move to more temporary and tenuous work relationships (e.g., the use of labor contractors). These changes have often clouded who is responsible for providing training to workers. It is also increasingly common for workers to hold a variety of jobs over their lifetimes. This is especially true for contingent or temporary workers, who may not only change jobs but also seek employment in different industries several times in the same year (O'Connor et al. 2011). Organizations charged with promoting OSH have to adapt to these changes if they hope to remain effective and relevant. Finding settings outside the worksite to provide training is one potential way to address the challenge presented by the changing nature of work. This will often result in workers from a variety of employers, jobs, or industries attending the same training. Therefore a second challenge is developing content that is general enough that it will be relevant to workers from a variety of settings and will provide individuals with transferable safety skills if they switch jobs or industries.

Addressing Barriers.   Traditionally, training has focused on transferring specific knowledge and skills from the trainer to the employees and convincing them that it is important to do things safely. The underlying assumption of this model is that if the workers know how to work safely and want to work safely, they will. Conversely, unsafe behaviors or incidents on the job are sometimes perceived to be the result of workers not knowing how to work safely or not choosing to work in a safe manner. This has become known as the "blame the worker" perspective. However, as mentioned above, there are a variety of reasons why workers feel pressured to work in an unsafe manner. Neal and Griffin (2004) suggest that while individual workers have a role to play in maintaining a safe workplace, it is often the attitudes and policies of the employer that have a greater impact on how work is performed. These barriers ultimately suggest the need for long-term social, political, and legal changes. Public policy research to identify problems, create potential remedies, and find effective ways of implementing these changes is essential to these efforts but can take a long time to enact (see Siquiera et al. 2011). In the meantime workers need to be given the tools to recognize and minimize, if not overcome, barriers to working safely while simultaneously advocating for these barriers to be eliminated. Training is essential, but not sufficient, to overcome all the barriers to safety that workers may experience. However, those providing safety training must do a better job of responding to the lived reality of workers by acknowledging the barriers that exist, providing practical ways to address these situations, and improving their access to resources such as legal consultation that can aid them in responding to unsafe situations. Increased access to resources is particularly important for immigrant workers, who are often unaware of the regulatory structure in the United States and how to access it. They may also fear approaching institutions for help as a result of their immigration status. Partnerships between OSH organizations and community/advocacy organizations in the immigrant community are one important way of improving access to resources for immigrant workers.

Documenting occupational health disparities for immigrant workers and investigating why these disparities exist are essential research tasks, but will be purely academic if this knowledge is not used to develop effective interventions that help prevent injuries and reduce disparities. While much of this work can be carried out by community groups and activists, researchers are needed to develop and evaluate theory-based interventions rooted in the lived experience of workers so that effective replicable models can be developed and disseminated.

PRACTICAL CONSIDERATIONS

This section discusses some key considerations that we have found helpful in our research on occupational health and immigrant workers. Some of the challenges and benefits discussed here are unique to research on occupational safety and health, while others apply to research in all areas. This is not meant to be an exhaustive account but rather some tips we have discovered over the years.

Issues Unique to OSH

Unlike public health research on other topics, occupational health not only deals with issues related to the individual's health but also directly involves their livelihood. This can present methodological and ethical challenges. Workers are often reluctant to divulge information about problems with safety at work for fear their employer will find out and retaliate against them. This can lead to a range of problems, from incomplete data to job loss if respondents cannot be assured their information will be confidential. Most institutional review boards require standard methods to ensure that the data are not traceable to the individual. However, one potential weak link may be other research participants breaking confidentiality, intentionally or otherwise. For example, if two employees of the same company were to participate in the same focus group, one might reveal information damaging to his or her coworker by repeating comments heard in the group. This is a particular concern when research is conducted in smaller immigrant communities or in a particular worksite or industry where the potential pool of respondents is relatively small. Researchers must find ways to minimize these risks for the safety of the respondents and the quality of the data. Some suggestions could include ensuring that all focus group participants are employed by different companies or conducting individual interviews.

Another ethical concern involves protecting respondents who do not have documents allowing them to legally work in the United States. There are at least two major ethical concerns related to collecting data on undocumented status. The first is ensuring that these highly sensitive data remain confidential. There are several techniques, such as using pseudonyms, eliminating or not collecting other personally identifiable information, and building a series of firewalls in the recruiting process to ensure that there is no way of tracking the data back to specific individuals (Nuñez and Heyman 2007; Eggerth and Flynn 2010). The second concern is that by addressing undocumented status with individuals, they are being conditioned to openly discuss a topic that could be highly detrimental were they to disclose it under different circumstances. Contrary to popular belief, we have found that participants will often freely discuss their undocumented status during focus groups and interviews, even when they are not asked about it directly. Because the future behavior of respondents is beyond the control of the researchers, this concern is more difficult to address than the first. One remedy we have used is to caution participants about revealing their status under different circumstances. Another has been to partner with grassroots immigrant advocacy groups to help recruit study participants. These groups are generally involved in promoting the rights of immigrants and frequently hold workshops for the community regarding their rights when interacting with law enforcement personnel or other government officials. Data collection frequently takes place in their facilities, and literature on the services they provide is made available to participants. Undocumented status is an overarching concern for many immigrants; thus researching this aspect of their lives is important and consistent with good professional ethics, if the correct care and consideration is taken.

While research on occupational health has some additional challenges, it also has at least one significant advantage. Unlike many other public health issues, the prevention and treatment of occupational injury and illness in the United States and many countries has a significant legal component. Generally speaking, employees, regardless of immigration status, are entitled to safe working conditions, the necessary knowledge and equipment to be safe on the job, and compensation for work-related injury or illness. This means that workers have concrete legal rights to resources aimed at preventing and treating work-related injuries and illnesses. While there can be barriers to accessing these protections, it is important to remember that they do exist and even more important to find effective ways to leverage these resources and ensure immigrants' access to them.

General Issues

Effective research generally involves working closely with the community. Therefore, one of the most important decisions for a researcher is choosing the right community partners (Eggerth and Flynn 2010). As has been mentioned previously, immigrant communities are frequently heterogeneous, and social divisions (i.e., race, class, regionalism, etc.) are often unrecognized by researchers who are not intimately familiar with the community. It is therefore essential to be aware of the role and reputation potential research partners (individuals or organizations) have in the immigrant community. Unfortunately, it is common for researchers to assume that because someone can speak the language or shares the same race or ethnicity, he or she will automatically be an effective partner (O'Connor et al. 2011). More care must be taken to understand the social position of your partners in relation to your research participants and how this may impact their effectiveness in brokering the relationship with the community. While there is no simple, sure-fire way to vet potential partners, there are some general practices that may help identifying potential blind spots or prejudices of individuals involved in the project. First, remember that communities are diverse and this diversity often results in institutionalized power relationships. Second, discussing experiences of power, privilege, and oppression is often uncomfortable. Make a concerted effort to discuss these topics with all individuals involved in the project, including individuals from the immigrant community, when selecting team members, and throughout the research project. Finally, as with any potential employee, get referrals from a variety of community organizations when considering hiring someone. That being said, properly vetted members of the particular immigrant group are invaluable in research efforts and it is highly recommended that they form part of the research team.

Cross-cultural research on health disparities in general and OSH research in particular primarily focuses on documenting and understanding the minority group, such as immigrant workers. What is frequently ignored is that the researchers bring perspectives, prejudices, and assumptions to the project that are rooted in their own cultural backgrounds and social positions (O'Connor et al. 2011). If left unevaluated, the perspectives of the researchers can become the de facto norms for the study. This can lead to misunderstandings of core concepts of the study, which in turn can result in erroneous data and false conclusions. Unchecked assumptions can have more dire consequences as well. For example, a well-intentioned campaign encouraged immigrant workers who were injured on the job to report to their doctor that the accident was work related. However, the developers of the campaign did not consider the fact that many undocumented immigrants do not use their real names at work. This led to an individual losing his job because the name on the workers' compensation claim did not match his employer's records and he was suspected of working with fraudulent documents.

This example highlights the need for formative research and the strong involvement of community representatives in any research effort. Several methods for understanding the community's perspective and involving community members in the research process are described at length in other chapters of this book. One technique we have found to be particularly useful is cognitive interviewing (Willis 1999). Cognitive interviewing (or testing) refers to a series of related methods where the basic goal is to ensure that the researcher and the participants understand a particular concept, question, statement, or image in the same way. This technique has proven equally useful with translated materials, such as previously developed instruments, including "off-the-shelf" validated surveys, as well as original materials developed by native speakers of the target language. In short, since occupational health research has traditionally favored quantitative methods and so little is known about OSH and immigrants, it is important to emphasize the need for increased use of qualitative methods in all areas of investigation with immigrant workers. Simply put, in many circumstances, it is premature to go directly into quantitative data collection as we don't know the questions we should be asking or what any answers might mean.

CONCLUSION

Labor migration to the United States and across the globe is a central characteristic and result of the global economy. In this chapter, we have argued that gaining a better understanding of the types and rates of injuries suffered by immigrants, contributing factors to these injuries, and improved prevention measures, will not only aid in protecting some of the most vulnerable workers in any society but will also reduce the economic burden for occupational injury and illness on society as a whole. However, in order to reach these goals most effectively, researchers will need to be flexible enough to collaborate with community partners on research design and goals, as well as enlisting their support with participant recruitment and data collection. Researchers also need to recognize their own cultural biases and recognize they may have cultural "blind spots." Finally, it is of the utmost importance that any interventions proposed and/or developed can be implemented and sustained by existing community resources, long after the artificial influx of grant dollars is gone.

REFERENCES

Ahonen, E. Q., F. G. Benavides, and J. Benach. 2007. "Immigrant populations, work and health—A systemic literature review." *Scandinavian Journal of Work, Environment and Health* 33(2):96–104.

Antshel, K. M. 2002. "Integrating culture as a means of improving treatment adherence in the Latino population." *Psychology, Health and Medicine* 4(4):435–49.

Azaroff, L. S., C. Levenstien, and D. H. Wegman. 2002. "Occupational injury and illness surveillance: Conceptual filters explain underreporting." *American Journal of Public Health* 92:1421–29.

Baron, S., J. Cone, and K. Souza, eds. 2010. "Special Issue: Occupational Health Disparities." *American Journal of Industrial Medicine* 53:81–215.

Caban-Martinez A. J., D. J. Lee, L. E. Fleming, K. L Arheart, W. G. Leblanc, K. Chung-Bridges, et al. 2007. "Dental care access and unmet dental care needs among U.S. workers: The National Health Interview Survey, 1978 to 2003." *Journal of the American Dental Association* 138:227–30.

Centers for Disease Control and Prevention (CDC). 2008. "Work-related injury deaths among Hispanics—United States, 1992–2006." *Morbidity and Mortality Weekly Report* 57(22):596–600.

Center to Protect Workers' Rights (CPWR). 2004. *Spanish-speaking construction workers discuss their safety needs and experiences: Residential construction program training program evaluation report.* Silver Spring, MD: CPWR.

Cole, B. L., and M. P. Brown. 1996. "Action on worksite health and safety problems: A follow-up survey of workers participating in a hazardous waste worker training program." *American Journal of Industrial Medicine* 30:730–43.

Connell, J. 1993. "Kitanai, kitsui, and kiken: The rise of labor migration to Japan." *Economic and Regional Restructuring Research Unit*. Sydney: University of Sydney.

Dong, X., and J. W. Platner 2004. "Occupational fatalities of Hispanic construction workers from 1992 to 2000." *American Journal of Industrial Medicine* 45:45–54.

Eggerth, D. E., S. C. DeLaney, M. A. Flynn, and C. J. Jacobson. 2012. "Work experiences of Latina immigrants: A qualitative study." *Journal of Career Development* 39(1):13–30.

Eggerth, D. E., and M. A. Flynn. 2010. "When the Third World comes to the first: Ethical considerations when working with immigrant workers." *Ethics and Behavior* 20(3):229–42.

Filios, M., M. Attfield, J. Graydon, S. Marsh, S. Nwlin, J. Sestito, et al. 2008. "The case for collecting occupational health data elements in electronic health records." Accessed 22 February 2012. http://www.cste.org/dnn/Portals/0/The%20Case%20for%20Collecting%20Occ%20Health%20Data%20Elements%20in%20EHRs.pdf.

Fleming, L. E., O. Gomez-Marin, D. Zheng, F. Ma, and D. Lee. 2003. "National Health Interview Survey mortality among US farmers and pesticide applicators." *American Journal of Industrial Medicine* 43:227–33.

Flynn, M. A. 2010. "Undocumented status and the occupational lifeworlds of Latino immigrants in a time of political backlash: The workers' perspective." Master's thesis, University of Cincinnati, Cincinnati, Ohio. Retrieved 22 December 2011. http://etd.ohiolink.edu/view.cgi?acc_num = ucin1280776817.

Gany, F., R. Dobslaw, J. Ramirez, J. Tonda, I. Lobach, and J. Leng. 2011. "Mexican urban occupational health in the US: A population at risk." *Journal of Community Health* 36(2):175–79.

Garcia, A. M., M. J. Lopez-jacomb, A. A. Agudelo-Suarez, C. Ruiz-Frutos, E. Q. Ahonen, and V. Porthe. 2009. "Condiciones de trabajo y salud en inmigrantes (Proyecto ITSAL): Entrivistas a informes claves." *Gac Sanit* 23(2):91–99.

Gomberg-Muñoz, R. 2010. "Willingness to work: Agency and vulnerability in an undocumented immigrant network." *American Anthropologist* 112(2):295–307.

Goodman, L. A. 1961. Snowball Sampling. *Annals of Mathematical Statistics* 32:148–70.

Health Foundation of Greater Cincinnati. 2006. 2005 Greater Cincinnati Hispanic/Latino Health Survey. Cincinnati, OH: HFGC.

Heckathorn, D. D. 1997. "Respondent-driven sampling: A new approach to the study of hidden populations." *Social Problems* 44:2.

Hudson, K. 2007. "The new labor market segmentation: Labor market dualism in the new economy." *Social Science Research* 36:286–312.

International Labor Organization (ILO). 2009. "International labor migration and employment in the Arab region: Origins, consequences and the way forward." Accessed 16 February 2012. http://www.ilo.org/public/english/region/arpro/beirut/downloads/aef/migration_eng.pdf.

International Migration Institute (IMI). 2006. "Towards a new agenda for international migration research." James Martin Twenty-First Century School, University of Oxford. Accessed 16 February 2012. http://www.imi.ox.ac.uk/pdfs/a4-imi-research-agenda.pdf.

Krieger, N., P. D. Waterman, C. Hartman, L. M. Bates, A. M. Stoddard, M. M. Quinn, G. Sorensen, and E. M. Barbeau. 2006. "Social hazards on the job: Workplace abuse, sexual harassment, and racial discrimination—A study of black, Latino, and white low-income women and men workers (US)." *International Journal of Health Services* 36:51–85.

Landsbergis, P. A., J. G. Grzywacz, and A. D. LaMontagne. 2011. "Work organization, job insecurity and occupational health disparities." Issue paper presented at the Eliminating Health Disparities at Work Conference, 14 September 2011, Chicago.

Leigh, J. P. 2011. "Economic burden of occupational injury and illness in the United States." *Milbank Quarterly* 89(4):728–72.

Loh, K., and S. Richardson. 2004. "Foreign-born workers: Trends in fatal occupational injuries, 1996–2001." *Monthly Labor Review* (June):42–53.

National Research Council (NRC). 2003. "Executive Summary." In *Safety is seguridad*, 1–32. Washington, DC: National Academies Press.

Neal, A., and M. A. Griffin. 2004. "Safety climate and safety at work." In J. Barling and M. R. Frone, eds., *The psychology of workplace safety*, 15–34. Washington, DC: American Psychological Association.

Nuñez, G. G., and J. M. Heyman. 2007. "Entrapment process and immigrant communities in a time of heightened border vigilance." *Human Organization* 66:354–65.

O'Connor, T., M. A. Flynn, D. Weinstock, and J. Zanoni. 2011. "Education and training for underserved populations." An issue paper presented at the Eliminating Health Disparities at Work Conference, 14 September 2011, Chicago.

O'Connor, T., P. Gildner, and M. Easter. 2000. "Immigrant workers at risk: A qualitative study of hazards faced by Latino immigrant construction workers in the Triangle Area of North Carolina." Durham: North Carolina Occupational Safety and Health Project. Accessed 5 January 2014. http://coshnetwork6.mayfirst.org/sites/default/files/cpwrstudy.pdf.

Okechukwu, C., K. Souza, K. Davis, and B. de Castro. 2011. "Discrimination, harassment, abuse, and bullying in the workplace: Contribution of workplace injustice to occupational health disparities." Issue paper presented at the Eliminating Health Disparities at Work Conference, 14 September 2011, Chicago.

Orrenius, P. M., and M. Zavodny. 2009. "Do immigrants work in riskier jobs?" *Demography* 46(3):535–51.

Passel, J. S., and V. D. Cohn. 2009. "A portrait of unauthorized immigrants in the United States." Washington, DC: Pew Hispanic Center.

Pew Hispanic Center. 2005. "The new Latino South: The context and consequences of rapid growth." Washington, DC: Pew Research Center.

Pew Hispanic Center. 2008. "U.S. population projections: 2005–2050." Washington, DC: Pew Research Center.

Pew Hispanic Center. 2009. "Statistical portrait of Hispanics in the United States, 2009." Washington, DC: Pew Research Center.

Pew Hispanic Center. 2011. "Country of origin profiles." Washington, DC: Pew Research Center. Accessed 28 December 2011. http://www.pewhispanic.org/2011/05/26/country-of-origin-profiles/.

Porthe, V., E. Ahonen, M. L. Vazquez, C. Pope, A. A. Agudelo, A. M. Garcia, et al. 2010. "Extending a model of precarious employment: A qualitative study of immigrant workers in Spain." *American Journal of Industrial Medicine* 53:417–24.

Quandt, S. A., T. A. Arcury, C. K. Austin, and L. F. Cabrera. 2001. "Preventing occupational exposure to pesticides: Using participatory research with Latino farmworkers to develop an intervention." *Journal of Immigrant Health* 3(2):85–96.

Quandt, S. A., J. G. Grzywacz, A. Marin, L., Carrillo, M. L. Coates, B. Burke, and T. A. Arcury. 2006. "Illness and injuries reported by Latino poultry workers in Western North Carolina." *American Journal of Industrial Medicine* 49:343–51.

Quinlan, M., and R. K. Sokas. 2009. "Community campaigns, supply chains, and protecting the health and well-being of workers." *American Journal of Public Health* 99 (Suppl. 3):S538–46.

Richardson, S., R. Ruser, and P. Suarez. 2003. "Hispanic workers in the United States: An analysis of employment distributions, fatal occupational injuries, and non-fatal occupational injuries and illnesses." In *Safety is seguridad,* 43–82. Washington, DC: National Academies Press.

Ruser, J. W. 2008. "Examining evidence on whether BLS undercounts workplace injuries and illnesses." *Monthly Labor Review* 131:20–31.

Schenker, M. B. 2010. "A global perspective on migration and occupational health." *American Journal of Industrial Medicine* 53:329–37.

Siqueira, C. E., M. Gaydos, C. Monforton, K. Fagen, C. Slatin, L. Borkowski, et al. 2011. "Effects of social, economic, and labor policies on occupational health disparities." Issue paper presented at the Eliminating Health Disparities at Work Conference, 14 September 2011, Chicago.

Smith-Nonini, S. 2003. "Back to 'The Jungle': Processing migrants in North Carolina meatpacking plants." *Anthropology of Work Review* 24:14–20.

Souza, K., L. Davis, and J. Shire. 2011. "Occupational and environmental health surveillance." In B. S. Levy, D. H. Wegman, S. L. Baron, and R. K. Sokas, eds., *Occupational and environmental health: Recognizing and preventing disease and injury.* 6th ed. Oxford: Oxford University Press. 55–68.

Souza, K., A. L. Steege, and S. L. Baron. 2010. "Surveillance of occupational health disparities: Challenges and opportunities." *American Journal of Industrial Medicine* 53:84–94.

Steege, A. L., S. Baron, and X. Chen. 2009. "Occupational health of hired from workers in the United States: National agricultural workers' survey occupational health supplement, 1999." DHHS (NIOSH) publication no. 209–119. Washington, DC: DHHS.

Striffler, S. 2007. "Neither here nor there: Mexican immigrant workers and the search for home." *American Ethnologist* 34(4):674–88.

Stuesse, A. C. 2009. "Race, migration, and labor control: Neoliberal challenges to organizing Mississippi's poultry workers." In M. E. Odem and E. Lacy, eds., *Latino immigrants and the transformation of the U.S. South,* 91–111. Athens: University of Georgia Press.

Walter, N., P. Bourgois, L. H. Loinaz, and D. Schillinger. 2002. "Social context of work injury among undocumented day laborers in San Francisco." *Journal of General Internal Medicine* 17:221–29.

Willis, G. B. 1999. *Cognitive interviewing and questionnaire design: A training manual.* Washington, DC: Office of Research and Methodology, National Center for Health Statistics. Centers for Disease Control and Prevention, Department of Health and Human Services.

21

Methodological Recommendations for Broadening the Investigation of Refugees and Other Forced Migrants

Andrew Rasmussen

INTRODUCTION

Immigrant subpopulations are usually defined by emphasizing their particular contexts of entry or the phenomena that influence their immigration to a particular country—that is, their "pull factors." Thus undocumented immigrants are defined primarily by their illegal migration process and entrepreneurial immigrants by the economic pull of a favorable business climate. Refugees and other forced migrants are distinguished almost entirely by emphasis on the premigration factors that force them from their countries of origin—that is, their "push factors." This emphasis on premigration factors is reflected in the refugee health literature by the large number of studies that report high rates of psychiatric disorders (e.g., Fox and Tang 2000; Holtz 1998; Jaranson et al. 2004; Keller et al. 2006; Mollica et al. 1992; Shresta et al. 1998) and health problems (e.g., Forrest 1999) related to premigration trauma. Although emphasizing push factors is understandable given that they distinguish forced migrants from other, "voluntary," migrants, it is also likely to mask considerable variance within the population related to a number of other relevant factors. Emphasizing trauma history may come at the expense of emphasizing narratives that display resilience. Focusing on premigration events may distract from important aspects of the forced migration process, such as patterns of migration and resettlement.

This chapter presents a critical review of the definitions that have been commonly used to define sample frames in the refugee literature, three proposals for new directions for the field, and a few cautionary notes drawn from a decade of experience doing research with forced migrant populations. The purpose is not to review for the sake of drawing conclusions about refugees or to minimize the importance of any of the literature to this point, but rather to encourage social science and health researchers to build upon the largely policy-driven categories that have guided the field and to provide suggestions regarding the types of research methodologies that may prove most useful in studying refugee populations through prisms other than the premigration trauma paradigm. I draw heavily from the refugee mental health literature (because that is what I know best), but contend that the issues are likely applicable to research in medicine, public health, and economics as well.

DEFINITIONS AND DIVERSITY ACROSS FORCED MIGRATION

The "first generation" refugee health literature, which dates back to the early 1980s, grew out of political concerns and human rights ideals, specifically those established in the United Nations Charter on Refugees in 1951. Prior to the UN charter refugees occupied no special place within the health literature. The UN charter defines a refugee as someone who

> owing to well founded fear of being persecuted for reasons of race, religion, nationality, membership of a particular social group or political opinion, is outside the country of his nationality and is unable or, owing to such fear, is unwilling to avail himself of the protection of that country; or who, not having a nationality and being outside the country of his former habitual residence as a result of such events, is unable or, owing to such fear, is unwilling to return to it. (UNHCR 2010a: 14)

The UN charter's emphasis on the violation of individual rights paved the way for the health literature to focus on premigration trauma by providing an etiology for refugee health problems.

The UN charter has formed the basis for defining forced migrant subpopulations. Practical descriptions of these are presented in Table 21.1. Categories are mutually exclusive, with their subtypes indented below them. Differences between these subpopulations are primarily legal. For example, technically refugee status is designated when persons displaced by a conflict cross a national border. This makes them legally eligible for assistance provided under the aegis of the UN. Depending on services and protections provided in their home country, experientially this may or may not make a difference to the health status of the displaced persons in question (which may be reflected in health research).

The number of research studies using sample frames aligned with the definitions presented in Table 21.1 is, in general, negatively associated with the number of individuals represented within each category. This is because of the geographical distance and political barriers between the various populations and well-resourced

TABLE 21.1 Forced Migrant Subpopulations

Subpopulation	Description	Population worldwide (UNHCR 2010b)
Internally displaced persons (IDPs)	A group of individuals that flee their homes but do not leave their country in order to seek safety from political violence or persecution	14.7 million
IDPs returned home	Returned to their homes without coercion	2.9 million
Refugees	Displaced persons that cross a national border to seek safety; they are designated as refugees by the UNHCR, who negotiates protection for them in the immediate host country	10.6 million
Voluntarily repatriated	Returned to their home countries without coercion	197,600
Locally integrated	Integrated into economies and political structures of immediate host nations	Unknown
In protracted refugee crises	Refugees living in groups of 25,000 people or more and for more than five years	7.2 million
In third countries of resettlement	Resettled from immediate host countries to (usually) wealthier countries by resettlement workers sanctioned by UNHCR	206,800 new cases; approximately 2 million living as refugees
Asylum seekers	Individuals that flee across national borders to seek safety, usually to a wealthier, industrialized country; asylum seekers that claim refugee status without being formally recognized by UNHCR, usually through host nation's immigration processing systems (e.g., immigration court in the US)	837,500 new claims; less than 1.5 million involved in asylum proceedings

NOTE: UNHCR = United Nations High Commissioner for Refugees.

researchers. For example, for researchers the approximately 2 million Darfur internally displaced persons (IDPs) living in Sudan are harder to reach than their 230,000 refugee compatriots across the border in eastern Chad, who are in turn harder to reach than those few Darfur refugees and asylum seekers who have resettled in the United States and Britain. This negative relationship between the number of research studies and population size likely has consequences for health services insofar as how service providers conceptualize the problems of forced migrants is influenced by the research available to them. For example, disaster relief seems appropriate for IDPs in immediate disaster settings; however, there is little research on acute needs of IDPs, which leaves service providers to rely on research done in resettlement contexts, where disaster relief is less relevant.

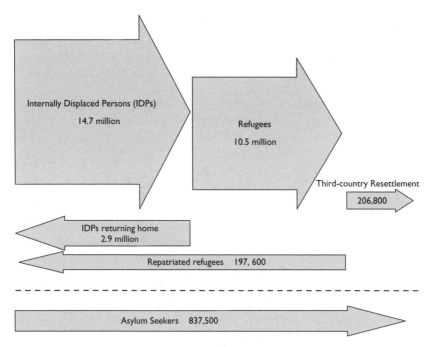

FIGURE 21.1. Forced migrant populations in 2010. (UNHCR 2010.)

Each subpopulation presented in Table 21.1 is described below in terms of likely health-related concerns, and, consistent with the purpose of this handbook, methodological issues. Figure 21.1 provides a graphical representation of the forced migration process. IDPs are individuals who have fled their homes and resettled within the confines of their home country (hence "internally displaced"). IDPs are the largest group of forced migrants worldwide; in 2010, large numbers existed within Colombia, the Democratic Republic of Congo, Somalia, Iraq, and Afghanistan (UNHCR 2011). The refugee literature's emphasis on push factors is likely most relevant for these forced migrants, as (1) their experiences of violence and persecution are most proximal in time and (2) they have engaged in limited migration. Relevant issues for IDPs usually fall under the rubric of disaster relief more than migration concerns. Disaster relief involves access to basic needs such as shelter and food, acute health care, and psychological first-aid. As IDPs are by definition displaced within their home countries, the health policies and protection of home countries are central to their well-being. Home country protection is also a concern for researchers, as governments that are hostile to IDPs are likely to be hostile to foreign researchers working with IDPs. Hence IDPs in Myanmar (Burma) have been the subject of few research projects, as the Myanmar government has been (until recently) hostile toward outsiders in general. In contrast there are many research studies that have taken place with IDP samples in northern Uganda (e.g., Roberts et al. 2008; Verdeli et al. 2008), where the government has welcomed humanitarian relief agencies and the researchers that often accompany them.

Once IDPs cross national borders they become refugees. This group worldwide is the second largest population of forced migrants, with the largest populations in 2010 being 2.9 million Afghanis in Pakistan and Iran and 1.8 million Iraqis in Syria, Jordan, and elsewhere throughout the Middle East (UNHCR 2011). Because refugees are usually further removed from their push factors than IDPs, relevant issues have less to do with disaster relief and more to do with chronic public health issues brought about by displacement, a lack of economic opportunity in host countries, and significant cultural differences between home and host countries. The term "refugee" is used to describe two distinct groups: refugees in countries of immediate resettlement who have resettled in neighboring countries, and refugees in third countries of resettlement who have been resettled by international non-governmental organizations (NGOs) from these immediate resettlement contexts to a UN charter signatory nation that has agreed to accept them. Refugees in countries of immediate resettlement are by far the larger group (80%), and are dealt with first; refugees in third countries of resettlement are then addressed. However, I begin by addressing sampling issues common to IDPs and both types of refugees.

SAMPLING REFUGEES AND IDPS

Apart from political issues that influence access to participants, methodological issues surrounding IDP and refugee sample frames in countries of immediate resettlement are similar. Many IDPs and refugees in countries of immediate resettlement congregate in camps. These refugees and IDPs are thus concentrated in relatively well-delineated areas, and constructing reliable epidemiological sample frames is thus not logistically complicated. A commonly used sampling technique in both IDP and refugee camps has been to sample households and interview those who are present. This has been done through a number of techniques, from cluster sampling, which often begins by spinning a pen (or stick, or some object that points in a particular direction) to determine initial seed households (e.g., Bolton et al. 2004), to random sampling of digitized households via satellite imagery (e.g., Green and Kloos 2008).

Although sampling households is thought to be sufficient given the assumption that IDPs and refugees are usually prohibited from engaging in local economies, mobility in and out of these settlements may present problems for representation. Most studies that report high response rates have focused on cluster sampling of households in camps, in which researchers interview a member of the household who is present. It is unclear to what extent household sampling biases camp samples. Using United Nations High Commissioner for Refugees (UNHCR) camp records to survey individuals in two Darfur refugee camps in Chad, my colleagues and I found that almost half of our simple random sample could not be contacted because they were not home when researchers arrived (Rasmussen and Annan 2010). Sampling households alone would have missed these individuals. Mobility is not incidental to health. One of the earliest studies in the refugee health literature reported that those refugees who were involved in the informal economy surrounding the camp were more likely to report fewer psychiatric symptoms (Mollica et al. 1993). Given that mobility likely differs between refugee crises (due to varying political and economic factors), researchers using spatial sampling techniques should be prepared to do research on mobility patterns before they decide what sampling methods to employ.

Although common images of refugees and IDPs involve camps, there is increasing evidence that forced migrants are more and more likely to resettle in urban areas (Spiegel et al. 2010). Urban refugee populations are more dispersed than those in camps, making them less accessible to humanitarian relief agencies and researchers alike. With a plurality of refugees now living in urban areas, ignoring urbanization likely results in mischaracterizing refugees as a whole. Problems with identifying refugees and IDPs in large urban centers where they may or may not be readily distinguishable from local populations (e.g., Iraqis in Amman, Jordan) lessens the utility of cluster sampling in favor of chain sampling models, such as snowballing or respondent-driven sampling (see chapter 7, by Johnston and Malekinejad, in this volume). These methods can be facilitated by working with identified community leaders; for example, work with Darfur refugees living in Cairo suggests that such strategies are useful for conducting health services research (Meffert and Marmar 2009). Whether such techniques result in representative samples of urban refugees is an empirical question worthy of exploration.

REFUGEES IN THE LONG TERM: DURABLE SOLUTIONS

UNHCR proposes three "durable solutions" for refugees in countries of immediate resettlement: voluntary repatriation, local integration, and third-country resettlement. Although there is a large literature using samples in third-country resettlement contexts, there is almost no research on voluntary repatriation or local integration. Refugees who are voluntarily repatriated and IDPs who return home constitute relatively small numbers worldwide, and these numbers have been decreasing over the past decade (UNHCR 2011). A review of the refugee health literature suggests that returnees should be worse off than their compatriots who do not return (Porter and Haslam 2005). Unfortunately, no direct comparison studies have been attempted. Comparison studies would likely be challenging, as they would by definition be multinational and probably expose researchers to substantial risks. However, the implications of such studies would be far-reaching insofar as they would directly inform a key policy platform of the international refugee regime—that displaced persons are best off returning to their homes.

Local integration involves the economic and political integration of refugees stuck in "protracted refugee crises" into the host country population. UNHCR defines protracted refugee crises as crises that involve the displacement of 25,000 people or more and continue for more than five years. As repatriation numbers are relatively small, and third-country resettlement accounts for less than 20% of refugees worldwide, local integration is UNHCR's plan for most refugees. A recent example of local integration is the 2009 naturalization of 155,000 Burundians in Tanzania.

By UNHCR's own admission, measuring the number of successfully integrated refugees remains a challenge (UNHCR 2010b). Local integration is largely a development issue, with primary challenges being economic sustainability on the part of refugees—that is, removing refugees from international donors' aid rolls—and integration into local political and health care structures. Even though over half of all refugees worldwide are slated for local integration, there has been virtually no published research in this area. Suffice it to say that multiple challenges exist when populations that have been dependent on international aid agencies for many years are removed from their rolls and local populations are told that they must now share resources with their former guests. Any researcher desiring to make a substantial contribution to refugee well-being would do well to describe and examine local integration projects. Although in the absence of data any methods would likely provide useful information, research strategies that involve long-term engagement, such as ethnography or carefully structured longitudinal surveys, would be most useful. As international NGOs are sometimes brought in to facilitate local integration projects, program evaluation involving case studies and randomized control trials would serve to further intervention aims and might be useful to NGOs seeking funding in this area.

Popular conceptions of refugees in North America and Europe are associated most closely with third-country resettlement, in which UN charter signatory nations take in individuals from refugee crises to become residents. The host nations then determine how these individuals are integrated. If refugees are allowed to adjust their immigration status to other, more permanent, statuses, they are no longer counted as refugees by UNHCR. Although during the Cold War (1945–1991) several refugee populations were resettled en masse (e.g., Vietnamese in the late 1970s and 1980s), currently most major host nations set annual limits on the number of resettled refugees they are willing to receive from around the world. Host nation governments weigh history, media attention, perceived threats within refugee populations, and need (as defined by the 1951 UN charter) in making their decisions. Need is further attenuated by limits on the proportion of "vulnerable cases"—individuals with serious medical and mental health conditions—within a refugee population. Currently the US is home to about three-quarters of individuals who have ever been resettled as refugees (US Department of State 2010).

Third-country resettlement begins with interviews and documentation undertaken in camp and urban refugee populations by resettlement workers who are NGO personnel charged with identifying individuals who meet UN criteria for resettlement. This process has implications for the composition of resettled populations and thus has consequences for resettled refugee sample frames. Once refugees have been selected to begin the resettlement interview process, they are faced with multiple rounds of interviews and considerable wait times, during which resettlement workers investigate claims. In 2011 Eskinder Negash, the director of the Office of Refugee Resettlement in the Obama administration, reported that the average wait to be resettled to the US for Somalis from the Dadaab refugee camp in Kenya was seventeen years; he noted that those who had the determination to wait seventeen years to resettle were likely to be particularly resilient (September 15, 2011; Migration Policy Institute). The hardiness of resettled refugees is likely to extend to physical health as well as mental health, aided by host nations' limits on the proportion of vulnerable cases. But conjectures such as these are as-of-yet unanswered empirical questions; to date there has been no systematic research on the differences between refugees who are and are not resettled to third countries of resettlement, or even good descriptive work on the resettlement selection process. A few strong studies comparing refugees selected for resettlement to those remaining in initial resettlement contexts could have an enormous impact on refugee policy worldwide. Such research might begin with qualitative work identifying the unofficial factors that determine if and when refugees are first scheduled for resettlement interviews and the pressures placed upon resettlement workers to process cases quickly. Ideally a random sample of refugees, some of whom would be resettled and others who would not be resettled, would be followed longitudinally to examine the preexisting factors associated with identification and successful resettlement over time.

RESETTLED REFUGEES AND ASYLUM SEEKERS

Refugees resettled in North America, Europe, and Australia are the forced migrant subpopulation about which most is known, due largely to their proximity to well-resourced researchers. For these forced migrants, relevant issues include access to health care, economic opportunity, and acculturation. Although much of the health and mental health research on resettled refugees acknowledges these issues, most studies still focus on the effects of premigration factors alone, particularly the effect of premigration trauma. Premigration trauma may account for a quarter of the variance in trauma-related mental health symptoms (e.g., Steel et al. 1999). Although not a small effect, that it is limited to a quarter suggests that push factors are not the only phenomena influencing postmigration well-being. This topic is discussed in detail below, in the discussion of proposed directions in forced migrant research.

Asylum seekers are forced migrants who claim refugee status in third countries of resettlement without being formally resettled. In contrast to refugees, who are designated as refugees by UNHCR before they arrive, asylum seekers attempt to designate themselves and are therefore subject to host countries' legal processes to prove that they would be harmed if they returned to their home countries. Asylum seekers are the smallest subpopulation of official forced migrants. There is considerable variation in their migration history: some travel through refugee camps prior to claiming asylum, some travel circuitous routes through several countries before arriving in their destination country, some pay to be smuggled into potential host nations, and some travel directly. As they choose their potential host country, pull factors are likely very important in determining their migration. Once asylum seekers arrive in their selected host countries they face a diversity of challenges. In the US, claiming asylum can result in being detained for several months if asylum is claimed at an airport or border crossing, or simply an appointment with an immigration official if asylum is claimed after the asylum seeker successfully makes it past border officials.

Research on asylum seekers has shed considerable light on the effects of asylum policy. Not surprisingly, being detained often has negative consequences for asylum seekers' mental and physical well-being (Keller et al. 2003; Steel et al. 2004, 2006; Venters and Keller 2009). Asylum claims can extend for years; during this time access to health care and employment is severely limited, both by law and by fear of negatively impacting legal outcomes. Also not surprisingly, obtaining asylum has a strong effect on asylum seekers' psychological well-being (Raghavan et al. 2013). Although there is literature on the health consequences of detention for asylum seekers in the US and Australia, in general there has been little investigation of the other sources of variance (i.e., migration pathways and contexts of entry) particular to asylum seekers. Most research treats asylees as if they were resettled refugees and focuses on premigration trauma. But "self-resettlement" is likely to be an important marker of hardiness, while the lengthy liminal immigration status of asylum seekers is likely associated with important psychosocial stressors not faced by officially resettled refugees.

A number of challenging research issues arise concerning asylum seekers. The first concerns sample frames. Because asylum seekers usually resettle to urban areas, researchers face the same challenges with sampling as they do with urban refugee populations. If researchers limit their sample frames to those refugees who have already applied for asylum, it might be possible to work with immigration officials to identify asylee sample frames. This approach would, of course, depend upon finding an ethical means to work around legal barriers set up to protect the privacy of individuals involved in legal proceedings (a decidedly nontrivial issue among individuals fleeing persecution). Most studies of asylum seekers come from health clinics and advocacy organizations designed to respond to asylum seekers in need (e.g., Keller et al. 2006). Sample frames from clinics are undoubtedly biased in terms of severity of the cases seen, and those focusing on legal advocacy are likely biased toward more complex and less easily substantiated asylum claims. The reliance on biased convenience samples would seem to call for using alternative sampling methods. As with urban refugee populations, chain sampling methods may be effective in constructing representative samples.

Qualitative narrative research may be especially relevant to identifying the variety of pathways and contexts of migration faced by asylum seekers. Although subject to the standard limits of retrospective data, a thorough documentation of the variety of asylum histories would provide a platform on which to build prospective longitudinal studies in the future. When in the asylum process such data would be collected makes a difference. Narratives taken before asylum applicants are granted asylum are likely to be influenced by the demand characteristics of the asylum process itself (see below for more on demand characteristics of refugee research), but waiting until after asylum decisions risks losing a substantial proportion of the sample to deportation.

OTHER FORCED POPULATIONS NOT DEFINED LEGALLY

Other forced migrant populations are those that do not fit into the preceding categories but may nevertheless have migrated for political violence or other persecution-related push factors. For example, among the estimated 3 million Zimbabweans living without legal status in South Africa in 2010, there were many that had been subject to human rights violations, and yet very few had been designated as refugees. Similarly, among nonrefugee Latino immigrants presenting to primary care clinics in Los Angeles, California, researchers found that half had a history of exposure to political violence and 8% reported experiences consistent with torture (Eisenman et al. 2003). These findings suggest that the definitions arising from the UN charter are subject to political and cultural considerations that prevent appropriate identification of forced migrants, and researchers who use those definitions to guide their sample frames should be aware that they may easily fall victim to the same biases. Refugee and immigrant researchers in general might subvert these biases by inquiring about push factors that indicate "forcedness"—persecution, war, and official harassment—rather than relying on immigration status or the legal intentions of their subjects.

PROPOSED DIRECTIONS IN FORCED MIGRANT HEALTH RESEARCH

Comparison Groups

Comparison is one of the basic methodological tools that health and social science researchers use to identify factors that are specific to particular groups of people. In the refugee health literature comparison has been woefully underutilized. Notable exceptions appear in a small but growing clinical intervention literature, which includes randomized control trials in refugee and IDP camp settings (e.g., Bolton et al. 2007; Meffert et al. 2011; Neuner et al. 2004, 2008). But comparison has been almost completely absent in basic literature on forced migrants. Included here are two suggestions for using comparison groups to further forced migrant health research: across stages and migration pathways in the forced migration process and between forced and voluntary migrants within the same ethnocultural groups.

Comparison across the Forced Migration Process.   When IDPs, refugees, and asylum seekers leave their homes they enter into a process, a narrative of flight and resettlement. This process, presented graphically in Figure 21.1, has multiple pathways and distinct stages, the entry into each defining the subpopulations referred to above. However, few refugee health researchers have conceptualized forced migration as a process, instead either focusing on descriptive characteristics at a given stage or premigration factors alone. Comparison studies of participants at each stage of the forced migration process is needed to better identify the particular needs associated with the different subpopulations. In a given conflict, who is forced to leave home and who is not forced to leave is presumably not random, but the current research acknowledges only those who are forced to leave as a population of interest. Who is later resettled and who is not is similarly nonrandom. And yet most studies that refer to forced migrants at various stages of the forced migration process do not acknowledge that the history of their migration may have effects on the conclusions that can be drawn about forced migration in general. Research designs that compare those who advance along the forced migration process to those who do not would be a substantial contribution to the refugee health and services literatures alike.

Comparison of Forced and Voluntary Migrants within Ethnocultural Groups.   Comparison between forced migrants and others in resettlement contexts has been largely limited to comparisons between refugees or asylum seekers and native-born populations (e.g., comparing Kurdish children to Swedish children; Sundelin-Wahlsten et al. 2001). Although such research is useful in highlighting disparities, it does not say much about forced migration in particular. Forced migrants are immigrants, and immigrants from particular ethnocultural communities, and as such forced migrants should be compared to voluntary immigrants within their own communities. Without designs that account for these factors, the etiology of health outcomes among forced migrant families is unclear. Are challenges facing forced migrants primarily due to past persecution, are they challenges common to low-income immigrants in general, or are they better conceived of as the results of some interaction between trauma, migration context, and adjustment? Examining differences and similarities between forced and voluntary migrants from the same cultural groups would allow practitioners to draw upon the larger literature related to voluntary migrants in order to adapt intervention strategies for forced migrants (and might provide further information about additional issues facing voluntary migrants as well). The one study (to date, 2011) comparing forced and voluntary migrants from the same ethnocultural background, Steel and colleagues' (1999) study of trauma, migration, and posttraumatic stress in Tamil communities in Australia, has shown that although there are clear differences in severity, substantial distress is common to both forced and voluntary migrants.

Studies that compare forced and voluntary migrants may be rare because of the relative scarcity of migrant populations that include both. Many conflicts are defined by whole ethnic groups being persecuted, and therefore research comparing forced and voluntary migrants is simply not possible. Among Somali immigrants, for instance, voluntary migrants are few and far between. A similar situation arises with groups whose ethnicity is profoundly defined by their collective experience of forced migration. Tibetans in India are often identified as forced migrants because of the history of cultural suppression in Tibet by Chinese authorities. Although there is considerable variance in persecution experiences (Sachs et al. 2008), few would identify themselves as strictly voluntary. In these instances it may be feasible to find a voluntary migrant comparison group from a similar cultural background. Cervantes and colleagues (1989) compared war-affected Central American immigrants to Mexican immigrants to the US, and found that rates of PTSD among the Central Americans were twice that of Mexicans.

Accounting for Culture

The refugee health literature is woefully uninformed about how culture affects measurement, outcomes, and the delivery of services. The emphasis on individual human rights violations that is central to the UN charter means that shared experiences of persecution across refugee populations are privileged over differing cultural interpretations of the consequences of that persecution. This has implications for how researchers select their constructs of interest and how they select their measures. In addition, ignoring culture has led them to ignore research questions that may be central to particular refugee groups' social structures.

Measuring Health and Illness across Cultures.   Culture influences the way individuals and groups express distress and conceptualize health problems. Measures that are constructed for refugee populations may account for some of the common variance of persecution, but do not account for particular expressions or conceptualizations of specific cultural groups. The implications of this are perhaps most obvious in refugee mental health research (though culture-related variation is in no way limited to psychological phenomena). For instance, in Mandinka medicine—prevalent throughout several conflict regions in West Africa—there are four separate emotional-cognitive states that can result from trauma (Fox 2003). Although each of these includes elements of what North American and European psychologists would call posttraumatic stress disorder (PTSD), they also overlap with other psychological problems (e.g., depression and panic disorder). Thus the common practice of using a PTSD questionnaire to assess refugee mental health does not fully capture the construct associated with posttraumatic stress among Mandinka forced migrants. These differences may seem somewhat esoteric at first, but they may have important health implications. In addition to being more sensitive to the way that refugees discuss their distress, measures of culturally specific constructs are generally more highly associated with measures of functional impairment (e.g., Jayawickreme et al. 2012; Kohrt and Hruschka 2010; Rasmussen et al. 2011), suggesting that these distinctions have treatment implications as well.

There is little methodological reason why researchers should not develop culturally specific measures in refugee settings where such measures have not yet been developed. Methods for rapid development of measures of local health constructs have been established in emergency settings (Bolton et al. 2004), and medical anthropology resources are often available. Using a combination of free listing followed by key informant interviews ("quick ethnography"; Handwerker 2001), several studies led by Paul Bolton have shown that such techniques can produce measures that are internally reliable (Bolton et al. 2004) and consistent with local mental health constructs (Betancourt et al. 2009; Bolton and Tang 2004). Such measures can also account for substantial variance in functional impairment (Bolton et al. 2002) and be effectively utilized to evaluate psychological interventions (Verdeli et al. 2008). Variations on this approach include using pile sorts of common symptoms to identify implicit categories of illness (e.g., Rasmussen et al. 2011) and integrating preexisting anthropological evidence to verify these categories (e.g., Kaiser et al. 2013). If time is available, more intensive ethnographic approaches may be used to build more reliable measures (Jayawickreme et al. 2012; Tol et al. 2010).

A related issue concerns response bias differences between ethnocultural groups. Studies using scaled responses presume that response bias within a sample is randomly distributed across participants, thus allowing researchers to treat response bias as "random error." However, cultural norms for expressing distress introduce nonrandom error into this equation. This has been recognized in social psychology for some time (e.g., Chen et al. 1995; Grimm and Church 1999; Hui and Triandis 1989; Zax and Takahashi 1967). When clinical scales developed for one cultural group are administered to another group, it becomes difficult to interpret the meaning of scale scores. For example, cultural norms toward keeping positive feelings private may lead to relatively more severe depression scores on tests that incorporate positively worded items (e.g., the CES-D; Noh et al. 1992).

Response bias has received scant attention in the refugee health literature, resulting in substantial clinical confusion. Research on Tibetan refugees using the Harvard Trauma Questionnaire (HTQ) displays the problem of response bias well. Multiple reports have documented severe traumatic events in Tibet against Tibetans at the hands of Chinese police and military. However, studies with Tibetan refugees report mean scores on PTSD measures well below what is seen in other similarly persecuted populations. In a convenience sample of the 769 Tibetans entering a refugee reception center in India, Sachs and colleagues (2008) found only one individual who met the 2.5 screening score for probable PTSD on the HTQ. Keller and colleagues reported that in their sample of patients at a US torture treatment center, Buddhists, almost all of whom were Tibetan, reported HTQ scores well below those of Muslims and Christians, who were from Europe, Africa, and Latin America. Lhewa and colleagues (2007) addressed the issue of response bias directly by comparing HTQ scores to clinical diagnoses of PTSD (made by a Tibetan psychiatrist) and found that sensitivity of the HTQ was perfect at a cutoff score of 1.9, well below the suggested 2.5 (Lhewa et al. 2007)—a response bias toward the low end of the HTQ's response scale among Tibetans. Trauma and suffering among Tibetans exists, but the tendency to express emotions in relatively mild terms means that researchers should recalibrate their thresholds. Unfortunately, such research is rare in the refugee health literature. If standardized measures like the HTQ must be used in cross-cultural research settings, sufficient pretesting should be done to identify valid clinical cutoffs.

Cultural Practices as Moderating Forced Migration Processes.   Integrating culture into research designs means integrating cultural practices that may be at odds with researchers' own culture. For example, recent conflicts producing large numbers of forced migrants—Iraq, Afghanistan, Somalia, Syria—have all occurred in societies in which polygamy is not uncommon. Although there is a rich advocacy and research literature on sexual- and gender-based conflict and refugee women, virtually none of this literature addresses dynamics within polygamous families. Polygamy has been shown to have public health consequences (e.g., in HIV/AIDS; Nyindo 2005), and it may be central to understanding how forced migrants allocate resources and support each other in disaster settings. Among Darfur refugees ($N = 848$) the number of wives that men had was positively correlated with their ratings of distress, but negatively correlated with their wives' ratings of distress (Rasmussen et al. 2007). These findings were interpreted with respect to culturally proscribed gender roles in which men with more wives are responsible for more people. By integrating culturally specific features into research designs, refugee health researchers who consider such factors make it more likely that their outcomes will be relevant to the populations they study.

Improved Modeling of the Social-Ecological Damage That Occurs during Forced Migration

The same events that affect forced migrants individually also damage their social support systems. This suggests that researchers interested in modeling forced migrant health and well-being should utilize social-ecological perspectives in designing their studies. Social-ecological approaches acknowledge that multiple hierarchically arranged settings affect individuals (Bronfenbrenner 1979; Sameroff and MacKenzie 2003). Miller and Rasco (2004) identify seven micro-, meso-, and macro-systemic stressors set in motion by war-related forced displacement: loss of social networks and roles, unemployment, loss of environmental mastery, discrimination, separation from loved ones, and differing intergenerational rates of acculturation. Each influences individual, family, and community well-being simultaneously. Political violence sets in motion a series of daily stressors associated with economic and social losses, and these have an additive degenerative effect on health; that is, distress is mediated through these secondary sequelae (Miller and Rasmussen 2010). Researchers interested in informing interventions in host countries need to focus on these mediating factors.

Qualitative methods are often rich approaches to describing social ecology. An excellent example from the refugee literature is Hampshire and colleagues' (2008) study of social interactions in a Liberian refugee camp in Ghana. Triangulating in the best tradition of qualitative inquiry, the authors use focus groups, individual interviews with residents and camp authorities, field note observations, diaries by refugees themselves, and administrative records to describe a situation in which established councils of elders have lost their authority over young people. Hampshire and colleagues (2008) provide a rich picture of the refugee experience as an exercise in "liminality" (p. 34). Another excellent example of using qualitative research to identify intervention-relevant social-ecological data is a study with Bosnian families resettled in Chicago (Weine et al. 2006). Qualitative designs such as narrative analysis and case study might be used to provide data about social-ecological phenomena across the forced migration process as well.

Another promising method for social-ecological research is social network analysis (SNA). SNA involves visual and statistical mapping of social networks, allowing for analyses of individuals within networks (e.g., their centrality), of the influence of the types of ties they have to others within their networks (e.g., the structures of their immediate surroundings), and of networks in their entirety (e.g., centralized vs. dispersed network structure). Network characteristics can also be used to predict individuals' and groups' well-being in standard variance-based statistical models (e.g., ANOVA). Social networks have been linked to multiple health outcomes among native-born populations (Christakis and Fowler 2008; Juster et al. 2009), and although deemed fairly important in the immigration health literature (Bertrand et al. 2000; Kuo and Tsai 1986; Leclere et al. 1994), SNA has yet to be used in the forced migrant literature. It is easy to see how the stressors associated with political violence and displacement should be ameliorated by social networks that include material supports and reliable sources of information about direct services and affiliative ties to community institutions. Differences between forced and voluntary migrant social networks might provide important evidence of the differences between the two.

The refugee intervention literature has been ahead of research in addressing higher-level (i.e., non-individual-level) migration stressors. Williams and Berry (1991) addressed "acculturative stress" among refugees and psychologists' attempts to ameliorate this in the pages of the *American Psychologist* in 1991, and the extensive work of Boothby argued for addressing psychosocial stressors at an even earlier date (Boothby 1992; Ressler et al. 1988). The popularity of psychosocial or "multimodal" (Nickerson et al. 2011) interventions among relief organizations that serve displaced and war-affected populations is an acknowledgment that there are stressors beyond premigration trauma that influence forced migrants' mental health. Goodkind (2005, 2006) has developed an entirely acculturation-based intervention for refugees that builds supportive networks postmigration by connecting refugee families with trained undergraduate students for a year. Goodkind has run these "mutual learning circles" with Hmong communities in Michigan and in a multinational group of refugees in New Mexico. Quantitative and qualitative evidence supports the contention that this intervention decreases forced migrants' subjective distress by providing them with an informed advocate in interactions with public institutions, from schools to hospitals to women and infant children (WIC) offices. Although higher-level factors related to refugee well-being have been introduced into the literature of late, they are still far too infrequent, particularly in the lower and middle-income settings where most forced migrants reside (Reed et al. 2012).

CAUTIONARY NOTES

This chapter concludes with a few cautionary notes related to doing research with people in need. These issues are not limited to forced migrants, but likely extend to other populations in which individuals feel some sense of desperation (e.g., undocumented migrants). In the language of the conservation of resources theory

(Hobfoll 1989, 2001), forced migrants have all experienced some degree of loss and they are searching for ways to compensate for that loss by marshaling whatever resources they can find. Refugee health researchers are often perceived of as likely sources of resources. Thus there are certain demand characteristics inherent in research interviews with forced migrants. The strength of these demand characteristics may vary between populations and across forced migration stages, but any researcher who has asked refugees or asylum seekers questions about any aspect of their well-being is familiar with the feeling that their subjects are trying to convince them that their particular plight is worthy of his or her attention. The pressure on forced migrants to portray themselves as deserving of researchers' charity is as powerful as it is understandable. At worst the research interview replicates resettlement or asylum interviews, in which forced migrants must convince an official that they are in need of protection; at best the demand characteristics driven by perceived differences in wealth between researchers and participants are still likely to have some influence on responses, and the researchers (to date) have no way of measuring it.

There are several consequences of these demand characteristics of which researchers should be aware. The first and perhaps most obvious are falsehoods and exaggeration. Currently falsehoods and exaggeration are discussed in the research literature only in limitations sections, dutifully stated among a number of factors that may limit results' reliability. As there is no published research on falsehoods and exaggeration among forced migrants, estimates of how much they influence our knowledge come from anecdotes in journalism and reports from service providers. A 2011 *New York Times* article on immigration lawyers suggested that lying in order to gain asylum was widespread (Dolnick 2011). It is common knowledge among refugee resettlement workers that different refugees sometimes report identical narratives of persecution, suggesting that refugees share (and perhaps even sell) stories they think will make them eligible for resettlement. Such reports suggest that falsehoods and exaggeration exist and that there is good reason to believe that they may affect what forced migrants say to people from potential host countries, but they give researchers little to go on concerning the extent and effect that such fraud would have on results.

The lack of reliable data on falsehoods and exaggeration has a direct effect on policy debates. To date concern about falsehoods and exaggeration has been voiced primarily by those who would restrict immigration, and refugee health researchers have little to rely on to show immigration officials that their participants are not lying. This is not to say that immigration officials have not sought out scientific means of determining this information. From 2009 to 2011 the United Kingdom tested the "Human Provenance Pilot Project," a £190,000 program that used DNA testing to determine whether asylum seekers were from the national group they claimed. The program proceeded despite being roundly criticized by geneticists from the start because nationality is not a genetic construct (Travis 2011). That such "scientistic" policies are taken seriously evinces the level of hunger on the part of policy makers that would be satisfied by even small advances in research related to detecting falsehoods or exaggeration. Such advances might be obtained by applying forensic research approaches that define malingering within given populations. Identifying what characterizes malingerers within different forced migrant populations would necessarily involve estimating culturally influenced response bias (see above) as well as the bias displayed by malingerers.

The issue of falsehoods and exaggeration is complicated by the fact that their existence may not be simply a matter of forced migrants intending to falsely represent themselves. Anecdotes from forced migrant researchers suggest that in some forced migrant populations there is a narrative of collective persecution that is at odds with the individual experiences valued by most social science researchers. A colleague who has worked with IDPs in Uganda tells a story in which a research assistant appeared on a radio program to discuss his own violent victimization by the Lord Resistance Army—this despite the fact that he did not live in the conflict zone during the war years. When asked directly about the inconsistency, the research assistant told the researcher that although it was true that he had not personally experienced the things he reported, what he had reported were important stories that had happened to people and needed be told. A Mauritanian leader of an ethnically based organization in New York City told me that he advised people to seek asylum based on stories of others who had not been able to flee so that "their place" among those seeking justice would not be lost. Individuals represent their communities, and their experiences may be superseded by the narratives of their people. Here again, discussion of this phenomenon in the research literature is woefully lacking. Methods that identify and account for these phenomena would provide forced migrant researchers with tools for better estimating individual- and community-level effects on their participants' well-being.

The second, less obvious consequence of the demand characteristics inherent in forced migrant research concerns the effect of engaging in research on participants who may be completely truthful but are unable to provide reliable information due to their psychological reactions to their trauma experiences. Because of the potential gain perceived to be the outcome of participating in research, forced migrants may feel the need to recount their persecution experiences even when they are overwhelmed by them emotionally, and despite researchers ethically holding fast to participants' right to discontinue research. Although recounting traumatic events is not likely to lead to permanent damage (evidence on "retraumatization" during research studies suggests that this concern is not empirically supported: Griffin et al. 2003; Legerski and Bunnell 2010; Orth and Maercker 2004), participants who recount traumatic experiences can become temporarily overwhelmed, and their distress may have effects on the reliability of their responses. When recounting stressful events participants may temporarily have problems with concentration and memory. The demand characteristics of the researcher-forced migrant interaction may thus cloud findings for participants that have no intention of reporting falsehoods or exaggerating.

The issue of adverse effects of research brings to the fore ethical standards of care for forced migrants with traumatic events in their past. There is recent evidence from neurological research that recounting potentially traumatic events involves producing neuronal structures associated with the environment immediately following that in which recounting is done (Debiec and LeDoux 2006; Nader et al. 2000). The immediate postrecounting environment is important because of a window of memory reconsolidation that lasts between approximately thirty minutes and six hours after reexposure to the trauma memory (this window is based on the time needed for protein synthesis to occur in neurons) (Nader et al. 2000). Although recent and still largely limited to animal models, findings from reconsolidation research may have ethical implications for how researchers design their protocols. Designs that involve the potential for recounting traumatic events should include provisions for participants' comfort following research interviews to maximize the likelihood that participants reconsolidate their trauma memories with less distress than they had previously. Although trauma research does not increase the likelihood of subsequent PTSD, it might be designed so as to decrease it.

CONCLUSIONS

This chapter presents an overview of research with forced migrant populations and provides recommendations about the topical areas and research methodologies that researchers might consider in order to move the field forward. Conceptual issues discussed include considering pull factors as well as push factors, addressing the role of culture, and investigating the social-ecological damage that occurs during the forced migration process. Methodological issues addressed include more attention to sampling, increased attention to comparison group approaches and longitudinal designs across the forced migration process, and the development of methods that estimate the systematic error in findings due to the demand characteristics inherent in the field. Each of these suggestions should be placed within its appropriate context. Building representative samples, for instance, might not be as important for some research questions as it is for others. But all researchers working with forced migrants would be well advised to consider these suggestions when designing their research in order to ensure that their work moves the field beyond the single-storyline findings of the first-generation literature and toward sophisticated and policy-relevant research.

REFERENCES

Bertrand, M., E. F. P. Luttmer, and S. Mullainathan. 2000. "Network effects and welfare cultures." *Quarterly Journal of Economics* 115(3): 1019–55.

Betancourt, Theresa, Judith Bass, Ivelina Borisova, Richard Neugebauer, Liesbeth Speelman, Grace Onyango, and Paul Bolton. 2009. "Assessing local instrument reliability and validity: A field-based example from northern Uganda." *Social Psychiatry and Psychiatric Epidemiology* 44(8): 685–92.

Bolton, Paul, Judith K. Bass, Theresa S. Betancourt, Liesbeth Speelman, Grace Onyango, Kathleen Clougherty, Richard Neugebauer, Laura Murray, and Helen Verdeli. 2007. "Interventions for depression symptoms among adolescent survivors of war and displacement in Northern Uganda." *Journal of the American Medical Association* 298(5): 519–27.

Bolton, Paul, Richard Neugebauer, and Lincoln Ndogoni. 2002. "Assessment of depression prevalence in rural Uganda using symptoms and function criteria." *Social Psychiatry and Psychiatric Epidemiology* 39: 442–47.

Bolton, Paul, and A. M. Tang. 2004. "Using ethnographic methods in the selection of post disaster, mental health interventions." *Prehospital Disaster Medicine* 19(1): 97–101.

Bolton, Paul, Christopher M. Wilk, and Lincoln Ndogoni. 2004. "Assessment of depression prevalence in rural Uganda using symptom and function criteria." *Social Psychiatry and Psychiatric Epidemiology* 39(6): 442–47.

Boothby, Neil. 1992. "Displaced children: Psychological theory and practice from the field." *Journal of Refugee Studies* 5(2): 106–22.

Bronfenbrenner, U. 1979. *The ecology of human development: Experiments by nature and design.* Cambridge, MA: Harvard University Press.

Cervantes, Richard C., V. Nelly Salgado de Snyder, and Amado M. Padilla. 1989. "Posttraumatic stress in immigrants from Central America and Mexico." *Hospital and Community Psychiatry* 40(6): 615–19.

Chen, Chuansheng, Shin-ying Lee, and Harold W. Stevenson. 1995. "Response style and cross-cultural comparisons of rating scales among East Asian and North American students." *Psychological Science* 6: 170–75.

Christakis, N. A., and J. H. Fowler. 2008. "The collective dynamics of smoking in a large social network." *New England Journal of Medicine* 358: 2249–58.

Debiec, Jacek, and Joseph E. LeDoux. 2006. "Noradrenergic signaling in the amygdala contributes to the reconsolidation of fear memory: Treatment implications for PTSD." *Annals of the New York Academy of Sciences* 1071: 521–24.

Dolnick, Sam. 2011. "Asylum ploys play off news to open door." *New York Times,* 12 July.

Eisenman, David P., Lillian Gelberg, Honghu Liu, and Martin F. Shapiro. 2003. "Mental health and health-related quality of life among adult Latino primary care patients living in the United States with previous exposure to political violence." *Journal of the American Medical Association* 290(5): 627–34.

Forrest, D. M. 1999. "Examination for the late physical after effects of torture." *Journal of Clinical Forensic Medicine* 6(1): 4–13.

Fox, Steven H. 2003. "The Mandinka nosological system in the context of post-trauma syndromes." *Transcultural Psychiatry* 40(4): 488.

Fox, Steven H., and S. S. Tang. 2000. "The Sierra Leonean refugee experience: Traumatic events and psychiatric sequelae." *Journal of Nervous and Mental Disease* 188: 490–95.

Goodkind, Jessica R. 2005. "Effectiveness of a community-based advocacy and learning program for Hmong refugees." *American Journal of Community Psychology* 36 (3–4): 387–408.

Goodkind, Jessica R. 2006. "Promoting Hmong refugees' well-being through mutual learning: Valuing knowledge, culture, and experience." *American Journal of Community Psychology* 37(1–2): 77–93.

Green, Eric P., and B. Kloos. 2008. *Using remote sensing and GIS to develop a sampling frame in a setting of internal displacement.* Columbia: University of South Carolina.

Griffin, M. G., P. A. Resick, A. E. Waldrop, and M. B. Mechanic. 2003. "Participation in trauma research: Is there evidence of harm?" *Journal of Traumatic Stress* 16(3): 221–27.

Grimm, Stephanie D., and A. Timothy Church. 1999. "A cross-cultural study of response biases in personality measures." *Journal of Research in Personality* 33(4): 415–41.

Hampshire, Kate, Gina Porter, Kate Kilpatrick, Peter Kyei, Michael Adjaloo, and George Oppong. 2008. "Liminal spaces: Changing inter-generational relations among long-term Liberian refugees in Ghana." *Human Organization* 67(1): 25–36.

Handwerker, W. P. 2001. *Quick ethnography.* Lanham, MD: AltaMira Press.

Hobfoll, S. E. 1989. "Conservation of resources: A new attempt at conceptualizing stress." *American Psychologist* 44(3): 513–24.

Hobfoll, S. E. 2001. "The influence of culture, community, and the nested-self in the stress process: Advancing conservation of resources theory." *Applied Psychology: An International Review* 50(3): 337–421.

Holtz, T. 1998. "Refugee trauma versus torture trauma: A retrospective controlled cohort study of Tibetan refugees." *Journal of Nervous and Mental Disease* 186: 24–34.

Hui, C. Harry, and Harry C. Triandis. 1989. "Effects of culture and response format on extreme response style." *Journal of Cross-Cultural Psychology* 20(3): 296–309.

Jaranson, James M., James Butcher, Linda Halcon, David Robert Johnson, Cheryl Robertson, Kay Savik, Marline Spring, and Joseph Westermeyer. 2004. "Somali and Oromos refugees: Correlates of torture and trauma history." *American Journal of Public Health* 94(4): 591–98.

Jayawickreme, Nuwan, Eranda Jayawickreme, Pavel Atanasov, Michelle A. Goonasekera, and Edna B. Foa. 2012. "Are culturally-specific measures of trauma-related anxiety and depression needed? The case of Sri Lanka." *Psychological Assessment.* Online first publication. doi: 10.1037/a0027564.

Juster, R. P., B. McEwen, and S. J. Lupien. 2009. "Allostatic load biomarkers of chronic stress and impact on health and cognition." *Neuroscience and Biobehavioral Reviews* 35: 2–16.

Kaiser, Bonnie N., Brandon Kohrt, H. Keys, N. M. Khoury, and A. Brewster. 2013. "Strategies for assessing mental health in rural Haiti: Local instrument development and transcultural translation strategies." *Transcultural Psychiatry* 50: 532–58.

Keller, Allen S., Dechen Lhewa, Barry Rosenfeld, Emily Sachs, Asher Aladjem, Ilene Cohen, Hawthorne Smith, and K. Porterfield. 2006. "Traumatic experiences and psychological distress in an urban refugee population seeking treatment services." *Journal of Nervous and Mental Disease* 194(3): 188–94.

Keller, Allen S., Barry Rosenfeld, Chau Trinh-Shervin, Chris Meserve, Emily Sachs, Jonathan A. Leviss, Elizabeth Singer, Hawthorne Smith, John Wilkinson, Glen Kim, Kathleen Allden, and Douglas Ford. 2003. "Mental health of detained asylum seekers." *Lancet* 362(9397): 1721–26.

Kohrt, Brandon, and Daniel Hruschka. 2010. "Nepali concepts of psychological trauma: The role of idioms of distress, ethnopsychology and ethnophysiology in alleviating suffering and preventing stigma." *Culture, Medicine and Psychiatry* 34(2): 322–52.

Kuo, W. H., and Tsai Y. 1986. "Social networking, hardiness, and immigrant's mental health." *Journal of Health and Social Behavior* 27(2): 133–49.

Leclere, F. B., L. Jensen, and A. E. Biddlecom. 1994. "Health care utilization, family context, and adaptation among immigrants to the United States." *Journal of Health and Social Behavior* 35(4): 370–84.

Legerski, John-Paul, and Sarah Bunnell. 2010. "The risks, benefits, and ethics of trauma-focused research participation." *Ethics and Behavior* 20(6): 429–42.

Lhewa, Dechen, Sophia Banu, Barry Rosenfeld, and Allen S. Keller. 2007. "Validation of a Tibetan translation of the Hopkins Symptom Checklist-25 and the Harvard Trauma Questionnaire." *Assessment* 14(3): 223–30.

Meffert, Susan M., Akram Osman Abdo, Omayma Ahmed Abd Alla, Yasir Omer Mustafa Elmakki, Afrah Abdelrahim Omer, Sahar Yousif, Thomas J. Metzler, and Charles R. Marmar. 2011. "A pilot randomized control trial of interpersonal psychotherapy for Sudanese refugees in Cairo, Egypt." *Psychological Trauma: Theory, Research, Practice, and Policy.* Advance online publication. doi: 10.1037/a0023540.

Meffert, Susan M., and Charles R. Marmar. 2009. "Darfur refugees in Cairo: Mental health and interpersonal conflict in the aftermath of genocide." *Journal of Interpersonal Violence* 24(11): 1835–48.

Miller, Kenneth E., and L. M. Rasco. 2004. *The mental health of refugees: Ecological approaches to healing and adaptation.* Mahwah, NJ: Erlbaum.

Miller, Kenneth E., and Andrew Rasmussen. 2010. "War exposure, daily stressors, and mental health in conflict and post-conflict settings: Bridging the divide between trauma-focused and psychosocial frameworks." *Social Science and Medicine* 70: 7–16.

Mollica, R. F., Y. Caspi-Yavin, P. Bollini, T. Truong, S. Tor, and J. Lavelle. 1992. "The Harvard Trauma Questionnaire: Validating a cross-cultural instrument for measuring torture, trauma, and post traumatic stress disorder in refugees." *Journal of Nervous Mental Disorders* 180: 111–16.

Mollica, R. F., Karen Donelan, Svang Tor, James Lavelle, Christopher Elias, Martin Frankel, and Robert J. Blendon. 1993. "The effect of trauma and confinement on functional health and mental health status of Cambodians living in Thailand-Cambodia border camps." *Journal of the American Medical Association* 270(5): 581–86.

Nader, Karim, Glenn E. Schafe, and Joseph E. LeDoux. 2000. "Fear memories require protein synthesis in the amygdala for reconsolidation after retrieval." *Nature* 406: 722–26.

Neuner, Frank, Patience Lamaro Onyut, Verena Ertl, Michael Oldenwald, Elisabeth Schauer, and Thomas Elbert. 2008. "Treatment of posttraumatic stress disorder by trained lay counselors in an African refugee settlement: A randomized controlled trial." *Journal of Consulting and Clinical Psychology* 76(4): 686–94.

Neuner, Frank, Margarete Schauer, Klaschik Christine, Unni Karunakara, and Elbert Thomas. 2004. "A comparison of narrative exposure therapy, supportive counseling, and psychoeducation for treating posttraumatic stress disorder in an African refugee settlement." *Journal of Consulting and Clinical Psychology* 72(4): 579–87.

Nickerson, Angela, Richard A. Bryant, Derrick Silove, and Zachary Steel. 2011. "A critical review of psychological treatments of posttraumatic stress disorder in refugees." *Clinical Psychology Review* 31(3): 399–417.

Noh, S., W. R. Avison, and V. Kaspar. 1992. "Depressive symptoms among Korean immigrants: Assessment of a translation of the Center for Epidemiologic Studies-Depression Scale." *Psychological Assessment* 4(1): 84–91.

Nyindo, M. 2005. "Complementary factors contributing to the rapid spread of HIV-I in Sub-Saharan Africa: A review." *East African Medical Journal* 82(1): 40–60.

Orth, Ulrich, and Andreas Maercker. 2004. "Do trials of perpetrators retraumatize crime victims?" *Journal of Interpersonal Violence* 19(2): 212–27.

Porter, Matthew, and Nick Haslam. 2005. "Predisplacement and postdisplacement factors associated with mental health of refugees and internally displaced persons: A meta-analysis." *JAMA: Journal of the American Medical Association* 294(5): 602–12.

Raghavan, Sumi, Andrew Rasmussen, Barry Rosenfeld, and Allen S. Keller. 2013. "Correlates of symptom reduction in treatment seeking survivors of torture." *Psychological Trauma: Theory, Research, Practice, and Policy* 5: 377–83.

Rasmussen, A., and J. Annan. 2010. "Predicting stress related to basic needs and safety in Darfur refugee camps: A structural and social ecological analysis." *Journal of Refugee Studies* 23(1): 23–40.

Rasmussen, Andrew, Basila Katoni, Allen S. Keller, and John Wilkinson. 2011. "Posttraumatic idioms of distress among Darfur refugees: Hozun and majnun." *Transcultural Psychiatry* 48(4): 392–415.

Rasmussen, Andrew, Leanh Nguyen, and John Wilkinson. 2007. "Polygamy in conflict settings: Distress and marriage among Darfuri refugees." In *22nd annual meeting of the International Society for Traumatic Stress Studies.* Hollywood, CA.

Reed, Ruth V., Mina Fazel, Catherine Painter-Brick, and Alan Stein. 2012. "Mental health of displaced and refugee children resettled in low and middle-income countries: Risk and protective factors." *Lancet* 379(9812): 250–65.

Ressler, Everett M., Neil Boothby, and Daniel J. Steinbock. 1988. *Unaccompanied children: Care and protection in wars, natural disasters, and refugee movements.* New York: Oxford University Press.

Roberts, B., K. Felix Ocaka, J. Browne, T. Oyok, and E. Sondorp. 2008. "Factors associated with the health status of internally displaced persons in northern Uganda." *Journal of Epidemiology and Community Health* 63: 227–32.

Sachs, Emily, Barry Rosenfeld, Dechen Lhewa, Andrew Rasmussen, and Allen S. Keller. 2008. "Entering exile: Trauma, mental health, and coping among Tibetan refugees arriving in Dharamsala, India." *Journal of Traumatic Stress* 21(2): 199–208.

Sameroff, A. J., and M. J. MacKenzie. 2003. "Research strategies for capturing transactional models of development: The limits of the possible." *Development and Psychopathology* 15: 613–40.

Shresta, N. M., B. Sharma, M. van Ommeren, S. Regmi, R. Makaju, I. Komproe, G. B. Shresta, and J. T. V. M. de Jong. 1998. "Impact of torture on refugees displaced within the developing world: Symptomatology among Bhutanese refugees in Nepal." *Journal of the American Medical Association* 280(5): 443–48.

Spiegel, Paul B., Francesco Checchi, Sandro Colombo, and Eugene Paik. 2010. "Health-care needs of people affected by conflict: Future trends and changing frameworks." *Lancet* 375(9711): 341–45.

Steel, Z., S. Momartin, C. Bateman, A. Hafshejani, D. M. Silove, and N. Everson. 2004. "Psychiatric status of asylum seeker families held for a protracted period in a remote detention centre in Australia." *Australian and New Zealand Journal of Public Health* 28: 527–36.

Steel, Z., D. Silove, Kevin Bird, Patrick McGorry, and P. Mohan. 1999. "Pathways from war trauma to posttraumatic stress symptoms among Tamil asylum seekers, refugees, and immigrants." *Journal of Traumatic Stress* 12(3): 421–35.

Steel, Z., D. Silove, Robert Brooks, S. Momartin, Bushra Alzuhairi, and Ina Susljik. 2006. "Impact of immigration detention and temporary protection on the mental health of refugees." *British Journal of Psychiatry* 188: 58–64.

Sundelin-Wahlsten, V., A. Ahmad, and A. L. Von Knorring. 2001. "Traumatic experiences and post-traumatic stress reactions in children from Kurdistan and Sweden." *Acta Paediatrica* 90: 563.

Tol, Wietse A., Ria Reis, Dessy Susanty, and Joop T. V. M. de Jong. 2010. "Communal violence and child psychosocial well-being: Qualitative findings from Poso, Indonesia." *Transcultural Psychiatry* 47(1): 112–35.

Travis, John. 2011. "UK abandons study of Nationality testing using DNA and isotopes." *Science Insider,* 17 June.

United Nations High Commissioner for Refugees (UNHCR). 2010a. *Convention and protocol relating to the status of refugees.* Geneva: United Nations.

United Nations High Commissioner for Refugees (UNHCR). 2010b. *UNHCR statistical yearbook 2009.* Geneva: United Nations.

United Nations High Commissioner for Refugees (UNHCR). 2011. *UNHCR stastistical yearbook 2010.* Geneva: United Nations.

US Department of State. 2010. *Proposed refugee admissions for Fiscal Year 2011.* Washington, DC: Government Printing Office.

Venters, H., and Allen S. Keller. 2009. "The immigration detention health plan: An acute care model for a chronic care population." *Journal of Health Care for the Poor and Underserved* 20(4): 951–57.

Verdeli, Helen, Kathleen Clougherty, Grace Onyango, Eric Lewandowski, Liesbeth Speelman, Theresa S. Betancourt, Richard Neugebauer, Traci R. Stein, and Paul Bolton. 2008. "Group interpersonal therapy for depressed youth in IDP camps in northern Uganda: Adaptation and training." *Child and Adolescent Psychiatric Clinics of North America* 17(3): 605–24.

Weine, Stevan, K. Knafl, S. Feetham, Y. Kulauzovic, A. Klebic, S. Sclove, S. Besic, A. Mujagic, J. Muzurovic, and D. Spahovic. 2006. "A mixed methods study of refugee families engaging in multiple-family groups." *Family Relations* 54: 558–68.

Williams, Carolyn L., and J. W. Berry. 1991. "Primary prevention of acculturative stress among refugees: Application of psychological theory and practice." *American Psychologist* 46(6): 632–41.

Zax, Melvin, and Shigeo Takahashi. 1967. "Cultural influences on response style: Comparisons of Japanese and American college students." *Journal of Social Psychology* 71(1): 3–10.

22

Working Internationally

Carol Camlin
David Kyle

INTRODUCTION

Working abroad will be a feature of many studies of migration and health and is worth considering as its own challenge. The introductory chapters to this volume detail the definitions of migration and mobility commonly used in migration studies, while chapters 4 through 17 describe strategies for identifying and gathering systematic samples of migrant populations. Chapters 18 through 25 describe special issues in working with hidden and hard-to-reach populations of migrants, for example, those who lack legal citizenship or residency status and those who are refugees or were forcibly displaced; these populations are not only migrant but also highly mobile. The issues and challenges to researchers in identifying, sampling, and involving migrants as participants in research, described across previous chapters, are in many ways magnified for researchers working in countries other than their own.

Local, national, and international politics can often interfere with the success of research projects, especially those involving migrant populations. Language and cultural barriers can impede the researcher's understanding of the populations and phenomena under study. To the array of unequal power relationships that may distance an investigator from his or her research participants (due to differences across social class, gender, or race) are added the dynamics of global power and wealth inequalities (between the global North and South, or the developed-versus-developing country divide). That inequalities are often felt or observed more keenly by those less empowered in these relations is often underappreciated by the novice investigator working in developing country settings. There are many such class and

TABLE 22.1 Two Phases of Research Planning and Execution in International Settings

Phase 1

Getting situated	Recover from jet lag and initial culture shock.
	Acclimate to culture, food, language, weather.
	Set up living and work settings (without getting to wedded to initial arrangements).
	Hire language interpreter if needed.
Getting connected	Gain entrée to communities in which you'll be working by making connections with a wide range of contacts, formally and informally.
	Learn about current social and political issues via local media and conversations.
Staying informed	Identify and make connections to key informants.
	Identify stakeholders for your research, and actively involve them in your plans.
	Read more literature about your topic.
	Find out who is doing what in the local community.

Phase 2

Getting down to work (and play)	Make friends, socialize, and engage in community activities.
Revising plans and starting preliminary research	Assess feasibility and get local input into your research plans.
	Revise and refine plans, methods for reaching study populations, and study instruments.
	Carry out preliminary research and/or pilot-testing.
Managing operations, expectations, and team members	Hire and train research team members, in collaboration with local partners.
	Begin the work, building in a process for getting iterative feedback from research team members.

social identity issues that one must confront, often connected to a soul-searching period of making appropriate choices sensitive to local norms and one's own values. Gender, sex, and religious values and expectations present challenging themes for researchers of migration and health, topics that typically intersect with such values. While these higher-order considerations will present the researcher at multiple times with very local and personal decisions, this chapter offers some practical advice for the novice researcher working internationally along some common, if not generic, pathways to getting to work in a foreign country and culture.

We first outline two phases (see table 22.1) of the first six months or so of field research such that the novice researcher can develop and execute a feasible research plan given "facts on the ground." The first phase concerns getting situated, connected, and informed about current issues and sensitivities. The second phase addresses the transition from the relative chaos of phase 1 to getting down to work, including the importance of continuing flexibility, maintaining high standards, cultivating local collaborations, and engaging in a social life (which may provide data and contacts). We describe the authors' first several months on field research as a graduate student (Kyle) and postdoc (Camlin) beginning work in Ecuador and Kenya, respectively. In addition, while many of the features of our work internationally may characterize a wide range of field research abroad, we highlight aspects particular to migration and health studies.

THE FIRST SIX MONTHS: TWO PHASES OF RESEARCH PLANNING AND EXECUTION

In the first phase of entering into work abroad, one can think of three significant areas that will need to be attended to, even while the many details of the trip and living abroad will be overwhelming. In fact, we offer these themes as a guard against the feeling of being overwhelmed, by both normalizing them and reminding the reader to keep the big picture in mind, thinking in terms of a dynamic process leading to producing usable and even significant research that is of interest to readers and that has practical local applications. It's useful to think of three areas of unfolding development in the first phase: getting situated, staying connected, and becoming informed. The difference between this way of structuring your thinking and simply being told to "be flexible" is that this approach can help you to build the structure and stability needed for work at a time in which "flexibility" will be forced upon you. This more structured approach will be invaluable, as you will likely have little control over many aspects of your life, or, perhaps better stated, the illusion of control will likely evaporate before you've made it through customs. We assume that while you may have some familiarity with the country you will be working in, possibly even having visited during shorter trips, you are embarking on a significant period of working and living abroad on the order of a year or more, typical of field research for a dissertation.

Phase 1: Getting Situated

Before you get on the airplane, it is useful to think of what you will need to "get situated"—a general description of several things big and small covered by many books on traveling and living abroad. The idea for us as researchers, however, is that you keep your eye on getting comfortably situated rather than being too wedded to a particular kind of housing, neighborhood, office space, and other amenities needed for living. Your safety should come first, though being minimally comfortable—a personal assessment—will be important to maintaining your balance and resilience in the months ahead. Before you leave for a significant period abroad, planning and procuring satisfactory living arrangements may prove more or less difficult, depending on communications, norms around contracts, and contacts you or others may have in the destination region.

There is also an emotional dimension to getting situated that can start prior to the trip, as social relationships and the stress of the event will start to shape your ability to work and plan. After arrival, you may experience the well-known phenomenon of culture shock and the accompanying frustration as you realize that "normal" strategies for making things happen are not working, and the alternatives are not obvious.

The first few days for the new investigator in a new research setting in a country other than his or her own are inevitably bewildering. The novice is well advised to allot time to simply acclimate: absorb the new time zone, climate, and local diet before attending to the matters of establishing professional and social relationships in the research setting. The sense of disorientation will pass, especially as you make more local connections with people who can help you navigate local pathways and cultures of bureaucracy. However, the acclimatization process for researchers who cannot communicate fluently in local languages is lengthier; researchers who can fluently speak at least the dominant professional-culture language in a country or region are at a distinct advantage. Depending on your funding levels, research design needs, and local norms, you may need to consider early on hiring a professional translator (useful for initial meetings and the review of any written documents, including survey instruments) and a language instructor—sometimes embodied in a single person.

Getting Connected.   The period of recovery from jet lag and initial culture shock usually culminates in a refreshed state of alertness and curiosity toward the new research setting, especially if you have the time and ability to start socializing and making professional contacts. At this point, the first order of business is to gain entrée to the communities in which you plan to work and to cultivate local partnerships for refining plans and carrying them out, especially if you do not have prior contacts or experience in the setting. Your plans and research design may be impeccable on paper, but in reality they will only get you out of the gate. To be successful, you will need to make contact and build relationships with gatekeepers, both formal and informal, and follow local customs of respect and reciprocity that are needed to work in their communities. Taking time to identify gatekeepers, any local conflicts or alliances that could affect those relationships, and following the official channels that may govern your actions as a foreigner will be well worth your time as the study progresses. This is why socializing and making friends with those not critical to your project is extremely useful in helping you navigate the social networks and cultural and political sensitivities important to helping or hindering your work. Getting connected initially to a wide range of people without spending too much time with just a couple of people or families (invitations will likely ensue) may be challenging but will lay the foundation for becoming and staying informed in ways directly relevant to your research plans.

Staying Informed.   While preparation for a new research study inevitably involves establishing relationships with local organizations and individuals, that process accelerates dramatically once you arrive in the research setting. Such relationships are crucial, and not only because local organizations and individuals tend to be relied upon to implement research plans. Early in the research process, such plans will need to be discussed with and vetted by local "key informants" (Patton 1990)— knowledgeable, articulate individuals who can help you understand what is happening in the setting you've chosen for your research. The selection of key informants is a mainstay of qualitative research, but quantitative researchers will also be well served by identifying and making contact with key informants. For newcomers to a setting, relying on the advice and opinion of a single key informant, or even a select two or three, can be counterproductive and even risky; it's not uncommon that people will seek you out with their agendas early on, when you do not have the capacity to fully vet their proposals and information and you are desperate to begin work. The first few weeks is a tricky time in which caution and triangulation of information is critical. Actively seek out multiple points of view and sources to avoid becoming unduly influenced by the views of one or two individuals who, because of their gate-keeping role, may also close some doors even while they are opening others.

It is much better to actively seek out the critiques, questions, and alternative perspectives of local informants at the very outset of the research process, rather than to discover later that one's underlying assumptions about critical aspects of the research plan were incorrect. This is the time to get one's "ear to the ground": to learn about unforeseen sensitive political or cultural issues that may impinge on the research, become informed about the preoccupations of local press and public discourse related to the research topic, and identify the key stakeholders for the research (i.e., the individuals or groups who share your goals, who have the most to gain or lose, or are likely to be affected in some way by the research findings). Actively involving stakeholders as local collaborators at the planning stages of the research process builds buy-in and may be absolutely necessary (see next section, on Kyle's experience in Ecuador). It also serves to distribute accountability and responsibility for successful outcomes through a network of individuals.

After these initial steps of acculturating and getting the lay of the land through conversations with key informants, you should review additional literature on the research topic, finding out about programmatic work being carried out in the research setting and often conducting exploratory research.

It is expected that you conducted a thorough review of the literature on the migrant population and health issues before you left home in order to formulate the research hypotheses that undergird your plans. However, once you are in the research setting, issues often arise from conversations with key informants, and additional review is undertaken. It may be surprising to find that you often need to spend time researching and reading additional material based on what you are hearing and learning through new relationships and the local press. Of course, such a review usually requires Internet and electronic library access, as well as adequate bandwidth for viewing and downloading articles. Infrastructure barriers to technologies are to be expected in many settings, but as of this writing these barriers are being dismantled in even the poorest developing country settings. Time spent reading and reviewing literature on the research topic both before and after arrival in the research setting is well spent as it may help you guard against making a critical error early on. Learn from others' mistakes. Most importantly, you are now reading with more focus and scanning for details that will directly shape your actual research plans.

Similarly, taking the time to find out about any programmatic work by state agencies, nongovernmental organizations (NGOs), or the communities themselves in the research setting yields dividends: programs or services targeted to the migrant population you wish to study will certainly have an impact on your research plan and will provide extremely valuable information about what can and cannot be done and how it can be successful. You are now seeking details of any existing projects and sensitivities that you must be aware of as you proceed. If the planned research is intended to lead to (or is comprised of) a policy or health intervention, plans must account for the potential synergies or conflicts between the research and other efforts under way in the population.

Phase 2: Getting Down to Work (and Play)

The second phase of the research process, a transitional period between getting situated and actually carrying out the planned, official data collection phase, will typically be longer than the first; however, there is no clear demarcation between them as our "phases" are for helping you keep a big picture perspective about the course of work in the context of your own developing comfort with the setting. You may realize very early on, for example, that one or more planned parts of your research will simply not be feasible, and you will start to consider revisions. For several reasons, recognizing a "phase 1" period helps prevent you from feeling too impatient and making important decisions before you are ready to do so. When you have gotten situated, established some trusted contacts—including local friendships, key informants, and critical gatekeepers—and have started to feel culturally competent, you will be ready to start considering any revisions to the planned research design and formulating the details of the operational plan for carrying out the research.

Revising Plans and Starting Preliminary Research.   Using the cumulative information gathered from conversations, review of literature, garnering of feedback, and sometimes an exploratory research study, you begin to refine the overall research plan. In phase 2, you define and refine research questions, rethink definitions and methods for reaching populations of interest, and develop the final plans for sampling and data collection methods. Revisions of data collection instruments may also be undertaken at this stage as long as they do not lead to major deviations from protocols approved by committees for ethical research in human subjects. If that is the case, revised protocols, interview guides, or survey instruments need to be submitted to these review groups (usually in the host country as well as your institution of origin), and approval must be obtained before data collection can begin.

Preliminary or exploratory research is often necessary to determine whether the research plans and methods are feasible in the research setting and are acceptable to the migrant population intended for participation. Pretesting not only is sound on scientific grounds to hone the survey instrument or other data collection methods, but also allows you to work out operational details.

Managing Operations, Expectations, and Team Members.   Field research team members may need to be hired and trained at this stage, including interviewers, interpreters or translators, and data entry or transcription personnel. The process of working with research teams to carry out research across languages and cultures involves hiring, training, and supervising (or arranging the supervision of) local research team members, but also working collaboratively in the data analysis and knowledge production phases of the research. Working in close collaboration with local academic researchers and institutions can result in much higher quality research than if you "go it alone," and can help you lay the groundwork for continued and expanded research activities at the site.

The Fine Line between Work and Play Abroad.   It may be tempting to think that once you've started to conduct some preliminary research, your life will be all business. This will likely not be the case, nor should it be, for sound, practical reasons useful for your research. Socializing with others and engaging in activities that are entertaining and fulfilling will be critical to keeping you healthy and for continuing many of the benefits outlined in phase 1. The fact is that you never know how or where you will learn about a relevant opportunity or challenging hurdle; most importantly, you will be learning about the social context and cultural and political systems impacting the subjects of your study. Thus, socializing with friends outside of an official work frame will give you critical insights and may even end up being "qualitative data" discussed in your writing and analysis. A daily log, jottings, or diary will be helpful especially after you have left the country and are trying to remember details of the setting or useful quotes from local friends and key informants.

Finally, data collection begins and you are on your way to working internationally as a professional researcher. Our experiences with these processes are detailed next in the following two case studies of international research projects with migrant populations.

PRACTICAL EXAMPLES FROM TWO STUDIES OF MIGRATION AND HEALTH

Ecuador

This section describes David Kyle's experiences in the early 1990s as a graduate student conducting research on two relatively new cases of transnational mobility from Cuenca and Otavalo, in southern and northern Andean Ecuador, respectively (Kyle 2000). The first case began as a study of HIV health care capacity and sexual education in Cuenca, as well as an overall assessment of the prevalence of HIV among returning migrants who had been living in New York City, including neighborhoods such as Jackson Heights, Queens, which has some of the highest HIV incidence rates in the US (Kyle and Sawyer 1993). That study, conducted during a preliminary three-month trip to Ecuador, evolved into an initial component of a larger study of transnational mobility comparing two regions with distinct "transnational economic strategies" abroad (labor vs. commercial activities) carried out over a year of living in Ecuador. Thus, we describe two episodes: first, what Kyle learned during the initial health study in Cuenca and how it developed into the final, broader research design after first overcoming a gender-based research challenge and, second, a significant hurdle encountered in Otavalo concerning the ability to carry out survey research.

Kyle first traveled to Cuenca to attend a public health conference as a graduate student after a mostly touristic visit to the capitol, Quito. At the conference, he was surprised to learn about a large-scale migration to New York City that had rapidly developed during the 1980s. There had been no systematic studies of migration from Ecuador at that time; it was also clear that the health implications for the region were significant, as returning migrants were shuttling back and forth in ways that Kyle and then others began to characterize as "transnational." He immediately began to consider a dissertation plan and a return trip. Returning the following summer for three months allowed for both exploratory research and a stand-alone study of HIV awareness and health care capacity.

Though that initial research experience led Kyle to radically change the research design into a comparative study of two disparate Andean regions, two features of this initial study were challenging and illustrative of topics discussed in the previous sections. First, Kyle's initial stay in Cuenca, to conduct research among medical and social science professionals, connected him to very elite networks that were both useful and also somewhat of a barrier to the full comparative study on transnational mobility that he later conducted. During the initial research trip, which could be considered part of phase 1, Kyle sought out professional social scientists and medical researchers who might have an interest in his research goals. However, this led to befriending and acculturating to the highest strata of Cuenca elite families, whose social position made them extremely useful as gatekeepers to many aspects of local life; however, they were not the subjects of the study and had somewhat condescending attitudes toward the mostly rural, much lower class, migrants.

Thus, networks afforded some opportunities but closed off others. Kyle began to realize that these social contacts also skewed his information and perception of the phenomenon he sought to study. Most importantly, through social contacts not obviously connected to the research goals as originally planned, information and opportunities with networks led to the inspiration for planning a more ambitious study of two distinct regions. Interestingly, playing music locally in homes led to a friend of a friend inviting him to play in a folkloric musical group, which unintentionally became a significant opportunity for the later study (see Kyle 2000).

When he returned for a full year the following fall, phase 2 could begin much more quickly, though getting situated, connected, and informed was still very much a part of that final year as well. The study design called for a combination of ethnographic research and survey research in four rural communities, two in each region. While ethnographic research often proceeds and builds through trusted contacts and has its own trade-offs regarding the networks one chooses to explore, in-person survey research requires careful consideration of the household, community, and regional politics around ethnicity, gender, and other attributes of the investigator.

In the Cuenca region, Kyle was unable to enter the homes of families in which the men were abroad and the women had been "left behind." Given the patriarchal norms and the local surveillance of women by relatives and friends of men living in New York City, there was a well-founded fear that domestic violence might occur months later if a husband returning from abroad learned that a male had spent an hour or more alone in a house with his wife. Kyle was able to hire a female anthropologist to overcome this barrier in one community with high levels of male migration. This had the added benefit of allowing the women to discuss features of their own planned migrations, even in the face of discouragement from husbands. During the course of the study, a handful of women left using the services of "coyotes," or smugglers, while several more were planning an upcoming trip. This was novel for the community and reflected the desperation to be reunited, dead or alive, with their male counterparts. Many expressed anger at the men who had migrated, including one woman who exclaimed: "He's going to return with me even if I have to burn his body and take it back in a box." The most sensitive aspect of the women's planning for the journey was that many were starting to take birth control pills, fearing that they might be raped en route—a very real prospect. It is doubtful that these women would have shared this fact with Kyle if he had not collaborated with a female anthropologist.

A significant snag in the survey research was also encountered when Kyle learned from local researchers in Otavalo, mostly anthropologists who had been working there for years or decades in some cases, that no one had ever successfully conducted a survey of an Otavalan community (there are sixty or so). In fact, after several months of living in Ecuador Kyle had still not read or heard about the "famous story" from the early 1800s in which census takers were drawn and quartered and their bodies were guarded by Otavalan women for several days as an additional warning of what would happen to all census takers in this fiercely independent region. Local foreign researchers who had been in and out of the region for years recounted this historical detail with near glee, while emphasizing that small-scale ethnographic research was the only method available to social scientists. The mere mention of survey research raised eyebrows; the fact that Kyle actually planned to conduct a "census" was considered laughable by many.

Kyle did conduct the first survey research in the region. How Kyle came to conduct this type of research in Otavalan communities speaks to the need to be flexible and informed while keeping a bird's-eye view on what was important to the study. First, after being initially discouraged and made to feel fearful of being able to conduct a census survey, at no time did he seriously consider abandoning the survey component in Otavalo, a critical part of his overall comparative design. The new information about possible local resistance did mean that the timing and planning of the survey would have to shift to the very end of the year, a delay that would provide the time needed to prepare a new plan. By learning as much as possible about the target communities through friendships and contacts outside and within the communities, Kyle learned about the needs and interests of community leaders and considered what he could provide to them in terms of data that would be useful. Simply offering any other resources (e.g., an economic incentive), even if that had been desirable, would have been dismissed out of hand. Neither the community leadership nor the community as a whole would want to be the first to "sell out" a regional norm for a price. As the region was partially financed by considerable outside aid from foreign governments and NGOs, Kyle realized that data about their community could be extremely useful for funding proposals submitted to such entities. Months of discussion with leaders ensued about the possibility of providing useful data and training members of the community to be survey researchers. Kyle also promised to provide the training needed to make the data most useful and to provide community reports before he left Ecuador. After community meetings debating whether to break such a long-standing norm against the taking of a census, community leaders agreed to this reciprocal arrangement. Thus, while the overall features of the research design remained, the operational plan and details of when, how, and who would administer it had to be completely changed.

Kenya

This section describes Carol Camlin's experience as a postdoctoral fellow carrying out a pilot research project in 2009–2010 on the HIV prevention needs of female migrants in the Kisumu area of Nyanza Province in western Kenya (Camlin et al. 2013, 2014). This experience, and the findings of the pilot research, provided the foundation she needed to successfully apply for a larger research grant for a five-year program of research on gender, migration, and HIV in western Kenya, the ultimate aim of which is to develop an effective HIV prevention intervention for female migrants. The rationale for the study stems from literature showing (e.g., in Camlin et al. 2010) that female migrants are a population at high risk of both HIV acquisition and HIV transmission, but the social contexts and migration processes that facilitate these risks in women are not well understood.

To carry out this research, Camlin assembled a research team in collaboration with a Kenyan research institution and sought the advice, guidance, and "buy-in" from senior-level faculty at both her home institution and the Kenyan institution before embarking on the work. This step is typical for postdoctoral fellows and early career faculty: both the guidance of faculty mentors and the research infrastructure they can offer are critical elements to laying the groundwork for the successful launch of a research program. In Camlin's case, faculty mentors in the US and Kenya led to her initial contact with a Kenyan co-investigator with whom she still works closely on most all aspects of her research, and resulted in the provision of office space, computers, and other institutional support in the field site that allowed her to hire and support a team of local researchers with whom she carried out her research.

In her initial pilot study in Kenya, Camlin worked with the research team to collect extensive ethnographic data over several months in 2010. The pilot study had these main aims: to characterize forms and patterns of migration and mobility among women in the Kisumu area of Nyanza Province, Kenya; to describe the spatial and social features of key destinations of female migrants and highly mobile women; and to describe the contexts and social processes that facilitated HIV infection and transmission risks among migrant and highly mobile women. She and her team used two qualitative research methods to conduct this study (which are described in chapter 14, by Aguilera and Amuchástegui, in this volume): (1) participant observation (Bernard 1994) in selected common migration destinations for women in the Kisumu area and (2) in-depth semistructured interviews (Chase 2008) with female migrants selected from these key destinations using theoretical sampling techniques (Strauss and Corbin 1998). The research team also carried out interviews with men in order to explore their perspectives on findings that emerged from daily debriefing and preliminary reading of women's interviews in the same locations.

Before they began data collection, Camlin and her Kenyan co-investigator conducted interviews with key informants, including government officials, representatives of NGOs, including many women's NGOs, other academic researchers working in the same research setting, and female migrants themselves, identified through initial contacts with NGO representatives. From these initial interviews the research team identified potential typologies of female migrants and highly mobile women, and garnered information about their potential migration destinations. They then visited each potential setting, selected exemplary destinations (e.g., those representative of small, medium, and large beach villages that attract female migrants, and the largest market in western Kenya, which is the key site of small-scale trade and a locus of activity for highly mobile female traders), and requested permission from local authorities in each setting to return and carry out further research.

This experience is also typical for research in international settings: multiple levels and stages of permission to carry out research are required, beginning with formal reviews and approvals by committees for human subjects research at academic institutions (in the US and in the field site), moving to the next level of informal but politically essential approvals to carry out research in specific settings (e.g., at each of the beach villages in Kenya, a local governance unit called a "Beach Management Unit" gave permission for the research team to visit and carry out its research in the setting). Finally, informed consent to participate in research must be given by individuals who opt to participate in the research.

After selecting sites and obtaining local permissions, Camlin and her team began the first phase of the data collection, using participant observation. Participant observation involves an immersion in local cultural worlds in order to learn about what people do and what it means to them, while also attending to the ways in which social and cultural factors shape and constrain individual and group practices (Bernard 1994). As described in chapter 14 of this handbook, it is an ideal method for building an understanding of hard-to-reach and mobile populations and understudied groups. Participant observation of the settings in which female migrants and highly mobile women live and work allowed Camlin and her research team to directly observe the social processes that are ongoing in the social contexts of female migrants in order to help them to construct an understanding of how these contexts influence HIV risks.

In classic anthropological research, participant observation has a true participation element: the researcher takes on a social role in a community, settles in, and takes part (e.g., serves as an apprentice to a local healer to assist and learn her practices, or volunteers in a local carpentry shop, etc.). The method conventionally presupposes that the researcher works solo and also lives in the given community over an extended period of time. However, researchers in public health involved in studies of migrant populations may not be able to follow this model of participant observation. Both funding and time constraints limit our ability to move into a community for an extended period of time, and the objectives of our research often require that we work in several settings, not just one. In Camlin's case, there were these hurdles and more: while she spoke rudimentary Kiswahili, she spoke no Dholuo, the dominant language in the settings in which she planned to work. To gain fluency in Dholuo would have required a relocation to western Kenya, but, having returned to the US after a two-year research stint elsewhere in Africa, and with a young child, she wanted to remain based in the US but carry out the research over several trips to Kenya (a two-month long trip, followed by three shorter trips). Her solution to the conundrum was to hire and train two local research assistants (RAs) in Kenya to carry out the participant observation, and later to conduct in-depth interviews, with the guidance and supervision of Camlin and her Kenyan co-investigator.

Neither of the RAs had previous experience working on a research study; one had earned a baccalaureate degree from a four-year university in the area, and the other had completed only primary-level education. Camlin and a colleague trained both RAs in qualitative data collection methods, but only the college-educated RA had the skills and training necessary to use a computer to type up her field and interview notes. Yet both of the RAs played a critical role in conducting the research: the older, less-educated RA was an extremely savvy, vibrant, and socially aware local trader, similar in many ways to many of the participants in terms of her background and life history, with intimate knowledge of the local settings for the research. She established instant rapport with key informants in the field research sites, identified individuals who were eligible to participate in the study, and facilitated entrée and social connections in the research sites to the younger, more educated RA. Moreover, this team-based approach, with both the elder RA and the younger RA in the sites, provided a modicum of social protection and physical security to the younger RA.

This arrangement had many benefits: the two research assistants were welcomed and quickly integrated into the settings chosen for participant observation. They did not stand out as foreigners in the settings, they interpreted what they observed in those settings with in-depth and swift understanding, and they easily established rapport with individuals whom they later screened and invited for participation in in-depth interviews. At the end of each day, the research assistants prepared field notes focused on their observations of the environment, social actors, and social relations within the migration destinations selected for participant observation. Camlin and the team discussed these field notes on a daily basis, and later the "data" from these notes were analyzed in conjunction with data from the in-depth, semi-structured interviews.

The participant observation continued and was interspersed with periods of in-depth interviewing carried out by the more highly educated RA. The Kenyan co-investigator of the study was also based locally, and conversant in the local languages, but like Camlin, he did not directly carry out the participant observation and interviewing. Given the dynamics of both gender and social class, it would have been difficult for the Kenyan male PI to engage female study participants and make them feel comfortable in disclosing sensitive, potentially stigmatizing behaviors, life events, thoughts, and opinions in interviews and conversations. His very presence in the research site, as an authoritative academic wearing a professional man's clothing, affected the social dynamic of those settings in a way in which the presence of the female RAs alone did not. Camlin's presence in the same settings was likely, given that she is a white, female, native English-speaking foreigner affiliated with an American university, to have been even more disruptive of the normal social ebb and flow. She could have chosen to directly carry out interviews with participants with the aid of an interpreter, and the Kenyan co-investigator could have interviewed the women, but they chose not to work that way in order to minimize the extent to which participants might be intimidated by the interview process.

This research study was accomplished through careful attentiveness to the politics of field research in a developing country context, as well as to the power dynamics of gender, race, and nationality. Such attentiveness was particularly necessary given the nature of the research topic, involving, as it did, highly emotionally charged issues related to the HIV/AIDS epidemic, sexuality and morally sanctioned and socially stigmatized sexual behaviors (such as transactional and commercial sex), cultural practices surrounding marriage, cohabitation, and household arrangements, and the recalling of the sometimes traumatic events that precipitated migration. With training and supervision from the PIs, the female RAs were able to elicit open and frank discussions with the female migrants who participated in the study.

Here we want to be very clear that we draw a distinction between the types of multinational research carried out under the rubric of social science and public health, involving short-term interactions between strangers, and the very different tradition of anthropological research in developing country settings. In the latter case, the longer term social immersion of the solo "stranger" in a community setting, and the process of his or her becoming known to members of the community (as well as her or his knowing others), may permit greater ease and facility in overcoming the barriers of nationality, race, gender, and class that we describe here. While such power dynamics can never be wished away, the intimacy and local knowledge that develops over time in anthropological field research can facilitate the sharing of social meanings across these differences, and permit a depth of investigation not typically possible in the context of grant-funded public health and social science research. However, greater social intimacy may also increase social desirability bias, as issues of social reputation, interdependence, and the desire for approval enter into relationships between researchers and participants.

Public health research is subject not only to time and funding constraints, but also to the ethical obligations of crafting timely solutions to urgent public health problems. Hence, the methods used for this study were designed to attend to the real barriers to knowledge production resulting from global and local power inequalities, despite typical time and logistical constraints—via use of a diverse, team-based approach involving local researchers who were socially connected and culturally similar to the population of people who participated in the research. The involvement of the RAs in data collection was crucial, but their involvement in data analysis was also necessary for accurate interpretation and in-depth understanding of the data.

The local dissemination of research findings also provided a crucial validation check of the interpretations the research team brought to the data collected from participant observation field notes and interview transcripts. Camlin, the Kenyan co-investigator, and the RAs presented the findings of the research in a workshop with local stakeholders, including the key informants initially interviewed as well as many of the study participants. As this program of research continues, Camlin plans an iterative process of discussion with the same group of stakeholders. As of this writing, she plans to develop a set of options for an HIV prevention intervention with female migrants on the basis of the cumulative findings of the research program, involving the group of local stakeholders in an assessment of the acceptability, relevance, and feasibility of the options for the local context. She anticipates that this process will culminate in the design, implementation, and evaluation of such an intervention.

CONCLUSIONS

This chapter has explored the cultural, political, and social questions that may be usefully considered when you are planning and conducting research internationally. We described the opportunities and challenges inherent in what we conceive as two phases in the process of carrying out international research with migrant populations. We believe that keeping a bird's-eye view of the process even while engaging in the daily struggle of appointments, transportation, and writing will help new investigators prepare emotionally for the challenges they will face when working internationally, and suggest strategies for managing or avoiding many of the most common problems that befall the novice (these are things we keep in mind when encountering a new project). We also described the processes and challenges encountered in carrying out our research as young scholars with migrant populations in Ecuador and Kenya, two very different regional settings of South America and sub-Saharan Africa, to give the reader a feel for how actual research unfolds in settings in which the researcher is, typically, not entirely culturally competent, socially connected, and completely informed. It is this dual process of both conducting useful research and, simultaneously, learning about a new culture based on new friendships, that makes working internationally so challenging and rewarding.

REFERENCES

Bernard, H. R. 1994. *Research Methods in Anthropology: Qualitative and Quantitative Approaches.* Thousand Oaks, CA: Sage.

Camlin C. S., V. Hosegood, M. L. Newell, N. McGrath, T. Bärnighausen, and R. C. Snow. 2010. "Gender, Migration and HIV in Rural KwaZulu-Natal, South Africa." *PLoS ONE* 5(7): e11539.

Camlin, C. S., Z. K. Kwena, and S. Dworkin. 2013. "Jaboya vs. Jakambi: Status, Negotiation and HIV Risks among Female Migrants in the 'Sex-for-Fish' Economy in Nyanza Province, Kenya." *AIDS Education and Prevention* 25: 216–31.

Camlin, C. S., Z. A. Kwena, S. Dworkin, C. Cohen, and E. Bukusi. 2014. "'She mixes her business': HIV Transmission and Acquisition Risks among Female Migrants in Western Kenya." *Social Science and Medicine* 102: 146–56.

Chase, S. E. 2008. "Narrative Inquiry: Multiple Lenses, Approaches, Voices." In *Collecting and Interpreting Qualitative Materials,* edited by N. K. Denzin and Y. S. Lincoln. Thousand Oaks, CA: Sage. 57–94.

Kyle, David. 2000. *Transnational Peasants: Migrations, Networks, and Ethnicity in Andean Ecuador.* Baltimore: Johns Hopkins University Press.

Kyle, David, and Ann Sawyer. 1993. "The Health Impact of Return Migration from New York City to Ecuador." *Migration World* 21: 39.

Patton, Michael Q. 1990. *Qualitative Evaluation and Research Methods.* 2nd ed. Thousand Oaks, CA: Sage.

Strauss, A., and J. Corbin. 1998. *Basics of Qualitative Research: Techniques and Procedures for Developing Grounded Theory.* 2nd ed. Thousand Oaks, CA: Sage.

23

Binational Collaborative Research

Sylvia Guendelman

INTRODUCTION

I first started working on United States–Mexico immigration studies in the mid-1980s. At the time the foreign-born Mexican population living in the United States was growing very rapidly mostly due to the surge in unauthorized immigration that had started in the 1970s. Undocumented immigrants openly crossed the border in search of work opportunities and better lifestyles in California. As a public health scholar interested in the health of women, children, and families, I considered this influx an exciting opportunity to study many relevant public health issues.

One issue that caught my attention was that as the immigrant population grew in California, so did the use of health services among immigrants. Concern was growing among US policy makers that increasing access barriers to health services in Mexico were pushing people to seek care across the border, taxing California's health system beyond its capacity. Particularly noticeable was the increasing demand for obstetric care by low-income women. Evidence indicated that public hospitals and clinics in California were serving a greater number of Mexico-born women at greater health risk compared with a decade earlier; of particular concern was the large proportion of uninsured women seeking care. This raised an important policy question: were Mexican women crossing the border so that they could give birth to American babies and have access to free care? Although the research question referred to the utilization of health services in California, I decided to research this issue in Mexico for two important reasons. First, experts assumed that the population utilizing health services was undocumented, and we simply lacked population estimates that would have allowed us to generate a representative sample of undocumented women in California. Furthermore, we were skeptical that immigrants interviewed in California would give honest responses to delicate questions.

I partnered with a researcher at Colegio de la Frontera Norte (COLEF) and with a local primary care clinic in Tijuana, Mexico, that had trained health promoters to provide care in the surrounding shantytowns. Together we built a strong partnership with low-income communities throughout the city and developed a sound multimethods project. We first designed a community household survey of binational health service utilization of 660 randomly selected households in Tijuana, including 1,162 household adult members who reported having used health services in the US and/or Mexico in the six months prior to the interview. The study found that among border residents, 7% had sought services in the US and 93% had sought services only in Mexico (Guendelman 1991). A follow-up survey among border resident women showed that while one out of ten women had crossed over to give birth in the US, the rate among upper- and middle-income sector women was one out of six (Guendelman and Jasis 1992). Follow-up focus groups with women stratified by socioeconomic level indicated that border women who delivered in California were not indigent, undocumented patients. Contrary to popular belief, border women giving birth in California tended to be upper-middle class and to have a history of close contact with the US, as demonstrated by their legal documentation for crossing the border, English-language skills, and for almost half of the sample, a history of living in the US prior to the pregnancy. Similar to other Mexican nationals using health services in the US, most women sought maternity care in the private sector and paid for these services primarily out of pocket or with private insurance, representing a low burden on publicly funded health care in California. Among women who delivered in the US, 47% expected to obtain citizenship for their children or families. Another 45% responded that they crossed the border because they were offered better attention or technology in the US. Only 8% reported that they chose US care to obtain special benefits such as food coupons or a comfortable hospital stay.

At the time of this study, one out of three births in California was of Latino origin. Yet, as our project demonstrated, the majority of Tijuana's non-affluent residents did not deliver babies in California. The increasing birth rates to Mexican mothers in California were largely explained by the higher fertility rate of Mexican immigrants already living in the state (Hamilton et al. 2003), which underscored the relevance of examining birth outcomes to Mexican immigrant mothers. Mexican immigrants tend to have low educational attainment, high rates of poverty, and delayed access to health care—traditionally all risk factors for adverse birth outcomes in other populations. To what extent did Mexican immigrant mothers have favorable birth outcomes such as term deliveries, normal birth weight, and low infant mortality?

This time, I set out to address these questions by collaborating with US researchers and using data collected in the US. Over the years, we conducted several quantitative and qualitative studies that used community surveys, analyses of statewide birth and administrative records, and focus groups to document what was observed (Guendelman and English 1995; Guendelman et al. 1990, 2001, 2005, 2006). The studies quite consistently found that compared to white non-Latina women, Mexican immigrant women were healthier and gave birth to healthier infants. Unfortunately, some of our studies also showed that the initial health advantage of immigrant mothers displayed at the time of arrival eroded with duration of US residence and with generational changes (Guendelman and English 1995; Guendelman et al. 1990). The erosion was reflected in deteriorating maternal health behaviors such as tobacco and alcohol consumption, poor dietary intake, and teen pregnancy, as well as in deleterious infant health outcomes, including fetal deaths, low birth weight, and morbidities during the first year of life. However, similar to others, my studies lacked a comparison group of mothers in Mexico. Without this population, we were unable to accurately assess the effects that exposure to the US environment has on health because mothers who immigrate to the US could have been favorably (or unfavorably) selected for health reasons before migration. Over time I learned to appreciate the need for binational health studies that went beyond binational exchanges of ideas or procurement of study sites in Mexico or the US and began to develop a research methodology that would allow us to collect and examine data on the heterogeneous Mexican-origin population living in both countries.

My first attempt began in 2002. I established collaboration with research partners at the Instituto Mexicano de Servicio Social (IMSS), one of the largest public health providers in Mexico. Our objective was to conduct a study of maternal morbidities during labor and delivery, focusing on serious obstetric complications that burden mothers and can result in poor pregnancy outcomes. We aimed to compare differences in morbidities among mothers living in Mexico, Mexico-born mothers living in California, and US-born mothers of Mexican origin living in California. We were hoping that evidence from this study would shed light on the puzzle about the favorable pregnancy outcomes of Mexican immigrant women. With approval from the California Committee for the Protection of Human Subjects to use linked hospital discharge-birth records for California, we were poised to link our data with maternal health data from an IMSS sample. It took months of lengthy discussions with our colleagues in Mexico City to program the IMSS data using morbidity codes comparable to those used in the US records. Yet, when it was time for IMSS to release estimates to allow for comparisons with US estimates, our Mexican partners began to stall. The waiting turned into a war of attrition and eventually our team gave up. We will never know what caused the Mexican researchers' hesitance. We do know that it was not a problem of data measurement, since presumably standardized data had been analyzed in both countries. Our experience painfully brought to the fore some of the challenges of binational collaboration. International partnerships need to bridge cultural, political, organizational, and methodological issues, which at times can loom large, making these partnerships vulnerable to disruption.

In recent years, I have made renewed attempts to establish binational research collaborations focusing on another timely and critical policy and planning issue: the alarmingly high rates of overweight and obesity in the Mexican-origin populations living in Mexico and in the US. This time, research partnerships have proceeded smoothly and relied heavily on binational data and on binational interpretation of the findings. Capitalizing on the lessons learned, this chapter aims to describe the purpose, advantages, and challenges of using a binational research methodology and provides some key questions that an uninitiated researcher must consider before attempting to engage in binational research. It also provides a case study that illustrates the application of this methodology for investigating overweight and obesity among adults of Mexican origin living in Mexico and the US.

WHAT IS A BINATIONAL COLLABORATIVE RESEARCH METHODOLOGY?

Binational collaborative research is a methodology that allows for the simultaneous examination of health issues in populations residing in the country or region of origin and the destination country. The approach uses linked datasets to describe and compare populations both within and across countries. The methodology can help elucidate common and unique health characteristics of populations that are linked demographically, culturally, and economically through migration. By describing the prevalence of key health outcomes, establishing associations between specific social determinants and the health outcomes, and comparing disparities between and within populations, this methodology can much more effectively identify potential levers for change. Studies on immigration and health must include the source population, which is essential for understanding the health effects of immigration and of other social determinants such as acculturation or integration into the receiving society (Kley 2011; Crimmins et al. 2005; Van Hook et al. 2012; Ullmann et al. 2011).

Binational collaborative research has many useful functions. It can help clarify misconceptions that are common in immigration studies, such as whether immigrants have better or worse health as a result of im/migration, and can lead to new insights about what factors predispose immigrants to be healthy/unhealthy. Binational collaborative research is also critical to building strong partnerships that allow us to tackle public health inequalities within and across countries, using the best available evidence. Strong collaborations encourage mutual learning, improve data collection, and enhance interpretation of findings. Evidence obtained from linked data can be synthesized and disseminated to key stakeholders in both countries to serve as a platform from which to draft more effective policy solutions and public health interventions.

ADVANTAGES AND CHALLENGES OF BINATIONAL COLLABORATIVE RESEARCH

International research on migration and health has been characterized by little synergy, and studies lack consensus on how to define immigrants and the social determinants of immigrants' health. For instance, a recent systematic review conducted to compare the rate of adverse perinatal outcomes between immigrants and host populations living in western industrialized countries, including the US, could draw only limited conclusions because most studies were so heterogeneous that the only common identifier that could be used to define the immigrant population was "foreign birth" (Merry et al. 2011). Immigrants in the US comprise a wide range of national origins, ethnicities, languages, socioeconomic status, lifestyles, and settlement patterns. These factors are considered important social determinants of health insofar as they are indicators of conditions in which people are born, grow, live, work, and/or age that reflect their social position in the hierarchy of power, prestige, and resources (Marmot and the Commission on Social Determinants of Health 2008). A growing body of research has focused on the relationship between social determinants and health status of immigrants, especially Mexican immigrants in the US. Nonetheless, evidence from these studies is often inconsistent because studies use very heterogeneous samples and methodologies, making it difficult to draw conclusions. Research tools and standardized approaches to collect immigration-related variables are needed to improve monitoring of immigrant health.

Traditionally health studies on Mexican immigrants to the US have been circumscribed to specific settings or communities in the Southwest, and many have employed small convenience samples. Large binational studies are few, and the most recent efforts have often focused on the border, such as the study by Diaz-Kenney et al. (2010), a representative diabetes study along the entire border begun in 2010. US-Mexico border studies are important because the largest concentrations of Mexican-origin populations in the US live close to the border. However, border studies are unique insofar as the populations residing on the US side of the border tend to be socioeconomically disadvantaged compared to other populations in the US, whereas those residing on the Mexican side of the US-Mexico border tend to be more affluent compared to populations residing in other regions of Mexico. Between 1996 and 2003, the Latino population in the US began to disperse at a very quick pace and immigrants almost doubled in new growth communities in the Southeast, central plains, mountain regions, and the Pacific Northwest (Cunningham et al. 2006). The increasing dispersion of Mexican immigrants and their influx into new communities began to underscore the need to shift research on Mexican immigration and health from one focused exclusively on regional contexts to one that took into account a national context.

Binational studies that engage in cross-national comparisons using nationally representative samples are very scarce. Since primary data collection is expensive, it is more feasible to link available nationally representative surveys, vital records, or administrative data from each country to create a binational dataset. Surveys that oversample study populations of interest such as immigrants, or that allow for pooling of data from several survey waves to obtain a sufficiently large sample, frequently yield sufficient power to compare groups of interest. Availability of uniform fields is critical, because uniformity allows for comparison of within-society determinants of an outcome and between-society determinants of health outcomes, which can help deepen our appraisal of contextual influences. For example, by disaggregating the population living in Mexico according to the propensity to migrate (Van Hook et al. 2012), or according to past migration history, and similarly, by disaggregating the population living in the US according to broad measures of acculturation or integration into US society—such as first or second generation—binational research better examines pivotal social determinants of health, using both within- and between-country comparisons. When specific migration status measures are not available, other indicators can be used in conjunction with each other, such as language proficiency, socioeconomic status, and legal status.

Binational collaborative research can also be useful for testing critical hypotheses that can advance our understanding of social determinants of health, two of which are key: immigration and acculturation. There are at least three hypotheses that can benefit from this approach:

1. The health of Mexican immigrants is initially better than that of the US-born population and of the source population in Mexico. This health advantage is due to selection factors associated with a "healthy immigrant effect" that exerts influence on newcomers at the time of arrival into the US.
2. The health advantage of immigrants erodes over time as migrants become more integrated with the US environment and/or occupy inferior socioeconomic positions. Whether this is a result of adoption of cultural norms, values, and behaviors prevailing in the US, or of socioeconomic influences (or a combination of both) is not well understood.
3. The health status of immigrants (also defined as first generation) is worse than the health status of comparable populations residing in Mexico or of US-born Mexican Americans due to increased vulnerability among immi-

grants, who have to face challenges of adapting to a new society such as living without legal documentation, in segregated neighborhoods, and in disadvantaged socioeconomic conditions (Van Hook et al. 2012).

The main disadvantage of using population studies is that they are often based on national surveys that rely on self-reported information and may lack clinical depth. Furthermore, linkage of national datasets can be time-consuming and constraining since at the moment, national surveys that can be linked offer limited common and compatible fields that can be used for comparisons.

Despite these limitations, binational collaborative research can be useful in broadening the viewpoint from which to evaluate the health consequences of migration. By examining the effects of immigration in the communities left behind in Mexico as well as in the communities of settlement, researchers can examine both sides of the issue and get a more balanced perspective. For example, in a study that utilized data from the Mexican Migration Project, researchers found that men who migrated to the US had better early life health than those who remained in Mexico, but had higher prevalence of heart disease, emotional/psychiatric disorders, obesity, and smoking upon returning to Mexico than nonmigrants (Ulmann et al. 2011). Finally, binational collaborative research can be an important vehicle for generating critical evidence for identifying and tailoring solutions to the issues that may be common and unique to each population. As such, a binational collaborative research methodology can be readily applied toward translational research—allowing for more accurate and targeted policy or programmatic decisions that address the core issues affecting the populations under study.

INITIAL GUIDELINES FOR THE UNINITIATED BINATIONAL RESEARCHER

Below are some important considerations that a researcher should ponder prior to engaging in binational collaborative research.

Form Partnerships

How do you construct a research team that involves a site in another country? Make sure that you draw on the most suitable members, those who have the particular expertise needed for your project, understand the issues from the standpoint of the respective country's sociopolitical/organizational reality, and who are ready to work collaboratively and show commitment to carrying out various aspects of the project. If your team is multidisciplinary, make sure to develop a common language and research culture for the project, so that if disagreements arise on how to frame the study, select a study design, collect data, or interpret findings, these disagreements can be overcome. It is sometimes helpful to have a bilingual coordinator or a cultural "broker" who can help should disagreements or cultural questions arise. Ask yourself whether there are important cultural differences that can be addressed up front. Identify early the most effective communication strategies, research reporting strategies, and deadlines that need to be met, and make sure that these are agreed upon by your team. Keep in mind that some flexibility is very helpful on the part of each team member in adapting to expectations as the research progresses. It helps to clarify publication expectations, roles, and styles from the onset. Also ensure that the team acknowledges and respects policies and rules particular to each research institution. These should be shared among the research team members at the outset of the project.

Evaluate Study Question(s)

Is the question really binational? Ensure that your project addresses a critical health issue or problem that is relevant to both countries and reflected in the populations to be compared in each country. Have ample discussions with your team on how to frame the problem, the key research questions that you want to address, the significance of this project, and the expected contribution or value that your project will add to science or policy. Also consider that policy implications might be different for each of the countries participating in the research.

Define Purpose of Study

Consider that possible purposes of the study may be influenced by the objectives of your binational team and their respective institutions. Which of the following do you aim to accomplish?

- describe a problem or health outcome (e.g., what is the health-seeking behavior of undocumented pregnant women?)
- monitor trends over time (e.g., does the rate of change in obesity differ between people living in Mexico and the US?)
- identify mechanisms or pathways that cause a problem or establish associations with the problem or health outcome (e.g., do obese women have worse pregnancy outcomes than non-obese women, and does poverty, depression, or risky behaviors such as drinking or smoking mediate that relationship?)
- evaluate the health consequences of a problem or health outcome
- apply the evidence gained toward solutions/interventions or action steps
- all of the above

Select One or More Outcome Measures

Will your data allow you to focus on specific outcomes of interest? Are these outcomes uniform and comparable across the linked datasets? Are they accurately measured?

Select One or More Exposures

What are the key determinants or factors that are likely to cause, prevent, or treat the problem? Are the exposures uniform and comparable across datasets? Are they accurately measured?

Select Study Design

A variety of qualitative and quantitative methodologies can be employed depending upon various factors (e.g., availability of datasets, financial resources, and nature of the research question, to name a few). Some key questions to address in planning a study are as follows: Will the study be population based or community based? Will the sample be representative of the binational populations or communities? Will you use a cross-sectional, longitudinal, or retrospective study design? Will you combine multiple methods for data collection and analysis, or will you rely on a strictly quantitative or qualitative approach? Will the data be obtained from interviews and questionnaires, laboratory assessments, administrative records, vital records, or other sources? How good is the overall quality of the data? Are they valid and reliable? What are some of the limitations of your study design? Can you overcome some of these limitations?

In the next section I describe a case study in binational research. It describes the collaborative partnership, the methodological approach, and how the dataset was constructed while also highlighting key findings and implications for research, policy, and programmatic interventions.

THE BIG FAT PROBLEM

The US and Mexico have among the highest overweight and obesity rates in the world (OECD 2011). Obesity is commonly measured using body mass index (BMI), a measure that considers weight and height (kilograms/meters squared). A BMI of over 25 is considered overweight, and a BMI of over 30 is considered obese. In the US in 2010, the prevalence of overweight and obesity (OO) among all adults over the age of twenty was 69%, but among Mexican Americans it was 80% (Flegal et al. 2012). In Mexico, the most recent estimates of OO from 2006 show a prevalence at approximately 70% for adults over the age of twenty (Barquera et al., 2009). Steep increases in OO over the last three decades occurred in both countries, creating a substantial public health threat (Ogden et al. 2012; Olaiz-Fernández et al. 2006). OO puts individuals at risk for chronic diseases. Diabetes, hypertension, coronary heart disease, high LDL cholesterol, stroke, nonalcoholic fatty liver disease, gallbladder disease, osteoarthritis, sleep apnea and other breathing problems, some cancer (breast, colorectal, endometrial, and kidney), and menstrual irregularities are all linked to OO (NIH 1998). Obesity is also associated with excess deaths due to these morbidities, and to enormous health care costs (Flegal et al. 2007; Tsai et al. 2011).

IT IS NOT JUST ABOUT ETHNICITY

In the US, obesity is often studied and spliced into different ethnicities, with results showing differentials in adult OO prevalence for non-Latino whites (68.0%), non-Latino blacks (76.6%), and Latinos (77.3%) (Flegal et al. 2012). Other estimates that take ethnicity into account show important trends over time. For example, in the US, during the twelve-year period from 1999 to 2010, obesity did not increase significantly for women overall, but increases were statistically significant for non-Latino black and Mexican American women (Flegal et al. 2012). While the role of ethnicity has received considerable attention in public health research, far less emphasis has been placed on country of birth as a social determinant of OO. This is surprising considering that one-third of Mexican Americans are born in Mexico (Pew Hispanic Center 2009). Even fewer studies have examined the social and cultural determinants of OO comparing the Mexican-origin populations living in the US and in Mexico.

WHY BINATIONAL RESEARCH

By looking at Mexican Americans simultaneously in the US and Mexico, epidemiologists can compare social, cultural, and behavioral factors, as well as perceptions and practices, that determine body weight within each society. While food production and marketing, access to fresh foods, parks and public transportation, and socioeconomic conditions such as food insecurity have been found to be important social determinants of obesity (Keegan et al. 2012; Durand et al. 2011; Strasburger et al. 2011), factors such as dietary intake and physical activity/inactivity stand out as the strongest and most proximal determinants of excess weight (Sharma 2007; US HHS 2010). Public health experts in both countries have launched campaigns that address obesity prevention and reduction, but despite sharing a sizable population, there is little inter-country collaboration. Effective campaigns to curb obesity and to tackle inequalities require evidence-based information that can identify populations at high risk for excess weight and for poor weight control, and can identify important social determinants that can act as potential levers for change. As a first step, researchers must work together to link population-based data that accurately measure the same indicators using standardized modules.

Fortunately, population-based samples that include standardized modules on weight and weight control behaviors are available in both the US and Mexico. In the US, the National Health and Nutrition Examination Survey (NHANES 2012) is a nationally representative survey that collects comprehensive nutrition and health information through surveys and physical examinations (http://www.cdc.gov/nchs/nhanes). Approximately 5,000 people are selected to be surveyed and examined each year, including an oversample of Latinos. In Mexico, the Mexican National Health and Nutrition Survey (ENSANUT) collects information on almost 48,600 households (in 2006 there were anthropometric measurements for 33,784 adults) regarding health and nutrition (Olaiz-Fernández et al. 2006). Both surveys use complex stratified multistage probability cluster sampling design to select participants from the noninstitutionalized population.

CASE STUDY: WEIGHT PERCEPTION AMONG MEXICAN ADULT WOMEN IN MEXICO AND THE UNITED STATES

Building a Collaborative Binational Team and Identifying a Research Focus

To begin to address information gaps in binational research on OO, we partnered with Martha Kaufer-Horwitz, a researcher in medical sciences at the Obesity and Eating Disorders Clinic at the Instituto Nacional de Ciencias Médicas y Nutrición Salvador Zubiran (INNSZ), one of the National Institutes of Health in Mexico. With her help we accessed ENSANUT data that were not readily available to the public at that time. Her contacts with other Mexican researchers working with ENSANUT data allowed us to assess the validity, accuracy, and comparability of the survey fields, and her professionalism and command of English helped us identify and bridge important cultural gaps. Lia Fernald, an associate professor in the School of Public Health at UC Berkeley who had previously evaluated the impact of Oportunidades, a large-scale poverty alleviation program in Mexico, and Miranda Ritterman-Weintraub, a doctoral epidemiology student focusing on how inequalities and variations in socioeconomic status contribute to adverse nutritional outcomes, also joined the team. I was the principal US investigator, bringing expertise on social determinants of Latino health. Together, we forged a strong collaborative partnership bolstered by the funding that we received from PIMSA, the research arm of the Health Initiative for the Americas, a UC Berkeley program that works with Latino health stakeholders in the US and Mexico.

While there is a significant body of work in Mexico and the US focusing on actual weight in the Mexican-origin population, information on perceptions surrounding weight is sparse. Weight perception is key in weight control and in the motivation to change behaviors—individuals who perceive their weight accurately are more likely to engage in weight management behavior (Dorsey et al. 2010). Weight perception can be influenced through many avenues, but one critical method is through health care screening for overweight and obesity.

We honed in on specific research questions:

1. To what extent do weight perceptions vary among overweight and obese women? Are women in Mexico more likely to misperceive their weight? These critical questions could elucidate which women are at greater risk of not participating in healthy weight loss behavior simply due to the fact that they lack awareness of their own weight and their weight's health implications.

2. To what extent are women screened for overweight and obesity by their health providers in the US and Mexico? This question, never before examined in a binational context, could help answer which women need to be targeted by public health programs to ensure appropriate weight information and advice is delivered by a respected and trained professional.

We focused on women due to the higher prevalence of obesity observed among women in Mexico and among Mexican American women (Flegal et al. 2012; Olaiz-Fernández et al. 2006) and because research, albeit limited, suggests that risk factors associated with obesity might differ by gender (Ogden et. al 2010; Guendelman, Fernandez, et al. 2011; Barquera et al. 2009).

We used data from 855 Mexican American adult women aged twenty to fifty-nine who participated in the NHANES waves 2001–2006 and 9,527 women of the same age who were part of ENSANUT in 2006. In both studies, weight and height were obtained by trained health professionals, so the BMI measurements are accurate and comparable. In addition, both studies queried women about their perceived weight before being weighed: Did the respondent consider herself to be underweight, overweight, or just right? A comparison of actual and perceived weight allowed us to assess whether weight perceptions were accurate or inaccurate.

Women in the Two Countries Had Similar Prevalence of OO but Differed on Their Weight Perceptions

We found no significant difference between prevalence of OO in Mexican (72%) and Mexican American (71%) women. However, Mexican women were less likely to be extremely obese—obese subclass 2 (BMI 35–40) and 3 (BMI 40). The main difference between the two populations was in perception. Only 50% of Mexican women perceived themselves as overweight or obese, versus 70% of Mexican American women. In addition, the prevalence of normal weight in both groups was approximately 25%; however, 42% of Mexican women placed themselves in that category as opposed to only 27% of Mexican American women (Guendelman, Ritterman-Weintraub, et al. 2011).

As shown in Figure 23.1, among OO women specifically, 86% of Mexican Americans perceived themselves accurately as OO, versus only 64% of Mexican women—revealing stark differences between the two cultures. Furthermore,

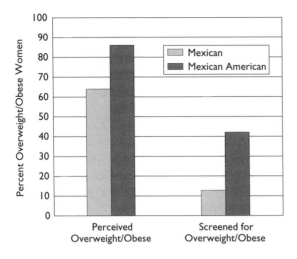

FIGURE 23.1. Perceived body weight among overweight and obese (OO) Mexican-origin women living in Mexico and the US. SOURCE: National Health and Nutrition Examination Survey (NHANES 2012) 2001–2006 and ENSANUT 2006. (Olaiz-Fernández et al. 2006.)

among OO women, 42% of Mexican American women had been screened by a provider for OO, compared to only 13% of Mexican women. In both countries, women who had been informed by a health professional that they were OO had an increased odds (OR = 5.3, 95% CI 3.8–7.3) of perceiving themselves as OO (Guendelman, Ritterman-Weintraub, et al. 2011).

Why Such Different Perceptions among Overweight and Obese Women in Each Country?

As our study shows, among the OO, accuracy in weight perceptions is closely linked to receiving information and advice from a health provider about weight status. Increased screening by health providers is needed in Mexico to improve weight perceptions and to motivate women to control their weight. Only 13% of OO women had ever been told by a health provider that they had excess weight, suggesting much room for improvement. Evidence indicates that provider encouragement, even brief advice, can promote health behavior change (Nguyen et al. 2011; Heaton and Frede 2006). Increased screening and advice by health providers is also needed among Mexican American women in the US. Only 40% of OO Mexican American women reported having been screened by a health provider, suggesting missed opportunities for intervention. Although these rates of screening are higher than those received by women in Mexico, they still corroborate evidence that immigrants and people with limited education have a lower likelihood of receiving physician screening and advice that promotes healthy behaviors (US Prevention Task Force 2003; Alexander et al. 2007). Since Mexican Americans overall have low access to health care and to educational, economic, or informational resources (Vargas Bustamante et al. 2010; Kirby et al. 2006), they may be showing delayed adoption of healthy dietary and lifestyle behaviors. Differences in perception could also be a result of fewer public health campaigns designed to raise awareness of obesity in Mexico compared to the US.

Next Steps

Outreach and education to providers concerning culturally appropriate counseling, as well as improved monitoring of screening in both the US and Mexico, is required. Acknowledgment of this need can serve as a first step from which to develop binational interventions for improving weight control behaviors among Mexican-origin women.

Body size has been shown to increase as immigrants adapt to the social-cultural environment in the US and incorporate the societal norms, dietary, and other lifestyle behaviors driving the obesity epidemic (Sundquist and Winkleby 2000; Barcenas et al. 2007). However, other studies have shown the reverse: that less acculturated, rather than more acculturated, Mexican Americans tend to be more obese (Hazuda et al. 1988; Espinosa de Los Monteros et al. 2008; Ahluwalia et al. 2007). In another study using NHANES waves 2001–2006, we found that Mexican American women born in the US but who speak only Spanish had on average higher age-standardized BMIs compared with both Mexican immigrants and Mexican American women born in the US who spoke at least some English (31.3 kg/m² vs. 29.3 kg/m² vs. 28.3 kg/m², respectively) (Guendelman, Fernandez, et al. 2011). This would suggest that being born in the US but not fully acculturating is associated with increased BMI, whereas being an exclusively English speaker is associated with lower BMI. The jury is still out on how acculturation (a term encompassing social and cultural determinants of health) affects the obesity epidemic among Mexican-origin women.

Currently our binational team is addressing selection issues by comparing Mexican immigrants who have arrived in the last five years with women living in Mexico. So far the team has found no significant differences in BMI. This would suggest that there is no selection occurring based on BMI, and that differences between countries and between populations in each country might be explained by social-cultural and structural factors within the context of each country.

Study Limitations

We were unable to make causal inferences, because our analyses are based on cross-sectional data. Furthermore, we did not measure many critical, within-country contextual, community, or environmental factors. The surveys asked respondents whether they had ever been told by a health provider that they were OO, and these questions may have been subject to recall bias. Weight perceptions were compared to BMI; comparisons with other measures such as waist circumference might yield different results (Yaemsiri et al. 2010). In NHANES, though, BMI has been found to correlate highly with percentage body fat as measured by dual x-ray absorptiometry (Flegal et al. 2012). To our study's benefit, we were able to use population-based estimates and relied on BMI measured by health technicians to ensure measurement accuracy. BMI is considered a valuable tool to provide a standardized definition of obesity, which allows for international comparisons (Flegal et al. 2010).

Many questions still remain unresolved. Why are more Mexican American women obese subclass 2 and 3 compared to women in Mexico, even though they have more access to health care providers and have a more accurate perception of their weight? What, aside from perception and lack of screening, are the specific risk factors that contribute to high rates of overweight and obesity among Mexican-origin women? Do Mexican-origin men exhibit different weight patterns, perceptions, and provider screens? Obviously obesity is a very complex problem, and no single solution or intervention will solve it. This study is a first step in generating useful comparisons for understanding obesity from a binational perspective.

CONCLUSION

Evidence obtained from binational collaborative studies can raise awareness of shared problems and critical social and cultural determinants of health, and provide potential collaborative solutions to these problems. Although this chapter has focused on US-Mexico migration, it can be applied in other countries that are joined by migration. Binational research allows collaborating investigators to observe beyond their own border—a much needed methodology in a world that is ever more globally connected.

ACKNOWLEDGMENT

I would like to thank Shayla Livingston for her help editing and researching sections of this chapter.

REFERENCES

Ahluwalia IB, ES Ford, M Link, and JC Bolen. 2007. "Acculturation, weight, and weight-related behaviors among Mexican Americans in the United States." *Ethnicity and Disease* 17(4): 643–49.

Alexander SC, T Ostbye, KI Pollak, M Gradison, LA Bastian, and RJ Brouwer. 2007. "Physicians' beliefs about discussing obesity: Results from focus groups." *American Journal of Health Promotion* 21(6): 498–500.

Barcenas C, A Wilkinson, S Strom, et al. 2007. "Birthplace, years of residence in the United States, and obesity among Mexican American adults." *Obesity* 15: 1043–52.

Barquera S, I Campos-Nonato, L Hernández-Barrera, M Flores, R Durazo-Arvizu, R Kanter, and JA Rivera. 2009. "Obesity and central adiposity in Mexican adults: Results from the Mexican National Health and Nutrition Survey 2006." *Salud Pública de México* 51(4): S595–S603.

Crimmins E, J Soldo, K Kim, and D Alley. 2005. "Using anthropometric indicators for Mexicans in the United States and Mexico to understand the selection of migrants and the 'Hispanic Paradox.'" *Social Biology* 52(3–4): 164–77.

Cunningham P, M Banker, S Artiga, and J Tolbert. 2006. "Health coverage and access to care for Hispanics in 'new growth communities' and 'major Hispanic centers.'" Kaiser Commission on Medicaid and the Uninsured. Menlo Park, CA.

Diaz-Kenney RV, R Ruiz-Holguín, FG de Cosío, et al. 2010. "A historical overview of the United States-Mexico border diabetes prevention and control project." *Revista Panamericana de Salud Pública* 28(3): 143–50.

Dorsey RR, MS Eberhardt, and CL Ogden. 2010. "Racial and ethnic differences in weight management behavior by weight perception status." *Ethnicity and Disease* 20: 244–50.

Durand CP, M Andalib, GF Dunton, J Wolch, and MA Pentz. 2011. "A systematic review of built environment factors related to physical activity and obesity risk: Implications for smart growth urban planning." *Obesity Review* 12(5): e173–82.

Espinosa de Los Monteros K, LC Gallo, JP Elder, and GA Talavera. 2008. "Individual and area-based indicators of acculturation and the metabolic syndrome among low-income Mexican American women living in a border region." *American Journal of Public Health* 98(11): 1979–86.

Flegal KM, MD Carroll, BK Kit, and CL Ogden. 2012. "Prevalence of obesity and trends in the distribution of body mass index among US adults, 1999–2010." *Journal of the American Medical Association* 307(5): 491–97.

Flegal KM, M Carroll, C Ogden, and L Curtin. 2010. "Prevalence and trends in obesity among US adults, 1999–2008." *Journal of the American Medical Association* 303: 235–41.

Flegal KM, BI Graubard, DF Williamson, et al. 2007. "Cause-specific excess deaths associated with underweight, overweight, and obesity." *Journal of the American Medical Association* 298(17): 2028–37.

Guendelman S. 1991. "Health care users residing on the Mexican border: What factors determine choice of the U.S. or Mexican health system?" *Medical Care* 29(5): 419–29.

Guendelman S, and P English. 1995. "Effect of United States residence on birth outcomes among Mexican immigrants: An exploratory study." *American Journal of Epidemiology* 142: S30–S38.

Guendelman S, A Fernandez, D Thornton, and C Brindis. 2011. "Birthplace, language use, and body size among Mexican American women and men: Findings from the National Health and Nutrition Examination Survey (NHANES), 2001–2006." *Journal of Health Care for the Poor and Underserved* 22(2): 590–605.

Guendelman S, J Gould, M Hudes, and B Eskenazi. 1990. "Generational differences in perinatal health among the Mexican American population: Findings from HHANES 1982–84." *American Journal of Public Health* 80(suppl): 61–65.

Guendelman S, and M Jasis. 1992. "Giving birth across the border: The San Diego-Tijuana connection." *Social Science and Medicine* 34(4): 419–25.

Guendelman S, C Malin, B Herr-Harthorn, and PN Vargas. 2001. "Orientations to mother-hood and male partner support among women in Mexico and Mexican-origin women in the United States." *Social Science and Medicine* 52: 1805–13.

Guendelman S, ML Ritterman-Weintraub, LCH Fernald, and M Kaufer-Horwitz. 2011. "Weight perceptions among overweight and obese women: A US-Mexico binational perspective." *Obesity* 13(1): 169–80.

Guendelman S, D Thornton, J Gould, and N Hosang. 2005. "Social disparities in maternal morbidity during labor and delivery between Mexican-born and US-born white Cali-fornians, 1996–1998." *American Journal of Public Health* 95(12): 2218–24.

Guendelman S, D Thornton, J Gould, and N Hosang. 2006. "Mexican women in California: Differentials in maternal morbidity between foreign and US-born populations." *Paedi-atric Perinatal Epidemiology* 20(6): 471–81.

Hamilton BE, PD Sutton, and SJ Ventura. 2003. "Revised birth and fertility rates for the 1990s and new rates for Hispanic populations, 2000 and 2001: United States." National vital statistics reports 51(12). Hyattsville, MD: National Center for Health Statistics.

Hazuda HP, SM Haffner, MP Stern, and CW Eifler. 1988. "Effects of acculturation and soci-oeconomic status on obesity and diabetes in Mexican Americans: The San Antonio Heart Study." *American Journal of Epidemiology* 128(6): 1289–1301.

Heaton P, and S Frede. 2006. "Patients' need for more counseling on diet, exercise, and smoking cessation: Results from the National Ambulatory Medical Care Survey." *Jour-nal of the American Pharmacists Association* 46: 364–69.

Keegan TH, S Hurley, D Goldberg, et al. 2012. "The association between neighborhood characteristics and body size and physical activity in the California teachers study cohort." *American Journal of Public Health* 102(4): 689–97.

Kirby J, G Taliaferro, and S Zuvekas. 2006. "Explaining racial and ethnic disparities in health care." *Medical Care* 44(5)suppl.: 1–64–1–72.

Kley S. 2011. "Explaining the stages of migration within a life-course framework." *European Sociological Review* 27(4): 469–86.

Marmot R, and the Commission on Social Determinants of Health. 2008. "Closing the gap in a generation: Health equity through action on the social determinants of health." Final report of the Commission on Social Determinants of Health. Geneva: World Health Organization.

Merry L, A Gagnon, I Hemlin, H Clarke, and J Hickey. 2011. "Cross-border movement and women's health: How to capture the data." *International Journal for Equity in Health* 10: 56.

National Health and Nutrition Examination Survey (NHANES). 2012. "About the National Health and Nutrition Examination Survey: An Introduction." Accessed February 27, 2012. http://www.cdc.gov/nchs/nhanes/about_nhanes.htm.

National Institutes of Health (NIH). 1998. "Clinical guidelines on the identification, evalu-ation, and treatment of overweight and obesity in adults." NHLBI Obesity Education Initiative. Accessed March 20, 2012. http://www.nhlbi.nih.gov/guidelines/obesity/ob_gdlns.pdf.

Nguyen H, K Markides, and M Windleby. 2011. "Physician advice on exercise and diet in a U.S. sample of obese Mexican-American adults." *American Journal of Health Promotion* 25: 402–9.

OECD. 2011. "Health at a Glance 2011: OECD Indicators." OECD Publishing. Accessed March 10, 2012. http://dx.doi.org/10.1787/health_glance-2011-en.

Ogden, CL, MD Carroll, BK Kit, and KM Flegal. 2012. "Prevalence of obesity in the United States, 2009–2010." NCHS data brief no 82. Hyattsville, MD: National Center for Health Statistics.

Ogden, CL, MM Lamb, MD Carroll, and KM Flegal. 2010. "Obesity and socioeconomic status in adults: United States 1988–1994 and 2005–2008." NCHS data brief no 50. Hyattsville, MD: National Center for Health Statistics.

Olaiz-Fernández G, J Rivera-Dommarco, T Shamah-Levy, R Rojas, S Villalpando-Hernández, M Hernández-Avila, and J Sepúlveda-Amor. 2006. "Encuesta nacional de salud y nutrición 2006." Cuernavaca: Instituto Nacional de Salud Pública.

Pew Hispanic Center. 2009. "Mexican immigrants in the United States, 2008." Accessed March 18, 2012. http://www.pewhispanic.org/2009/04/15/mexican-immigrants-in-the-united-states-2008/.

Sharma M. 2007. "Behavioural interventions for preventing and treating obesity in adults." *Obesity Reviews* 8: 441–49.

Strasburger, VC, and Council on Communications and Media. 2011. "Children, adolescents, obesity, and the media." *Pediatrics* 128(1): 201–8.

Sundquist J, and M Winkleby. 2000. "Country of birth, acculturation status and abdominal obesity in a national sample of Mexican-American women and men." *International Journal of Epidemiology* 29: 470–77.

Tsai AG, DF Williamson, and HA Glick. 2011. "Direct medical cost of overweight and obesity in the USA: A quantitative systematic review." *Obesity Reviews* 12(1): 50–61.

Ullmann SH, N Goldman, and DS Massey. 2011. "Healthier before they migrate, less healthy when they return? The health of returned migrants in Mexico." *Social Science and Medicine* 73(3): 421–28.

US Department of Health and Human Services (US HHS). 2010. "The surgeon general's vision for a healthy and fit nation." Rockville, MD: U.S. Department of Health and Human Services, Office of the Surgeon General.

US Preventive Service Task Force. 2003. "Screening for obesity in adults: Recommendation and rationale." Accessed April 10, 2012. http://www.uspreventiveservicestaskforce.org/3r_duspstf/obesit.htm.

Van Hook J, E Baker, C Altman, and M Frisco. 2012. "Canaries in a coalmine: Immigration and overweight among Mexican-origin children in the US and Mexico." *Social Science and Medicine* 74: 125–34.

Vargas Bustamante AS, J Chen, H Rodríguez, J Rizzo, and A Ortega. 2010. "Use of preventive care services among Latino subgroups." *American Journal of Preventive Medicine* 38(6): 610–19.

Yaemsiri S, MM Slining, and SK Agarwal. 2010. "Perceived weight status, overweight diagnosis, and weight control among US adults: The NHANES 2003–2008 study." *International Journal of Obesity* 35(8): 1063–70.

24

Ensuring Access to Research for Nondominant Language Speakers

Francesca Gany
Lisa Diamond
Rachel Meislin
Javier González

INTRODUCTION

Migrant populations enrich the societies into which they settle, bringing new perspectives, revitalizing neighborhoods, and enhancing the tax base (Rex 1995). Despite their many contributions, immigrants and migrants often face barriers to ethical participation in research. When these barriers are not adequately addressed, health disparities can result. This chapter will review the demographics of limited-English-speaking populations in several large English-speaking countries, address the need to develop an inclusive research infrastructure, and discuss the considerations in implementing research across languages.

The aim of this chapter is to help enable researchers to increase equity in research and improve outcomes for limited English proficient (LEP) populations in English-dominant societies. To accomplish this we will

- describe LEP populations and their unique challenges in accessing health services,
- demonstrate the ethical imperative for truly engaging LEP participants in research and the additional care that should be taken for their meaningful participation, and
- guide researchers on the inclusion of LEP participants in research activities, including needs assessment, development of study materials and instruments, translation, recruitment and retention, interpretation, and adverse events reporting.

Cultural and linguistic barriers are prevalent in a number of research settings, and they present important challenges. Patients in language-discordant encounters, where the provider speaks a language different from that of his or her patient, face poorer health indicators, even when adjusting for socioeconomic status: diminished access to mental health, pediatric, and adult health services, and health insurance (Perkins 2003), fewer health care visits and screenings (Kim et al. 2011; Javier et al. 2010; Toppelberg and Collins 2010; Leng et al. 2010; Papadopoulos et al. 2004), and difficulty communicating with the providers when at these visits (Derose and Baker 2000; Thornton et al. 2009; Ngo-Metzger et al. 2003). Access to research also suffers, resulting in data that do not adequately reflect, and are thereby not necessarily applicable to, the needs of the broad population. Research populations need to represent the increasing diversity of the United States (USCB 2010), and of migrant-recipient countries across the globe (Somerville et al. 2009; Crush 2008; Inglis 2002; Challinor 2011), so that results are generalizable. Without this, health equity cannot exist.

A COMPARISON OF LEP POPULATIONS IN SELECTED ENGLISH-SPEAKING COUNTRIES

The United States, Canada, the United Kingdom, South Africa, and Australia, among many other countries, have seen large influxes of immigrants and/or shifts of internal populations. This chapter will focus on LEP populations, although the principles will be applicable to most language-discordant research settings.[1]

United States

The 2010 United States Census describes the growing population of Americans for whom English is not their primary language. Almost 21% of the US population five years of age or older speaks a language other than English at home. This is an increase from the 2000 census, in which 18% were found to speak a language other than English, up from 14% in 1990 and 11% in 1980 (Shin and Bruno 2003). There are four census categories for people to describe their English-speaking ability: Very Well, Well, Not Well, and Not at All. Those who speak English less than "Very Well" are considered to have limited English proficiency (Karliner et al. 2008). Of the US population, 8.7% speak English "less than very well" (ACS 2010) and hence are limited English proficient; this percentage is up from 8.1% in 2000 and 6.1% in 1990 (Shin and Bruno 2003). The three most widely spoken non-English languages are Spanish, Chinese, and Tagalog (ACS 2010).

In the United States, the LEP population is protected under Title VI of the 1964 Civil Rights Act, which states that nobody should be denied access to federal services on the basis of race, sex, religion, or national origin (Levy 2009). Those with limited English proficiency are considered in this context to be a subset of national-origin minorities and are protected as such. In 2000, Executive Order 13166, "Improving Access to Services for Persons with Limited English Proficiency" was issued. This order sought to facilitate access to services provided by federally funded agencies for LEP persons, reinforcing compliance with Title VI regulations. The order states: "The Executive Order requires Federal agencies to examine the services they provide, identify any need for services to those with limited English proficiency (LEP), and develop and implement a system to provide those services so LEP persons can have meaningful access to them. It is expected that agency plans will provide such meaningful access consistent with, and without unduly burdening, the fundamental mission of the agency. The Executive Order also requires that the Federal agencies work to ensure that recipients of Federal financial assistance provide meaningful access to their LEP applicants and beneficiaries" (Clinton 2000: 50121).

Human subjects in research are strictly protected by international guidelines that emerged as a response to a history of unethical experimentation. In the United States, Title 45 Code of Federal Regulations, Part 46, protects human research participants. The law includes instructions for institutional review boards and informed consent processes and defines protections for especially vulnerable populations. The Office for Human Research Protections (OHRP), the federally funded agency overseeing human research, delineates the guidelines for obtaining informed consent from LEP patients (OHRP 2012).

Australia

The 2006 countrywide census in Australia found that 21% of the population spoke a language other than English at home, an increase from 18% ten years prior. Additionally, 17% of all speakers of languages other than English spoke English "not well" or "not at all" (AG 2008). In Australia, the most common languages after English are Italian, Greek, and Cantonese (AG 2008).

In 1975, the Australian government issued the Race Discrimination Act, which made discrimination based on race, color, descent, or national or ethnic origin illegal and promoted equality for all (AG 2011). In 2005, the Charter of Public Service in a Culturally Diverse Society was enacted to ensure that government services are provided in a manner that is sensitive to the language and cultural needs of all Australians (ADIMA 2005).

The National Statement on Ethical Conduct in Human Research, issued by the Australia National Health and Medical Research Council (ANHMRC) in 1999 and revised in 2007, is a series of ethical guidelines concerning human subjects research in Australia (ANHMRC 2007, 1999). It mandates the creation of ethics committees and review procedures, and the protection of vulnerable populations (ANHMRC 2007, 1999; Ballantyne et al. 2008). The ANHMRC has also prioritized the inclusion of minorities, including limited English speakers, in research (ANHMRC 1999).

Canada

In Canada, there are two official languages, English and French. The 2006 Statistic-sCanada Survey found that 20% of the population has a first language that is neither English nor French, an increase from 18% allophone in 2001. Chinese is the third most common language in Canada after French and English, and the most common new languages are from Asia and the Middle East (StatisticsCanada 2007).

Canada's policies for ethical research practices are provided by the joint efforts of three separate research councils through the *Tri-Council Policy Statement: Ethical Conduct for Research Involving Humans (TCPS)* (CIHR et al. 2010) There are specific provisions for conducting research across a language barrier: "When language barriers necessitate the assistance of an intermediary for communication between the research team and participants, the researcher should select an intermediary who has the necessary language skills to ensure effective communication (see Article 4.1)"[2] (CIHR 2010). These agencies will only grant funding to those researchers who follow these provisions.

South Africa

South Africa has eleven official languages, and most health care providers speak only one or two of them. This commonly results in a lack of language concordance between doctor and patient (Schlemmer and Mash 2006). Internal migration between regions of South Africa, where dominant languages differ, accentuates this problem (Deumert 2010). In one study of the Xhosa-speaking population, a minority language among the eleven official languages, language barriers to health care were found to be more of an issue than structural and socioeconomic barriers (Levin 2006).

The Pan South African Language Board (PanSALB) mandated the passage of the Pan South African Language Board Act 59 of 1995, promoting multilingualism and the equal representation of all of its eleven languages within South Africa. PanSALB also promotes and ensures the respect of languages used for religious purposes, including Hebrew and Arabic (PanSALB 2011).

The National Health Research Ethics Council (NHREC) was established under National Health Act No. 61 of 2004. It provides guidelines for the ethical research of human subjects and, similar to other ethics committees, promotes informed consent and works to minimize discrimination (RSA 2004).

UK

Prior to the 2011 census, there was no official national data source in the United Kingdom on the proportion of the population with English as a second language (Aspinall 2007, 2005). The 2011 census, for the first time, included a question on English proficiency, asking "How well do you speak English?" (White and McLaren 2009). It also surveyed migration status and included additional response choices for ethnic minority. At the time of this writing, results from this survey were not yet available. However, a recent academic study estimates the number of people with LEP in the UK at 400,000 to 1.2 million (Gill et al. 2009).

Lack of LEP data has made it difficult for health care providers to gauge their patients' language services needs. The National Health Service provides telephone interpretation whenever required, both for clinical encounters and for obtaining consent for research (Robinson 2010). In-person, face-to-face interpretation is granted on a case-by-case basis (MacFarlane et al. 2009). The Health Research Authority (HRA) is a recently established (2011) organization of the National Health Service whose purpose is to protect the interests of those involved in health research (Wilson et al. 2005). One of the first initiatives of the HRA has been to oversee the National Research Ethics Service (NRES). The NRES reviews research proposals that include human subjects to ensure their safety and ethical treatment (Wisely 2011).

HEALTH LITERACY

Immigrants with limited English proficiency in the United States are more likely to have lower health literacy than English speakers (Wilson et al. 2005). Health literacy refers to one's capacity to understand medical information and directions (Wilson et al. 2005; Sudore et al. 2009). Higher health literacy is associated with increased preventive care, better communication with physicians, and better utilization of health services (Todd and Hoffman-Goetz 2011; Kreps and Sparks 2008; Jonkers et al. 2011; Tieu et al. 2010). The National Assessment of Adult Literacy (NAAL) found that over one-third of Americans would have difficulty with common health tasks such as following directions on a prescription drug label. Lower health literacy may impede investigators from effectively communicating with their LEP participants. Limited health literacy affects adults in all racial and ethnic groups (USDHHS 2008).

In a cross-sectional study in Australia, low functional health literacy was common, and was significantly associated with being born outside of Australia, New Zealand, the United Kingdom, and Ireland (Adams et al. 2009). A recent study in South Africa found that there are 7.3 million people twenty years of age and older who are functionally illiterate, and recommends that research instructions should be in plain language, concordant with any of all eleven official languages as needed, and include pictorial aids and graphics (Dowse and Ehlers 2004).

ETHICAL IMPERATIVES FOR INCLUSION OF NONDOMINANT LANGUAGE SPEAKERS IN RESEARCH

There is an ethical imperative to include nondominant language speakers in a manner that (1) is sensitive to their abilities to communicate and understand the research process, and (2) addresses its cultural and linguistic barriers to meaningful participation. Underrepresentation of the LEP population in research not only denies the benefits of individual participation in research, including access to cutting-edge treatments in clinical trials, but also presents a barrier to the generalizability of clinical research findings (Glickman et al. 2011, 2008; Giuliano et al. 2000).

Serious and effective measures to regulate the research environment are in place, and they should be communicated widely. In the United States, the Belmont Report provides the ethical backbone for clinical research (NC 1979). It outlines three basic ethical principles: respect for persons, beneficence, and justice (Bustillos 2009; Jacobs et al. 2001). The ethical research practices that have come forth as a result of the Belmont Report and in response to historical injustices such as the Tuskegee experiment are also in effect in the UK and Ireland, Australia, Canada, and South Africa (ANHMRC 1999; SADH 2004; DH and NHS 2005).

Respect for Persons

The principle of respect for persons concerns the autonomy of individuals. It recognizes that people are autonomous agents whose decision making and capacity for self-determination should be heeded. It includes the protection of persons of limited autonomy. To ensure respect for persons, the enrollment of study participants should occur with no coercion, that is, with the participants' full understanding of the risks and benefits of participation, and the decision to participate should be made freely in the context of this full understanding. To ensure this full understanding, communication barriers must be eliminated. In this chapter we will describe strategies to enable full understanding in the context of language discordance.

Beneficence

Research with human subjects should maximize the benefits to an individual while minimizing the risks. Generally, this means protection from harm. Steps should be taken in research with LEP participants to provide all information so that it is comprehensible, in the participant's own language, and at the participant's reading level. Participants need to be able to recognize adverse events as such and to receive prompt, linguistically appropriate attention should these occur.

Justice

Justice is the principle concerning fairness and equity in research. There are both risks and benefits associated with research, and all people should share in both. Unfortunately, there is demonstrated evidence of the exclusion of limited English populations from research (Glickman et al. 2011). Given the growth of limited-English-speaking populations in English-dominant countries worldwide, researchers should emphasize the fair recruitment of these populations.

This chapter will share strategies to overcome language-based gaps in adherence to these three principles.

NEEDS ASSESSMENTS

Needs assessments can help guide the entire research process. Once the researcher has determined that participants with limited English proficiency are either the primary focus of the research or a population for inclusion, a needs assessment can define the target population's languages and health literacy levels, the needs for translation of documents and other study materials, the need for interpretation services, and the associated costs (which could inform budgets in advance). The regions from which the population migrated, the length of time since migration, dialect(s), reading levels, and needed resources for participation should guide the study design, instruments, and materials. Researchers should avail themselves of templates/checklists that address the aforementioned areas of consideration. The National Cancer Institute, for example, has published a set of guidelines for adapting research programs for different populations (NCI and SAMHSA). At minimum, special consideration should be given to (1) native and primary language (or preferred or dominant language); (2) country of origin and length of time since migration; and (3) educational attainment and literacy. Information on these topics should enable researchers to determine translation and interpretation needs and level of readability of the study materials as well as the need for cultural adaptations.

Assessment of Language Proficiency and Health Literacy

Establishing the level of English proficiency of the target population is essential. False fluency—*the illusion that one is fluent in a language*—has been reported not only among researchers and other personnel, including clinicians, but also among study participants (Shi 2011; Zun et al. 2006). A commonly employed strategy to *estimate* English language proficiency is the use of the question from the US Census survey, "How well do you speak English?" Those who answer "Less than very well" are considered limited English proficient (Karliner et al. 2008; Wilson et al. 2005). This question is not an indicator of language fluency or of health literacy, however.

Factors affecting individuals' willingness to declare fluency levels may present as barriers to eliciting objective responses and are not specific to English. Let us consider the cases below:

- In New York City, a relatively recent influx of Quechua-speaking Ecuadoreans started to appear during Sunday morning tuberculosis screenings at a Catholic church in Queens. The bilingual research team started to notice that a significant number of the participants were not fluent in Spanish. Many had self-declared their fluency, but were in fact falsely reporting fluency. Indigenous languages such as Quechua had sometimes been stigmatized in Ecuador. The awareness of the actual languages of the participants required modification of the study approach and the training of personnel on issues particular to this emerging population.

- Acknowledging that one is illiterate may be hard and hence not revealed. Some patients have been noted, in fact, to say that they left their glasses at home or that someone else will read their instructions at home instead of acknowledging that they are unable to read (Hornberger and Coronel-Molina 2004; Weiss 2007).

It is essential to keep in mind that as with participants, bilingual research personnel, oftentimes composed primarily of heritage speakers, may not possess full language fluency. Heritage speakers are individuals who are raised in a household where the language spoken is different from the dominant language spoken in the country (HJ 2008). While heritage speakers in the United States may be bilingual in the oral language, many do not have a formal education in the non-English language and therefore present special challenges. This is especially true of, but certainly not limited to, speakers of languages that do not use the Roman alphabet, such as Chinese, Arabic, Russian, Vietnamese, and Tagalog (HJ 2008).

Thus it is imperative to test the language skill of any member of the study team who self-declares fluency in any given language and will have contact with the study participants. There are several methods to assess language fluency. One is to enlist the help of fully bilingual personnel whose dominant language is the target language and who have demonstrated fluency. These personnel may conduct a structured bilingual interview to assess the oral skills of the individual and determine the level of oral fluency. At minimum, the interviewer should engage in a conversation in the target language and discern (1) the individual's native and primary languages, (2) his or her country of origin and length of time since migration, (3) where the majority of his or her education took place, and (4) if the individual is able to discern and produce different levels of nuance in both languages. To assess written skills, this person may have the individual compose a page on a specific subject or have him or her do a translation. This ad hoc method, however, may fail to truly establish thresholds of fluency and usability of language skills. For this reason, researchers should consider the use of professional assessment services whenever possible. There a number of reputable agencies that conduct foreign language testing in the United States, such as ALTA Language Services (2012) or groups recommended by local chapters of the American Translators Association (ATA 2012).

In terms of literacy, health literacy in English can be measured using the Test of Functional Health Literacy in Adults (TOFHLA), the Short Test of Functional

Health Literacy in Adults (STOFHLA), and the Rapid Estimate of Adult Literacy in Medicine (REALM) (Parker et al. 1995; Davis et al. 1993; Wallace 2006). Other tests for literacy may be utilized, but these tests measure health literacy specifically.

The REALM is administered in 1–5 minutes and tests word recognition and pronunciation but does not test comprehension. TOFHLA tests the ability to both read and comprehend and takes 20–30 minutes to complete. The STOFHLA is the first two paragraphs of the TOFHLA and is highly correlated with the entire assessment; it takes 5–7 minutes to administer. One major drawback to using these exams is that they test written language skills but not oral competency (Wallace 2006).

TRANSLATION AND INTERPRETATION

Translation

Translation is the *written* rendition in one language (the target) of what has been written in another language (the source). The overall objective of translation is the achievement of equivalence between two languages and cultures (Lee et al. 2009; Brislin 1970; Jones et al. 2001; Weeks et al. 2007).

Translation is a process of considerable complexity, depending on the linguistic register—*or level of sophistication of the language*—of the source document (document to be translated). The ideal for translation is to produce a text that is faithful to the content and the style of the original text. Translated questionnaires/instruments, surveys, and brochures must have a high degree of readability *(easy for the research participants to read and understand),* with the content simply conveyed to the participant (while maintaining the intended objective and eliciting the research question).

A recent literature review highlighted four guidelines to help ensure quality medical translations (Garcia-Castillo and Fetters 2007): (1) including experts highly fluent in both the source and target languages, (2) using experts on the content of the material being translated, (3) ensuring the necessary cultural equivalences are in place in the translation, and (4) keeping a documentation trail. We address these four points below.

Who Should Translate?

Choosing the team to accomplish the translation task is the first step in the process. In the United States, the American Translators Association (ATA) is a certifying body for translators. Individuals who take the ATA certification exam must be ATA members for at least four weeks and must provide proof that they meet the educational and experience prerequisites prior to registering for the exam (ATA 2012). Prerequisites include having accreditation or certification by a member association of the Fédération Internationale des Traducteurs; or having an advanced degree or approved translation and interpreting certificate; or having a bachelor's degree with at least two years of work experience as a translator or interpreter; or for those with less than a bachelor's degree, at least five years of work experience as a translator or interpreter (ATA 2012).

It is worth noting that ad hoc translation is an unfortunate, though prevalent, practice. Researchers may resort to personnel who declare their own bilingual capacities and are often allowed to translate without rigorous confirmation of their expertise (Lee et al. 2009; Flores 2005). Many of those providing ad hoc translations are heritage speakers.

A quality assurance program should have a validated method to test staff who are said to be bilingual, examining the individual's translation skills. In contrast to interpreting, which will be discussed later in this chapter, translation requires a high level of reading comprehension and writing skill. Bilingualism is a necessary though not sufficient skill for the process.

When credentialed translators are unavailable or outside of a study's budget, a rigorous screening interview for potential translators should be employed to examine the main skill areas that translators should possess. In a report entitled *A Guide to Understanding Interpreting and Translation in Healthcare*, published by the National Health Law Program, the following skill areas are identified (NCIHC and ATA 2009):

1. reading comprehension and written ability (including a high level of grammar in both languages)
2. knowledge of specialized terminology
3. proofreading skills and the ability to work in a team (for quality assurance purposes)
4. access to dictionaries, forums, and experts in the subject

A study by Eberle et al. (2012) illustrates the use of culturally appropriate translations (see sidebar 24.1).

There are several methods and approaches for translation. Below we present those most pertinent to the needs of researchers. This list, however, is not exhaustive.

Emphasizing Cross-cultural Adaptation

The utilization of a review panel of researchers, physicians, public health officials, and community leaders is recommended. The panel can examine both source and translated documents and make recommendations prior to pilot testing, such as alternatives for English colloquialisms or inaccessible language. In a study entitled "Methods for Translating Survey Questionnaires" the authors examined a five-step quality control process for translating a tobacco-related questionnaire into Mandarin, Korean, Cantonese, and Vietnamese. The five steps included translation,

SIDEBAR 24.1 SHORT CASE STUDY: CULTURALLY APPROPRIATE TRANSLATIONS

In Eberle et al.'s (2012) study of ethnic disparities in employment status and medical outcomes among breast cancer survivors, study materials were translated into Korean, Mandarin, and Spanish. The study hoped to identify baseline clinical, social, and employment characteristics that mediate differences in employment outcomes. Survey questions were reviewed by bilingual research staff, vetted by bilingual experts, and piloted with patients.

Experts identified cultural discrepancies, including grade levels in the Korean education system and colloquial English terms requiring clarification, such as "sick leave" in Spanish. Patients with LEP who were interviewed about the survey uncovered comprehension issues, such as differentiating between "somewhat agree" and "definitely agree" in Chinese Likert scales. They also found some socioeconomic variables relevant to immigrants that were missing, such as owning a business as a wage category and Emergency Medicaid as an insurance type.

In this study, in addition to survey translation, vetting by bilingual experts and LEP patients was necessary to ensure the accuracy of linguistically, culturally, and socioeconomically targeted data collection.

review, initial adjudication, cognitive interview pretesting, and final review and adjudication to achieve a translation that was believed to be effective and faithful to the English source (Forsyth et al. 2007).

It is admittedly labor-intensive to translate study instruments. As with most other research documents, study instruments deserve special scrutiny in terms of linguistic nuance and cultural equivalency. One way to reduce both money and time spent on translation is to use validated, translated scales when they are available. In addition to being cost-effective, such instruments can be used with more confidence, as they have already been validated. Importantly, there is a difference between validated scales that have been translated and translated scales that have been validated in the target language.

Forward Translation

Simple forward translation involves a single translator rendering the source document into a target language document. The translation is usually checked for accuracy by a different translator or by a back translation (described below). The method to be used depends on the level of complexity of the document to be translated.

A more robust model encompasses a team or teams of translators and bilingual subject matter experts. At minimum, two translators and one subject matter expert should comprise the team. More translators or subject matter experts can be added based on the volume and the level of sophistication or difficulty of the materials. In this approach, one translator in the team will execute the first translation and a second will thoroughly and independently review it, line by line, for accuracy. The translator doing the review should copiously note every error or question and have a one-on-one reconciliation meeting with the first translator. Errors in translation can be categorized as errors of (1) form (style) and (2) content (meaning). Errors of content can be further categorized as (1) omissions, (2) additions, (3) substitutions, or (4) editorializing. Once reconciliation occurs and a final first version is produced, the translation is given to the subject matter expert. The role of the subject matter expert is to proof the translation for specialized terminology or jargon embedded in the document. For example, if the English document to be translated into Spanish is a questionnaire about eating habits, the subject matter expert should be a bilingual nutritionist whose dominant language is Spanish. He or she will review the translation and note any jargon or other specialized terminology that is problematic and issue a report with detailed notes and recommendations. The translation team may want to discuss any questions or discrepancies with the subject matter expert, after which the translation team will produce the final draft. The subject matter expert should be selected carefully and instructed about all of the objectives of the source documents, including the characteristics of literacy, speech community (*a group of people who share norms and other language characteristics*), whether documents will be self-administered or not, any language that was challenging in English, and any other questions the researchers may have that may pose as concerns regarding the clarity of the written material. The final step in this method should invariably be to arrive at a consensus in terms of the accuracy of the document translated, the content and the style used, the lexicon, and the specialized terminology or jargon. This last step in the process is known as synthesis. It is also important to note that translators should involve the authors of the source document whenever a doubt exists. Moreover, translators often serve as the ultimate editors/proofreaders of the source document (Canino and Bravo 1994; Acquadro et al. 2008).

Back Translation

Back translation involves having a different translator or team of translators translate the translation rendered in the target language (the *forward translation*) back into the source language from which it was originally translated (Brislin 1970). Back translation is often used as a way to check the quality of the forward translation (Downing and Bogoslaw 2003). For example, if a pamphlet originally written in English is translated into Mandarin, the pamphlet written in Mandarin should then be back-translated into English. The English translation is then compared to the original English-written source document and any inaccuracies brought to the attention of the translators. The translator conducting the back translation should be blind to the original document (Brislin 1970; McDermott and Palchanes 1994).

Back translation is often but not always used. Some have found the forward-backward standard of translation to be awkward (King et al. 2011) because the translators who execute the forward translation and those who do the backward, in addition to perhaps having distinct styles, are also working in the context of reversed source and target linguistic/cultural systems. For example, the concept of a nurse practitioner is relatively new in the United States and is rare or may not even exist in Spanish-speaking cultures. A translator may convey this concept by providing an explanation in the Spanish target (e.g., a nurse that is highly specialized and can prescribe). The resulting Spanish text may mislead the reader in the apparent lack of terminological precision because it will read as "a nurse that is highly specialized and can prescribe" versus "a nurse practitioner." Whenever a back translation is performed, the forward and the back translators should meet to discuss problematic areas, if possible involving the creator of the source document, and ideally come to a consensus.

Linguistic and cultural differences cannot be completely addressed by a back translation, so bilingual/bicultural specialists are recommended to work together to negotiate such differences. Ultimately, whether back translation is implemented will depend on the purpose and nature of the documents (Acquadro 2008). For example, if the study relies on surveys that need to be completed by the participants themselves, simple forward and back translation will not be sufficient.

Localization and Transcreation

Translation alone is not always enough. "Localization," a term borrowed from the marketing industry, describes adjusting the language to the needs of the target speech community—*a group of people who share norms and other language characteristics*. In practice, a translating team is tasked with writing a text that responds to the particular linguistic needs of the speech community to which the translation is targeted. If the target population is mostly made up of Spanish speakers from Guatemala, then the translation team should develop a plan to ensure that all idioms and jargon used conform to the lexicon of the specific population. Alternatively, if the Spanish-speaking population is diverse, then the localization team should make sure that the language used is neutral.

In transcreation, the source text is completely rewritten from scratch in the target language to convey the concepts and achieve the aims of the source text while accounting for both language and cultural considerations (Macario 2007). For example, for a nutrition study interested in the dietary habits of a group of recently arrived Tibetan immigrants, the food options used to survey middle-class white Americans would not be meaningful. Therefore, rather than using the English source as a model for direct translation, the document should be written anew in the target language. The merit of this method is that the text is rendered using the same process as it was rendered in English, where readability, literacy, and cultural appropriateness are part of the initial process. The person executing the transcreation should be screened for writing skill and should have an excellent understanding of the study's objectives. The writer and other investigators should meet to discuss the challenges, if any, concerning style, culture-bound concepts *(or ideas that are particular to the culture at stake)*, readability, and other content as dictated by the study needs (e.g., foods). As discussed later in this chapter, the writer and the study team should field-test their assumptions in terms of the content, word choice, literacy level, and so forth, through interviews or focus groups using community members of the target language. We describe the most common field-testing methods below.

Field Testing: Focus Groups and Pilot Testing

One way that localization *(adjusting the needs to the targeted speech community)* can be implemented successfully is through the use of focus groups. During focus groups, the research team meets with representative members of the specific speech community. The facilitator of the group queries participants on the language in question, including all difficult words identified in the English source document (or in the document written anew in the target language), checks for understanding, and asks for alternate word choices as needed. Once changes are made to the document, a second focus group should be conducted with different participants from the same community to check specific language and comprehensibility.

Studies have shown that words that are thought to be of a low register—that are colloquial in nature—may present great difficulty when translated into other languages. For example, consider the issue of the self-reporting of health status. It has been found that LEP Spanish speakers. compared to non-LEP patients, self-rate their health as worse (Jimenez-Garcia et al. 2008; Franzini and Fernandez-Esquer 2004). These results seem more than plausible considering the many barriers to good health status that this population faces. However, a recent study found that one reason that Spanish-speaking LEP individuals are more likely to rate their health status as "fair" is because the word "fair" in Spanish has a more positive connotation than it does in English (Viruell-Fuentes et al. 2011). While this does not necessarily invalidate the research on perceived health status, it does illuminate the need for a greater awareness in approaching instrument translation.

Focus groups can also be used to test the study instrument type used and the question format (e.g., Likert scale versus multiple choice). Survey questions/guides should be tested for questions/formats that may work in English but not in other language groups, especially for individuals with a lower literacy level. The Likert format, for example, is often used in English but may pose difficulties for a non-English-speaking target population (D'Alonzo 2011). In some cases the original English questionnaire may need to be modified or even redeveloped (Yu et al. 2004; Hilton and Skrutkowski 2002).

Researchers should pilot-test the questions and topic guides to be used prior to conducting an interview, as unforeseen cultural issues and/or word choices could disrupt the dynamic. For example, researchers conducting qualitative research in mainland China found that certain groups were more resistant to discussing topics in detail or divulging personal experiences, and that taking time in the beginning of an interview to build trust was of invaluable help (Smith et al. 2008).

One overall approach to pilot testing uses cognitive testing approaches (Jabine et al. 1984; Willis 2005) to determine whether or not respondents understand questions consistently and in the way researchers intended, and whether respondents have the information/experiences needed to answer the questions and are able to provide meaningful answers given the response tasks provided. We administer surveys accompanied by a series of questions and probes to assess respondents' understanding, perceptions of what we are asking, and difficulties in fitting their experiences and responses into the survey options/formats. Both "talk out loud" (having respondents explain their thinking and impressions as they respond to particular questions) and structured follow-up and reflection ("How easy was that to answer? What made it difficult? What were you thinking about? What do you think this phrase meant?") approaches are used. At the end of this process, having gone through the full survey, respondents are debriefed—asked about their overall experience of the survey, suggestions and feedback for improvement, and sense of the goals of the survey.

Translation does not always occur with English as its source. In the next section we examine the considerations that need to be taken into account when translation occurs from the target language into English.

Qualitative Research Translation into English

There are many similarities in the tasks of translation of quantitative and qualitative research. Unique to qualitative research, including narrative interviews and focus groups, is the need to translate the responses of the participant into a form that is understandable by the researcher, unless the researcher speaks the language of the participants, which is always preferable (Esposito 2001). Cross-language qualitative research requires systematic strategies and methodologies to obtain valid results (Squires 2009). Unlike quantitative research, which often relies on validated questionnaires with standardized responses, focus groups and interviews present a more fluid dynamic in eliciting narrative data. Unfortunately this also leaves room for more mistakes in translation and interpretation (Esposito 2001).

As mentioned earlier, focus groups are often used to acquire knowledge in cross-cultural, cross-linguistic research studies (Minkler 2004). Customarily, when focus groups are conducted in the native language of the participants, the transcribed content is translated into English for English-speaking researchers to review. Importantly, researchers working with LEP populations should be able to discern the complexity and nuance expressed in the subjects' narratives once translated, as they do when conducting focus groups in English-speaking populations. Translation is accomplished by audio-recording the focus group and then either first transcribing the conversation and then translating into English (two steps) or translating directly from the audio (one-step) (Esposito 2001; Willgerodt 2003). The two-step scheme is the established method. In another method, the researcher can participate in the focus group with a simultaneous interpreter.

Keeping a Documentation Trail

It is key to keep detailed notes of all document drafts and procedures used during the materials development process. This enables the research team to go back to problem areas, assess the discussion/procedures related to their resolution, and move forward with a clear understanding of the reasons behind technique, word, and phrase choice.

INTERPRETATION

Interpretation is the rendering *orally* in one language of what is said in another language, expressing the message faithfully, accurately, and objectively (NCIHC and ATA 2009). Medical interpreting can be either consecutive or simultaneous. In consecutive interpreting, the interpreting occurs after the speaker has completed speaking, necessitating that the speakers pause for the interpreter. In simultaneous interpreting, interpreting occurs at the same time as the original speech. Interpreting can also be proximate or remote. Proximate interpreting involves an interpreter who is physically present at the encounter. In remote interpreting, the interpreter is outside the room of the encounter. Medical interpreting is usually proximate consecutive (PCMI) or over-the-telephone consecutive—remote consecutive medical interpreting (RCMI); less commonly utilized is the newer method of remote simultaneous (United Nations style) medical interpreting (RSMI) (Gany et al. 2007a).

When done appropriately, consecutive interpreting can be accurate, as can be simultaneous. To be accurate in consecutive, interpreters need to pace their interlocutors or take notes. Generally, attempting to consecutively interpret passages that are longer than three long ideas is risky. Studies have shown that in these cases, interpreters tend to summarize the information (Gany et al. 2007b). Note taking is a good strategy, but it should be exercised with caution and parties should be consulted for approval. It is important to consider that in some settings, for example, where the participants are refugees or asylum seekers, note taking may elicit memories of surveillance.

Generally, it is useful to think of interpreters in terms of their role as a conduit (or a black box that simply repeats everything said without any filtering whatsoever), but also in terms of their inevitable omnipresence. In our research, the role of the interpreter is fluid. Interpreters should indeed be as invisible as possible to approximate a same-language encounter and should help foster a relationship between interlocutors (investigator/provider and research participant). However, in this model, interpreters may identify moments in which they need to be more present, perhaps to aid either party in clarifying a perceived misunderstanding. This intervention should be done with caution; the interpreter should not speak for either party. The role of the provider/investigator is to elicit the point of view of the research participant and not that of the interpreter (NCIHC and ATA 2009). The choice of an interpreter and mode of interpretation, and an awareness of the legalities, ethics, and costs involved in the provision of interpreting services to LEP participants, are important considerations in conducting research across language discordance.

Who Should Interpret?

As with translation, interpreting is a skill that requires professional training; bilingualism is necessary but not sufficient to interpret in the research setting. Training programs for interpreters vary in duration and quality.

US Guidelines. Medical interpreting is a relatively nascent profession in the United States and there is a wide range of professionalism in how it is delivered. Using ad hoc bilingual individuals is not uncommon, but it is an unacceptable practice. The National Council on Interpreting in Health Care (NCIHC) releases national standards for health care interpreting education courses, which are available on their website (http://ncihc.org). Interpreters should have completed coursework in accordance with NCIHC recommendations, including instruction on the ethics involved in interpreting.

The Certification Commission for Healthcare Interpreters (CCHI) is a nonprofit organization that supplies certification of medical language interpreters (Yu et al. 2004). To qualify to take the CCHI certification examination, an interpreter must (CCHI 2011)

1. demonstrate proficiency in English and in the second language,
2. be at least eighteen years of age,
3. possess a high school diploma or equivalent, and
4. have undergone at least forty hours of interpreter training.

The CCHI requirements are also endorsed by the NCIHC.

Australia Guidelines.   Australia has similar guidelines for medical interpreting, issued through its National Accreditation Authority for Translators and Interpreters (NAATI). NAATI is the national body that standardizes the translating and interpreting professions (Israel et al. 1998). Australia's medical interpreters are certified by this agency (ADIC 2010). Moreover, due to the universality of health insurance and the centralization of care in Australia, there is a nationalized Translating and Interpreting Service (TIS National) available. TIS provides free medical interpreting services to both Australian citizens and permanent residents (ADIC 2010).

How to Work with an Interpreter

The role of the interpreter should essentially be to serve as an invisible vehicle through which the researcher can elicit the participant's point of view and share information accurately. Working with a trained interpreter should be straightforward, as the interpreter should have been trained in the following standards of practice: impartiality, confidentiality, accuracy, respect, cultural awareness, and professionalism (NCIHC 2005).[3] Interpreters should also be aware that they must feel free to ask for clarification in case of jargon or other unfamiliar language. Interpreters should use the first person and avoid eye contact with the researcher or the participant. Importantly, the researcher should speak directly to the study participant and not to the interpreter (CDC 2006).

Sight Translation

In sight translation, an interpreter reads the source document and then translates orally in the target language. A unique skill set is required for sight translation, as the translator must be able to both read and comprehend the written text as well as to render an oral translation. In health care, this type of interpretation is subject to professional training and accreditation (NHeLP et al. 2010). Much of the health care information available to research participants is provided in written form— including brochures, questionnaires, and discharge instructions. If these documents have not been translated, which is not recommended, an interpreter trained in sight translation should be employed. Otherwise, the researcher or a member of the team should explain the areas that need to be rendered orally and the interpreter can interpret them.

RECRUITMENT AND RETENTION

Study recruitment of LEP individuals is most effective with a community-engaged approach (Israel et al. 1998). While specific strategies may differ by culture, several broad, effective strategies emerge for recruiting participants in an outpatient setting (Maxwell et al. 2005; Mendez-Luck et al. 2011; Yancey et al. 2006; Kreuter et al. 2003; Baumann et al. 2011):

- Reach out to local leaders to learn about the community.
- Work in partnership with these leaders, who will introduce researchers to potential study subjects and help researchers tailor recruitment materials and plan events, such as health fairs.
- If brochures and flyers are distributed, the translation should be appropriate and written in a way that it is culturally relevant to the needs of the target population.

Whether recruiting in a hospital or in the surrounding community, it is crucial to explain the study in the individual's language and to ensure that it is comprehensible.

Our experience has been positive when we have used native speakers and/or same-ethnicity researchers to recruit study participants. A language-concordant interaction between research assistant and individual establishes trust and rapport, facilitating empowerment of the research participant. This type of relationship can prevent the participant from feeling like a test subject and more like a participant in knowledge-gathering efforts.

Because of potential low literacy levels, study participants may need help beyond a translated form, and integral to recruitment and retention is the informed consent process. In the next section, we examine this process with its many intricacies.

INFORMED CONSENT FOR LEP POPULATIONS

Obtaining informed consent from a participant is more than just acquiring a signature—it is a process through which the individual learns about the study and what will be required of him or her, and through which the person's autonomy is respected, as described in the section on research ethics. In the United States, the Office for Human Research Protections (OHRP) protects the rights and well-being of human research subjects and provides specific guidelines for enrolling LEP individuals in research studies. The consent document must be provided in a language understandable to the subject, as per 21 CFR 50.20. A copy of the translated document, in the case of non-English-speaking participants, must be provided (USFDA 2011).

According to the OHRP, if the consent is not available in the language of the research subject, the consenting professional may provide an oral presentation of the informed consent along with a written document (referred to as the short form) that states the aspect of the consent that has been rendered orally and a summary of what has been said orally (Clark et al. 2011). During this process, an interpreter should be present to interpret the oral presentation, along with a bilingual person who can sign as the witness (OHRP 1995).

There is, however, no federal mandate for the use of a professional interpreter during this process. Given the above-described issues with ad hoc interpretation, these guidelines should be considered the minimum standard required by law, albeit insufficient due to this issue (Clark et al. 2011).

The National Council on Interpreting in Health Care (NCIHC) has issued recommendations on the provision of informed consent: only a person who is a qualified health care interpreter, or someone on the research staff who is certified as fluent in that language, should be allowed to obtain consent, and all informed consent printed materials must be in the research participant's language (DH and NHS 2005). The NCIHC recommends printing the translated materials at no higher than a sixth-grade reading level (Jacobs et al. 2001). We would also add that experts should review the translated document after back translation to replace inappropriate jargon and to ensure cross-cultural equivalence.

NAVIGATING RESEARCH PARTICIPANTS THROUGH STUDIES

Employing research navigators to guide research participants through the various points of the study can help ensure optimal communication, participant retention, and reporting of adverse events. In health care, patient navigation through medical treatment has helped to ameliorate disparities in treatment. Such navigation can be effectively transposed to clinical research (Gany et al. 2011). As in navigation through care, researchers can aid participants to follow up with research study requirements (Nguyen et al. 2006; Freund et al. 2008; USDHHS et al. 2004).

ADVERSE EVENTS REPORTING

As part of the protection of research participants from risk, there are regulations in place that enable participants to report adverse events that may arise during a study. Depending on the study, an adverse event can be a deleterious change in one's health as a result of a clinical protocol, or a less serious and transient side effect. Adverse events are considered a serious and reportable event in every country mentioned in this chapter (ANHMRC 2007; Jacobs et al. 2001; Parker 2011). Additional protections for recognition and reporting of adverse events should be provided to LEP participants. For instance, the NCIHC recommends that LEP study participants be able to call someone in their language at any time (Jacobs et al. 2001). Further, in the event that the principal investigator notes an adverse event that requires reporting, the patient should be notified in his or her language.

COSTS

There are potentially additional monetary costs of including nondominant language speakers in research. However, lack of inclusion can be costly in the longer term. The costs involved with translation will vary based on the complexity of the task, including the following:

1. Target language: Spanish and other languages that use the Roman alphabet tend to be less expensive to translate than other languages.
2. Subject matter: The complexity of the document to be translated can affect costs, for example, a brochure for recruitment may be less expensive to translate than a study instrument.
3. Deadlines: A short turn-around time for translation may be more expensive than providing ample time.

Forward translation with one translator only may be the least expensive method, but it is generally improper practice. Rigorous back translation, panel review, and pilot testing are key. It is advisable to undertake the more costly approach and obtain reliable results than to get potentially invalid data or costly adverse events.

There are a growing number of organizations in the United States that provide translation and interpreting services in the community. Consulting the NCIHC's website may provide helpful ideas on government and community resources. It is helpful to account for all language expenses during budget planning, including language access resources as line items on grant budgets.

Education and advocacy should be considered to increase funding specifically for translation and interpretation services.

SUMMARY

In this chapter, we provide a guide for increasing equity in research through increased enrollment of people with limited English proficiency and increased protection and retention of those enrolled. Cross-cultural awareness is a vital part of conducting research with LEP populations. High-quality translation and interpretation, while potentially costly and time-consuming, are crucial to ensuring valid and reliable data.

NOTES

1. For a glossary of terms, see *The Terminology of Health Care Interpreters: A Glossary of Terms,* from the National Council on Interpreting in Health Care (NCIHC 2008).

2. Article 4.1 is based on the principle of justice. It imposes a duty on researchers not to exclude individuals or groups from participation for reasons that are unrelated to the

research. This duty is explicitly stated because groups have been inappropriately excluded from participation in research on the basis of attributes such as gender, race, ethnicity, age, and disability (CIHR et al. 2010).

3. The NCIHC's (2005) national standards of practice can be easily accessed as a PDF file from its website (http://www.ncihc.org/mc/page.do?sitePageId = 98592&orgId = ncihc). The report expands upon the listed standards of practice and includes related ethics examples.

REFERENCES

Acquadro, C., et al. 2008. "Literature review of methods to translate health-related quality of life questionnaires for use in multinational clinical trials." *Value in Health* 11(3): 509–21.

Adams, R. J., et al. 2009. "Risks associated with low functional health literacy in an Australian population." *Medical Journal of Australia* 191(10): 530–34.

ALTA Language Services. 2012. Language Testing Services. http://www.altalang.com/language-testing/.

American Community Survey (ACS). 2010. *Selected social characteristics in the United States: 2010 American community survey 1-year estimates.*

American Translators Association (ATA). 2012. *A guide to ATA certification.* http://www.atanet.org/.

Aspinall, P. J. 2005. "Why the next census needs to ask about language—Delivery of culturally competent health care and other services depends on such data." *British Medical Journal* 331(7513): 363–64A.

Aspinall, P. J. 2007. "Language ability: A neglected dimension in the profiling of populations and health service users." *Health Education Journal* 66(1): 90–106.

Australia Department of Immigration and Multicultural Affairs (ADIMA). 2005. "The charter of public service in a culturally diverse society." In *Access and equity annual report 2005.* http://www.immi.gov.au/about/reports/access-equity/access-equity-2005/.

Australian Department of Immigration and Citizenship (ADIC), National Communications Branch. 2010. *Australian immigration fact sheet 91—Translating and Interpreting Service (TIS).* Canberra.

Australian Government (AG). 2008. *The people of Australia: Statistics from the 2006 census.* Canberra.

Australian Government. 2011. *Act no. 52 of 1975*, in C2011C00852 Com Law. http://www.comlaw.gov.au/Details/C2011C00852.

Australia National Health and Medical Research Council (ANHMRC). 1999. *National statement on ethical conduct in research involving humans.* http://www.nhmrc.gov.au/_files_nhmrc/publications/attachments/e72.pdf.

Australia National Health and Medical Research Council (ANHMRC). 2007. *National statement on ethical conduct in human research 2007.* http://www.nhmrc.gov.au/_files_nhmrc/publications/attachments/e72_national_statement_131211.pdf.

Australia National Health and Medical Research Council (ANHMRC). 2009. *NHMRC Australian Health Ethics Committee (AHEC) position statement: Monitoring and reporting of safety for clinical trials involving therapeutic products.* http://www.alfredresearch.org/ethics/NHMRC%20Position%20Statement%20AE%20Reporting.pdf.

Ballantyne, A.J., et al. 2008. "Fair inclusion of men and women in Australian clinical research: Views from ethics committee chairs." *Medical Journal of Australia* 188(11): 653–56.

Baumann, A., M. D. Rodriguez, and J. R. Parra-Cardona. 2011. "Community-based applied research with Latino immigrant families: Informing practice and research according to ethical and social justice principles." *Family Process* 50(2): 132–48.

Brislin, R. W. 1970. "Back-translation for cross-cultural research." *Journal of Cross-Cultural Psychology* 1(3): 185–216.

Bustillos, D. 2009. "Limited English proficiency and disparities in clinical research." *Journal of Law Medicine and Ethics* 37(1): 28.

Canadian Institutes of Health Research (CIHR), National Sciences and Engineering Research Council of Canada, and Social Sciences and Humanities Research Council of Canada. 2010. *Tri-council policy statement: Ethical conduct for research involving humans.* http://pre.ethics.gc.ca/pdf/eng/tcps2/TCPS_2_FINAL_Web.pdf.

Canino, Glorisa, and Milagros Bravo. 1994. "The adaptation and testing of diagnostic and outcome measures for cross-cultural research." *International Review of Psychiatry* 6(4): 281–86.

Centers for Disease Control and Prevention (CDC). 2006. *National Health and Nutrition Examination Survey (NHANES): Interpretation guidelines.* http://www.cdc.gov/nchs /data/nhanes/nhanes_07_08/Interpretation_Guidelines.pdf.

Certification Commission for Healthcare Interpreters (CCHI). 2011. *Credentials and eligibility.* http://www.healthcareinterpretercertification.org/images/pdf/Eligibility.pdf.

Challinor, A. E. 2011. *Canada's immigration policy: A focus on human capital.* Washington, DC: Migration Policy Institute. http://www.migrationinformation.org/Profiles/display. cfm?ID=853..

Clark, S., et al. 2011. "The informed consent: A study of the efficacy of informed consents and the associated role of language barriers." *Journal of Surgical Education* 68(2): 143–47.

Clinton, William J. 2000. "Executive Order 13166—Improving access to services for persons with limited English proficiency." Department of Justice. *Federal Register* 50121–50122.

Crush, Jonathan. 2008. *South Africa: Policy in the face of xenophobia.* Washington, DC: Migration Policy Institute. http://www.migrationinformation.org/USfocus/display .cfm?ID=689.

D'Alonzo, K. T. 2011. "Evaluation and revision of questionnaires for use among low-literacy immigrant Latinos." *Revista Latino-Americana de Enfermagem* 19(5): 1255–64.

Davis, T. C., et al. 1993. "Rapid estimate of adult literacy in medicine: A shortened screening instrument." *Family Medicine* 25(6): 391–95.

Department of Health (DH) and National Health Service (NHS). 2005. *Research governance framework for health and social care.* http://www.dh.gov.uk/prod_consum_dh/groups /dh_digitalassets/@dh/@en/documents/digitalasset/dh_4122427.pdf.

Derose, K. P., and D. W. Baker. 2000. "Limited English proficiency and Latinos' use of physician services." *Medical Care Research and Review* 57(1): 76–91.

Deumert, A. 2010. "'It would be nice if they could give us more language'—Serving South Africa's multilingual patient base." *Social Science and Medicine* 71(1): 53–61.

Downing, B. T., and L. H. Bogoslaw. 2003. "Effective patient-provider communication across language barriers: Focus on translation." http://www.slideserve.com/plato/effective-patient-provider-communication-across-language-barriers-focus-on-translation.

Dowse, R., and M. Ehlers. 2004. "Pictograms for conveying medicine instructions: Comprehension in various South African language groups." *South African Journal of Science* 100(11–12): 687–93.

Eberle, Carolyn, et al. 2012. "Optimizing self-reported data in a study of employment in low-English proficiency breast cancer survivors." In *Memorial Sloan Kettering Clinical Research Professionals Week Poster Session*. New York.

Esposito, N. 2001. "From meaning to meaning: The influence of translation techniques on non-English focus group research." *Qualitative Health Research* 11(4): 568–79.

Flores, G. 2005. "The impact of medical interpreter services on the quality of health care: A systematic review." *Medical Care Research and Review* 62(3): 255–99.

Forsyth, B. H., et al. 2007. "Methods for translating an English-language survey questionnaire on tobacco use into Mandarin, Cantonese, Korean, and Vietnamese." *Field Methods* 19(3): 264–83.

Franzini, L., and M. E. Fernandez-Esquer. 2004. "Socioeconomic, cultural, and personal influences on health outcomes in low income Mexican-origin individuals in Texas." *Social Science and Medicine* 59(8): 1629–46.

Freund, K. M., et al. 2008. "National Cancer Institute patient navigation research program methods, protocol, and measures." *Cancer* 113(12): 3391–99.

Gany, F., et al. 2007a. "Patient satisfaction with different interpreting methods: A randomized controlled trial." *Journal of General Internal Medicine* 22: 312–318.

Gany, F., et al. 2007b. "The impact of medical interpretation method on time and errors." *Journal of General Internal Medicine* 22: 319–23.

Gany, F., et al. 2011. "Targeting social and economic correlates of cancer treatment appointment keeping among immigrant Chinese patients." *Journal of Urban Health–Bulletin of the New York Academy of Medicine* 88(1): 98–103.

Garcia-Castillo, D., and M. D. Fetters. 2007. "Quality in medical translations: A review." *Journal of Health Care for the Poor and Underserved* 18(1): 74–84.

Gill, P. S., et al. 2009. "Access to interpreting services in England: Secondary analysis of national data." *BMC Public Health* 9: 12.

Giuliano, A. R., et al. 2000. "Participation of minorities in cancer research: The influence of structural, cultural, and linguistic factors." *Annals of Epidemiology* 10(8): S22–S34.

Glickman, S. W., et al. 2008. "Challenges in enrollment of minority, pediatric, and geriatric patients in emergency and acute care clinical research." *Annals of Emergency Medicine* 51(6): 775–80.

Glickman, S. W., et al. 2011. "Perspective: The case for research justice: Inclusion of patients with limited English proficiency in clinical research." *Academic Medicine* 86(3): 389–93.

Hablamos Juntos (HJ). 2008. "Language testing options 2008." Princeton, NJ: Robert Wood Johnson Foundation. http://www.hablamosjuntos.org/newsletters/2008/june/pdf/lang-testingoptions 06–23–08.pdf.

Hilton, A., and M. Skrutkowski. 2002. "Translating instruments into other languages: Development and testing processes." *Cancer Nursing* 25(1): 1–7.

Hornberger, Nancy H., and Serfain M. Coronel-Molina. 2004. "Quechua language shift, maintenance, and revitalization in the Andes: The case for language planning." *International Journal of the Sociology of Language* 167: 9–67.

Inglis, Christine. 2002. "Australia's increasing ethnic and religious diversity." *Migration information source.* http://www.migrationinformation.org/Feature/display.cfm?ID = 72.

Israel, B. A., et al. 1998. "Review of community-based research: Assessing partnership approaches to improve public health." *Annual Review of Public Health* 19: 173–202.

Jabine, T. B., et al., eds. 1984. *Cognitive aspects of survey methodology: Building a bridge between disciplines.* Washington, DC: National Academies Press.

Jacobs, Elizabeth, Wilma Alvarado-Little, and Eric Hardt. 2001. "Recommendations for the ethical involvement of limited English-speakers in research." National Council on Interpreting in Health Care Working Papers Series 7. Washington, DC.

Javier, J. R., et al. 2010. "Children with special health care needs: How immigrant status is related to health care access, health care utilization, and health status." *Maternal and Child Health Journal* 14(4): 567–79.

Jimenez-Garcia, R., et al. 2008. "Ten-year trends in self-rated health among Spanish adults with diabetes, 1993–2003." *Diabetes Care* 31(1): 90–92.

Jones, P. S., et al. 2001. "An adaptation of Brislin's translation model for cross-cultural research." *Nursing Research* 50(5): 300–304.

Jonkers, M., et al. 2011. "Severe maternal morbidity among immigrant women in the Netherlands: Patients' perspectives." *Reproductive Health Matters* 19(37): 144–53.

Karliner, L. S., et al. 2008. "Identification of limited English proficient patients in clinical care." *Journal of General Internal Medicine* 23(10): 1555–60.

Kim, G., et al. 2011. "Limited English proficiency as a barrier to mental health service use: A study of Latino and Asian immigrants with psychiatric disorders." *Journal of Psychiatric Research* 45(1): 104–10.

King, K. M., et al. 2011. "Examining and establishing translational and conceptual equivalence of survey questionnaires for a multi-ethnic, multi-language study." *Journal of Advanced Nursing* 67(10): 2267–74.

Kreps, G. L., and L. Sparks. 2008. "Meeting the health literacy needs of immigrant populations." *Patient Education and Counseling* 71(3): 328–32.

Kreuter, M. W., et al. 2003. "Achieving cultural appropriateness in health promotion programs: Targeted and tailored approaches." *Health Education and Behavior* 30(2): 133–46.

Lee, C. C., et al. 2009. "Ensuring cross-cultural equivalence in translation of research consents and clinical documents: A systematic process of translating English to Chinese." *Journal of Transcultural Nursing* 20(1): 77–82.

Leng, J. C. F., et al. 2010. "Detection of depression with different interpreting methods among Chinese and Latino primary care patients: A randomized controlled trial." *Journal of Immigrant and Minority Health* 12(2): 234–41.

Levin, M. E. 2006. "Overcoming language barriers." *South African Medical Journal* 9(10): 1058.

Levy, Martin L. 2009. *Civil Rights Act of 1964.* New York: Oxford University Press.

Macario, Everly, Jennifer Isenberg, and Ileana Quintas. 2007. "Drugs + HIV: Learn the Link Campaign: How IQ solutions and the National Institute on Drug Abuse (NIDA) adapted a television PSA for Hispanic teens." *Cases in Public Health Communication and Marketing*, June.

MacFarlane, Anne, Carrie Singleton, and Eileen Green. 2009. "Language barriers in health and social care consultations in the community: A comparative study of responses in Ireland and England." *Health Policy* 92(2–3): 203–10.

Maxwell, A. E., et al. 2005. "Strategies to recruit and retain older Filipino-American immigrants for a cancer screening study." *Journal of Community Health* 30(3): 167–79.

McDermott, Mary Anne Nelson, and Kathleen Palchanes. 1994. "A literature review of the critical elements in translation theory." *Journal of Nursing Scholarship* 26(2): 113–18.

Mendez-Luck, C. A., et al. 2011. "Recruitment strategies and costs associated with community-based research in a Mexican-origin population." *Gerontologist* 51: S94–S105.

Minkler, M. 2004. "Ethical challenges for the "outside" researcher in community-based participatory research." *Health Education and Behavior* 31(6): 684–97.

National Cancer Institute (NCI) and the Substance Abuse and Mental Health Services Administration (SAMHSA). *Guidelines for choosing and adapting programs, in research-tested intervention programs (RTIPs)*. http://rtips.cancer.gov/rtips/reference/adaptation_guidelines.pdf.

National Commission for the Protection of Human Subjects of Biomedical and Behavioral Research (NC). 1979. *The Belmont report: Ethical principles and guidelines for the protection of human subjects of research*. http://ohsr.od.nih.gov/guidelines/belmont.html.

National Council on Interpreting in Health Care (NCIHC). 2005. *National standards of practice for interpreters in health care*. http://www.ncihc.org/assets/documents/publications/NCIHC%20National%20Standards%20of%20Practice.pdf.

National Council on Interpreting in Health Care (NCIHC). 2008. *The terminology of health care interpreters: A glossary of terms*. http://www.ncihc.org/mc/page.do?sitePageId = 98592&orgId = ncihc.

National Council on Interpreting in Health Care (NCIHC) and American Translators Association (ATA). 2009. *What's in a word? A guide to understanding interpreting and translation in health care*. National Health Law Program. http://www.ncihc.org/mc/page.do?sitePageId = 98592&orgId = ncihc.

Ngo-Metzger, Q., et al. 2003. "Linguistic and cultural barriers to care." *Journal of General Internal Medicine* 18(1): 44–52.

Nguyen, T. T., et al. 2006. "Community-based participatory research increases cervical cancer screening among Vietnamese-Americans." *Journal of Health Care for the Poor and Underserved* 17(2): 31–54.

Office of Human Research Protections (OHRP). 1995. *Obtaining and documenting informed consent of subjects who do not speak English*. http://www.hhs.gov/ohrp/policy/ic-non-e.html.

Office for Human Research Protections (OHRP). 2012. "Obtaining and documenting informed consent of subjects who do not speak English." http://www.hhs.gov/ohrp/policy/ic-non-e.html.

Pan South African Language Board (PanSALB). 2011. *PanSALB annual report 2010/11*. http://www.pansalb.org.za.

Papadopoulos, I., et al. 2004. "Ethiopian refugees in the UK: Migration, adaptation and settlement experiences and their relevance to health." *Ethnicity and Health* 9(1): 55–73.

Parker, Lucy. 2011. *Recording, managing and reporting adverse events in the UK,* July14, 2011. https://workspace.imperial.ac.uk/clinicalresearchgovernanceoffice/Public/JRO_SOP_001%20Safety%20Reporting%20FINAL%2014.07.2011.pdf.

Parker, R. M., et al. 1995. "The test of functional health literacy in adults—A new instrument for measuring patients' literacy skills." *Journal of General Internal Medicine* 10(10): 537–41.

Perkins, Jane. 2003. "Ensuring lingusitic access in health care settings: An overview of current legal rights and responsibilities." The Kaiser Commission on Medicaid and the Uninsured, Washington, DC. 1–37.

Republic of South Africa (RSA). No. 61 of 2003: National Health Act, 2004. 2004. *Government Gazette* 469. Cape Town, SA. http://www.info.gov.za/view/DownloadFileAction?id=68039.

Rex, John. 1995. "Ethnic identity and the nation state: The political sociology of multi-cultural societies." *Social Identities* 1(1): 21.

Robinson, James. 2010. "Interpreting and translation in NHS Lothian: Policy for meeting the needs of people with limited English proficiency." http://www.nhslothian.scot.nhs.uk/YourRights/TICS/Documents/InterpretingTranslationPolicy.pdf.

Schlemmer, A., and B. Mash. 2006. "The effects of a language barrier in a South African district hospital." *South African Medical Journal* 96(10): 1084–87.

Shi, Lu-Feng. 2011. "How 'proficient' is proficient? Subjective proficiency as a predictor of bilingual listeners' recognition of English words." *American Journal of Audiology* 2(1): 19–32.

Shin, Hyon B., and Rosalind Bruno. 2003. "Language use and English-speaking ability: 2000." Washington, DC: US Census Bureau. http://www.census.gov/prod/2003pubs/c2kbr-29.pdf..

Smith, H. J., J. Chen, and X. Y. Liu. 2008. "Language and rigour in qualitative research: Problems and principles in analyzing data collected in Mandarin." *BMC Medical Research Methodology* 8: 44.

Somerville, Will, Dhananjayan Sriskandarajah, and Maria Latorre. 2009. "United Kingdom: A reluctant country of immigration." *Migration Information Source.* http://www.migrationinformation.org/feature/display.cfm?ID = 736.

South Africa Department of Health (SADH). 2004. *Ethics in health research: Principles, structures and processes.* http://www.nhrec.org.za/wp-content/uploads/2008/09/ethics.pdf.

Squires, A. 2009. "Methodological challenges in cross-language qualitative research: A research review." *International Journal of Nursing Studies* 46(2): 277–87.

StatisticsCanada. 2007. *The evolving linguistic portrait, 2006 census.* http://www.12.statcan.ca/census-recensement/2006/as-sa/97–555/p3-eng.cfm.

Sudore, R. L., et al. 2009. "Unraveling the relationship between literacy, language proficiency, and patient-physician communication." *Patient Education and Counseling* 75(3): 398–402.

Thornton, J. D., et al. 2009. "Families with limited English proficiency receive less information and support in interpreted intensive care unit family conferences." *Critical Care Medicine* 37(1): 89–95.

Tieu, Y., C. Konnert, and J. L. Wang. 2010. "Depression literacy among older Chinese immigrants in Canada: A comparison with a population-based survey." *International Psychogeriatrics* 22(8): 1318–26.

Todd, L., and L. Hoffman-Goetz. 2011. "A qualitative study of cancer information seeking among English-as-a-second-language older Chinese immigrant women to Canada: Sources, barriers, and strategies." *Journal of Cancer Education* 26(2): 333–40.

Toppelberg, C. O., and B. A. Collins. 2010. "Language, culture, and adaptation in immigrant children." *Child and Adolescent Psychiatric Clinics of North America* 19(4): 697–717.

US Census Bureau (USCB). 2010. *2010 census shows America's diversity.* Public Information Office: http://2010.census.gov/news/releases/operations/cb11-cn125.html.

US Department of Health and Human Services (USDHHS). 2008. "America's health literacy: Why we need accessible health information." http://www.health.gov/communication/literacy/issuebrief/.

US Department of Health and Human Services (USDHHS), National Institutes of Health (NIH), and National Cancer Institute (NCI). 2004. "Patient Navigation Research Program." http://crchd.cancer.gov/pnp/pnrp-index.html.

US Food and Drug Administration (USFDA). 2011. "A guide to informed consent—Information sheet: Guidance for institutional review boards and clinical investigators." http://www.fda.gov/RegulatoryInformation/Guidances/ucm126431.htm.

Viruell-Fuentes, E. A., et al. 2011. "Language of interview, self-rated health, and the other Latino health puzzle." *American Journal of Public Health* 101(7): 1306–13.

Wallace, Lorraine. 2006. "Patients' health literacy skills: The missing demographic variable in primary care research." *Annals of Family Medicine* 4(1): 85–86.

Weeks, A., H. Swerissen, and J. Belfrage. 2007. "Issues, challenges, and solutions in translating study instruments." *Evaluation Review* 31(2): 153–65.

Weiss, Barry. 2007. "Removing barriers to better, safer care. Health literacy and patient safety: Help patients understand." Chicago: American Medical Association's Health Literacy Educational Toolkit.

White, Ian, and Elizabeth McLaren. 2009. "The 2011 census taking shape: The selection of topics and questions." *Population Trends* 135: 8–19.

Willgerodt, M. A. 2003. "Using focus groups to develop culturally relevant instruments." *Western Journal of Nursing Research* 25(7): 798–814.

Willis, G. B. 2005. *Cognitive interviewing.* Thousand Oaks, CA: Sage.

Wilson, E., et al. 2005. "Effects of limited English proficiency and physician language on health care comprehension." *Journal of General Internal Medicine* 20(9): 800–806.

Wisely, Janet. 2011. "NRES proposals ahead of planning for further service improvement and evaluation." Yarrow, UK: NRES Management Group and HRA Interim Board, December 1.

Yancey, A. K., A. N. Ortega, and S. K. Kumanyika. 2006. "Effective recruitment and retention of minority research participants." In *Annual Review of Public Health.* Palo Alto: Annual Reviews. 1–28.

Yu, D. S. F., D. T. F. Lee, and J. Woo. 2004. "Issues and challenges of instrument translation." *Western Journal of Nursing Research* 26(3): 307–20.

Zun, Leslie S., Tania Sadoun, and LaVonne Downey. 2006. "English-language competency of self-declared English-speaking Hispanic patients using written tests of health literacy." *Journal of the National Medical Association* 98(6): 912–17.

25

Extended Case Study

A Mixed-Methods Approach to Understanding Internal Migrant Access to Health Care and the Health System's Response in India

Bontha V. Babu

Anjali B. Borhade

Yadlapalli S. Kusuma

INTRODUCTION

Migration has taken place throughout human history and currently represents an important livelihood strategy, mainly for the poor in many of the world's developing countries. The Human Development Report of the United Nations Development Program (UNDP) estimated that there are approximately 740 million internal migrants and 214 million international migrants (UNDP 2009). UNDP defined internal migrants as those individuals who move within the borders of a country, usually measured across regional, district, or municipal boundaries, resulting in a change of usual place of residence. In India, internal migration is a common phenomenon, with the National Sample Survey Organization (NSSO) of India estimating that in 2007–2008 there were 326 million internal migrants (i.e., 28.5% of the population) (NSSO 2010). Bhagat and Mohanty (2009) found that internal migration contributed substantially to the 9.2% urban growth rate in the decade 1991–2001.

There has been increased attention to migrant health as illustrated by a World Health Organization (WHO) resolution calling upon member states to promote migrant-sensitive health policies, equitable access to health promotion, and disease prevention and health care programs for migrants. That resolution also called for the establishment of health information systems to assess and analyze trends in migrant health and for the disaggregation of health information by migrant-relevant categories (WHO 2008). Subsequently, the WHO developed a framework for migrant-sensitive health systems (WHO et al. 2010).

Although a high proportion of migrants in India are represented by higher income quintiles, there is a substantial number of poorer migrants involved in low-wage jobs, principally in the informal sector. This population also suffers from various deprivations and handicaps that have to do with the nature of urban policies and the absence of employer support (Srivastava 2011) for health and health care. This lack of support leads to disparities in terms of inequities in health and health care access. In this study, the term "migrant" refers to socioeconomically disadvantaged urban migrants.

MIGRANTS: A VULNERABLE POPULATION ESSENTIAL FOR CITIES

The benefits of internal migration are often not recognized despite the fact that migrants are a necessity for developmental activities in cities. Since migrants form a considerable and essential group in cities, meeting their basic needs, including providing better access to health care services, is the Indian health system's responsibility. It is a prerequisite for the system to recognize migrants as a vulnerable group that needs targeted interventions for improving health care access.

In India, rural-urban migration is on the rise due to rural impoverishment, rapid industrialization, and a strong desire for upward economic mobility. However, it appears that migrants are having difficulty coping with urban living and are becoming vulnerable in the new environment. Vulnerability here is defined as a state of being exposed to or susceptible to neglect or abuse. This vulnerability leads to less control over the resources that are meant for all communities, including migrants. It is obvious that urban migrants are affected by livelihood insecurity, negligence, and alienation in the new sociocultural environment. This situation impedes the integration of migrants into the local population. Not much is yet known about health care access for migrants except for some micro studies that have highlighted migrant vulnerabilities in terms of health status and poor access to health care (Swain and Mishra 2006; Borhade 2007, 2011; Babu et al. 2010; Kusuma et al. 2009a, 2009b, 2010, 2013; Saggurti et al. 2011). Unfortunately, there are no nationwide data on migrants' health and health care access. Hence, there is a need for additional data on these issues to substantiate evidence-based policies.

THE NEED FOR FOCUSED STUDIES ON MIGRANTS' HEALTH CARE

Since access improves if health care services become better aligned with people's needs and resources, it is important to know both the migrants' perspectives as well as the health system's response. It is documented in the preliminary studies cited above that disparities in health care access for migrants exist, and health officials are concerned that gaps may widen further if appropriate steps are not taken. Given this background, innovative approaches are needed to better align health care services with migrant needs, expectations, and resources. The Indian Council of Medical Research has initiated a countrywide study looking at these issues in thirteen cities (six metro/major cities and seven small, fast-growing cities) spread across ten states of India.

The authors of this case study are all involved in the project. Dr. Babu is the national program officer for the study, and Drs. Kusuma and Borhade are principal investigators of Delhi (a metro) and Nasik (small, fast-growing city), respectively. The authors, along with principal investigators from the other cities, constituted a task force to carry out the study and engaged in extensive discussions about which methodologies to use. The study has been initiated with a formative phase where the objectives are to assess health care access for migrants in the context of migration and livelihood insecurity and to identify key points for developing an intervention strategy to improve health care access for socioeconomically disadvantaged migrants in Indian cities. The subsequent steps of the project will be to develop, implement, and evaluate an innovative strategy to improve migrants' access to health care.

CONCEPTUAL FRAMEWORK

Many of the factors influencing migrants' health status and utilization of health services have to do with social circumstances; hence, it is important to understand migrant health care access in the broader social context of development, livelihood insecurity, and vulnerability (Obrist et al. 2007). We used the existing health access livelihood framework of Obrist et al. (2007) and the WHO's health systems responsiveness framework (de Silva 2000) to develop a methodological framework for investigating the issues of migrant access to health care and the health system's responsiveness to migrant health needs.

Fiedler (1981) and Anderson's (1995) social determinants models, which consider access as a general concept summarizing a set of more specific dimensions including availability, affordability, accessibility, adequacy, and acceptability, can be applied to the utilization of health care services among migrants. Access can be viewed as the interplay between the availability of health care services and the status of the community in the context of vulnerability (Obrist et al. 2007).

Peters et al. (2003) opined that the large number of people migrating into urban slums requires local authorities to focus on the delivery of essential public health services with the active support of both state and federal governments. Responsiveness is one of the goals of the health system as stated in the WHO's framework on health systems performance assessment (Murray and Frenk 2000). Responsiveness is defined as how well the health system meets the legitimate expectations of the population for the non-health-enhancing aspects of the health system. It includes seven elements: dignity, confidentiality, autonomy, prompt attention, social support, basic amenities, and choice of provider (Darby et al. 2000). Thus, the WHO's health system's responsiveness framework helps us to understand the system-related factors that have a bearing on access. Combining these two frameworks leads to a holistic understanding of factors from both sides. This understanding is necessary to the design of health care delivery that is accessible even to new migrants, and it is essential for developing policy interventions that ameliorate the barriers to accessing services.

METHODOLOGY

The methodological framework for the project is based on a mixed-methods approach. We adopted this approach because of the specific strengths of quantitative and qualitative methods and the insights they can bring when combined. A mixed-methods approach facilitates a holistic understanding of the problem. This mixed methodology is most appropriate here as the quantitative aspects facilitate generalizations and highlight the issues of greatest concern to large numbers of migrants, while the qualitative research, whose design is flexible, opportunistic, and heuristic in nature, facilitates in-depth understanding and aids in identifying specific means to achieve the project goals.

STUDY DESIGN

It was decided to select migrant households that had migrated to the current city of residence within the last ten years, but not less than thirty days, through cluster random sampling. (Generally six months is considered as the minimum period of stay in a place in the Census of India and National Sample Surveys; however, we kept the minimum at one month so as to capture seasonal/circular migrants.)

A major challenge was to locate and identify widely dispersed migrants who met the defined criteria. It was decided to identify certain high-concentration clusters where approximately 15–20% of the households were newer migrants. Initially, researchers visited several slums, slum-like areas, resettlement colonies, habitations along railway tracks and overpass bridges (where people set up temporary tents and huts to live), newer habitations near existing slums, and habitations near footpaths, roadsides, and construction work sites. Information was gathered through talking informally with residents and community leaders regarding how long people had been staying in the area, and if there were any people who had joined recently (i.e., within the last ten years).

Most people were very helpful in providing information and, additionally, they often informed us about specific areas where the newly migrated tended to live.

Thus, clusters to be considered for inclusion were identified and care was taken to include clusters from all parts of each city included in the study. For qualitative research, participants were selected based on availability and the project's information needs. All clusters were considered for selecting key informants, focus group participants, and other community-level participants. Key informant selection was an ongoing process from the project's inception.

Talking to various people helped us in identifying key informants, and sometimes they suggested themselves as people who could provide good information. For focus group discussions (FGD), respondents were selected based on the criteria developed for each type of FGD. Sometimes, local health workers were helpful in organizing focus groups; however, our experience in Delhi showed that having researchers identify the participants resulted in very good focus groups, with enthusiastic participants who were highly interested in the discussion.

The surveys, interviews, and discussions were conducted at times that were convenient for participants. For example, in Nasik, interviews were mainly conducted in the evenings between 7 and 9 P.M.; in contrast, evening interviews proved problematic in Delhi. There, women wouldn't consent to evening activities, suggesting that researchers avoid evening visits as the atmosphere in the clusters was not congenial to research, with several men often drunk and likely to play pranks and tease participants. At construction work sites in Delhi, work site managers often cooperated with researchers and allowed the interviewing of workers during lunch break and even during working hours, as long as it did not interfere with the work of other workers. Off-work times were found more suitable for conducting interviews with those working in shops, factories, and so forth. Interviews were timed in coordination with the people's daily routines in each area; for example, we avoided the time of water supply (which is typically intermittent through public taps or through water tankers). In Delhi, women, who mainly are homemakers, were generally free by 11 A.M. after completing their cooking and other household chores, and again in the afternoon between 3 and 5 P.M. Generally interviews and discussions lasted for one to two hours, with some variation depending on location (i.e., rarely two hours in Delhi, while in Nasik, the focus group discussions were often two to three hours in duration).

One particular challenge was getting people interested in the study, with quite a few individuals questioning the benefits of participating. However, once the purpose of the study was explained, a majority became interested enough to share their views. It was made clear to them that we were collecting this data for research purposes and were interested in knowing about their opinions and experiences with health care. We informed them that their participation was completely voluntary and that by participating they could be helpful in developing solutions to health problems in their communities.

Often people asked for information about their own health problems and they wanted to know about health facilities where they might receive treatment. They also wanted to know what kinds of procedures they might benefit from and how to obtain ration and the government health cards that are issued to India's poor to fund medical treatment. The research team provided information on these topics whenever possible, but at times we had to admit we did not know the answers. In such instances, we said that we would try to get the information and provide it on the next visit. We observed that people became more enthusiastic after we listened to their questions and were then more willing to cooperate until the end of the interview.

Other issues arose related to focus group participation and the need to include more representatives from local institutions in the study. During focus groups, it was expected that discussions would take place freely among participants; however, in many of the groups, the moderator had to repeatedly encourage participants to express themselves and discuss topics in greater detail. Select personnel from municipal administrations, health institutions of various categories, and nongovernmental organizations (NGOs) were initially selected based on their proximity to the study areas. But then after deciding that cities as a whole would constitute the unit of study, we used a snowballing technique to identify additional relevant officials for inclusion in the study.

Another challenge was that in certain areas, particularly the slums that are not recognized as slums by the government, people had expectations that the research team would immediately do something about their specific problems. For example, we were asked to get electricity, improve water supplies, provide ration cards, set up a new dispensary, bring a mobile van for providing health care services, and so forth. In such cases, we admitted our limitations and explained that we were trying to understand the situation through the study and hoped that the research would lead to improvements in the future.

SAMPLE SIZE ESTIMATION

The required sample size for quantitative data was calculated according to the formula $n = z^2_{1-\alpha/2} (1-P)/\varepsilon^2 P$ (Lwanga and Lemeshow 1991). The prevalence of utilization of government health care services (P) was estimated at 15% (based on an ongoing study in Delhi [Kusuma, personal communication]), with 10% relative precision and 95% confidence interval. A design effect (DEFF) of 1.7 and a 5% nonresponse rate were estimated. A sample size of 3886 was finalized for each city. The selection of samples for qualitative studies was purposive, and the number of each type of interview/discussion was flexibly determined and based upon reaching saturation of data. Since qualitative research is iterative in nature, it was decided to review interviews on a daily basis to arrive at a better understanding of the issues as well as to identify new issues. If new issues needed to be explored, we interviewed additional relevant personnel using the same or a different method (or a combination of methods).

SOURCE OF DATA AND DATA COLLECTION

We decided to use both quantitative and qualitative research methods; however, questions concerning which method to use for what sort of data and where data could be obtained through both approaches arose. As noted, the specific objectives for this phase of the study were based on the health access livelihood and health system's responsiveness frameworks. After the specific objectives were finalized, a methodology matrix (see table 25.1) was constructed based on each specific objective. Under each specific objective, a list of variables/issues to be studied was prepared. For each variable, the sources of information (e.g., head of household, key informant, medical officer at dispensary, etc.) and corresponding methods of data collection (e.g., quantitative household survey, in-depth interview, etc.) were identified. After the matrix was finalized, lists of variables/issues for each source of information by type of data collection were prepared. Usually for each variable, more than one source/method of data collection that combined both quantitative and qualitative methods was adopted. In the end, a list of quantitative and qualitative surveys (methods) along with the source of information (participants) was made.

A multiphase process was used to develop the questionnaires and guides/checklists to ensure that they were culturally and linguistically appropriate. The questionnaires were prepared initially in English and translated into the languages of the study cities. The translated questionnaires were further reviewed for linguistic reliability and correctness by the study staff. Later the questionnaires were piloted to check the appropriateness and clarity of the questions among respondents in each cluster; those individuals who participated in the pilots were not included in the actual survey. In addition, piloting provided practice for the research staff, who then collected data using these questionnaires and qualitative tools. The responses to questions, which were in many languages, were translated back into English by translators who were not otherwise involved in the study to ensure semantic and content validity.

The quantitative methods included an interviewer-administered questionnaire for heads of households and another interviewer-administered questionnaire for mothers who had delivered during the last twelve months. Most of the issues derived from the frameworks were quantifiable and covered by these methods. The quantitative surveys collected information on (1) basic demographics, household composition, migration history and pattern, access to basic amenities, social care, and so on; (2) illness experiences of household members (excluding pregnancy and delivery), episodic illnesses in the past six months, hospitalizations in the past year, and chronic illnesses, as well as treatment-seeking behavior and treatment costs and the means of payment; and (3) health care access and responsiveness. The access and responsiveness domains were derived from the WHO's

TABLE 25.1 Research Methods Matrix

Objective	Variable	Source	Method
1. Demographic and socioeconomic characteristics of migrant communities			
a. Migration history/duration of migration	Place of origin, last place of residence, duration of stay in present city, reasons for migration, language used with neighbors/with family members	Head of household (HoH), wife of the HoH, any adult member of household (HH)	Quantitative household survey (QHS)
b. Age and gender; educational, occupational, religious, ethnic, social networks of the migrants/migrant communities; access to social welfare schemes	List of HH members by marital status, education, occupation, income, religion, caste	HoH, wife of HoH, any adult HH member	QHS
	Possession of ration or government health card		
	Living conditions: type of house, ownership, electricity, gas connection, toilet, number of rooms, etc.	Observations of researcher Any adult HH member	Observation, QHS
	Who brought you to this city? Existence of relatives/villagers in this area; social/ethnic networks	HoH	QHS
	Help-seeking behavior in difficult situations such as serious illnesses	HoH/mothers	In-depth interview (IDI)
c. Formal and informal processes of decision making related to health care issues (at HH level and community level)	Decision making regarding treatment of family member who is ill	Mothers of ill children/ mothers who had experienced delivery problems	Semistructured interview (SSI)/IDI
	Community-level decision making	Community key informants (KIs)	IDI
d. Organizational capacity of the migrant groups to negotiate for better services	Existence and functioning of groups such as community-based organizations, women's groups, committees, etc.	Community KIs, members of committees/groups	IDI, focus group discussion (FGD)

(Continued)

TABLE 25.1 Continued.

Objective	Variable	Source	Method
e. Communication channels and their utilization pattern	Viewership of TV, radio, means of getting to know the news (TV/radio/interpersonal/ print media)	HoH; KI	QHS; IDI
2. Assessing availability, accessibility, adequacy, affordability, and acceptability of existing system of health care delivery to migrants, in view of distinct features of migrants	Availability of primary health care services (government/other) in or near community Type of services: prenatal, child delivery, postnatal, child health (immunizations, treatment for diarrhea, acute respiratory infections [ARIs], etc.) provided by these facilities; visits by health workers	HoH, KIs; community members, top-level health officer from municipal/state government	QHS, IDI, FGD, SSI
	Accessibility: distance from place of residence, mode of commuting, time taken, opening hours	KIs; community	IDI, FGD
	Adequacy: supply of drugs, diagnostic services, presence of providers, time schedules, adequacy of waiting space and hours, basic amenities	HoH, KIs, community, health care providers	QHS, IDI, FGD, IDI
	Affordability: availability of money, health insurance, costs (direct and indirect)	HoH, KIs	QHS, IDI
	Acceptability: health provider behavior, satisfaction with the services, privacy, consultation time, doctor-patient communication	HoH, KIs, community	QHS, IDI, FGD
a. Assessing felt health care needs, utilization, and perceived relevance of available health care services by migrants	Health problems perceived by community, what health care services people need for their area	KIs, community (including mothers)	IDI, FGD

Objective	Topics	Respondents	Method
b. Eliciting migrants' subjective assessment of quality of health care	Utilization: prenatal care services, delivery, postnatal care, immunization, child health care (diarrhea, ARI), care sought for illness experienced in the past three months	Mothers	SSI/IDI
	Quality of care in terms of availability of services, opening hours, waiting time, perceived competence of health care providers, behavior of health care providers, basic amenities, availability of drugs, diagnostic services, etc.	HoH, any adult HH members	QHS, SSI/IDI
c. Identifying perceived roles of community and health system in improving provision of health care services	Suggestions for improvement of health care by knowing roles of community and health system	KIs from community; community members	IDI, FGD
3. Identifying the demand-side barriers deterring migrants' access to health care services	Health facility hours, linguistic barriers, economic barriers, apprehensions about health providers and nonavailability of medicine at facility, cost of consultancy and treatment, perceived efficacy of the treatment regimen	Adult HH members	IDI
4. Identifying the difficulties and bottlenecks of government health services in delivering health care service to migrants	Community's felt needs, illness recognitions/ perceptions/knowledge, awareness of facilities	KIs, community	IDI, FGD
	Availability of people to deliver services; follow-up health care of mothers/children	Health care providers; public health officials, etc.	IDI
	Problems pertaining to the delivery of services to the community		
5. Exploring governmental process of identifying new areas/settlements and process of placing health infrastructure and personnel to cater to those areas by health system	Existence of officers at city level to look after the following:		

(Continued)

TABLE 25.1 Continued.

Objective	Variable	Source	Method
	Slums in general	Municipality	IDI
	Health of slum dwellers	Director of health services	IDI
	Migrants, specifically	Records	Review
	Existence of specific health programs for slum dwellers:	Program officers in municipality	IDI
	Mechanism of identifying newer settlements /habitations, legalization (notification) process	Top-level officers of municipality	IDI
	Process of placing health infrastructure /manpower	Top-level municipal health officers	IDI
	Intersector coordination with other departments (revenue, land, corporation etc.) to identify new areas/settlements	Municipal officers, health officers	IDI
		Records	Review
	Programs that cater to new/temporary slums not recognized as slums by the government	New settlement Officers of health, municipality	Case studies IDI
6. Understanding exclusion of migrants from provision of health care services given background of alienation and nature of mobility	Reasons for not including their area/people for services like schooling, health care, water, etc.	KIs	IDI
	Social aspects, stigma, language, barriers, alienation, etc.	Community	FGD
	Case studies with reference to health care programs such as immunization and reproductive and child health (RCH) activities, when intentionally/unintentionally excluded	Community	Case studies

7. Reviewing existing modes of communication and information, education, and communication (IEC) strategies by health system to identify strengths and gaps in reaching migrant communities	Source of information on availability of health services to slum dwellers with reference to pulse polio, immunization, and RCH activities	KIs	IDI
	Existing mode of communication/IEC targeting: (a) general public in the city, (b) slum/migrant population specifically	Officers from health services	IDI
8. Reviewing existing policies and regulations with regard to health care provided to migrants and slum population	State's health policies specific to slums	State/municipality officers	IDI
	Details of budgetary allocations for slum development and specifically for health of slum dwellers	Records	Review

health system responsiveness module, and the questions were devised to capture the subjective assessment of the participants pertaining to the domains of dignity, autonomy, confidentiality, prompt attention, access to social support networks during care, quality of basic amenities, and choice of care provider/institution. Qualitative methods included in-depth interviews with key informants, household heads, and recently delivered mothers, and focus group discussions with community members. These methods were used to understand the community/ migrant's perspective concerning perceived needs, barriers, and facilitators in accessing health care services and in identifying the existing communication channels and their utilization pattern among migrants.

Thus, the present study used a mixed-methods approach by combining quantitative and qualitative methods to gain a better understanding of the issues that influence access to health care services in the vulnerability context of poverty and migration. Combining the health access livelihood framework of Obrist et al. (2007) and the WHO's health system responsiveness framework (de Silva 2000) facilitated a more holistic understanding of the issues that influence health care access for migrants who are vulnerable due to socioeconomic disadvantage and migration. Further, adopting these two frameworks facilitated an understanding of the issues from both sides, that is, the client's (migrants) and the system's (here the Indian health care system). Quantitative surveys facilitated the quantification and generalization of issues such as illness experiences, utilization of health care services, and other factors pertaining to access; they also provided quantifiable data on the sociodemographic profile of migrants. Qualitative techniques helped in identifying and understanding issues that were not well captured quantitatively. These techniques were used to develop a deeper understanding of several key issues under investigation. In addition, qualitative research methods facilitated good rapport with participants, helped generate interest in the study, and provided people with a feeling of responsibility to share their views and discuss their problems.

To understand factors related to the health care system, in-depth interviews with health care providers at various levels and with municipal authorities were conducted with a focus on outreach services, the system's preparedness to provide services to the ever-increasing migrant population, barriers and facilitators (related to financial resources as well human resources), infrastructure, modes of communication and health service delivery, and behavior-related issues for the provision of services to migrant communities. Health care policy makers and providers from the public sector primary health care services (various types of health care facilities, including mobile health care units, health and family welfare centers, government dispensaries, hospitals working under state/federal governments, industries, and municipal corporations) were identified for in-depth interviews. Developmental activities undertaken specifically among the migrant population as case studies. Case studies of certain activities like sanitation campaigns, prenatal care programs, immunization programs, family planning programs, and so on, were undertaken to identify the processes of these ongoing activities and to assess the involvement of the government and NGOs. Case studies of slums/settlements with both better and poorer amenities were conducted to identify the elements that contributed to the success/failure of the interventions.

In the study, several issues were explored using both quantitative and qualitative approaches, which allowed for the triangulation of the data and the various methods employed. We are continuing to assess which method was most effective in generating the data needed to address specific issues (i.e., quantitative or qualitative; within qualitative, which specific methodology was most appropriate for which type of data and which issues; which method revealed more reliable information and yielded a more in-depth understanding, etc.). Continued research and analysis of the issues that were explored using multiple techniques may lead to an even better understanding of the limitations and strengths of the methods used and result in a deeper understanding and appreciation of the mixed-methods approach for conducting research among migrant populations.

REFERENCES

Anderson, RM. 1995. "Revisiting the behavioral model and access to medical care: Does it matter?" *Journal of Health Social Behaviour* 36: 1–10.

Babu, BV, BK Swain, S Mishra, and SK Kar. 2010. "Primary healthcare services among a migrant indigenous population living in an eastern Indian city." *Journal of Immigrant and Minority Health* 12: 53–59.

Bhagat, RB, and S Mohanty. 2009. "Emerging patterns of migration and contribution of migration in urban growth in India." *Asian Population Studies* 5: 5–20.

Borhade, AB. 2007. "Addressing the needs of seasonal migrants in Nashik, Maharashtra." Health and Population Innovation Fellowship Programme. Working paper no. 2. New Delhi: Population Council.

Borhade, AB. 2011. "Health of internal labour migrants in India: Some reflections on the current situation and way forward." *Asia European Journal* 8: 457–60.

Darby, C, N Valentine, CJL Murray, and A de Silva. 2000. "World Health Organization: Strategy on measuring responsiveness." GPE discussion paper series no. 23. Geneva: World Health Organization.

de Silva, A. 2000. "A framework for measuring responsiveness." GPE discussion paper series no. 32. Geneva: World Health Organization.

Fiedler, JL. 1981. "A review of the literature on access and utilization of medical care with special emphasis on rural primary care." *Social Science and Medicine* 15C: 129–42.

Kusuma, YS, SK Gupta, and CS Pandav. 2009a. "Migration and hypertension: A cross-sectional study among neo-migrants and settled-migrants in Delhi, India." *Asia Pacific Journal of Public Health* 21: 497–507.

Kusuma, YS, SK Gupta, and CS Pandav. 2009b. "Knowledge and perceptions on hypertension among neo- and settled-migrants in Delhi, India." *CVD Prevention and Control* 4: 119–29.

Kusuma, YS, R Kumari, CS Pandav, and SK Gupta. 2010. "Migration and immunization: Determinants of childhood immunization uptake among socioeconomically disadvantaged migrants in Delhi, India." *Tropical Medicine and International Health* 15: 1326–32.

Kusuma, YS, SK Gupta, and CS Pandav. 2013. "Treatment seeking behavior in hypertension: Factors associated with awareness and medication among socioeconomically disadvantaged migrants in Delhi, India." *Collegium Antropologicum* 37: 717–22.

Lwanga, SK, and S Lemeshow. 1991. *Sample size estimation in health studies: A practical manual.* Geneva: World Health Organization.

Murray, CJL, and J Frenk. 2000. "A framework for assessing the performance of health systems." *Bulletin of the World Health Organization* 78: 717–31.

National Sample Survey Organization (NSSO). 2010. *Migration in India (2007–2008). NSS 64th ROUND (July 2007–June 2008).* New Delhi: National Sample Survey Office, Ministry of Statistics and Programme Implementation, Government of India.

Obrist, B, N Iteba, C Lengeler, A Makemba, C Mshana, R Nathan, S Alba, A Dillip, MW Hetzel, I Mayumana, A Schulze, and H Mshinda. 2007. "Access to health care in contexts of livelihood insecurity: A framework for analysis and action." *PLoS Medicine* 4: 1584–88.

Peters, DH, KS Rao, and R Fryatt. 2003. "Lumping and splitting: The health policy agenda in India." *Health Policy and Planning* 8: 249–60.

Saggurti, N, S Nair, A Malviya, MR Decker, JG Silverman, and A Raj. 2012. "Male migration and HIV among married couples: Cross-sectional analysis of nationally representative data from India." *AIDS and Behavior* 16: 1649–58.

Srivastava, R. 2011. *Internal migration in India: An overview of its features, trends and policy challenges.* New York: Social and Human Sciences Sector, UNICEF.

Swain, BK, and S Mishra. 2006. "Immunization coverage among migrant tribal children in slums of Orissa." *Indian Pediatrics* 43: 1011–13.

United Nations Development Programme (UNDP). 2009. *Human development report 2009: Overcoming barriers: Human mobility and development.* New York: UNDP. Accessed October 12, 2010: http://hdr.undp.org/en/media/HDR_2009_EN_Complete.pdf.

World Health Organization (WHO). 2008. "The 61st World Health Assembly, migrants health." Accessed November 12, 2010: http://apps.who.int/gb/ebwha/pdf_files/A61/A61_R17-en.pdf.

World Health Organization (WHO), International Organization for Migration, and Government of Spain. 2010. *Health of migrants—The way forward: Report of a global consultation of World Health Organization, International Organization for Migration and Ministry of Health and Social Policy of Spain at Madrid, Spain, March, 3–5 2010.* Geneva: World Health Organization.

CONTRIBUTORS

VOLUME EDITORS

MARC B. SCHENKER, MD, MPH, is Distinguished Professor of Public Health Sciences and Medicine at UC Davis School of Medicine and, since July 2012, Associate Vice Provost for Outreach and Engagement in the Office of University Outreach and International Programs. He is Founding Director, Migration and Health Research Center, Western Center for Agricultural Health and Safety, and Center for Occupational and Environmental Health. He is codirector of the Migration and Health Center of Expertise, University of California Global Health Institute. Dr. Schenker served as Department Chair of Public Health Sciences from 1995 to 2007.

Associate Vice Provost Schenker provides leadership for UC Davis outreach and engagement efforts at the state, national, and international levels. He received his BS from UC Berkeley, his MD at UC San Francisco, and his MPH from Harvard University. Dr. Schenker is board certified in internal medicine (pulmonary disease) and preventive medicine (occupational medicine). Before coming to UC Davis in 1983, Associate Vice Provost Schenker was Instructor of Medicine at Harvard from 1980 to 1983.

XÓCHITL CASTAÑEDA, PHD, has been Director of the Health Initiative of the Americas at the School of Public Health, UC Berkeley, since 2001. A medical anthropologist by training, she was educated in Guatemala and Mexico. She did a postdoctoral fellowship in reproductive health at UC San Francisco. She also received postdoctoral training in social science and medicine at Harvard University and Amsterdam University.

For over seven years, she was Professor of Public Health Sciences and a principal investigator researcher at Mexico's National Institute of Public Health, where she directed the Department of Reproductive Health. In 1999, she received the National Research Award on Social Science and Medicine. In 2010, the California Latino Legislative Caucus awarded her with the National Spirit Award for her leadership in initiatives to improve the quality of life of Latino immigrants in the US. She has published over 120 manuscripts and has served as a consultant for more than thirty national and international institutions.

Her vision and commitment have led to the creation of binational health programs. Under her direction HIA has coordinated Binational Health Week for ten consecutive years, one of the largest mobilization efforts in the Americas to improve the well-being of Latin American immigrants. Through these strategies, hundreds of thousands of Latinos have received medical attention and been referred to public and private agencies to obtain services. She has twice been elected to be an advisor to the Institute for Mexicans Abroad (IME), for which she has served as the National Coordinator of the Health Commission in the US.

ALFONSO RODRIGUEZ-LAINZ, PHD., DVM., MPVM, is a Senior Fellow at the Centers for Disease Control and Prevention (CDC) Division of Global Migration and Quarantine. Dr. Rodriguez's main responsibilities include acting as a liaison, coordinator, planner, and project lead for domestic migrant health activities for the division, across the CDC, and in collaboration with national and international partners. In that role, he has designed, implemented, and analyzed multiple health studies targeting migrant populations in the US and Mexico. Prior to joining the CDC, Dr. Rodriguez was the Senior Epidemiologist for the California Office of Binational Border Health, California Department of Public Health. He has extensive experience in coordinating cross-border surveillance and public health projects between California, Mexico, and Latin America.

Dr. Rodriguez received his PhD in epidemiology and master's in preventive veterinary medicine from UC Davis, and his DVM from the School of Veterinary Medicine in Cordoba, Spain. He has coauthored many peer-reviewed publications and several border and migrant health reports. He also teaches courses on migrant health, global surveillance, and international epidemiology at San Diego State University Graduate School for Public Health.

CHAPTER AUTHORS

ROSA MARÍA AGUILERA is a Level C Researcher in Medical Sciences at the Mexican National Institute of Psychiatry. She is the Project Manager of the Mental Health Migration section between Mexico and the US. She has a degree in psychology from the Universidad Iberoamericana (UIA, Mexico City) and also holds a master's in health science with a major in public mental health from the National Autonomous University of Mexico. She is currently a PhD candidate in social sciences at the Mexican Metropolitan Autonomous University. In the early 1990s, she worked at the UN High Commissioner for Refugees (UNHCR) and at several NGOs promoting community development projects with Guatemalan refugees in Chiapas, Mexico. She has led various research projects and participated in two binational research efforts on migration and mental health. She has an extensive record of publications in international journals and has published book chapters in several scientific volumes.

ANA AMUCHÁSTEGUI, PHD (Goldsmiths College, University of London), is Professor in the Department of Education and Communication in the Universidad Autónoma Metropolitana-Xochimilco, Mexico City. She is the author of "Virginidad e iniciación sexual en

México: Experiencias y significados" (EDAMEX) and numerous articles in both national and international journals such as *Debate Feminista, Sexualities, Reproductive Health Matters,* and *Men's Studies.* Her most recent publications are "Body and Embodiment in the Experience of Abortion for Mexican Women: The Sexual Body, the Fertile Body, and the Body of Abortion," in *Gender, Sexuality and Feminism* (2013), and, with Rodrigo Parini, "Normalized Transgressions: Consumption, the Market, and Sexuality in Mexico," in *Understanding Global Sexualities* (2012), edited by Peter Aggleton et al. She is currently leading a research-action project on women as peer counselors in HIV health services in conjunction with the Mexico City HIV/AIDS Program and collaborating NGOs.

BONTHA V. BABU is currently Scientist-F (Senior Grade Deputy Director General) in the Health Systems Research Division of the Indian Council of Medical Research, New Delhi, India. He obtained master's and doctoral degrees in anthropology from Andhra University, India. He is a health social scientist who focuses on community-based interventions for health promotion and disease prevention. Currently, he is on the WHO's Experts Panel on Parasitic Diseases (filarial infections). He has published approximately 130 papers in national and international journals, and about a dozen book chapters. Presently, he is coordinating a collaborative intervention study on migrants' access to health care in thirteen Indian cities.

BONNIE BADE is a medical anthropologist at California State University, San Marcos. Her work focuses on farmworker health, health care, California agriculture and farm labor, transnational migration, and ethnomedicine and ethnobotany with peoples indigenous to Oaxaca, Mexico. Dr. Bade has worked specifically with Mixtec communities in California and Oaxaca for over twenty years. Dr. Bade earned her PhD in anthropology at UC Riverside in 1994. Her dissertation is entitled *Sweatbaths, Sacrifice, and Surgery: The Practice of Transnational Health Care by Mixtec Families in California.*

FERNANDO G. BENAVIDES, MD, PHD, is Professor and Director of the Centre for Research in Occupational Health at the Pompeu Fabra University (Barcelona, Spain) and an Adjunct Professor at the University of Texas School of Public Health (Houston). He has been Chairman of the Spanish Society of Epidemiology since 2009. Dr. Benavides holds a PhD in public health (University of Alicante, Spain) and is the author of more than 160 articles published in peer-reviewed scientific journals as well as numerous books and book chapters. He is the author of the widely used textbook *Manual de Salud Laboral,* now in its fourth edition. Dr. Benavides has participated in over twenty research projects with competitive funding, serving as principal investigator in sixteen such projects. From 1998 to 2005 he served as the director of the journal *Archivos de Prevención en Riesgos Laborales,* the only Spanish-language peer-reviewed journal in the field of occupational health. Dr. Benavides has been involved as a principal investigator in the Centroamerican Working Conditions Survey (Panama, Costa Rica, Nicaragua, Honduras, El Salvador, and Guatemala) and the Argentina Working Conditions Survey.

ANJALI BORHADE has been working with migrant populations in India for fourteen years. She has an MS in social work and public health from Tulane University, and she is a PhD research fellow at the University of Oxford. Her research is focused on developing plausible solutions for urban migrants for primary health care in India. She is currently working with the Indian Institute of Public Health as an Associate Professor, and she is a founding director of the pioneering Disha Foundation, an NGO that supports migrant rights, including health. In the last fourteen years she has been actively engaged in various interventions, research, and high-level advocacy initiatives to ensure the rights of migrants in India. She has published several articles on migrant rights and policy recommendations.

CAROL CAMLIN serves as Assistant Professor in the Department of Obstetrics, Gynecology, and Reproductive Sciences and at the Center for AIDS Prevention Studies at UC San Francisco. Her research focuses mainly on an underinvestigated aspect of gender, migration, and global health: the HIV prevention and care needs of female migrants. Her current work crosses the disciplines of social demography, sociology, and health behavior to examine the overlooked role that women's mobility plays in sustaining HIV epidemics in southern and eastern Africa. She has published about twenty peer-reviewed journal articles and book chapters on topics mostly related to mobility, global reproductive health, and HIV/AIDS.

HEIDE CASTAÑEDA is Associate Professor in the Department of Anthropology at the University of South Florida. She received a PhD in anthropology from the University of Arizona (2007), an MPH from the University of Texas (2002), and an MA from the University of Texas at San Antonio (2000). Her research activities focus on health inequalities related to unauthorized migration in Germany and the United States, especially the analysis of legal status and constructs of citizenship. Her work has appeared in the journals *Social Science and Medicine, Medical Anthropology Quarterly, Journal of Health Care for the Poor and Underserved, Medical Anthropology, Citizenship Studies, Health Promotion Practice, American Journal of Health Behavior, Human Organization,* and *Annals of Anthropological Practice,* among others. She has contributed to the books *The Deportation Regime: Sovereignty, Space, and the Freedom of Movement* (Duke University Press, 2010), *Gender and Illegal Migration in Global and Historical Perspective* (Amsterdam University Press, 2008), and *Transnational Migration to Israel in Global Comparative Context* (Lexington Books, 2007).

CHARLOTTE CHANG, DRPH, MPH, is Associate Project Scientist with the Labor Occupational Health Program at UC Berkeley. Dr. Chang has published several articles and book chapters on participatory research with a Chinese immigrant worker community in San Francisco. She conducts research on and evaluates programs that promote occupational safety and health and leadership capacity among vulnerable immigrant worker populations.

LISA DIAMOND, MD, earned her medical degree from the George Washington University School of Medicine and Health Sciences and her master's in public health from the Johns Hopkins School of Hygiene and Public Health. Currently, she is a member of the research faculty at Memorial Sloan-Kettering Cancer Center's Immigrant Health and Cancer Disparities Service. Dr. Diamond is the author of numerous publications in journals such as the *Journal of the American Medical Association* and the *Journal of General Internal Medicine.* Her research focuses on understanding how clinician non-English language proficiency affects the quality of care delivered to patients with limited English proficiency (LEP). Ultimately, she plans to use the results of her research to establish standards for the appropriate use of non-fluent non-English language skills by clinicians and to identify process and outcome measures that capture the quality of cancer care being delivered to LEP patients.

ELIZABETH DINENNO is a Behavioral Scientist with CDC's Division of HIV/AIDS Prevention, Behavioral, and Clinical Surveillance Branch. Since 2004, she has led behavioral research on high-risk populations for HIV, including leading the National HIV Behavioral Surveillance system (NHBS) from 2008 to 2011. Her current research focuses on best practices to ensure that high-risk persons are tested for HIV at appropriate intervals and that those testing positive are retained in medical care. Dr. DiNenno received her PhD in sociology from Temple University.

DONALD E. EGGERTH, PHD, is Senior Team Coordinator in the Education and Information Division of CDC/NIOSH, where he manages a portfolio of projects related to immigrant worker occupational safety and health. In addition, he is a Research Fellow with the Consortium for Multicultural Psychology Research at Michigan State University and an Affiliate Faculty Member with the Department of Psychology at Colorado State University. Dr. Eggerth received his degree in psychology from the University of Minnesota and is a Fellow of the American Psychological Association (Divisions 17 and 45).

EMILY FELT has been managing public health programs for the past six years as both policy analyst and program analyst with UC Berkeley and as a research manager with Pompeu Fabra University, Department of Experimental and Health Sciences, in Barcelona, Spain. She has coauthored numerous publications related to the health and well-being of migrants. She studied public policy at the Goldman School of Public Policy, UC Berkeley.

MICHAEL A. FLYNN is a Social Scientist with the National Institute for Occupational Safety and Health (NIOSH) Training Research and Evaluation Branch, where he serves as the Project Officer for a program of research to better understand and improve the occupational health of immigrant workers. Mr. Flynn also serves as the Assistant Coordinator for the Priority Populations and Health Disparities Program at NIOSH. He is the principal investigator for several multiyear field studies and is a member of the National Advisory Committee for the Ventanillas de Salud health promotion program, operating in Mexican consulates across the United States. Prior to coming to NIOSH, he worked for several nongovernmental organizations in Guatemala, Mexico, and the United States, focusing on a variety of issues ranging from rural development to human rights. Mr. Flynn has a master's degree in anthropology from the University of Cincinnati and is a Research Fellow of the Consortium for Multicultural Psychology Research at Michigan State University.

PATRICIA GABRIEL, MD, is a full-service family physician in British Columbia, Canada, and a clinical faculty member at the University of British Columbia, where she teaches evidence-based medicine and research skills in the international medical graduate residency program. She conducts primary care research in the areas of refugee health, language barriers, and mental health.

FRANCESCA GANY is the Founder and former Director of the Center for Immigrant Health, New York University School of Medicine, of the NYU Cancer Institute CORE Center (Cancer Outreach, Outcomes, and Research for Equity), and of the Health Promotion, Disease Prevention, and Human Migration concentration in the NYU Global Masters of Public Health Program. She is now the founding Chief of the Immigrant Health and Cancer Disparities Service and the Center for Immigrant Health and Cancer Disparities at Memorial Sloan-Kettering Cancer Center. She has served as the principal investigator on a number of pioneering immigrant health studies in the areas of language access and cultural responsiveness, cancer, immigration-associated alternative tobacco products, cardiovascular disease, technology and immigrant health, and health care access. She has led several studies in the Latino and Asian communities that have tracked thousands of participants and their health outcomes. She has set up a medical interpreting research lab to build the evidence base on linguistically competent research and care. Dr. Gany's research has led to the development of long-term policy and programmatic changes. Dr. Gany earned her Bachelor of Science from Yale University, her MD at Mount Sinai School of Medicine, and her MS in health policy at the Wagner Graduate School of Public Service at New York University.

JAVIER GONZÁLEZ, MFA, leads the Linguistic and Cultural Responsiveness Program at the Immigrant Health and Cancer Disparities Service at Memorial Sloan-Kettering Cancer Center. He has developed curricula in the areas of interpreting and translation in health care, including screening, testing and evaluation, training, and standards. He implemented the Remote Simultaneous Medical Interpretation (RSMI) Project at Gouverneur Hospital in New York City in 1999 and developed its training curriculum and quality control program. He directed the translation program at Hunter College Continuing Education and has created numerous nationally recognized videos and distance-learning modules. He currently directs the Program for Medical Interpreting Training and Education: PROMISE. He is advisor to the Certification Commission for Healthcare Interpreters (CCHI).

DAVID GRANT, PHD, is Director of the California Health Interview Survey (CHIS) at the UCLA Center for Health Policy Research. For more than twenty years, Dr. Grant has been involved in applied social research at academic and public agencies. He received his undergraduate degree at the University of Michigan and his master's and doctoral degrees in sociology at UCLA.

SYLVIA GUENDELMAN is Professor in the Division of Community Health and Human Development and Chair of the Maternal and Child Health Program at UC Berkeley. She has published extensively in the field of migration and health, with a special emphasis on US-Mexico migration, focusing on perinatal health, cross-border use of health services, and more recently on obesity among children and adults. Her work has been published in numerous public health and medical journals.

SETH M. HOLMES is a cultural anthropologist and physician whose work focuses broadly on social hierarchies, health inequalities, and the ways in which such inequalities are neutralized and normalized in society and in health care, especially in the case of indigenous Mexican migrant farmworkers. Dr. Holmes completed his PhD in anthropology at UC Berkeley, his MD at UC San Francisco, his Internal Medicine Residency at the University of Pennsylvania, and his Robert Wood Johnson Health and Society Scholars Program at Columbia University. An article from his research won the Rudolf Virchow Award from the Society for Medical Anthropology, and his book, *Fresh Fruit, Broken Bodies,* won the Society for Anthropology Work Book Award and the Society of Medical Anthropology New Millennium Book Award. Dr. Holmes is Martin Sisters Endowed Chair Assistant Professor in the UC Berkeley School of Public Health and the Graduate Program in Medical Anthropology. He is codirector of the MD/PhD track in medical anthropology, coordinated between UC San Francisco and UC Berkeley, and Director of the Berkeley Center for Social Medicine.

GUILLERMINA JASSO (PHD, JOHNS HOPKINS) is Silver Professor and Professor of Sociology at New York University. Professor Jasso has written extensively on international migration and longitudinal methods, including an article that recently won an award from the Population Section of the American Sociological Association. With Mark R. Rosenzweig, she coauthored *The New Chosen People: Immigrants in the United States*. Professor Jasso's contributions include estimating the family-reunification multiplier, the number of persons waiting for high-skill permanent visas, and the previous illegal experience of new legal immigrants, as well as deriving an empirically based point system for immigrant selection. Currently she is a principal investigator for the New Immigrant Survey, the first nationally representative longitudinal survey of legal immigrants in the United States. Professor Jasso's Erdös number is 3.

LISA JOHNSTON, MA, MPH, PHD, is an international independent consultant with affiliations at UC San Francisco, Global Health Sciences, and Tulane University School of Public Health and Tropical Medicine. Dr. Johnston has conducted hundreds of studies using respondent-driven sampling to sample migrants and other hidden and hard-to-reach populations. She has authored or coauthored roughly forty journal articles on surveys using adaptive sampling methods, written training manuals for planning and implementing RDS, and edited and cowrote the book *Applying Respondent Driven Sampling to Migrant Populations: Lessons from the Field*. Dr. Johnston also cofounded the Hard to Reach Population Methodology Research Group (www.hpmrg.org) to evaluate and improve RDS methodology and analysis. For more information and copies of some journal articles, please see her website at www.lisagjohnston.com.

PHILIP H. KASS is Associate Vice Provost for Faculty Equity and Inclusion at UC Davis and Professor of Analytic Epidemiology in the university's School of Medicine and School of Veterinary Medicine. He received his DVM, MPVM, MS (statistics), and PhD (epidemiology) at UC Davis, and completed a postdoctoral fellowship in epidemiologic methodology at the UCLA School of Public Health. He has authored/coauthored over four hundred peer-reviewed articles and book chapters on a diversity of topics related to epidemiology and evidence-based medicine, most recently a chapter on modern epidemiologic study designs in the authoritative *Handbook of Epidemiology*, 2nd edition (Springer, 2014). His research, spanning more than two decades, is focused on companion animal epidemiology, including adverse vaccine effects, cancer epidemiology, overpopulation, and syndromic surveillance methodology. His current interests also include studying the epidemiology of violence (particularly firearm) in communities and developing evidence-based methods to improve equity and diversity at his university.

YADLAPALLI S. KUSUMA is Additional Professor (anthropology) at the Centre for Community Medicine, All India Institute of Medical Sciences (AIIMS), New Delhi, where she teaches health social and behavioral sciences. Her doctorate in anthropology was earned from Andhra University in 1999, based on her work on the cultural epidemiology of blood pressure among socioeconomically disadvantaged populations of Andhra Pradesh. Currently, she is conducting research among socioeconomically disadvantaged migrants on various public health issues, including social and behavioral aspects of hypertension, health care access, health insurance, and women's health. She has published about sixty research papers, including several book chapters.

DAVID KYLE is Associate Professor of Sociology, former UC Davis Faculty Director for the UC Global Health Institute, and former Director of the Gifford Center for Population Studies. Professor Kyle earned his PhD from Johns Hopkins University. He recently cofounded the Mercury Project: Mobility, Health, and Habitat in a Warming World as a multidisciplinary research network. His current research agenda explores the social management of the imagination as a social institution, the sociology of creativity, and the relation of both to social change and creative agency. As a jazz pianist, he is also engaged in an interdisciplinary research agenda on improvisation and innovation in the arts and in social life. His past work has concerned why and how people move across state borders, pioneering the concepts of transnational migration, the migration industry, and cognitive migration. With Rey Koslowski he recently coauthored *Global Human Smuggling: Comparative Perspectives* (2nd ed., Johns Hopkins University Press, 2011), and he is author of *Transnational Peasants: Migrations, Networks, and Ethnicity in Andean Ecuador* (Johns Hopkins University Press, 2000).

REGINA DAY LANGHOUT received her PhD in community psychology from the University of Illinois at Urbana-Champaign. Currently, she is Associate Professor of Social Psychology at UC Santa Cruz. Her research examines educational access and inequality for students of color and working-class and working poor students. She has published over thirty articles and book chapters. Most recently, she has been using youth participatory action research to collaborate with Latinas/os from immigrant families to examine whether the creation of community-based murals on school grounds can alter student and family sense of belonging to their school.

KATIA LEVECQUE obtained her PhD in sociology from Antwerp University (Belgium) in 2007. Since then she has been working as a lecturer, researcher, and research manager at Ghent University in the Departments of Sociology and of Work and Organizational Psychology. Her research focuses on mental health and well-being and their social determinants as related to social inequality and diversity, work and employment, organizational structures, and welfare state arrangements. She has published in medical sociology, psychology, social psychiatry, and epidemiology journals. Much of her research includes a micro-macro perspective and cross-national comparisons of European countries.

LIN YU-CHIEH works as a Research Associate for the Survey Research Center (SRC) at the University of Michigan. Prior to joining the center, he was the survey methodologist for the California Health Interview Survey (CHIS) at the UCLA Center for Health Policy Research. Lin received double bachelor's degrees in economics and political science from National Taiwan University. He earned his first master's in international development from the Graduate School of Public and International Affairs (GSPIA) at the University of Pittsburgh and his second master's in survey methodology from the Institute for Social Research (ISR) at the University of Michigan.

MOHSEN MALEKINEJAD, MD, MPH, DRPH, is Assistant Adjunct Professor of Health Policy and Epidemiology at UC San Francisco, based in the Philip R. Lee Institute for Health Policy Studies (IHPS). Dr. Malekinejad completed his MD degree in Iran in 1999, received his MPH degree from UC Davis in 2003, and his DrPH from UC Berkeley in 2008. Mohsen has several years of research experience in the field of injection drug dependency, harm reduction, HIV/AIDS, global health, sampling of hard-to-reach populations, translational research, and advanced methods in systematic reviews. Dr. Malekinejad has several peer-reviewed publications in the area of drug users and respondent-driven sampling.

PROFESSOR ENRICO A. MARCELLI is a demographer at San Diego State University, where his research and teaching focuses on estimating (1) the number, characteristics, and economic effects of unauthorized US migrants; and (2) the economic, geographic, and social sources of health among immigrants and other hard-to-reach populations. Most of his work involves working directly with community-based organizations and students to design and implement random household surveys to study the behavioral and biological pathways through which various life domains and circumstances influence health. Dr. Marcelli offers courses in demography, statistics, survey methodology, applied econometrics, social epidemiology, and international migration. He has published more than fifty academic articles on health, international migration, and work, and is coeditor of *Informal Work in Developed Nations* (Routledge 2010).

DR. KONANE MARTINEZ is an applied medical anthropologist with over fourteen years experience working with Mixtec transnational immigrant communities in the US-Mexico border region and Oaxaca, Mexico. Dr. Martinez's expertise includes transnationalism, qualitative research methods, health disparities, disaster preparedness, and access to clinical health care. Collaborative research is at the heart of Dr. Martinez's research endeavors at California State University, San Marcos, where she is Associate Professor of Medical Anthropology.

RACHEL MEISLIN is a medical degree candidate at the New York University School of Medicine. She graduated cum laude from the University of Pennsylvania in 2009 with a BA in health and societies. She has researched with Dr. Francesca Gany in immigrant health and cancer disparities and recently completed a summer research fellowship at Bellevue Hospital in health disparities in obstetrics and gynecology. She has previously published research on Israeli health policy in the journal *Health Policy* and in *Six Countries, Six Reform Models: The Healthcare Reform Experience of Israel, The Netherlands, New Zealand, Singapore, Switzerland and Taiwan,* and is a volunteer in the free women's health clinic at the NYU School of Medicine.

RICHARD MINES, PHD (agricultural economics), has been a member of a group of researchers who over the last thirty years have altered the public perception of the characteristics of farmworkers in the United States. The availability of accurate information about farmworkers, based on his original survey research, changed the public's view of who farmworkers are, allowing for better design of programs for this community. While working at the US Department of Labor from 1988 to 1999, he initiated the ongoing National Agricultural Workers Survey (NAWS). He has published many articles on US farmworkers, rural development in Mexico, and technological change in agriculture.

MEREDITH MINKLER, DRPH, MPH, is Professor of Health and Social Behavior at the School of Public Health, UC Berkeley, and Director of the Community Outreach and Translation Core of the CHAMACOS project with immigrant farmworker families in the Salinas Valley. Dr. Minkler has coauthored or edited eight books, including the new edited volume *Community Organizing and Community Building for Health and Welfare* (Rutgers, 2012) and *Community-Based Participatory Research: From Processes to Outcomes* (with Nina

Wallerstein, 2008). She has also published close to 150 peer-reviewed articles. In addition to the CHAMACOS project, she has recently worked with immigrant Chinese restaurant workers in San Francisco, and currently works with Vietnamese youth and other populations on the Healthy Retail project in San Francisco's Tenderloin District.

ROYCE J. PARK is Assistant Director of Survey Planning and Operations for the California Health Interview Survey (CHIS) at the UCLA Center for Health Policy Research. With over a decade of survey administration experience, he currently contributes to the design, implementation, and operations of CHIS. In addition to population health and survey methodology, his previous survey research experience involved health disparities among underserved and immigrant populations, substance use/abuse, and HIV/AIDS risk behaviors. Park received his undergraduate degree from UCLA and studied epidemiology at George Washington University School of Public Health and Health Services.

ELENA RONDA-PÉREZ, PHD, MD, MPH, is currently Senior Lecturer in Public Health (University of Alicante, Spain) and a researcher at CISAL (Research Center in Occupational Health). She has been involved in the coordination of several projects related to the health of migrants and the link between migration, working conditions, and health in Spain and Europe. The results of this research have been published in more than twenty articles in peer-reviewed journals.

CLELIA PEZZI has worked for seven years in the Division of Global Migration and Quarantine at CDC, and currently serves as an epidemiologist on the division's Migrant Health Team. She has a BS in environmental studies and an MPH in epidemiology, both from Emory University. She has two publications to date with more in the pipeline. Her research focus has been on migrant and refugee health and communicable disease prevention.

KEVIN POTTIE is Associate Professor and practicing physician at the Departments of Family Medicine and Epidemiology and Community Medicine, and Principal Scientist at the Institute of Population Health, University of Ottawa. He is a member of the Canadian Task Force on Preventive Health Care and the GRADE Methods Working Group. He published the Canadian Immigrant Health Guidelines (CMAJ 2011), an international evidence-based series covering intestinal parasites, malaria, TB, posttraumatic stress disorder, child maltreatment, and other topics relevant to primary care. He has published over a hundred peer-reviewed articles and chapters, including "Migrant Health" in *Oxford Bibliographies Online*.

ANDREW RASMUSSEN, PHD, is Associate Professor of Psychology at Fordham University in New York. Dr. Rasmussen's academic work focuses primarily on the psychosocial needs and assessment of forcedly displaced populations. He received his doctorate in clinical/community psychology in 2004 from the University of Illinois at Urbana-Champaign, and has been awarded grants from the United States National Institutes of Health and the Foundation for Child Development. In addition to scholarly research, Dr. Rasmussen has been integrally involved in policy development and program evaluation of psychosocial programs serving trauma-affected populations around the world.

OLIVER RAZUM, MD, MSC, is a medical doctor and epidemiologist. He is Dean of the School of Public Health, Bielefeld University, Germany. He is also a full professor at the school and is heading the Department of Epidemiology and International Public Health. He has coauthored more than a hundred peer-reviewed papers and published numerous book chapters and books, mainly in the field of migrant health and social epidemiology. His current research interests comprise access to, and quality of, health care for immigrants, and the effect of contextual factors on the production of health inequalities.

SALAAM SEMAAN, MPH, DRPH, is Deputy Associate Director for Science, National Center for HIV/AIDS, Viral Hepatitis, STD, and TB Prevention, Centers for Disease Control and Prevention (CDC). As a Senior Scientist at CDC since 1996, Adjunct Associate Professor at Emory University Rollins School of Public Health since 2010, and Faculty Affiliate at Georgia State University School of Public Health since 2012, Dr. Semaan focuses on domains (e.g., epidemiology, biostatistics, behavioral and social sciences) that influence the validity of scientific results and their translation into programs, interventions, and national agendas. Dr. Semaan's experience covers developing scientific sampling methods for recruiting hard-to-reach populations, leveraging formative and qualitative research and health education, conducting systematic reviews and meta-analysis for evidence-based models, and developing and responding to relevant health policies. Dr. Semaan focuses on being sensitive to the needs of diverse communities and populations by building on extensive cross-cultural experience and travel (more than twenty-seven countries). Her work appears in federal publications and guidance, peer-reviewed journals, books, and textbooks. Dr. Semaan received her master's in public health from the American University of Beirut, Lebanon, and her doctorate in public health from the Johns Hopkins University.

GOPAL K. SINGH, PHD, MS, MSC, is Senior Epidemiologist with the Maternal and Child Health Bureau, Health Resources and Services Administration, US Department of Health and Human Services, in Rockville, Maryland. Dr. Singh is also Adjunct Professor, University of Southern California Keck School of Medicine, Department of Preventive Medicine. He has published over 125 peer-reviewed papers in the field of health inequalities; immigrant health, obesity, and physical activity; minority health; cancer epidemiology; and maternal and child health. His recent works on immigrant health have appeared in the *American Journal of Public Health, Public Health Reports,* and the *International Journal of Epidemiology.* Dr. Singh holds a doctorate in demography/sociology from the Ohio State University; a master's of science degree in population planning from the University of Michigan; a post-master's diploma in population studies from the International Institute for Population Sciences, Mumbai (Bombay); and a master's of science degree in statistics from India.

JACOB SPALLEK, DRPH, MSC (epidemiology), is an epidemiologist and public health researcher, Associated Professor of Social Epidemiology, and deputy head of the Department of Epidemiology at the School of Public Health, Bielefeld University, Germany. Dr. Spallek is also principal investigator of the migrant birth cohort BaBi-Study. He has expertise in both social epidemiology and migrant health and has published several books and scientific papers. Dr. Spallek is an expert in social epidemiology and prevention measures in the prenatal period and early childhood from a life course perspective.

COBURN C. WARD received his PhD in mathematics from the University of Chicago. He is a professor emeritus of mathematics from the University of the Pacific, Stockton. For a decade he has advised San Joaquin County General Hospital residency programs on experimental design and statistical analysis.

PATRICIA ZAVELLA is Professor in the Latin American and Latino Studies Department at UC Santa Cruz. Her work is at the intersection of feminist ethnography and Chicana/o studies and focuses on poverty, women's labor, family, sexuality, health, reproductive justice, and transnational migration by Mexicans to the United States. Her most recent book is *"I'm Neither Here nor There": Mexicans' Quotidian Struggles with Migration and Poverty* (Duke University Press, 2011).

HAJO ZEEB is Professor of Epidemiology at the University of Bremen (Germany) and department head at the Leibniz Institute for Prevention Research and Epidemiology. He has published widely on mortality and morbidity among migrants in Germany and is involved in epidemiologic and qualitative studies on prevention and health care for migrants.

INDEX